The Independent Tribunal into Forced Organ Harvesting from
Prisoners of Conscience in China

JUDGMENT

China Tribunal

Tribunal Members
Sir Geoffrey Nice QC (Chair)
Prof Martin Elliott
Andrew Khoo
Regina Paulose
Shadi Sadr
Nicholas Vetch
Prof Arthur Waldron

Date
1 March 2020

For over a decade the People's Republic of China has stood publicly accused of acts of cruelty and wickedness that match the cruelty and wickedness of medieval torturers and executioners.

If the accusations are true, then thousands of innocent people have been killed to order having their bodies – the physical integrity of their beings – cut open while still alive for their kidneys, livers, hearts, lungs, cornea and skin to be removed and turned into commodities for sale.

Those innocents were killed by doctors simply because they believed, for example, in truthfulness, compassion, and forbearance and lived lives of healthy exercise and meditation and because the way they lived was seen as dangerous to the interests and objectives of the totalitarian state of the People's Republic of China.

And yet the People's Republic of China has done little to challenge the accusations except to say that they were politically motivated lies.

Governments around the world and international organisations, all required to protect the rights of man, have expressed doubt about the accusations, thereby justifying their doing nothing to save those who were in due course to be killed to order.

If the accusations are proved, they will, inevitably, be compared to the worst atrocities committed in conflicts of the 20th century; but victim for victim and death for death, the gassing of the Jews by the Nazis, the massacre by the Khmer Rouge or the butchery to death of the Rwanda Tutsis may not be worse than cutting out the hearts, other organs and the very souls of living, blameless, harmless, peaceable people.

If the accusations are to be proved in this Judgment then the images above, and the words that describe them, must be minimised; priority must instead be given to the process where judgments can be made free of emotion and where universal principles of justice can be applied to that process in the interests of any who may be at risk.

Table of Contents

People's Tribunals

People's Tribunals are formed of citizens and make decisions about important issues that have not been, and are not being, dealt with by formal national or international judicial or similar bodies when, on some reckonings, they should be.

The several People's Tribunals that have operated over time[1] have determined their jurisdiction to act on different bases.

For example, the 'Comfort Women' Tribunal, the Iran Tribunal and the 'Indonesia' Tribunal, which all dealt with historic, concluded events for which there were still surviving victims, rooted their jurisdiction in the authority of victims:

The 'Comfort Women' Tribunal (Women's International War Crimes Tribunal For the Trial of Japan's Military Sexual Slavery):[2]

> *This is a Peoples' Tribunal, a Tribunal conceived and established by the voices of global civil society. The authority for this Tribunal comes not from a state or intergovernmental organisation but from the peoples of the Asia-Pacific region, and indeed, the peoples of the world to whom Japan owes a duty under international law to render account. Further*

---

[1]   See, for example:

1966/7: International War Crimes Tribunal, the 'Russell-Sartre Tribunal' (American foreign policy and military intervention in Vietnam)

2000: The Women's International War Crimes Tribunal on Japan's Military Sexual Slavery, the 'Comfort Women Tribunal' (Rape or sexual slavery, forcing women to sexually service Japanese soldiers)

2012: Iran Tribunal (Human rights violations and crimes against humanity in the Islamic Republic of Iran during the 1980s)

2017: International People's Tribunal (IPT) 1965 (Events of October 1965; 500,000 to 1,000,000 people accused of being members or supporters of the Communist Party of Indonesia (PKI) were murdered, detained without trial, or were exiled)

[2]   https://www.asser.nl/upload/documents/DomCLIC/Docs/NLP/Japan/Comfort_ Women_Judgement_04-12-2001_part_1.pdf

this Tribunal steps into the lacuna left by states and does not purport to replace their role in the legal process. The power of the Tribunal, like so many human rights initiatives, lies in its capacity to examine the evidence, develop an historical record and apply principles of international law to the facts as found. The Tribunal calls upon the government of Japan to realise that the greatest shame lies not in this recording of the truth about these crimes, but in its failure to accept full legal and moral responsibility for them. (para 8)

...This Peoples' tribunal acts out of the conviction that the cornerstone of the international domestic rule of law is legal accountability – the calling to account of individuals and states for polices that grossly violate established norms of international law. To ignore such conduct is to invite its repetition and sustain a culture of impunity. In part because of its failure to prosecute the Turkish officials for the genocide against the Armenians in the early 20th century, Hitler was emboldened to pursue his crimes against the Jews, communists, Roma, gays and others, in the belief that such crimes would not be punished...(para 9)

Iran Tribunal:[3]

The Tribunal's jurisdiction is the jurisdiction given to it by the Campaign and the Legal Steering Committee on behalf of those who have suffered horrific pain and injuries, both mental and physical as a result of the crimes alleged. The Tribunal was to exercise its jurisdiction by rendering a judgment based on the evidence presented. The integrity and independence of the Tribunal guaranteed the fairness and objectiveness of its final judgment.

International People's Tribunal on Crimes Against Humanity in Indonesia 1965:[4]

As a people's tribunal, the Tribunal derives its moral authority from the voices of victims, and of national and international civil societies. The Tribunal will have the format of a formal human rights court, but it is not a criminal court. It has the power of prosecution but no power of

---

[3]   http://irantribunal.com/index.php/en/

[4]   https://www.globalresearch.ca/the-1965-crimes-against-humanity-in-indonesia-final-report-of-the-international-peoples-tribunal-ipt/5537431

enforcement. The essential character of the Tribunal will be that of a Tribunal of Inquiry.

The International War Crimes Tribunal, the 'Russell-Sartre Tribunal' (into American foreign policy and military intervention in Vietnam),[5] dealt with an existing armed conflict, continuing at the time the tribunal was doing its work. The French philosopher, Jean-Paul Sartre, in his inaugural statement to the Russell Tribunal, looked back to the Nuremberg trials and forward, as he hoped, to the creation of a permanent successor to Nuremberg. He observed that, at that time: 'neither governments nor the masses are capable of forming one'.

Since then, despite Sartre's gloom, The Rome Statute was signed on 17 July 1998 and entered into force on 1 July, 2002 creating the International Criminal Court, no doubt thought by some as having universal jurisdiction.[6] In truth it is effective only over part of the world and some of its citizens. The treaty establishing the court was not ratified by the People's Republic of China or several other great powers.

Sartre, in his address, went on to speak of how easy it would have been to create a universal body:

> *It would have sufficed that the body created for the judgement of the Nazis had continued after its original task, or that the United Nations, considering all the consequences of what had just been achieved, would, by a vote of the General Assembly, have consolidated it into a permanent tribunal, empowered to investigate and to judge all accusations of war crimes...*

---

[5]   http://www.tuantran.org/russelltribunal/#3

[6]   The ICC – https://www.icc-cpi.int – is a court thought by some to be thwarted in the exercise of its powers by deference to manifest realpolitik of the kind that Lord Russell recognised was a part of the Nuremberg trials, however well conducted, when he said:
'Inevitably, the Nuremberg trials, supported as they were by state power, contained a strong element of realpolitik ...'
Today's realpolitik operates to block trials where inconvenient to the great powers, as evidenced by the caution with which the ICC has approached any investigation into the US, UK or Israel or the way reports of immense authority recommending referral to the ICC, such as the Kirby report to the UN into North Korea, get no further than to sit on a shelf: https://www.ohchr.org/EN/HRBodies/HRC/CoIDPRK/Pages/ReportoftheCommissionofInquiryDPRK.aspx

Explaining how and why no such body had been created he suggested that:

> *There are, in fact, two sources of power for such a body. The first is the state and its institutions. However, in this period of violence most governments, if they took such an initiative, would fear that it might one day be used against them and that they would find themselves in the dock with the accused.*[7]

> *The other source is the people, in a revolutionary period, when institutions are changing. But, although the struggle is implacable, how could the masses, divided by frontiers, unite and impose on the various governments an institution which would be a true Court of the People?*

Speaking of the Russell Tribunal itself:

> *We are perfectly aware that we have not been given a mandate by anyone ... But, it [the Russell Tribunal] is not a substitute for any institution already in existence: it is, on the contrary, formed out of a void and for a real need ... The Russell Tribunal believes ... that its legality comes from both its absolute powerlessness and its universality...*

> *We are powerless: that is the guarantee of our independence. ... As we do not represent any government or party, we cannot receive orders. ....*

> *From the very fact that we are simple citizens, we have been able, in co-opting ourselves from all over the world, to give our Tribunal a more universal structure than that which prevailed at Nuremberg....*

Sartre connected the Russell Tribunal to what he detected as a universal spirit coming to life – a sadly short life, he feared at the time of the Nuremberg trials. That same universal spirit may, however, have been the driving force for all the informal, People's Tribunals that have been created since World War II when a world order was developing.

---

[7]   Prescient, almost, of the defensive approach taken by the US, for one, to the risk created for it by the ICC that came to exist contrary to the US's wishes: https://deythere.com/president-trump-us-one-icc-un-speech/; https://www.aljazeera.com/news/2018/09/full-text-john-bolton-speech-federalist-society-180910172828633.html

From 1993, various formal war crimes tribunals – for conflicts in the former Yugoslavia, in Rwanda and elsewhere – have been created, appropriate to the age and the problems they dealt with and inspired by that same spirit and the developing world order.

Informal People's Tribunals drew on changing social and political cultures, together with the world order that had created the formal tribunals, to express the same spirit of which Sartre spoke.

Introduction

1. This is the Judgment (Judgment) of a People's Tribunal, namely The Independent Tribunal into Forced Organ Harvesting from Prisoners of Conscience in China (Tribunal).

2. In the context of this Inquiry 'forced organ harvesting' means killing a person without their consent so that their organs may be removed and transplanted into another person.[8]

3. The term 'prisoners of conscience' was first defined in The Forgotten Prisoners, an article by UK barrister Peter Benenson published in The Observer newspaper on 28 May 1961[9], as: Any person who is physically restrained (by imprisonment or otherwise) from expressing (in any form of words or symbols) an opinion which he honestly holds and which does not advocate or condone personal violence.[10]

---

[8]   Other terms have also been used to describe such a practice, including 'organ pillaging'. Save where state authorised killings including any such practice could be legal because they are by way of executions for 'capital offences', such killings would clearly be murders. The term 'organ harvesting' may be thought inadequate to describe the realities of such a practice. However, the term has come into common use and will used throughout this Judgment.

[9]   Benenson also explained how the 'Appeal for Amnesty, 1961' campaign was the result of an initiative by a group of lawyers, writers and publishers who shared the underlying conviction expressed by Voltaire: 'I detest your views but am prepared to die for your right to express them.' A critical part of the definition is that 'Any person who is physically restrained … from expressing … an opinion which he honestly holds and which **does not advocate or condone personal violence**.'

[10]   Benenson's campaign led to the creation of the organisation Amnesty International. The London based organisation 'Prisoners of Conscience' was originally established in 1962 as the relief arm of Amnesty International but became a separate charity making grants specifically to prisoners of conscience, applying the Benenson definition of the term for those receiving grants. Sir Geoffrey Nice – see Footnote 17 – is a Patron of 'Prisoners of Conscience' https://www.prisonersofconscience.org

4.   Forced organ harvesting may be said to constitute the greatest possible breach of a person's 'human rights', a term that appears at various places in this Judgment. The term is used in much contemporary discussion concerning wrongdoing by states against people. Its origin may be found in the French Revolution's Declaration of the Rights of Man and of the Citizen.[11] Human rights were codified by the United Nations' 1948 Universal Declaration of Human Rights. That Declaration was drafted by a committee, initially of three persons, that happened to include Dr Peng-chun Chang of China[12]; and China was one of the 48 countries voting for the Declaration in 1948. In this Judgment the term 'human rights' refers to rights set out in the 1948 Declaration.[13]

5.   This Judgment is written and structured to be readily understood by readers with no background knowledge and no expert knowledge of China, human rights, law or medicine. It should not be necessary to read footnotes in order to follow the judgment itself.

How this Tribunal was Set Up

6.   This Tribunal was commissioned by The International Coalition to End Transplant Abuse in China (ETAC). ETAC is a not-for-profit coalition of lawyers, academics, ethicists, medical professionals, researchers and human rights advocates dedicated to ending what they assert to have been, and to be, the practice of forced organ harvesting in China.[14]

---

[11]   It can be traced back further by some scholars; but this is the moment most cited for creation of the modern concept.

[12]   Vice-Chair of the Commission on Human Rights; a playwright, philosopher, educator and diplomat, Dr Peng-chun Chang was able to explain Chinese concepts of human rights to the other delegates and creatively resolved many stalemates in the negotiation process by employing aspects of Confucian doctrine to reach compromises between conflicting ideological factions. He insisted, in the name of universalism, on the removal of all allusions to nature and God from the Universal Declaration of Human Rights:

      Dag Hammarskjöld Library http://research.un.org/en/undhr/draftingcommittee

[13]   https://www.un.org/en/universal-declaration-human-rights/

[14]   The International Coalition to End Transplant Abuse in China (ETAC) began in 2014 as a web platform providing a comprehensive information source on the issue of forced organ harvesting of prisoners of conscience in China. The website features independent reports, lectures, testimonies, government action, latest news, press coverage and videos. Its website says 'ETAC is an independent, non-partisan organisation. We are not aligned with any political

7.   A principal focus of ETAC's interest since its creation in 2014 has been the alleged suffering of practitioners of Falun Gong, a spiritual practice that involves performing meditative exercises and pursuing truthfulness, compassion, and forbearance – *Zhen, Shan, Ren* – in daily life to bring better physical health, mental well-being and spiritual enlightenment. Since 1999 these practitioners have been regarded by the People's Republic of China (PRC) as followers of an 'anti-humanitarian, anti-society and anti-science cult'[15] and were described by the PRC's then president, Jiang Zemin, as unprecedented in the country since its founding 50 years previously. Any person detained on grounds of being a Falun Gong practitioner qualifies for the definition of 'prisoner of conscience', given above.

8.   Uyghurs living in Xinjiang, while not ETAC's main focus, nevertheless feature significantly in this Judgment. Uyghurs are ethnically and culturally a Turkic people living in the area of Central Asia commonly known as East Turkistan that includes present-day Kazakhstan, Kyrgyzstan, Tajikistan, Turkmenistan Uzbekistan and, currently, the Xinjiang region of China, which officially became part of Communist China in 1949. Separatist Uyghur groups sought independence and in the 1990s, open support for independence increased after the collapse of the Soviet Union and the emergence of independent Muslim states in Central Asia.

9.   Tensions between the Uyghurs and the PRC escalated in 2009 with, by way of example, large-scale ethnic rioting in the regional capital, Urumqi, where some 200 people were killed in the unrest, most of them Han Chinese, according to PRC officials. In June 2012, six Uyghurs reportedly tried to hijack a plane from Hotan to Urumqi before they were overpowered by passengers and crew. There was bloodshed in April 2013 and in June that year 27 people died in

---

party, religious or spiritual group, government or any other national or international institution. Our members are from a range of backgrounds, belief systems, religions and ethnicities. We share a common commitment to supporting human rights and ending the horror of forced organ harvesting.' It is not an organisation of Falun Gong practitioners. None of its Advisory Board members is a Falun Gong practitioner. A minority of its committee members are practitioners. The site was originally named End Organ Pillaging (EOP): https://endtransplantabuse.org/

[15]   Document produced from the Embassy of the PRC in the Republic of Estonia – 'Falun Gong's anti-humanity, anti-science, anti-society nature denounced': www.chinaembassy.ee/eng/ztlm/jpflg/t112893.htm

There are similar documents published on the United States, Australian and other Embassy websites.

Shanshan county after police opened fire on what state media described as a mob armed with knives attacking local government buildings.

These accounts of possible violence by Uyghurs are only of relevance for this Judgment because the definition of prisoners of conscience, in its original form, includes a restriction that such people do not advocate or condone personal violence; the PRC may argue that Uyghurs seeking independence do use personal violence.

10. ETAC was asked by the Tribunal what was their position on Uyghurs being 'prisoners of conscience'. ETAC's China Tribunal Steering Committee stated: 'ETAC regards anyone who has been imprisoned/detained simply for being a member of the persecuted group in question as a prisoner of conscience. We therefore regard the vast number of Uyghur people in China who have been and are currently detained simply because they are Uyghurs, as prisoners of conscience. If individuals have been detained due to violent behaviour or incitement to violence each case would need to be judged in a court that abides by the principles of the rule of law, including the principle that no person, official, political party or government agency is above the law, to determine if that individual is guilty. Collective punishment on the basis of ethno-religious identity is a grave violation of fundamental human rights.'[16]

11. Although the evidence concerning Uyghurs has been far less in quantity than the evidence about Falun Gong practitioners, the Tribunal has approached those Uyghurs about whom evidence has been given on the basis that they are prisoners of conscience.

12. A minority of those working in and for ETAC are themselves Falun Gong practitioners. However, ETAC has campaigned to end forced organ harvesting throughout China and to protect the human rights of all prisoners of conscience who are at risk of having their organs forcibly extracted.

13. ETAC first asked Sir Geoffrey Nice in 2016 to write an opinion on the issues now before the Tribunal. He advised that it could be better to have a body composed of people from different disciplines to consider the facts and the law and this led to ETAC deciding to form a People's Tribunal.

---

[16]   See https://chinatribunal.com/

14. ETAC invited Professor Martin Elliott, Andrew Khoo, Sir Geoffrey Nice QC (Chairman), Regina Paulose, Shadi Sadr, Nicholas Vetch, and Professor Arthur Waldron to form the Tribunal.[17] All those invited – including those who accepted the invitation – were approached by ETAC from names provided to ETAC by several people[18] according to criteria of diversity.[19]

15. Once commissioned by ETAC, the Tribunal was asked specifically to consider the evidence regarding forced organ harvesting from prisoners of conscience in the PRC and to say what criminal offences (if any) have been committed by the PRC or by individuals, organisations, official or unofficial bodies in China that may have engaged in forced organ harvesting.[20]

---

[17]   **Professor Martin Elliott**; professor of cardiothoracic surgery at UCL, London and paediatric transplant surgeon.

    Andrew Khoo; Advocate and solicitor Kuala Lumpur; Co-Chair, Constitutional Law Committee, Bar Council Malaysia.

    Sir Geoffrey Nice QC; Barrister England and Wales; prosecutor UN Criminal Tribunal for former Yugoslavia 1998-2006.

    Regina Paulose; Attorney (US), Chair, World Peace through Law Section, WSBA

    Shadi Sadr; Iranian lawyer, Director of 'Justice for Iran'; judge of People's Tribunals on Indonesia and Myanmar.

    Nicholas Vetch; London Businessman; Trustee Fund for Global Human Rights.

    Professor Arthur Waldron; Lauder Professor of International Relations, University of Pennsylvania; specialist in China.

    Further details available on the China Tribunal website: https://chinatribunal.com

[18]   including Sir Geoffrey Nice, who took no further part in the invitation process

[19]   Charter of Tribunal:

'In order to provide a multi-disciplinary international approach to examining the evidence, members of the Tribunal shall be diverse in regard to professional background, gender, nationality and cultural background. The professional backgrounds of members of the Tribunal will include expertise in the Law, Human Rights, China Human Rights, Medicine, International Relations, Politics and Business. (In alignment with the Commissions of Tribunal and fact-finding missions on international human rights and humanitarian law – Guidance and Practice, 2015)': https://chinatribunal.com

[20]   Mandate of the Tribunal: The Members of the Tribunal are asked to consider the evidence regarding forced organ harvesting from prisoners of conscience in China and determine whether international crimes have been, and continue to be, committed. The Tribunal is asked to address and answer specific questions that arise from existing evidence of systematic, widespread forced organ harvesting from prisoners of conscience in the People's Republic of China:

    1. Given the available evidence about past and continuing forced organ harvesting from prisoners of conscience in China, have international crimes been committed?

16. The Tribunal was served by Counsel to the Tribunal, Hamid Sabi and Tabitha Nice.[21] Their role was to liaise as necessary with ETAC, including by preparing for evidence hearings and arranging for the attendance of witnesses. They were assisted at the evidence hearings and generally by volunteer lawyers from the UK and elsewhere.[22] This document was edited by Helen Davies[23].

17. All members of the Tribunal, Counsel to the Tribunal, volunteer lawyers and the editor of this Judgment have worked entirely *pro bono publico* (for the public good) which for those unfamiliar with the term or practice means completely without financial return of any kind[24] None of the members of the Tribunal, Counsel to the Tribunal, the editor or the volunteer lawyers working with Counsel to the Tribunal is a Falun Gong practitioner or has any special interest in Falun Gong. Two advantages flow from this: first,

---

2. If so, what legal and other actions should be taken by the international community? In responding to these questions, the Tribunal should consider the extent to which alleged perpetrators of forced organ harvesting can be named under relevant legislation and the effect of sovereign immunity on protecting wrongdoers from civil suits.

3. The Tribunal is also urged to consider the responsibilities of international hospitals, universities, doctors, professional societies, medical researchers, pharmaceutical and biotech companies, medical journals and publishers regarding collaboration with their Chinese counterparts and Chinese transplant professionals, whether such collaboration might amount to complicity in forced organ harvesting, what constraints should apply to any future collaboration and to make recommendations regarding existing or proposed professional and legal sanctions.

[21] Hamid Sabi; International arbitration lawyer; Counsel to the Iran Tribunal.

[22] Markus Findlay; Junior Counsel; Caseworker at Advocate, Bursary Officer of the Human Rights Lawyers Association.

Eleanor Stephenson; international arbitration and litigation lawyer working in London.

Eliah Alexander English; LLM in international criminal law, University of Amsterdam and Columbia Law School.

Tatiana Lindberg; international lawyer.

Adetokunbo (Toks) Hussein; Legal Intern at the United Nations International Residual Mechanism for ICTY

[23] Helen Davies; former Guardian subeditor

[24] In other parts of the world the term can have different meanings, some of which allow the person providing a *pro bono* service to be paid. For this Tribunal the UK model of *pro bono publico*, as regularly engaged in by UK lawyers and others, applies and the term means precisely what it says – for the public good and entirely without financial return

all those engaged on the work are completely free of any influence from Falun Gong practitioners; second, worthwhile work otherwise unaffordable is done. Where funds have been required, for hire of rooms for evidence hearings, travel to London of non-UK Tribunal members etc, these have been provided by ETAC.

The Fundamental Questions Asked of the Tribunal

18.   Investigations into transplantation of human organs in the PRC started as long ago as 2001. Those investigations led to allegations that prisoners sentenced to death in the PRC and prisoners of conscience were subject to forced organ harvesting almost always for profit.

19.   The principal detailed private investigations have been as follows:
2009 *Bloody Harvest* by David Matas and David Kilgour.[25]
2014 *The Slaughter* by Ethan Gutmann.[26]
2016 *Bloody Harvest/The Slaughter: An Update* by David Kilgour, Ethan Gutmann and David Matas (the Update).[27]

20.   Formal investigations and inquiries have included:

a.   2001 *Subcommittee on Trade of the House Committee on Ways and Means;* reciting evidence of Dr Wang Guoqi former doctor at a Chinese People's Liberation Army Hospital. Dr Wang spoke of organ and skin harvesting from prisoners 1990-1995.[28]

b.   2007 *UN Human Rights Council – Report of Manfred Nowak, the Special Rapporteur on Torture and other Cruel, Inhuman or Degrading Treatment or Punishment;* containing substantial detail by reference

---

[25]   Bloody Harvest: The Killing of Falun Gong for their organs, published by Seraphim Editions 2009. See also Appendix 3, Item 10.
      Appendix 3 of this judgment is a document, also posted on the Tribunal's website, identifying by number the documents that were part of the Tribunal members' pre-reading.
[26]   The Slaughter, published by Prometheus Books 2014. See also Appendix 3, item 4
[27]   The Update, published on the net: https://endtransplantabuse.org/wp-content/uploads/2017/05/Bloody_Harvest-The_Slaughter-2016-Update-V3-and-Addendum-20170430.pdf See also Appendix 3 item 7
[28]   Appendix 3, item 44

to hospitals, operatives etc. of organ harvesting and response of PRC saying it was false propaganda.[29]

c. 2008 November – UN Committee Against Torture Forty-First Session consideration of reports submitted by states parties under article 19 of the Convention; containing allegations of organ harvesting from Falun Gong prisoners.[30]

d. 2009 May – *Report of the UN Special Rapporteur on extrajudicial, summary or arbitrary executions;* containing accounts of deaths of Falun Gong in custody[31]

e. 2013 *European Parliament resolution of 12 December 2013 on organ harvesting in China;* referring to hearings of 21 November 2009, 6 December 2012 and 2 December 2013 by the Subcommittee on Human Rights and to the respective testimonies of former Canadian Secretary of State for Asia-Pacific David Kilgour and human rights lawyer David Matas on the large-scale organ harvesting carried out on unwilling Falun Gong practitioners in China since 2000.[32]

f. 2016 *US Subcommittee on Africa, Global Health, Global Human Rights; 114th Congress Second Session June 23, 2016, Organ Harvesting: an Examination of a Brutal Practice*[33]

g. 2016 European Parliament Written declaration on stopping organ harvesting from prisoners of conscience in China [34]

h. 2016 *H.Res. 343 — 114th Congress (2015-2016);* including calls on the People's Republic of China to allow a credible, transparent, and independent investigation into organ transplant abuses; and calling on the United States Department of State to conduct a more detailed

---

[29] Appendix 3, item 21

[30] Appendix 3, item 20

[31] Appendix 3, item 22

[32] Appendix 3, item 65

[33] Appendix 3, item 18

[34] Appendix 3, item 66

analysis on state-sanctioned organ harvesting from non-consenting prisoners of conscience in the annual Human Rights Report.[35]

i.   2018 *U.S. Commission on International Religious Freedom (USCIRF) Report*; documenting ongoing persecution of Falun Gong practitioners and discussing the Vatican summit including statements made by Huang Jiefu, (page 35).[36]

j.   2018 November – Australia House of Representatives Joint Standing Committee on Foreign Affairs, Defence and Trade, Human Rights Sub-Committee *Compassion, Not Commerce: An Inquiry into Human Organ Trafficking and Organ Transplant Tourism.*[37] This inquiry is considered in detail below at paragraphs 422 *et seq.*

21.   With the exception of the hearings mentioned above, at paragraph 20a, b, c, and d, all official bodies dealing with this issue have relied to some extent on the works of Matas, Kilgour and Gutmann.

22.   Matas, Kilgour and Gutmann have become certain of their conclusions about forced harvesting as a past and continuing activity of the PRC. Official bodies, including those in paragraph 20 above, on the other hand, have declined to express certainty that these conclusions are justified on the evidence. This has led Matas, Kilgour and Gutmann to believe, as Kilgour suggested in evidence to the Tribunal on 7 April 2019, that the facts revealed by their research are an 'inconvenient truth' for other countries (See Appendix 2A Witness 53). Countries are, it appears, reluctant to make adverse findings on issues such as these about other countries.

23.   There may be reasons for the disinclination of international bodies, states and state bodies (such as Congressional Committees) to confront and comment conclusively on the potential criminality of other states, especially if those other states, such as the PRC, are powerful. Dr Jacob Lavee, an Israeli heart and lung transplant surgeon and former chair of the Israel Society of Transplantation, who gave evidence to the Tribunal, provides an example of

---

[35]   Appendix 3, item 67

[36]   Appendix 3, item 14

[37]   https://www.aph.gov.au/Parliamentary_Business/Committees/Joint/Foreign_Affairs_Defence_and_Trade/HumanOrganTrafficking/Tabled_Reports)

how PRC pressure may be the direct cause of such disinclination. Lavee's concern about how organs in China were sourced was based on personal experience with one of his own patients; this led in 2007 to an international academic conference (hosted by Israel's National Transplant Centre and the Israel Society of Transplantation) on the ethical problems of organ transplants, where forced organ harvesting was to be discussed. The PRC successfully urged the Israeli Ministry of Health via the Israeli Ministry of Foreign Affairs to press for David Matas to be prevented from addressing the conference. The pressure was unsuccessful but the willingness of both ministries to yield to PRC pressure showed a disinclination by governments, as well as by professional bodies, to have this important issue properly confronted.[38]

24.   Other bodies, even NGOs and media outlets, may demonstrate similar reserve.[39] Yet there is no good reason for criminality in organ harvesting not

---

[38]   Appendix 2A, Witness 31 and Appendix 2B, item 31. Lavee and his fellow organisers were asked by the Israeli Ministry of Health to consider cancelling Matas' presentation in response to a request from the Chinese embassy to the Israeli Ministry of Foreign Affairs. This request was rejected. The Ministry of Health then requested Matas' presentation to be balanced with a presentation by a representative of the Chinese embassy in Israel in order to avoid diplomatic discomfort. The PRC's presentation that *was* allowed gave no account of the source of organs in the PRC while portraying the *Bloody Harvest* report as an attempt to slander China. The Chinese speaker was literally booed by the audience. Attendees included Professor Delmonico, then a special adviser on transplantation to the WHO and who is referred to below at paragraphs 405 *et seq.*

[39]   Amnesty International, the BBC and other press organisations were unwilling to review Ethan Gutmann's very extended notes of interviews that he found overcame his own scepticism: See https://chinatribunal.com/wp-content/uploads/2019/04/EthanGutmann.pdf and *The Slaughter* Appendix 3, item 4; Appendix 3, item 7 Gutmann p232) A somewhat determined disinclination by the UK Government is revealed at https://chinatribunal.com/wp-content/uploads/2020/03/InvitationsCorrespondence_withIndex_2020.pdf Pages 69-72. This comprises a short correspondence between a UK government Foreign and Commonwealth (FCO) Minister, Mark Field, and Counsel to the Inquiry Tabitha Nice and Professor Martin Elliott, a member of the Tribunal. Field was overheard by Nice and Elliott immediately after a 'Westminster Hall debate' on organ harvesting of prisoners of conscience speaking of the subject as 'such a relatively small thing'. The correspondence shows a determined unwillingness by Field, a minister of the UK Government, to face gross human rights abuses frankly. Overhearing a minister saying what was heard by Nice and Elliott – and neither denied nor given an alternative explanation – is something that the Tribunal considers it has a responsibility to record. From time to time public perceptions of developing tragedies of enormous proportions have been more acute than publicly expressed opinions of governments, whose disinclination to speak

to be identified and this Tribunal has no reason to be reluctant about making factual and mixed legal/factual findings on the subject.

25. It is clear that although some of the official bodies listed above considered and reached some conclusions about whether the practices revealed international criminal law offences, none pronounced on the criminality of the practices with any certainty.

26. It should be noted that if any official national or international body had pronounced authoritatively on the criminality of the organ transplant practices in the PRC then there would have been no reason for ETAC to commission the Tribunal, as it did, and the Tribunal members would not have accepted the commission.

27. The Tribunal considers that the fundamental questions asked of it are: whether, when, to what extent, and how, forced organ harvesting has been committed in the PRC; and, as outlined in paragraph 15 above, what criminal offences (if any) have been committed by the PRC, or by official or unofficial bodies, organisations or individuals in China that may have engaged in forced organ harvesting.

28. The Tribunal has to consider past and present practices. Past practices of the kind alleged (if proved) cannot be set aside as historic and more conveniently forgotten. The allegations made are of the gravest possible kind and should attract the maximum public censure if proved, whether or not the practices are continuing.

---

truth to *another* power has then allowed tragedy to continue or even to begin. This may be such an instance. These are not small things to be disregarded.

The Tribunal's Jurisdiction and Authority to Act

29. The source of the Tribunal's authority is straightforward. Although there are no direct victims to instruct the Tribunal because any such victims are dead, ETAC has a clear objective:

    The principal object for which the International Coalition to End Transplant Abuse in China (ETAC) has been established is to advance and promote the education of human rights and values with the goal of ending human rights violations associated with organ trafficking involving forced organ harvesting from prisoners of conscience in China and seeking justice for the victims of forced organ harvesting.[40]

30. These clear human rights interests and objectives can be seen against a significant number of well researched studies and reports by recognised and often very senior bodies referred to in paragraphs 19 and 20 above, which set out concerns – including of forced organ harvesting – that are appropriate for ETAC to deal with. ETAC's request for the Tribunal to perform the task asked of it is plainly within ETAC's authority, an authority the Tribunal entirely accepts.

31. Jurisdiction is an altogether different matter. The China Tribunal cannot found its jurisdiction in victims' authorisation because victims, if there have been any, would all be dead. Furthermore, the circumstance giving rise to the request by ETAC to act may be continuing. This circumstance – the concern about a past and continuing practice – may make the China Tribunal closer in function to the Russell Tribunal, the very first People's Tribunal, which dealt with the Vietnam War (see pages 6-7 above). The war was continuing when that Tribunal was designed, as Lord Russell said in his speech to

---

[40] https://endtransplantabuse.org/about-us/

fellow members of the Tribunal in November 1966, to *'prevent the crime of silence'*.[41]

32.   The China Tribunal's jurisdiction is expressly to be found in a gap left by the failure of any official body to pronounce on the criminality or otherwise of the PRC's organ transplant practices.

33.   The only official judicial body that might have been required to act, or to consider acting, to deal with the issue of criminality of individuals in any practice of forced organ harvesting is the International Criminal Court (ICC). However, for reasons explained in paragraph 35, it is manifestly powerless to deal with organ transplant practices in the PRC.

34.   Breaches of the Genocide Convention[42] as a way of holding the PRC – rather than individuals – to account for what may have happened can only be dealt with by the International Court of Justice (ICJ). It will be seen from paragraphs 114 *et seq* below that that it is almost impossible for the powers of the Court to be invoked in respect of these issues.

35.   It would require states other than the PRC to trigger the procedures of either of these courts – ICC or ICJ – and none of the states known to be aware of the forced organ harvesting allegations has shown any inclination or willingness to test the allegations at these courts, or by creating an *ad hoc* court of the UN.

36.   Founding its jurisdiction on the gap left by all other official bodies' failure to deal with the specific issue of criminality in the PRC's organ transplant practices imposes constraints on the Tribunal. Despite the instructions of ETAC, the Tribunal takes the view that it should not make policy, legislative or other broader recommendations[43] built on its own Judgment unless there is

---

[41]   http://www.tuantran.org/russelltribunal/#3

[42]   The Convention on the Prevention and Punishment of the Crime of Genocide, adopted by the United Nations General Assembly on 9 December 1948. The Convention, which defines genocide in legal terms, entered into force on 12 January 1951.

[43]   There may, for example, be many businesses and institutions – including schools and universities, orchestras and art galleries – likely to have policies related to China that could be the subject of recommendation. They are clearly capable of acting on available information about the PRC without a recommendation from a People's Tribunal

a gap in the ranks of politicians, civil society, NGOs and powerful individuals who can make their voices heard on issues to which the Judgment may relate – ie its recommendations should not invade the territory of others.

37.   Save for what is said above about the UK government (paragraph 24 and footnote 39 above), no significant evidence exists to suggest that these individuals and bodies would **not** now act on the basis of whatever judgment the Tribunal returns. In these circumstances – as further explained at paragraphs 124-126 and 497 *et seq* below – the Tribunal will go no further than to list concerns, already mentioned in other reports, that may be taken up in further actions by the bodies concerned. [44]

---

[44]   At paragraphs 410-413 below an implied recommendation is made in respect of The Transplantation Society (TTS) because, on the evidence considered by the Tribunal, that organisation has fallen short in doing what it manifestly should in respect of its member surgeons and there is no one else apart from the TTS to do what is considered as obviously necessary by the Tribunal.

The Proceedings

38. The Tribunals' evidence hearings were held between 8 and 10 December 2018 and 6 and 7 April 2019 at The Connaught Rooms in Holborn, London WC2. These sessions were open to the public.

39. The evidence before the Tribunal was in the first place as submitted by ETAC. Between and following the first and second evidence hearings, the Tribunal sought further factual evidence from ETAC and received advice from the legal experts (on the relevant issues of law) practising in different jurisdictions.

40. The Tribunal met, in person and online, on several occasions to discuss its Judgment.

41. All witnesses except two were heard in public and videos of their evidence are available on the China Tribunal website https://chinatribunal.com. Two witnesses and associated video footage were heard in private for security reasons. However, the substance of their evidence is set out at relevant points of the Judgment below.

42. Twenty-eight witnesses related their personal experience of events to the Tribunal. The remaining witnesses had investigated forced organ harvesting in China and gave analytical or expert evidence. Every witness produced in advance a witness statement, which greatly assisted the Tribunal in managing its proceedings. The testimonies were given in English, Mandarin or Uyghur, a variety of the Turkish language. One witness, speaking in Korean, produced an investigative documentary.

43. The Tribunal and members of the public who attended in person at the December hearings benefited from simultaneous interpretation of Chinese and Turkish into English, and *vice versa*. Sequential interpretation was used in the April 2019 hearings.[45]

---

[45] Witnesses' statements, with a summary in each case of the oral evidence given at the hearings, are at Appendix 1A. (fact-witnesses, 1-28) and Appendix 2A. (experts' and

44. The witnesses were not sworn (as it happens in courts of law) but were asked to confirm the truthfulness of their written statements and evidence.

45. An additional 16 witnesses provided statements to ETAC that duplicated evidence given by others. There was not time to call these witnesses but their statements are available on the Tribunal's website https://chinatribunal.com/wp-content/uploads/2019/08/Submissions_ NotCalled_FalunGongFactWitnesses_web.pdf. The Tribunal found no reasons from their statements to doubt what these witnesses wrote but, of course, did not have the advantage of seeing and testing them at a hearing.

46. Pre-reading materials submitted by ETAC and critically examined by members of the Tribunal, are listed in Appendix 3 of this Judgment, which can also be found at https://chinatribunal.com

Invitations to attend the proceedings, to participate in them and/or to make representations were sent by the Tribunal's Counsel Mr Hamid Sabi to the Ambassador to London of the PRC on five occasions (20, 26 Nov and 13 Dec 2018, 15 March and 2 April 2019); no reply was received to any of these invitations. Invitations were also sent to prominent transplant physicians in China and elsewhere to give their views and to give evidence about Chinese transplant activity, as well as to the past and current presidents of The Transplantation Society (TTS) and Declaration of Istanbul Custodian Group (DICG).[46] This correspondence is at the Tribunal's website https://chinatribunal.com/wp-content/uploads/2020/03/ InvitationsCorrespondence_withIndex_2020.pdf

47. None of those invited agreed to appear or submit a statement to the Tribunal.

48. Evidential material came to the Tribunal in other ways exhibits or further statements supplied by witnesses during evidence hearings; summaries and reports provided by ETAC; material provided voluntarily by individuals or

---

investigators' statements, 29-54). Appendix 3 contains "pre-reading materials" and Appendix 4 all other documents presented to the Tribunal. Videos recording of all proceedings are at https://chinatribunal.com Except for the two witnesses heard in private, and subject to a few instances of technical breaks in the video recordings

[46] On 29 October 2019, three members of the Tribunal (Elliott, Nice and Vetch) and Hamid Sabi held a constructive telephone conference with the Co-Chair of the DICG.

organisations, sometimes in response to invitation from ETAC at the evidence hearings.

Some organisations have produced more than one report – for example, the World Organisation to Investigate the Persecution of Falun Gong (WOIPFG)[47], which has prepared a great number of reports reflecting 15 years of research (available at https://chinatribunal.com or elsewhere on the internet). The Tribunal's assessment of the honesty of such organisations' witnesses, and the reliability of research, in respect of the particular reports dealt with at hearings has been applied for the work of the organisations generally in the absence of any reasonable doubt to do otherwise. For WOIPFG no such reason was indicated in any way or found by the Tribunal.

Most of this material is referenced in the Judgment, and full copies of the material cited and any material not referred to in the Judgment itself can be found in Appendix 4 and at https://chinatribunal.com[48]

49. Thus, all material available to and considered by the Tribunal – including video recordings of witnesses who gave evidence in person – is readily available to readers of this Judgment and to the public generally.

The Tribunal's Approach to Evidence and Decision-making

50. With the fundamental questions asked of the Tribunal identified, its authority and jurisdiction explained and the categories of evidence on which it has acted, listed, the Tribunal sets out what the route it has taken to reach a Judgment.

51. Some People's Tribunals referred to above equipped themselves with 'statutes' and adopted formal rules of procedure. Some have had 'prosecutors'. The China Tribunal, composed of people who were not

---

[47] Founding statement of WOIPFG, United States, January 20, 2003:

Our Mission Statement: 'To investigate the criminal conduct of all institutions, organizations, and individuals involved in the persecution of Falun Gong; to bring such investigation, no matter how long it takes, no matter how far and deep we have to search, to full closure; to exercise fundamental principles of humanity; and to restore and uphold justice in society.' World Organization to Investigate the Persecution of Falun Gong http://www.upholdjustice.org/node/38

[48] See ETAC Statement: Call for submissions process https://chinatribunal.com/wp-content/uploads/2019/09/ETAC_Statement_CallForSubmissionsProcess.pdf

operating as specialists but as 'jurors'. In considering evidence the Tribunal was only limited by its incapacity to compel witnesses. It needed no 'statute' as is required for national legal systems. And it had no formalised rules of courtroom practice and procedure that typically limit a judge's or jury's approach to evidence.

52.   Thinking of Tribunal members as jurors and having to meet a 'proof beyond reasonable doubt' test before making any judgment adverse to the PRC (see Standard of Proof paragraph 85 below), may explain why it was necessary for the Tribunal to do its work.

There have been other bodies and individuals, for example, WOIPFG (World Organisation to Investigate the Persecution of Falun Gong), Freedom House, The China Organ Harvest Research Centre (COHRC) and Victims of Communism (VOC), that have prepared full reports on relevant events, sometimes covering most, or nearly all, of the topics to be covered by the Tribunal. But they all operate with different approaches and according to their own 'disciplines'.

The Tribunal members, as 'jurors', started with no presumptions, no attitude towards the PRC allowing effect on their decision-making, almost no knowledge of the allegations (see paragraph 79 below) and no interest in the subject matter. They were able to approach witnesses of facts on the basis of there being no presumption of *dis*belief in what people say about facts, with experience of the need for caution wherever there is a *reason* for doubting some piece of evidence (the 'reasonable doubt') and allowing only limited reliance on expert opinions (see paragraph 57 below). So the judgment of this Tribunal of non-specialist, non-committed citizens may have function and impact that the other organisations cannot have.

53.   Ordinary citizens entrusted with serious questions to be answered by evidence are capable of acting without being subject to statute or courtroom practice and procedure. Nevertheless, the Tribunal's members have, as demonstrated below, applied the law on which they have been directed and applied well-known principles that underlie universally recognised norms of judicial procedure.

54.   Important decisions – including judgments by judicial or 'quasi-judicial' bodies such as People's Tribunals – are reached in many different ways. The Tribunal has had regard to some aspects of formal legal processes, and as an example:

55.   In jury trials of individuals in many countries, the jury is *directed* as to how to approach evidence, for example, by being told when certain inferences may be drawn, when they may not be drawn, if and when corroboration is required, and so on. The jury is sequestered (kept in isolation) to reach its decisions and its discussions are never revealed; it returns a decision (the verdict) without any accompanying written reasons and the verdict is accepted – subject to appeal – on the basis that the jury has understood the instructions and faithfully applied them.

56.   In formal international criminal courts and tribunals, by contrast, the judges apply certain rules of evidence and procedure that they may have developed in part by themselves, for example, when the factual decisions of one concluded trial may be adopted as facts and applied in another trial without all the same evidence being heard again (known as 'adjudicated facts'). The judges deliver very detailed written judgments identifying all evidence on which they have relied and showing where and how all their rules about evidence have been applied.

57.   Judges and juries hearing expert evidence in many jurisdictions, in criminal and non-criminal cases, may be required by the relevant rules of the jurisdiction concerned to work on the basis that they cannot rely on the opinion of experts on the *final issues* they have to decide, but can rely on their expertise for intermediate conclusions; the judge or jury have to form their final conclusions on all the evidence including the expert evidence, but limited by this rule.

58.   The Tribunal has also had regard to principles enshrined in the 1948 Universal Declaration of Human Rights, which deal in different ways with judicial processes applied to *individuals*. All members of the Tribunal live in countries where those principles – including the right to equality before the law and the right to a fair hearing – are instilled automatically in citizens' thinking, regardless of whether they are lawyers.

59.   The Tribunal has also had firmly in mind the obvious consideration that the more serious the issue, the greater care must be taken in reaching a decision and the greater caution shown in accepting evidence on which to make the decision.

60.   Although this Judgment will deal at appropriate places with the approach taken to particular pieces of evidence, some of the evidential issues that arise are worth setting out at the start:

61.   The opinions of the three best known and most often cited researchers –
       Matas, Kilgour and Gutmann – are to the effect that state-sponsored forced
       harvesting of organs from prisoners of conscience has been going on for a
       long time in the PRC. Their opinions are expressed as without doubt and
       arguably reinforced by the fact that no one, over the years, has produced a
       tenable argument to counter their conclusions. Does this mean the Tribunal
       can simply adopt as evidence, and rely on, their conclusions? Or should it
       review the evidence they have relied on, accept some of their conclusions
       where judged safe to do so, but always make its own judgment of the major
       questions facing the Tribunal? The latter is the Tribunal's position.

62.   Does the PRC's failure to reply to requests for engagement at various
       public hearings, or to respond to invitations to participate in the Tribunal's
       proceedings, or to answer its questions, allow the Tribunal to draw factual
       inferences that are adverse to the PRC? The Tribunal will not draw any such
       inferences.

63.   Does the PRC's failure to have reacted over many years to many reports
       of forced organ harvesting – to the expert reports of Matas, Kilgour and
       Gutmann and to the inquiries at high level of many governments – with
       an explanation that could eliminate all the concerns of those reports, have
       some consequences for the Tribunal's route to its judgment? This is a more
       difficult question and one the Tribunal addresses specifically at paragraphs
       434 – 447.

64.   But it may be worth noting at the start, that in the 'scales of justice' image,
       any weight of evidence deposited on one side of the scales where the other
       scale is completely empty will take the first scale down, so that a just decision
       would appear to be on that side. If – over the years of these allegations being
       made – the PRC has put nothing on the other scale, then all analysts' and
       experts' reports may be seen as bound to 'win' on any scales of justice test.
       But the Tribunal considers it must do what it can to consider possible counter
       arguments and explains where and when it does, in particular at paragraph
       194. And, in any event, the PRC *has* advanced counter arguments to a very
       limited extent as covered at paragraphs 422 and following.

65.   There has been no challenge to the evidence given by any witness beyond the
       questioning by the Tribunal's Counsel and by Tribunal members themselves.
       Their questions were asked without knowledge of what the PRC's position

would be on the evidence presented and without knowledge of whether contrary evidence existed to counter the evidence heard.

66.   Further, when a state's interests are at risk in court proceedings it is not unusual for the state to deploy secret intelligence it has about witnesses hostile to the state. The state's lawyers may be able to 'ambush' witnesses with material otherwise completely unknown to the court or to the party relying on the witness. The PRC took no steps to damage any witnesses by intelligence-based 'ambushes' at hearings or even in the media, as it might have done, despite not being represented before the Tribunal and, to this extent, the witnesses enjoyed 'easy rides'.

67.   To cope with this deficit in the testing of the evidence, the Tribunal will approach all evidence with a degree of scepticism, searching for weaknesses in the evidence and being alive to the risk of group enthusiasm operating on the minds of those witnesses who are Falun Gong supporters or practitioners.

68.   And finally, what weight should the Tribunal give to evidence from the pre-reading material where there has been no witness in person to give the evidence? As with any work of scholarship or research, or any detailed factual account, the underlying material supporting the document or video recording has to be explored in a search for reliability. The Tribunal's approach to individual documents of this kind is detailed when the documents are referred to.

69.   The Tribunal is also aware of how the human rights activities of its members could lead to concerns about their not being impartial. Members have sought to neutralise any such concern by limiting the evidence on any particular factual issue before them to what is strictly 'admissible' and relevant to that issue, and by reaching no conclusion until all evidence, and all arguments favourable to the PRC, have been considered.

The Tribunal's Relationship with ETAC

70.   ETAC and other NGOs associated with it are committed activists convinced in general of the matters that are the Tribunal's concern. The Tribunal members had, and have, no commitment as activists in the cause pursued by ETAC and are engaged simply to answer the question(s) asked of them.

To ensure Tribunal members retained their complete independence of thought at all times a barrier was created in the overall process between ETAC and The Tribunal. It was managed by Counsel to the Tribunal – Hamid Sabi and Tabitha Nice – through whom all inquiries and documents were channelled. The Chairman has been party to this process, sometimes out of necessity.

71. This process and the practices set out below are spelt out in detail because some readers of this Judgment may not be familiar with the open and public approaches to justice of the UK, the US, Malaysia, and other countries with which members of the Tribunal are acquainted. Using these mechanisms, the Tribunal has reached its Judgment purely on the basis of the factual, analytical and expert evidence presented to it, and on nothing else.

72. Furthermore, every step of the process has been explained by postings on the Tribunal website, along with all evidence presented to and acted on by the Tribunal. In this way the public may themselves engage in the same exercise of decision-making as the Tribunal has done.

Practices of the Tribunal

73. The Tribunal was composed of members from diverse backgrounds. To ensure all members were equal participants in decision-making, any who had special expertise, for example in law, China, or transplant surgery, understood at recruitment that they would be asked to deploy their expertise only to ensure that all members fully understood any technicalities of the evidence presented. This was particularly important for the lawyers who, coming from four different jurisdictions, would, as with other Tribunal members, accept incoming legal advice just as if they were jurors being instructed in the law by a judge before reaching a verdict.[49] In the event, it proved necessary, on occasion, for Professor Martin Elliott to add some medical expertise on non-contentious subjects. Otherwise all members of the Tribunal may be seen as jurors acting on evidence of fact and the expertise of others, including expertise about the law, to make their judgment.

---

[49] The most senior judge when sitting as a juror (on jury service) can, and does, accept the direction on law coming from the trial judge however junior she or he may be.

74. With no formal statute and no formal rules of procedure and evidence the Tribunal – as with other People's Tribunals – has made 'free evaluation' of evidence. For example, it has not imposed on itself any requirements of corroboration or counted as inadmissible hearsay evidence. However, it has kept in mind the additional caution that assessment of any evidence other than direct oral evidence may require, and has considered all possible objections to the accuracy of the evidence presented before accepting it.

75. The approach to evidence not given personally by witnesses at the Tribunal but which came in documents (including videos) is as it would be for any similar work of reportage, analysis, expert analysis, government committee report etc. Namely, the document is searched for internal inconsistencies and incompatibility with other material relied on by the Tribunal. It is checked for the nature and reliability of footnoted and other underlying material. Only when it has met these levels of checking has it been included or relied on in this Judgment, and with the proviso that material that has not been produced by witnesses heard by the Tribunal may have less value than evidence from witnesses in person.

76. The Tribunal has made all possible efforts to attend to the rule – enshrined in many legal systems as paramount in importance – of 'hearing the other side', by asking the PRC to make its case known, but with no success.

77. The Tribunal and ETAC have made contacts with all those who might be able to help with expressing views favourable to the PRC. They are dealt with in detail in paragraphs 404 to 408 below.

78. With the PRC failing to engage and there being no individual or official body to put forward any view that might count as the PRC position, the Tribunal considered asking a lawyer to operate as an *amicus curiae* (friend of the Tribunal) and to argue the presumed position of the PRC and cross-examine witnesses in accordance with that position. But the PRC's position has barely been articulated and any *amicus* engaged would have no access to individuals from the PRC to say what its position might be and no access to evidence that might be helpful to the PRC. It was decided that use of an *amicus* would not help decision-making and would run the risk of apparently bolstering evidence that may be adverse to the PRC because the *amicus* would simply not be able to argue much, if anything, beyond what the Tribunal members themselves would do in testing evidence presented.

The Human Rights Reputation of the People's Republic of China and the Presumption of Innocence

79.   Most members of the Tribunal had absolutely no knowledge of the allegations made about forced organ harvesting in the PRC until they were approached by ETAC.[50] This reflects the widespread ignorance of the allegations in citizens around the world who have no special interest in Chinese affairs.

80.   However, all members of the Tribunal were aware in general terms that the PRC had a reputation for abject failure to respect the 1948 Universal Declaration of Human Rights, and the evidence considered by Tribunal members overall left them certain that throughout the last 20 years the PRC has been in substantial breach of at least Articles 2, 3, 5, 6, 7, 8, 9, 10, 11, and 13 of the Declaration, and of Articles 6, 7, 9, 10, 12 and 14 of the International Covenant on Civil and Political Rights of 16 December 1966 (which the PRC signed in 1998 but has not ratified).[51] However, the Tribunal's certainty about these breaches has not, in any way, affected its decision-making process or its final judgment. Where these breaches may be relevant to the Tribunal's Judgment, it is explained, for example, in paragraph 459 below. Furthermore, where the Tribunal is certain these breaches are of no relevance, the 'presumption of innocence' has been applied. There is no presumption of innocence in the PRC.[52]

---

[50]   This reality was particularly surprising given that many activities of members of the Tribunal have been concerned with what are described as human rights issues. For some reason publicity has not been given to, or has not been effective for spreading information about, the many inquiries into the subject of forced organ harvesting in China.

[51]   https://wiki2.org/en/International_Covenant_on_Civil_and_Political_Rights#Parties_to_the_Covenant

[52]   Evidence from Clive Ansley (Appendix 2A, Witness 32), an expert on the laws of China, explains that there is no presumption of innocence in operation in trials in the PRC. Indeed, as Ansley makes clear at paragraphs 67-88 of his statement, the PRC applies no presumption of innocence – only a presumption of guilt. The purported introduction of a presumption of innocence, set out in the Revised Criminal Procedure Law of 1996, Article 12, was a sham – an attempt to mollify overseas critics and impress a foreign audience. It consists of the tautological assertion that: 'No person shall be found guilty without having been judged as such by a People's Court, in accordance with law.' Ansley observes, and this is consistent with evidence before the Tribunal, that the wording of the article does not actually address the issue of presumption of innocence, or the onus of proof to which the presumption gives rise.

81.   The Tribunal applies the presumption of innocence to its task by looking only at evidence it judges relevant to any decision it has to make. It reaches its decision on that evidence and nothing else. Thus, where breaches of the Universal Declaration of Human Rights, or of the International Covenant on Civil and Political Rights are of no relevance to a particular decision, the Tribunal has not allowed the breaches to prejudice the PRC; instead, it has behaved as if the evidence related to an imaginary country with the best human rights record.[53]

82.   Members of the Tribunal have set aside anything but evidence judged as admissible.[54]

83.   Applying the presumption of innocence, and other practices explained later, should allow those considering this Judgment to follow and to have confidence in the reasoning of the Tribunal.

Standard of Proof

84.   In daily affairs humans regularly use different terms to express the strength of any conclusion they make. From 'I think that' to 'I am absolutely certain that'. In legal processes judges and juries have to apply standard tests to the strength of their conclusions. In criminal trials of individuals there is a commonly used test of 'beyond reasonable doubt'. The Judgment of the Women's International War Crimes Tribunal on the Trial of Japan's Military Sexual Slavery ('Comfort Women' Tribunal, December 2000) deals with this issue (in the context of assessing culpability of individuals) as follows:

> *25. ... We note that under international law, the standard of proof is not specified in international legal instruments, with the exception of Article 66(3) of the Rome Statute of the International Criminal Court*

---

[53]   If imagining a purely fictitious country is not possible Denmark and New Zealand are examples of countries with high human rights rankings on some scales. See, for example, https://worldjusticeproject.org/sites/default/files/documents/WJP-ROLI-2018-June-Online-Edition_0.pdf

[54]   This may be difficult for people who live in the PRC to believe. The need to be able to do this is ingrained into the cultures of the countries where Tribunal members live. It is a matter of individual responsibility that each member of this Tribunal – just like any judge or juror in countries that operate the rule of law – can articulate a decision made by reference to admissible evidence and nothing else

which provides: 'in order to convict the accused, the Court must be convinced of the guilt of the accused beyond reasonable doubt.' While the post-war Tribunals did not often articulate the standard applied, we note that the Nuremberg Tribunal did so on occasion. For example, it found the defendant Schacht not guilty as charged because the evidence provided by the prosecution was not sufficient to establish his guilt 'beyond reasonable doubt' ...

26. The Human Rights Committee has subsequently affirmed, in General Comment 13, that, 'by reason of the presumption of innocence, the burden of proof of the charge is on the prosecution and the accused has the benefit of the doubt. No guilt can be presumed until the charge has been proved beyond reasonable doubt.'

Accordingly, this Tribunal adopts the position that, to find an accused guilty, it is necessary for the Prosecutors to prove 'beyond reasonable doubt' that the accused committed the necessary actus reus and possessed the necessary mens rea of the crimes alleged.

85. Recognising that the China Tribunal is not specifically concerned with potential criminality of *individuals,* and has had no prosecutor presenting evidence and argument but has proceeded on a more inquisitorial basis, it will nevertheless only make conclusions of certainty about the commission of (act of committing) crimes, whether by individuals or by the PRC itself, by applying this same test: 'proof beyond reasonable doubt' both to the thing done *(actus reus)* and mental state of the person or body doing it *(mens rea).* For any lesser degree of strength of conclusions, it will use non-legal terms.

Applicable Law

86. The applicable law in this case is the law relevant to international crimes and to the proof of crimes committed by individuals and states.

87. The Tribunal sought independent legal advice in order to fulfil part of its mandate, namely:

... The Tribunal is asked to address and answer specific questions that arise from existing evidence of systematic, widespread forced organ

harvesting from prisoners of conscience in the People's Republic of China:

... Given the available evidence about past and continuing forced organ harvesting from prisoners of conscience in China, have international crimes been committed?... '[55]

88. Legal Opinions and Advice were received from the following:
     Edward Fitzgerald QC of the UK Bar, dated 22 January 2019 (Appendix 4.14). Five members of the Tribunal had a video linked conference with Mr Fitzgerald on 21 May 2019, which was followed by a Supplementary Opinion dated 21 May 2019, and a further Supplementary Opinion dated 3 June 2019.
     Datuk N Sivananthan of the Malaysian Bar, dated 23 May 2019 (Appendix 4.21).

89. Both advisers are expert in the relevant law. They advised independently of each other but, since providing their Opinions and Advice, have reviewed each other's Opinions and been able to provide observations to cover any points of apparent difference between them and to deal with one other question, which had not been asked of them initially, about the International Court of Justice.

90. The Opinions and Advice given considered customary law, legal conventions and the law as codified in the Rome Statute of the International Criminal Court.[56] The ICC has international reach far beyond that of any of the *ad hoc* tribunals and its statute is generally regarded as authoritative and, thus, the most appropriate for present purposes whenever the Tribunal was considering the definition of international crimes applicable to individuals. The Genocide Convention[57] featured where the Tribunal was testing the liability of the PRC itself for breaches of that Convention, with customary law filling some gaps.

91. The central issue from the mandate was whether crimes have been committed. It was not whether any particular individual – or the PRC itself – should be subject to action by a particular court.

---

[55]   https://chinatribunal.com/tribunal-charter/
[56]   https://www.icc-cpi.int/resource-library/documents/rs-eng.pdf
[57]   https://www.ohchr.org/en/professionalinterest/pages/crimeofgenocide.aspx

92. This distinction may be understood further by considering the comparative ease with which the Tribunal may reach decisions of certainty about the fact that particular crimes have (or have not) been committed and the far greater difficulty of finding proved specific criminality by individuals or a state. In his Advice, Sivananthan makes the following critical point:

> As discussed above, care must be taken by the China Tribunal in considering the various elements of these international crimes and there must be proper justification that must be made before concluding that any of these crimes have been committed. _An important gap or weakness that currently exists in the proposed determination process of the China Tribunal is the lack of involvement of the accused and hence the lack of opportunity for the individuals accused of these crimes to defend themselves. This is especially important in situations where issues of criminality are raised._ (Para 52)

93. Absence of an accused individual or state from a process of inquiry may prove more difficult for People's Tribunals than for formal judicial processes because the latter have mechanisms and powers of enforcement of attendance and obtaining of documentation.

94. The Tribunal has had Sivananthan's advice much in mind and recognises that the comparative difficulty of reaching conclusions about specific criminality generally, is heightened where the crime of genocide is considered, given the very specific mental element – '_to destroy, in whole or part, a national, ethnical, racial or religious group, as such_' – that has to be proved. (See also paragraph 95 below.)

95. Recognising these limitations and being alive to other potential difficulties set out elsewhere in the Judgment, the Tribunal is, nevertheless, confident of its competence to do what is required of it in the application of relevant law.

96. The questions asked of the experts focused on the possible crimes of genocide, crimes against humanity and torture.

97. **Genocide** The law on genocide is complicated and is developing as cases in international courts are decided. There is no simple definition in law that could match the non-lawyer's understanding of genocide in the way that, for

example, legal definitions of crimes such as murder or dangerous driving may broadly match the non-lawyer's understanding. Genocide may be defined, in ordinary dictionaries, as 'the deliberate killing of a large group of people, especially those of a particular nation or ethnic group'. However, the very specific definition derived from the Genocide Convention, and always applied in any legal setting, is 'genocide means any of the following acts … committed *with intent* to destroy, in whole or in part, a national, ethnical, racial or religious group, as such.' Not only is this different in formulation, but the listed acts required as a part of any crime of genocide are not just killings and do not necessarily involve killing. This substantial difference may have led to a gap between the non-lawyer citizen's expectation of when the charge of genocide may be brought and what it is possible to *prove* in national and international courts, a gap that is not necessarily helpful or healthy, but is for the time being unavoidable. [58]

98. In their advice to the Tribunal, Fitzgerald and Sivananthan deal in different ways with the various component parts of the crime of genocide, as now

---

[58] There is a recurring issue with the use of the term genocide by those who have themselves personally suffered, or are concerned on behalf of those who have suffered, terribly at the hands of others. Believing that no suffering can match for gravity their suffering, such people often want the cause of the suffering labelled as 'genocide' on the basis that genocide is the worst of all possible crimes. This is a grave misunderstanding as there are many examples of crimes labelled in other ways that might be regarded as being as bad, or worse, than genocide. For example, the destruction of the Twin Towers in 2001 was no genocide. Should someone explode a nuclear device – or let off a 'dirty bomb' – in a multi-ethnic city it would not necessarily be genocide.

Genocide is a crime for which there has to be proof of a particular hostile state of mind in an individual or in a government body towards a group that qualifies under the Genocide Convention's or the ICC Statute's limited set of groups against whom genocide can be committed. The state of mind – hostility to a group simply because of who are in the group – is irrational or even mentally disturbed by today's standards. It is not *necessarily* more evil or wicked than would be a mental state driving a calmly calculated decision to commit the same acts but for a clearly non-genocidal reason – e.g. to slaughter a defined ethnic group of prisoners who might otherwise rise again as combatants. And as to the difficulties of any victim group being properly within the statutory definition, the limited category of qualifying groups is a matter of drafting of the Convention in 1948 and not now a matter for revision or even complaint.

In short, atrocities of concern not being labelled or proved as genocide but being cast as different crimes, for example crimes against humanity, in no way diminishes the gravity of those crimes.

regularly codified. But both experts agree that, based on the facts before the Tribunal, all bar one of the component parts of genocide are present – see Fitzgerald's Opinion, paragraphs 1-25 and Supplementary Opinion, and Sivananthan's Advice, paragraphs 9-21 (Appendix 4).

99. Sivananthan was much more cautious about the one outstanding component, namely the specific mental state (*mens rea*) required to prove genocide. He explains in the opening paragraph of his Advice:

> *The area of law in which this advice is sought upon is complex. As such, too much focus on simplifying the law for the purposes of this advice may run the risk of having important legal principles and legal thoughts on the subject matter overlooked in favour of simplicity, which in turn may result in an uninformed decision being made by the China Tribunal. The area of law is new and bridled with uncertainties, some of which have yet to be fleshed out by international jurisprudence.*

100. In his concluding remarks on genocide (his paragraph 26) he highlights some of the considerations and difficulties in deciding about 'intent'. On the possibility of relying on a 'knowledge-based' genocide he is firmly of the view:

> *An important point that must be noted by the China Tribunal is that an intention to forcefully harvest the organs for the sake of profit is not the same as an intention to forcefully harvest the organs to bring about the physical or biological destruction in part or in whole of a protected group. In deciding whether genocide has been committed, the China Tribunal must make this distinction carefully. One may seek to argue that even if the harvesting of the organs were done for the sake of profit, the perpetrators would have knowledge that their actions would bring about the destruction in part or in whole of the group. However, this argument is reliant on a knowledge-based approach that has yet to be supported by any court, rather than a purpose-based approach that has been adopted by the ICTY [International Criminal Tribunal for the Former Yugoslavia], ICTR [International Criminal Tribunal for Rwanda] and ICC. As such, it is highly unlikely that the perpetrators' knowledge <u>of the effect of their actions without any intention to cause such an effect would be sufficient to meet the requirement of intent under the Genocide Convention.</u>*

101. In his second Supplementary Opinion, having reviewed Sivananthan's Advice, and further evidence from the Tribunal, Fitzgerald is firmly of the view that the Uyghur population in China is likely to satisfy the requirement of being a 'substantial part' of the world Uyghur population, sufficient for the purposes of a genocide finding, if all other elements are established.

102. However he agrees with Sivananthan that there are serious issues with proving specific intent in relation to genocide of the Uyghurs, making the point, as he does, that harvesting organs for profit from Uyghurs is not the same thing as intending to bring about the physical or biological destruction of Uyghurs as a group (protected by the Genocide Convention) in whole or in part. Both experts explain that the evidence they have been shown by the Tribunal seems to indicate that the Chinese Government wishes to destroy Uyghurs as a separate cultural group, but not as a physical group. This aim would not meet the 'intent' requirement of the crime of genocide, since genocide, as Sivananthan points out (in his paragraph 23) involves physical or biological destruction of a group, and cultural destruction is different. To meet the requirement of intent in the case of the Uyghurs, the organ harvesting would either have to be on a massive scale, such that it would be liable to bring about the physical disappearance of a substantial part of the population of Uyghurs in China, or it would have to take place as part of a wider attempt to destroy the group, in which organ harvesting was combined with mass murder, deprivation of necessities of life, and other acts of genocide.

103. Fitzgerald does not think that the evidence presently available could support a case of genocide committed by China against the Uyghurs.

104. Armed with additional information about the evidence and Sivananthan's Advice, however, Fitzgerald considers genocide seems much stronger in the case of Falun Gong practitioners, particularly in relation to specific intent, in view of the existence of the 610 office (see paragraph 147 below) expressly dedicated to the destruction of Falun Gong, evidence indicating widespread and systematic use of Falun Gong prisoners for organ harvesting, and of the fact that all Falun Gong prisoners had blood samples taken as a matter of routine subsequent to their initial detention.

105. Fitzgerald considers that in the case of Falun Gong because of the context of a systematic attempt to destroy the group, the evidence of organ harvesting, if

accepted by the Tribunal as accurate, does, or certainly could, fulfil the legal definition of genocide.

106. On the sometimes troubling issue of whether Falun Gong could qualify as a religion for purposes of the crime of genocide, Fitzgerald finds his earlier positive opinion on the subject strengthened by the UK Supreme Court case of R(Hodkin) v Registrar of Births, Marriages and Deaths [2013] UKSC 77, which considers the definition of religion at paragraphs 31-64 of its judgment. In light of this authoritative ruling on the issue by the Supreme Court, both experts consider that it is beyond argument that Falun Gong is a religious group.[59]

107. Critical to the Tribunal's final conclusions is the manner in which it intends to deal with the *strength* of any judgment it makes – whether a matter is 'proved beyond reasonable doubt' or a conclusion of lesser strength is expressed in 'non-legal language'. In consequence, if it is unable to be certain about any component part of a crime it is considering, the Tribunal will only be able to express its conclusion about the commission of that crime in non-legal terms. For genocide, the Tribunal could find that all the component criminal acts have been proved – against named and unnamed individuals, and even the PRC itself – but conclusions of 'beyond reasonable doubt' are not possible so far as the complete offence of genocide is concerned without better evidence of the thinking processes of the individuals or state.

108. The Tribunal's conclusions in paragraphs 471-478 below, set out the elements of the offence of genocide of which it is certain, guided by the Opinions and Advice, together with its decision about genocidal intent and its overall conclusion about genocide.

109. **Crimes Against Humanity** In paragraphs 28-30 of his Opinion, Fitzgerald raises some concerns about whether forced organ harvesting, as evidenced, could constitute an 'attack', as defined in international humanitarian law. This issue was resolved in the video link conference between Tribunal members and Fitzgerald, and the necessary descriptors 'widespread' and 'systematic' are very clearly factual issues for the Tribunal, not ruled out on any technical grounds.

---

[59] The Tribunal was assisted in its deliberations by the letter from Professor Peter W Edge. And Dr Michael John-Hopkins. https://chinatribunal.com/wp-content/uploads/2019/06/Edge-and-John-Hopkins-letter.pdf]

110. Sivananthan lists, in paragraph 27 of his Advice, the 'prohibited acts' – proof of one or more of these would be essential to any finding that a crime against humanity had occurred. In paragraph 34 and paragraphs 37–30 he deals with the requirement of knowledge of an attack and the discriminatory element required for some acts, going on to caution about the term 'widespread'. He directs the Tribunal as to the best route to its judgment, which the Tribunal followed as shown later at paragraphs 479-484

111. Both the Opinions and the Advice deal with universal jurisdiction, where the courts of some countries are allowed by law to try anyone from any country for certain particular offences committed anywhere in the world, i.e. the alleged crime being without *any* connection to the countries exercising such jurisdiction. Some countries exercise such jurisdiction for offences of torture. Sivananthan notes that the definition of torture in the Convention Against Torture excludes 'pain or suffering arising from lawful punishment or incidental to it' but that the criteria for a finding of torture are clear and straightforward in light of the evidence heard and read by the Tribunal.

112. On the additional question of whether the International Court of Justice could be engaged, Fitzgerald notes that Article IX of the Genocide Convention provides that:

> *Disputes between the contracting parties relating to the interpretation, application or fulfilment of the present Convention, including those relating to the responsibility of a State for genocide or for any of the other acts enumerated in article III, shall be submitted to the International Court of Justice at the request of any of the parties to the dispute.*

113. Fitzgerald explains that although China is a party to the Genocide Convention it has entered a specific reservation in relation to Article IX, so a case against it in relation to an allegation of genocide cannot be referred to the International Court of Justice under the Genocide Convention itself.

114. Nor, he says, can the issue be referred to the ICJ by another country, bilaterally, outside the framework of the Convention, save in the extremely improbable event that China, now the PRC, agreed to such a reference, because the long-established jurisprudence of the ICJ is that its contentious jurisdiction under Article 36 of its Statute is founded upon the consent of

the parties (See e.g. *Corfu Channel (Preliminary Objections)* ICJ Reports 1948, p15).

115. In addition to its contentious jurisdiction (between parties in disagreement) under Article 36 of its Statute, the ICJ exercises an advisory jurisdiction under Article 65. This provides that:

116. *The court may give an advisory opinion on any legal question at the request of whatever body may be authorised by or in accordance with the Charter of the United Nations to make such a request.*

117. Thus, says Fitzgerald, the UN General Assembly can ask the ICJ for an advisory opinion, as, for example, in its recent Opinion on the Legal Consequences of the Separation of the Chagos Archipelago (25 February 2019), which was referred to the ICJ by a majority vote of the General Assembly, opposed by the United Kingdom which currently occupies the Chagos Islands. In the exercise of this advisory jurisdiction, unlike the ICJ contentious jurisdiction, there is no longer a rule that the affected states must consent to exercise of the advisory jurisdiction (see Western Sahara case, ICJ reports 1975, paragraph 12).

118. Moreover, he notes, there is no veto by permanent members of the UN Security Council in relation to resolutions of the UN General Assembly. So, it is therefore theoretically possible that the UN General Assembly could refer the issue of genocide by the PRC to the ICJ.

119. It is also arguable that such authorisation has also been given to the UN Human Rights Council by the UN Resolution which created that body (Resolution 60/251 of 15 March 2006), so it would seem theoretically possible that in a situation of widespread and intense international outrage at apparent genocide, the UN Human Rights Council might refer a question of possible genocide to the ICJ, which would then presumably rule on the legality of the reference, before moving on to rule on the substantive issue.

120. On the basis that the Tribunal finds that crimes have been committed in the course of forced organ harvesting, its mandate includes:

   ... 2. If so, what legal and other actions should be taken by the international community? In responding to these questions, the Tribunal

should consider the extent to which alleged perpetrators of forced organ harvesting can be named under relevant legislation and the effect of sovereign immunity on protecting wrongdoers from civil suits.

121. The Opinions and Advice identify jurisdictional possibilities and hurdles; possibilities include the exercise of universal jurisdiction of many countries for offences against customary international law, offences of genocide, crimes against humanity and torture; hurdles include the limitations effectively imposed by China not being a party to the Rome statute of the ICC and being able to veto reference to it in the Security Council and the possibility of the PRC exercising 'head of state immunity'.

122. Underlying the lawyers' words are the following realities confronting the citizen – and the China Tribunal is composed of citizens. (See Sartre on the powerlessness of a People's Tribunal, page 7 above.)

    No matter how grave atrocities elsewhere in the world may be, the non-politician citizen has no direct access to any empowered court to achieve action other than by writing to the Prosecutor of the International Criminal Court urging action or, in a democracy, pressing their representative in a parliament to encourage their government to take action.

    Government action in such matters *is* possible – by using universal powers established in national courts; by referring the gravest of breaches of Conventions to the International Court of Justice; by pressing for action by the International Criminal Court; or by doing the same at the UN or in the Security Council.

    The powers of government to initiate processes, at criminal courts or at the International Court of Justice, over atrocities believed to have been committed by other countries will always be subject to political considerations, which may result in, for example, a government refusing to face revealed realities, finding political justification for complete inactivity or 'foot dragging' once processes have been initiated.

123. These realities are not dealt with specifically in the Opinions or Advice but are matters of common knowledge and within the experience of members of the Tribunal.

124. In these circumstances, it may be futile for this Tribunal to press particular solutions when it would be entirely unrealistic to expect governments to act on the Tribunal's recommendations.

125. It may be better to note the possible courses of action that governments *could* take, and leave to citizens, activists and motivated politicians the task of pressing governments to do what may be thought their duty in the face of any revealed wickedness such as forced organ harvesting that has happened or is continuing to happen.

126. Guided by the Opinions and Advice, the Tribunal lists in paragraph 485 and following –without recommendations – possible courses of action that governments and others may take in light of findings made in paragraphs 448 – 484.

Evidence

127. The tribunal considered several categories of evidence, – for example, evidence of medical testing, evidence of incarceration and torture – confining its consideration of any particular category to that category and nothing else, and approaching its analysis, as noted above, on the basis that the evidence relates to an imaginary country that has a good human rights record. The Tribunal's conclusions are outlined in the final paragraphs of each category. In reaching these, the Tribunal has asked itself what, viewed in isolation, would the evidence tell us about the subject matter of the category, the imagined country and its relationship with a particular minority group? The purpose and value of this exercise emerges later in paragraph 453.

General Information Relating to Transplant Surgery[60]

128. The ability to transplant an organ from one human being to another may be considered a scientific and social triumph. It has been hailed as such in many societies and has been used as an indicator of the development of a state and a measure of its status. In many ways, organ transplantation represents the apotheosis of human generosity; one human thinking of another and, in mental preparation for death, having the generosity of spirit to offer one or more of their organs (after their own death) potentially to save the life of another (unknown) person.

129. An organ transplant is a surgical operation in which a failed or damaged organ is removed and replaced with one from another individual. Following improved understanding of immunology and tissue rejection (and its suppression), solid organ (eg heart, lung, liver, kidney) transplantation has evolved considerably over the last 70 years and procedures have been developed to permit transplantation of many organ types. Most people will

---

[60] Material under this heading should be non-controversial and can be sourced in the following textbooks. Textbook of organ transplantation, Eds. Kirk AD, Knechtle SJ, Larsen CP, Pearson TC, Madsen JC, Webber SA. Published 2014; John Wiley, UK

be familiar with kidney, liver, corneal, heart and lung transplantation, but over recent years, bowel, pancreas, uterus and even face transplants have become possible.

130. Integral to any form of transplantation is the principle of consent; of the organ donor and his or her family, and of the recipient. The family of the donor is important, because the members of that family have both to live on after the donor's death and to live with any decisions they make or support. Throughout most of the world, governance structures have evolved to ensure that transplantation is conducted against a set of strong ethical principles. Organs should only be removed from people who have either given consent or, in the case of countries legislating for an opt-out system, have not *objected* in advance to such removal. In either case, relatives should, after the death of the potential donor, have the right of veto. This is widely agreed throughout the world.

131. In most countries, organs can only be removed from people who are brain dead (DBD, donation after brain death).

132. The three findings essential to define brain death are coma, the absence of brainstem reflexes, and apnoea (absence of breathing). An evaluation for brain death should be considered in patients who have suffered a massive, irreversible brain injury of identifiable cause, including trauma. A patient determined to be brain dead is legally and clinically dead. More recently, donation after circulatory death (DCD)[61] has become possible because of advances in organ preservation, and this has resulted in a modest increase in the number of available donor organs[62].

---

[61] *'Donation after Circulatory Death (DCD), previously referred to as donation after cardiac death or non-heartbeating organ donation, refers to the retrieval of organs for the purpose of transplantation from patients whose death is diagnosed and confirmed using cardio-respiratory criteria.*

'There are two principal types of DCD, controlled and uncontrolled. Uncontrolled DCD refers to organ retrieval after a cardiac arrest that is unexpected and from which the patient cannot or should not be resuscitated. In contrast, controlled DCD takes place after death which follows the planned withdrawal of life-sustaining treatments that have been considered to be of no overall benefit to a critically ill patient on ICU or in the Emergency Department.' Source: https://www.odt.nhs.uk/deceased-donation/best-practice-guidance/donation-after-circulatory-death/

[62] Smith M, Dominguez-Gil B, Greer DM, Manara AR, Souter, MJ: Organ Donation after Circulatory Death; current status and future potential. Intensive Care Med (2019) 45:310–321

133. Demand for organ replacement far exceeds supply. Waiting times for organs are long and deaths of potential recipients occur while waiting for an organ to become available.

134. Without the principle of consent, organ donation has the potential to become coercive, either exploiting the poor (by trading in organs such as a kidney) or violating the human rights of individuals, as in the case of executed prisoners, extracting their organs either without any consent or under conditions of forced consent – contrary to Articles 3 of the Universal Declaration of Human Rights. It has been argued that a trade in organs, provided that it ensures that the seller is fully informed of all the consequences of donation, is a mutually beneficial transaction between consenting adults. A donation which unavoidably results in the death of the donor can in no way be considered mutually beneficial to both parties.

135. Live donation of blood, bone marrow, a kidney, part of a liver and part of a lung is possible without sacrificing the donor, who can return to a normal life. Most transplantation of solid organs, however, can only take place from a cadaver; it is not possible to continue living without, for example, a heart, lungs, whole liver or both kidneys.

136. Organ donation laws vary from country to country but are largely covered by the concepts of 'opt in' or 'opt out', summarised above. To opt in means that an individual adds their name to a voluntary organ donor list, usually maintained nationally. Opt-out systems mean that an individual will automatically be deemed a potential organ donor unless they register their wishes to opt out in advance. In both systems, the family of the donor has a say in whether organs can be used after death. The entire process is built on sound, well-established ethical foundations and considerable trust.[63]

137. Successful transplantation also requires the following:

- As close as possible tissue type matching between donor and recipient. This usually comprises matching ABO blood type and human leukocyte antigen (HLA) compatibility. If HLA antigens (which regulate the immune system) of the recipient are well matched with a donor organ,

---

63   Virtual Mentor. 2012;14(3):264-268. doi: 10.1001/virtualmentor.2012.14.3.mhst1-1203.

the possibility of donor organ rejection is minimised. Recently, molecular techniques have been developed for HLA DNA testing[64] which allow greater accuracy in testing. Once a donor has been identified, more detailed cross-matching may also be employed.

- Proof of the absence of other disease (usually infection or malignancy) in the donor.
- Appropriate organ size matching.[65]

138. Transplantation at national and international level (at scale) requires an infrastructure that matches potential recipients with the characteristics of a donor. The shortage of available organs in relation to the demand means that there exists in most countries a formal organ-allocation system, which varies according to organ.[66]

139. Organs are usually retrieved from donors at the hospital in which the donor is being cared for. Each country has an integrated system for organ retrieval, underpinned by strong ethical principles and robust quality – and clinical governance-support systems, which respect both the donor and their family's wishes.[67] A single donor may provide organs for several recipients, for example, one patient could donate heart, small bowel, pancreas, two kidneys, and two parts of a liver, and two lungs. Thus, nine patients who would otherwise die, may live because of one act of donation.

140. An effective transport and organ distribution system is necessary to create a well-functioning transplant system. To maintain clear ethical separation, the retrieval (donor) team is maintained as a separate entity from the recipient (transplant) team. The extracted organs are packed cold and transported to the recipient hospital as quickly and safely as possible.[68] Advances in organ preservation have meant that it is not necessary for donor and recipient to be in the same place.

---

[64]   https://doi.org/10.1016/B978-0-12-407821-5.00024-3

[65]   See footnote 60 supra.

[66]   By way of example for UK regulations and system see: https://www.odt.nhs.uk/ transplantation/tools-policies-and-guidance/ Details are beyond the scope of this Judgment.

[67]   For more information see: https://www.odt.nhs.uk/retrieval/retrieval-process

[68]   Recent developments mean that organs may be perfused warm in certain circumstances during transport

141.	Skilled trained teams of transplant surgeons, physicians, nurses and technicians are required. Transplantation is a highly integrated process requiring a broad range of expertise.

142.	Transplantation is built on trust, and proper governance structures are designed to underpin that trust. Removal of organs from a conscious and healthy person, without their consent, clearly constitutes murder if the organs are vital to life. If the organ can be spared, as in the case of a single kidney or part of a liver or lung, coerced or forced removal would in *any* system of law constitute a grave crime. Either coercive or forced transplantation clearly conflicts with the 'philosophy' inherent in medicine, wherever it is practised and regardless of political or religious beliefs.

143.	These understandings have assisted the Tribunal in its assessments of what normally happens in transplant surgery and to what extent this 'normal' background can inform the Tribunal's consideration of the evidence of what surgeons in the PRC may have done.

General Information about China

144.	China is one of the oldest continuous civilisations of the world. It is the world's third largest country geographically and its most populous country, with some 1.4 billion inhabitants. Since the Chinese Communist Party (CCP) came to power in 1949 the PRC has come to enjoy substantial economic advances, especially in recent decades.

145.	The people of China – its citizens – have lived under authoritarian communist governments since World War II. That may be significant for understanding the behaviour of some of the country's citizens in the events which are the subject of this Tribunal's inquiry. But there can be no suggestion that the people of China are in any way different, in essence, from other human beings, or entitled to rights different from those of other human beings. Indeed, the events in Tiananmen Square in 1989, or the subsequent willingness of individuals to protest for human rights causes in which they believe, show that the Chinese people's understanding of their rights as humans is no different from that of their fellow human beings living under different regimes around the world. Practitioners of Falun Gong, in particular, who have never been characterised as anything but entirely peaceful, and who at one stage were believed to number 70 million in China, are driven by the pursuit of truthfulness, compassion and forbearance. Their beliefs may be thought entirely compatible with universal human rights now, just as they were when a citizen of China contributed to the drafting of the 1948 Declaration of Human Rights.

146. The PRC is entitled to the respect that is due to an enormous and powerful state. Its citizens are entitled to the respect that is due to every citizen of the world. And that self-same respect is due to them *from* every citizen of the world, however near or far from China they may be.[69]

147. For a general account of relevant early history, the Tribunal has accepted as reliable the background sections of the Statement of Facts and Application to Law report prepared for the Tribunal by the COHRC (China Organ Harvest Research Centre), written by Grace Yin, David Li, Yiyang Xia, William H. Boericke, Ann F. Corson, Michel le Li, Huige Li.[70] (See excerpt below) Two of the authors, David Li and Dr Huige Li, spoke to the Tribunal as witnesses.[71] The Tribunal pays no regard to any conclusions drawn in the report about organ harvesting, – these conclusions are for the Tribunal to draw from all the evidence.

Excerpt from the COHRC report:

> *Since 2000, the Chinese government prioritized organ transplantation in its national strategy and continuously incorporated organ transplantation into its Five-Year Plans for multiple ministries. The government invested heavily in research, development, and personnel training in transplantation technology to meet the needs of this rapidly growing industry. A large number of organ transplantation projects developed as a result of funding from major national programs established by the ministries of health, science and technology, and education, as well as from other sources within the central government. The military and local governments invested heavily in domestic medical institutions to facilitate basic research and development in*

---

[69] These very general observations may be seen as particularly relevant when the Tribunal observations about actions to be taken by the citizen are considered at paragraphs 485 – 496

[70] Relevant history appears in many other documents the Tribunal has considered, usually backed by substantial research.

[71] Appendix 2A, Witness 36

organ transplantation and promote its industrialization. Prestigious universities and affiliated hospitals, as well as almost all military and civilian medical universities and their affiliated hospitals, rapidly developed their organ transplant research and received large amounts of funding. As a result, China's transplant centres made breakthroughs in key organ transplantation capabilities and technologies which have allowed the industry to become the most prolific in the world in just a few years. Beginning in 2000, [it leapt] from 'follower' to 'leader' of worldwide transplantation technology in recent years. These initiatives and developments happened before China piloted its first organ donation program in 2010.

[Indeed] China came to perform more transplants than any other country in the world in just a few years after 2000 despite the lack of an organ donation system.

After allegations of forced organ harvesting from prisoners attracted international scrutiny in 2006, the Ministry of Health established a new approval system that required hospitals to obtain permits from the Ministry to continue performing transplants after July 2007. Of the more than 1,000 hospitals that applied, 164 were given permits. This change created a false impression that most hospitals in China stopped performing transplants in July 2007. In fact, the large Ministry-approved institutions have continued to develop with full government support and expanded significantly with the addition of more beds and new wards, wings and buildings.

In response to international criticism since 2006, Chinese officials acknowledged that almost all transplant organs came from death-row prisoners but later, it was claimed, from voluntary donations.

Huang Jiefu, a critical figure to the early history[72] said in a CCTV

---

[72]   Current Chair of the PRC's National Organ Donation and Transplantation Committee; reported to have led the party committee in the Sun Yat-sen University studying anti Falun Gong literature. In May 2001 reported as saying the 'struggle against Falun Gong is a serious political campaign. We must have no mercy towards the few active members'; in September 2005 he ordered two spare livers of the required blood type from Guangzhou and Chongqing to do a demonstration transplant operation in Xinjiang province. The inference drawn is that two

interview in 2015 that China built up its organ donation and transplant framework in only a few years, whereas in other countries this process required decades. He further stated in 2017 that the difference between the Chinese model and that of the West is that China is the only country where a central government plays a leading role in developing organ donations and transplants.

Falun Gong is a Buddhist meditation practice based on ancient Chinese traditions of health and self-improvement, whose adherents seek to cultivate the qualities of truthfulness, compassion, and tolerance. By the end of the 1990s, the government estimated that over 70 million people in China were practicing Falun Gong, a figure also quoted by several Western news outlets. The former Communist Party leader Jiang Zemin saw the group's popularity and revival of traditional values as a threat to his rule and launched a violent campaign on July 20, 1999 to eradicate Falun Gong. Under direct orders from Jiang Zemin, the CCP Central Committee established a 'Central Leading Group for Handling the Falun Gong Issue' under which the '610 Office', an ad hoc agency named for the date of its founding, June 10, 1999, came into being. The 610 Office was built with a structure extending from top to bottom throughout the Party, government, and military. Jiang made a speech in Politburo Meeting on June 7 requiring that 'all CCP central departments, all ministries, all provinces, and all cities must cooperate with the 610 Offices very closely.' The 610 Office was endowed with extraordinarily broad and extra-legal power to systematically eradicate Falun Gong. However, its existence was kept a state secret until December 2013. Each level of the 610 Office can override other government organizations at the same level and reports directly to its next higher level. The 610 Office of the Central Committee has been approved neither by the

---

people were killed to order for the 'back up' livers – that were never used – to be available. In a January 2003 paper he had referred to 123 orthotopic liver transplantations performed at his centre with warm ischemia time between 30 seconds and 8 minutes – indicating death at the hospital site not at an execution site. A 2012 paper he co-authored an article recording … 10 liver pancreas transplants from voluntary donors with no heartbeats all aged between 21 and 41, consistent with livers coming from extrajudicial killings because voluntary donation had yet to start in the PRC; See several further references to Huang Jiefu below and https://chinatribunal. com/wp-content/uploads/2019/06/MagnitskySubmission_OfficialsSurgeons_Final.pdf, pages 29 *et seq.*

National People's Congress (NPC) nor by the State Council. Thus, it derives its power not from the law but rather the Chinese Communist Party itself. Most 610 Office orders are issued verbally, and those who receive the orders are forbidden to record them or write them down. 610 Offices on various levels are authorized to act outside the law. 610 Office agents can break into civil residences at any time without a warrant; they can ransack homes, conduct body searches, and make arrests without following any legal procedures; they can send people to prison and forced labour camps without judicial process; and they are not held responsible for using torture.

A collection of documents and notices issued around July 20, 1999, identifies the official start of the persecution of Falun Gong practitioners. The 'CCP Central Committee's Notice of Forbidding CCP Members to Practice Falun Gong' states that 'the transformation task for CCP members who practice Falun Dafa [= Falun Gong; an alternative name] must be accomplished.' It also defines the standard for 'transformation' as 'to voluntarily separate from Falun Gong organizations, to mentally sever the relationship with Falun Dafa, and to expose and criticize Falun Gong and its founder.' On August 24, 1999, Xinhua News Agency published a notice from the Office of CCP Central Committee and the State Council that extended the above policy from Party members to all Falun Gong practitioners 'to better accomplish the mission of transforming the majority of Falun Gong practitioners.' These documents emphasized that even for 'those who practice Falun Gong only for the purpose of health and fitness,' if they do not hold the 'correct opinion' and do not give up their faith, then they will not be treated as having been 'converted.' The documents instructed all offices and organizations 'to spy on and investigate Falun Gong practitioners and identify all un-transformed practitioners.' They demanded that 'for those un-converted Falun Gong practitioners (though they only practice at home), there is no exception but to send them batch-by-batch to the law education centres [brainwashing facilities – authors' note.] for transformation.' The documents also claimed that Falun Gong practitioners are 'specially treated' because they violated the laws. However, there is no law in China stating that practicing Falun Gong is illegal. The campaign to eradicate Falun Gong was thus launched by the personal will of Communist Party leader Jiang Zemin and has no legal basis. On

November 30, 1999, the Central 610 Office called more than 3,000 officials to the Great Hall of the People to address the campaign against Falun Gong. The head of Central Leading Group on Dealing with the Falun Gong Issue, Li Lanqing, announced Jiang's directives to 'ruin their reputations, break them financially, and destroy them physically.' The Party's policies were as follows: 'Party members are prohibited from practicing Falun Gong.' '100% transformation (renouncing the practice) with absolutely no exceptions.' 'Three terminations and one detention': being expelled from the party, removed from official posts, terminated from one's job, and detained. On August 21, 2000, the Ministry of Public Security held a nationwide telephone conference to relay new orders that the practice of Falun Gong was to be eradicated in three months.

In early September 2001, after being subjected to intense pressure from the international community, the Chinese judicial system ordered the release of illegally detained Falun Gong practitioners, especially those who were being held beyond their terms. However, Luo Gan, the head of the 610 Office, issued a secret order to all levels of the judicial system: 'Whoever is found to be practicing Falun Gong should be secretly arrested and sentenced to a life sentence until death. Police officers that do not arrest Falun Gong practitioners will be discharged from public service, and their permanent residency registrations will be revoked.' In the same month, Jiang Zemin issued another directive: 'Beating them to death is nothing. If they are disabled from the beating, it counts as their injuring themselves. If they die, it counts as suicide!' In March 2002, several directives were spread to all levels of the 610 Office: First, eradicating Falun Gong is an arduous political task; do not be afraid of bloodshed and Second, tightly conceal the deaths and prevent leaking of information, which could lead to negative international impact; Third, all levels of the prosecution and judiciary branches of the government should not conduct investigations into the deaths or injuries of Falun Gong practitioners. Everything should give way to the big picture.

In 2002, Jiang Zemin promoted Zhou Yongkang to be Minister of Public Security and Deputy Secretary of the Central Political and Legal Affairs Committee, which handles policy guidelines and directs the work of the Supreme People's Procuratorate, the Supreme People's

*Law, the Ministry of Justice, and the Ministry of Public Security.
Zhou made the eradication of Falun Gong a major focus of domestic
security work in China. He was further promoted to head the 'Central
Leading Group for Handling the Falun Gong Issue' and was placed on
the Party's highest strategic tier, the Politburo Standing Committee,
in October 2007. Du Daobin, a former Hubei provincial government
worker, also reported in May 2003 that the local 610 Office had received
instructions that stated, 'No law regulates the treatment of Falun Gong
practitioners' and 'deaths of Falun Gong practitioners from beating
are nothing and shall be counted as suicide; the bodies shall be directly
cremated without investigating the person's identification.' Numerous
cases of practitioners' bodies being cremated without the consent of
their families continue to be reported on Minghui.org.[73] According to
its website in 2004, the China International Transplantation Network
Assistance Centre (CITNAC), which focused primarily on foreign
patients, attributed its achievements to government support: 'To be
able to complete such a large number of organ transplant surgeries
every year, we need to give all of our thanks to the support given by
the government. In particular, the Supreme People's Court, Supreme
People's Procuratorate, Ministry of Public Security, Ministry of
Justice, Ministry of Health, and Ministry of Civil Affairs have jointly
promulgated laws to establish that organ procurement receives
government support and protection. This is one of a kind in the world.[74]*

148. This report by COHRC is very heavily footnoted and apparently well-researched, although not all of it is immediately accessible to English language readers.

---

[73] Minghui.org – from its website – is an all-volunteer organization that operates a website dedicated to reporting on the Falun Gong community worldwide. The focus of Minghui is reports from China. For more than a decade, Minghui editors have received scores of first-hand reports from across China every day – more than any other organisation in the world. Minghui offers the most direct and up-to-date window into the lives of Falun Gong practitioners across China and throughout the world. Minghui also serves as a central communication hub for Falun Gong practitioners around the world to share insights and ideas, expose the persecution faced inside China, and comment on its ramifications. It is the primary site read by Falun Gong practitioners. It is also watched closely by Chinese regime officials.

[74] https://chinatribunal.com/wp-content/uploads/2019/04/COHRC_SubmissionCover-Letter_COHRC-DavidLi.pdf

https://chinatribunal.com/wp-content/uploads/2019/04/COHRC_Independent-Tribunal-_Statement-of-Facts-Application-to-Law_20181128_Submited.pdf

Nothing in the report has been contradicted by the evidence from witnesses heard in person by the Tribunal; much of it has been directly confirmed.

149. The dramatic increase in hostility by the PRC towards Falun Gong practitioners after the various 1999 statements can be seen in documents provided by Hong Chen, a witness to the Tribunal (see paragraphs 192 and 216 below).

It may have been only in the early stages of the changed approach to Falun Gong practitioners that documents of any kind were provided – few witnesses who gave evidence to the Tribunal spoke of receiving any. Hong Chen's documents from 2000 may be seen as confirming other evidence about the determined, bureaucratic and unforgiving approach of the PRC to Falun Gong practitioners. On 2 November 1999 she had four books of Falun Gong beliefs withheld. On 13 March 2000, for breach of Communist Party discipline in going to a Falun Gong gathering, she was suspended from the Communist Party for one year – this was 'to allow her to re-educate herself'. On 28 April 2000, she was detained for a year for 're-education through labour'. The language of the order is revealing:

Upon investigation Hong Chen has the following illegal behaviours:

On the morning of 24 April 2000, Chen colluded with Shuping Zhang and intruded into Beijing, engaging in "Falun Gong" evil cult activities on Tiananmen Square, and was captured. After that, a large number of "Falun Gong" evil cult books, audio and video materials were found from Chen's home and confiscated.

During her detention by the Public Security Bureau, she still stubbornly stuck to her 'Falun Gong' evil cult's position and had bad attitude.

According to the State Council's relevant laws and rules on the issue of re-education- through-labour, it is now decided that Hong Chen will be re-educated through labour for one year (from 24 April 2000 to 23 April 2001).[75]

---

[75]   English translations of Hong Chen's documents can be found on the China Tribunal website or directly at:
https://chinatribunal.com/wp-content/uploads/2019/08/HongChen_Instructions-on-the-Handling-of-CHEN-Hong%E2%80%99s-Mistakes-English.jpg.pdf

On 24 May 2000 she was removed from Communist party membership.

150. Another witness, Yiyang Xia, spoke of a different report, prepared by The Human Rights Law Foundation (HRLF), a body entirely separate from COHRC (whose report is quoted in paragraph 147 above). The China Tribunal accepts as accurate the following narrative from the HRLF report and has no reason to doubt the reliability of the commentary made in the report about the period of relevant history. The report contains various documents, consistent with the COHRC report, that reveal Jiang Zemin's plan in his own words. Some of the things he said, mostly recorded in written communications, are included in the following excerpts:[76]

> *On April 27, 1999, the Office of the CCP Central Committee issued a 'Notice about Copying and Distribution of the "Letter from Jiang Zemin to Politburo Standing Committee Members and Other Related Leaders".' This notice ordered CCP leaders to study a letter written by Jiang Zemin on the night of April 25, 1999. It also ordered CCP leaders to implement the directives contained in the letter and report their progress in meeting those orders to the CCP's Central Committee. According to this notice, it was Jiang Zemin who personally decided to respond to Falun Gong adherents' peaceful appeal with a violent persecution. Jiang Zemin's letter and notice showed that he sought to impose his views on the top leadership of the CCP. (The notice ordered CCP leaders to study and implement the letter, rather than asking for suggestions and advice.)*
>
> *Jiang Zemin sent CCP leaders a few important signals in his letter: 'Was this [April 25 peaceful petitioning incident] related to overseas and the western countries? Were there "Master-hands" behind*

---

https://chinatribunal.com/wp-content/uploads/2019/08/HongChen_List-of-Withheld-Articles-English.jpg.pdf

https://chinatribunal.com/wp-content/uploads/2019/08/HongChen_InstructionsOnRemovingCHENHongsPartyMembershipEnglish.jpg.pdf

https://chinatribunal.com/wp-content/uploads/2019/06/HongChen_Decision-on-Re-education-through-Labour-English.pdf

[76] https://chinatribunal.com/wp-content/uploads/2019/04/April_HRLF_02-Exhibit-B-Jiang-Zemin.pdf (p3, paragraphs A,1a; A,1b; A,1c etc).

See also Appendix 2B, Item 40(b)

the scenes planning and directing?' The use of this aggressive and militaristic language against Falun Gong adherents was a signal for the launching of the violent crackdown, even before any investigation of the peaceful petitioning incident had been conducted.

'Can the Marxism, Materialism, and Atheism that we Communists have really not win over the theory that Falun Gong advocates? If that were true, it would be a real joke!

This incident showed how weak our ideological, political, and mass work has been in some areas and sections. We must insist on educating the cadres and general public with the right world outlook, philosophy, and values . . . Our leaders at all levels, especially at high levels, should be clearheaded now!' This may have indicated that the high level leaders in the CCP still did not want to comply with the crackdown. It was a personal order by Jiang Zemin. Thus, it became necessary to 'educate the cadres and general public' and to make sure that the high-level leadership was 'clearheaded' about Jiang Zemin's demand for their compliance in the persecution.

A second letter by Jiang Zemin (not available and only the subject of reports) was addressed to the members of the CCP's ruling 25-member Politburo. The content regarded how the CCP should 'deal with' what the letter described as a 'May 1, 2, and 3 Falun Gong practitioner gathering'. There has never been any Chinese or Western media report from any source about this 'gathering' and so it seems likely that Jiang Zemin was just using this as a further excuse to mobilize his persecution plan.

The second physically available document is the 'Notice about Printing and Distributing Comrade Jiang Zemin's Instructions to Politburo Members, the Offices of the Central Party Secretaries, and the [CCP's] Central Military Commission' by the Office of the Chinese Communist Party Central Committee' (Office of CCP Central Committee Official Document #19 [1999]). This document was officially sent out on May 23, 1999, based on Jiang Zemin's instructions regarding Falun Gong issued on May 8. The CCP's Provincial-level committees held meetings to study this document around May 28, 1999. So far, we do not have any original copies. The content of the document discusses how to secretly prepare for the persecution of Falun Gong (i.e., how severely to punish

Falun Gong adherents, what CCP resources to use for this purpose, and who should be in charge of implementing overall CCP orders regarding these tasks). This document was made available as evidence because it was incorporated into and referenced by an official document of the CCP Hebei Province Committee: (Hebei Official Document [1999] #21 'Seriously Following and Carrying out the Order of "the Office of CCP Central Committee Official Document [1999] #19"'). This document was exposed by Xu Xinmu, who worked for the Hebei provincial government. Due to exposing this secret document, Xu Xinmu and his collaborator in the exposure, Duan Rongxin,, were sentenced to four and eight years in jail, respectively. CCP media reported on the trial.

The third available document was also issued by the Office of the CCP Central Committee. This document ordered CCP leaders to study and implement 'Jiang Zemin's Speech in the Politburo Meeting about Paying Attention to Dealing with and Solving the Falun Gong Issue.' This document was dated June 7, 1999. The June 7 speech by Jiang Zemin directly ordered the establishment of the '610 Office' three days later on June 10 (that is also how '610 Office' was named). In the speech, Jiang Zemin said, 'the Falun Gong issue involved deep political and societal contexts and a complex international background. It was the most significant incident since the political turmoil in 1989. We must treat it seriously, do thorough research, and take effective countermeasures.' The speech equated Falun Gong adherents with the Tiananmen Square protestors in 1989, who were massacred for their nonviolent protests. This was another command by Jiang Zemin to mobilize the CCP to persecute Falun Gong.

In this speech, Jiang Zemin also announced that 'the central [CCP] authority has decided that Li Lanqing is going to lead the effort of establishing a "Leading Group" particularly for dealing with the Falun Gong issue. Li Lanqing will be the chief of the group. Ding Guangen and Luo Gan will be the deputy chiefs. Other group members will be the leaders from all related [CCP] departments. It will centralize all effort of discussing and implementing the detailed steps, tactics, and measures for solving the Falun Gong issue. The [CCP] Central Committee, and all [CCP] departments at the state level, provinces, municipal autonomous regions, and [other municipalities] must cooperate closely.' The leading group mentioned here was later called 'the Leading Group for Handling the Falun Gong Issue.' Its operating office was called 'the Office of the Leading Group for Handling the Falun Gong Issue,' which is also called the '610 Office.'

This speech indicates two important facts. The first is that establishment of the '610 Office' was Jiang Zemin's personal decision [and]Jiang Zemin's speech establishing a 'Leading Group' was just to tell the Politburo an already finalized decision, instead of proposing a motion. If the Politburo had already had a meeting on this subject before this meeting, it would be unnecessary for Jiang Zemin to tell the Politburo a decision they had made. If there was no meeting before that, it must have been Jiang Zemin's personal order.

In September 1999, at the APEC [Asia Pacific Economic Cooperation] meeting in New Zealand, Jiang Zemin made a very unusual move that was highly unprecedented at such gatherings. He gave leaders of all countries, including then-president Clinton, a book full of the CCP's anti-Falun Gong propaganda, including portrayals of Falun Gong adherents as dangerous and/or insane persons needing to be suppressed.

On October 25, 1999, before Jiang Zemin's state visit to France, he accepted an interview in written format by the French newspaper Le Figaro. Jiang Zemin attacked Falun Gong and called Falun Gong an 'evil cult,' before any documents or media controlled by the CCP had used the term. That again showed that it was Jiang Zemin who had personally made the decision for the crackdown and kept pushing it forward. Three days later, the CCP's official mouthpiece, the People's Daily, published special commentators' articles to echo Jiang's claim: 'Falun Gong Is A Cult.' Five days after Jiang's interview, the Standing Committee of People's Congress hurriedly passed the 'Decision to Ban Heretical Organizations [using the same phrase as 'Evil Cults.']'

In September 2000, Jiang Zemin was interviewed by CBS TV and made the following statement: 'after careful deliberations, we concluded that Falun Gong is an evil cult.'[77]

---

[77]   The complete HRLF report and its supporting footnotes can be found at Appendix 2A, Witness 40.

151. All witnesses have contributed to the Tribunal's overall understanding of the background. Witnesses making notably valuable contributions to the broad understanding of background include Edward McMillan-Scott[78], a former MEP (Member of the European Parliament) and an outside observer with many years' experience of the workings of China. He spoke of the non-violent nature of the practice of Falun Gong, and of the 70-100 million practitioners in 1999; and of the 25 April 1999 mass protest in Beijing as being peaceful. However, despite or because of his position, his own 2006 interviews with practitioners Cao Dong and Niu Jinping caused Cao Dong to be imprisoned.

152. His meeting and the meeting of the UN Rapporteur on Torture, Manfred Nowak, with human rights attorney Gao *Zhisheng* was followed by a traffic accident, injuring Gao, and believed to have been staged. This led Gao to send letters to the European Parliament and to the US Congress.[79] He was then imprisoned and tortured to such an extent that he attempted suicide. He is now reported to the 31st Session of the 2018 UN Universal Periodic Review (UPR) Working Group on China as an enforced disappearance.[80] McMillan-

---

The Report deals in some detail with the nature and various names of the 610 Office as follows:

The '610 Office' is an extrajudicial chain of command established for persecuting Falun Gong;

On June 10, 'the Leading Group for Handling Falun Gong Issues' was established. This office is formally known as 'The Office of the Leading Group for Handling Falun Gong Issues', also known as 'the 610 Office';

Since September 2000, it has sometimes also been referred to under the name of 'The Office for Preventing and Handling Cult-Related Issues of the State Council';

Since 2003, 'The Leading Group for Handling Falun Gong Issues' at all levels of the Party formally changed its name to

'The Leading Group for the Prevention and Handling of Cult-Related Issues' of the CCPCC.

This report also notes that in addition to domestic activities, the 610 Office has infiltrated Western countries.

[78] Appendix 2A, Witness 38

[79] https://gaoworks.wordpress.com/2015/10/07/gao-zhishengs-open-letter-to-the-united-states-congress-sep-12-2007/

[80] See: https://eeas.europa.eu/delegations/azerbaijan/62404/2018-human-rights-and-democracy-country-update---peoples-republic-china_zh-hans at paragraph 5

In August 2019 Amnesty International carried a report by a friend of Gao: 'In August 2017, Gao Zhisheng went missing again and has not been heard from since. His family and loved ones have never stopped worrying about him. We continue to look for Gao. We hope

Scott told of the consistency of accounts of Falun Gong practitioners concerning torture and of increased repression before the 2008 Olympics. Information he received from Special Rapporteurs Dr Nowak and Mrs Asma Jahangir suggested thousands were undergoing 're-education through labour' and gave accounts of later camps created for Uyghurs, as well as of medical testing of Falun Gong practitioners.

153. From a different angle, Matthew Robertson, a Chinese-speaking academic and researcher, spoke of how China's organ transplantation industry embarked on a period of rapid development post-2000, including the opening of new transplant wards, buildings, and research laboratories.[81] In that time, many hospitals performed their first liver, heart, and lung transplants, and thousands of new surgeons and nurses were trained and began publishing research. The state began to subsidise immunosuppressant research and manufacture and placed domestic immunosuppressants on health insurance subsidy lists. Many new organ transplant-related patents were registered; many more transplant-related medical papers were published. From official Chinese organ registry documents and clinical papers, it became clear that after the year 2000 there were numerous cases of transplants available *on demand*; hospitals regularly reported being able to perform transplants *within weeks*.[82]

154. Significantly, official explanations for organ sourcing in China have changed on several occasions. Prior to 2006, the official stance was that organs came from volunteers. In 2006, this shifted to all organs coming from death row prisoners. In 2015, it was claimed that only volunteers were used. Robertson explained that human rights research organisations and scholars are of the view that the number of death penalty executions declined almost every year

---

that we will soon find his gentle smile, his extraordinary strength, his unrelenting spirit in his fight for human dignity and his refusal to accept defeat.' https://www.amnesty.org/en/latest/news/2019/08/bravest-lawyer-china-gao-zhisheng/

[81]   Matthew Robertson is the former China News Editor for The Epoch Times. He was previously a reporter for the newspaper in Washington, D.C. In 2013 he was awarded the Society of Professional Journalists' Sigma Delta Chi award for coverage of the Chinese regime's forced organ harvesting of prisoners of conscience. Appendix 2A, Witness 34.

[82]   Incomprehensible, even to non-experts, who will be acquainted with systems elsewhere in the world that are dependent on voluntary donation and where waiting times, by common knowledge, are months or years.

from 2000 onwards, a view also found in Chinese-language judicial sources. Reforms to the review of death penalty cases in China included the Supreme People's Court's recentralised review authority beginning in 2007, which subjected each death sentence to a process of review and approval. This led, according to Chinese and foreign academic sources, to a significant decline in death penalty executions. The growth trajectory of the transplantation system is wholly incompatible with the trajectory of decline of death penalty executions. The Chinese government, Robertson explained, has provided no adequate explanation for the source of organs through most of this period (2000-present) given these opposite trajectories in transplant system growth and availability of the primary source of organs claimed to supply it.[83]

155.   A glimpse of background from a specialist viewpoint was provided by Wendy Rogers[84.] She is an ethicist and researcher into forced organ harvesting allegations. She is on the ETAC board of directors and is not herself a Falun Gong practitioner. She reported on how research papers prepared by PRC transplant bodies and professionals between 2000 and 2017 failed extensively to meet ethical standards. First, they failed to exclude all research based on organs from prisoners; second, they failed to provide evidence of consent by donors to the transplants detailed in the research. This may be a small piece of the overall picture, but the Tribunal must consider it odd that a country forging ahead with such an important – highly prized and public – element of medical work and research should fail in these respects without some good cause. By implication, the Tribunal is invited to conclude that there is no 'good cause' that could be made public and that the failings are indicative of a far darker reality. Rogers also points to a broader background noting that international inactivity may have served to encourage, and certainly not to discourage, the perpetuation of unethical, or worse, organ transplant practices in the PRC. The shortcomings of research papers may indeed point to this reality: it is not unusual for wrongdoers to fail to deal honestly, or at all, with something that would be damning if spelt out; in this case the source of organs. Rogers also comments on, and offers explanations for, the exculpatory approaches of a few transplant surgeons, notably from Australia, who give public support for China's organ transplant practices. This support has served to quell the worst of fears (at least as expressed) acknowledged in some inquiries by other countries. The response of some of those doctors

---

[83]   Appendix 2A, Witness 34

[84]   Appendix 2A, Witness 39

to requests from the Tribunal to answer reasonable questions and requests is dealt with at paragraphs 405 *et seq* below.[85]

156. The general approach of the PRC towards the practice of Falun Gong could hardly be clearer. Because they were seen to be a threat – however unintended – to the authority of the Communist Party, Falun Gong practitioners were to be subject to any process of physical harm and dehumanisation that might operate to eliminate Falun Gong thinking, and ultimately to extra-judicial killing.

157. The PRC's determination to eradicate the practice of Falun Gong was shown by the actions its embassy staff abroad were required to take. Chen Yonglin, a former diplomat from the Chinese Consulate in Sydney, Australia, revealed several secret internal documents of the Chinese Consulate in Sydney. These documents record detailed plans of how the Chinese Consulate in Sydney, acting in cooperation with the CCP, would spread hate propaganda outside of China and continue the persecution of Falun Gong abroad:

- *Edit and rewrite Chinese and English materials that criticize Falun Gong.*
- *Recommend articles that criticize Falun Gong from People's Daily and Xinhua News Agency to the overseas Chinese media.*
- *Compile articles criticizing Falun Gong combined with local situations and publish them on local Chinese media under the name of Consulate Speakers.*
- *Strictly block Falun Gong members from obtaining visas. Keep good record of the names and situations of those who applied for visas.*
- *Talk with Falun Gong member applying for a visa, try to learn information through these talks.*
- *Collect information on Falun Gong through known local Chinese people, especially any mentioning illegal crimes or harming their family.*
- *Distribute materials criticizing Falun Gong to the Chinese community, help overseas Chinese people hold seminars to slander Falun Gong, hold press conferences or release statements, and so on. Facilitate overseas Chinese to write to the New South Wales State, local governments, and Congress members to slander Falun Gong. On special occasions, initiate local Chinese go against Falun Gong.*

---

[85]   Ibid, Witness 39

- *Collect information on Falun Gong through known local Chinese people, especially any mentioning illegal crimes or harming their family.*
- *If possible, on some special occasions, to stir up overseas Chinese to fight Falun Gong.*
- *Actively introduce the [slanderous term omitted] nature of Falun Gong to students abroad, and invite them help spread propaganda in their institutions whenever there are any opportunities.*
- *Play criticizing Falun Gong films when playing a movie or video to students abroad.*
- *Provide criticizing Falun Gong materials to all institutions' Chinese Student Association.*
- *If possible, on special days (when Falun Gong has activities), deploy students to oppose their actions and fight with them. The students may help local Chinese people make banners and display boards to criticize Falun Gong.*

158. On the basis of the above evidence, viewed in isolation without regard to the direct evidence given to the Tribunal of torture and forced organ harvesting, the Tribunal concludes with certainty that since 1999 the PRC and the CCP regarded practitioners of Falun Gong as unworthy of any of those universal rights that attach to human beings by reason of their humanity. This view taken by the PRC and the CCP, and all that followed from it was simply to maintain the PRC's and CCP's power and authority over the Chinese people. And coinciding with an expansion of the persecution of practitioners of Falun Gong, there has been an enormous unexplained growth in the number of transplant hospitals – in the absence of a voluntary organ donor system.

Direct Evidence of Forced Organ Harvesting

159. 'Direct' evidence means statements from individuals to the Tribunal about personal involvement in forced organ harvesting, or statements coming by hearsay of other sorts from individuals whose evidence, if it were direct to the Tribunal, would be about their personal involvement. As far as possible, the evidence presented below is in chronological order, based on the year or years when the events described took place.

160. Forced organ harvesting means, as in paragraph 2 above, killing a person without their consent in order that their organs may be removed and

transplanted into another person. Technically, it can also refer to the forced harvesting of one organ (for example, a single kidney) or part of an organ (for example, part of a liver), where the 'donor' patient survives. However, there has been no evidence of this, and the entire focus of the Tribunal has been on forced organ harvesting that has been fatal.

161.   1978 – An expert witness, Dr Huige Li,[86] cited a paper of which he was a co-author:[87]

> *In 1978, Zhong Haiyuan, a schoolteacher from the Jiangxi Province, was sentenced to death for her "counter-revolutionary" thoughts. The execution was performed by three officers from the People's Armed Police Forces on April 30, 1978. Two officers restrained Zhong while the third officer put the gun against her back on the right side and fired the bullet.'* Years later, one of the officers told the book author Hu Ping that the order was not to kill Zhong immediately. *'The kidneys must be harvested before she dies',* because the army doctors wanted high quality kidneys, *'kidneys from a living person'.*

162.   1990s – Witness 26 (name withheld, see Appendix 1A), a medical intern at the time of which he spoke, gave an account to the Tribunal of organ and eyeball extraction from a soldier, killed to meet a need for a kidney. The man was seen to be tied up and injured after a gunshot was heard and was then dragged in conditions of extreme cruelty to have his organs extracted while still alive.[88]

163.   1990 and 1995 – Wang Gouqi, a physician from the PRC, said in evidence in 2001 to the US House of Representatives Committee on Ways and Means (Sub-Committee on Trade). that he was a specialist in burns at the Paramilitary Police General Brigade Hospital in Tianjin. His work involved the removal of skin and corneas 'from the corpses of over 100 executed prisoners and, on a couple of occasions, victims of intentionally botched executions'.

  He had researched the procedure in Beijing at the Beijing People's Liberation Army (PLA) Surgeons Advanced Studies School, a direct

---

[86]   Appendix 2A, Witness 37

[87]   Paul NW, Caplan A, Shapiro ME, Els C, Allison KC, Li H. Human rights violations in organ procurement practice in China. *BMC Med Ethics* 2017; 18(1):11 [http://rdcu.be/o617].

[88]   Appendix 1A Witness 26 – Name redacted.

subsidiary of the PLA. In Beijing, he and others would rush to the autopsy room to remove skin, kidneys, liver, bones and corneas from executed prisoners sent there rather than to the crematorium. The activity was commercial. The removal of skin could generate significant income, charged by the square centimetre to the recipient. He testified that the success of this programme for obtaining organs from prisoners led to the design of similar programmes, for example, in renal transplantation.

He recalled that, in 1990, four death row prisoners were assessed, and tissue-typed for potential donation, and one proved to be a good match for a recipient. He testified that on the day of execution, they arrived at the execution site in plain clothes and after the execution of the prisoner, the 'best urological surgeons' removed both kidneys while in the back of a waiting ambulance and rushed the organs to a nearby hospital. The skin and corneas of the other executed prisoners were removed as well.

Wang recounted another specific occasion in October 1995 when he was sent to Hebei province to extract kidneys and skin. Before the execution of a prisoner who had been sentenced to death, Wang injected heparin into him to prevent his blood clotting. The prisoner was told by police that it was a tranquiliser. The execution was botched, and the victim was still alive when the kidneys were removed. His heart was still beating. A potentially fatal second shot was denied, and he was left to die.[89]

164. 1995 – Enver Tohti (the first Tribunal witness to give evidence of personal involvement in forced organ harvesting), whose account dates from 1995, when he was a general surgeon (junior in some respect) at Urumqi Central Railway Hospital. Dr Tohti's account appeared in The Slaughter by Ethan Gutmann (2014).[90] He explained to the Tribunal that because, by chance, he had no scheduled surgery that day, he was ordered to go with two assistants, two nurses and two anaesthetists, and 'the largest mobile operation kit' to the Western Mountain Execution Grounds. He did not know why he was going.

At the execution grounds he heard the sound of multiple, simultaneous gunshots. Tohti then saw '10 or 20' executed prisoners, all but one of them shot in the head:

'Shaved heads with prison uniform, the foreheads were blown up, a police officer shouted at us: to the right, far right, the last one is yours.

---

[89]   Appendix 3, Item 44, page 13

[90]   Appendix 1A, Witness 13

Confused, why is ours? Not time for that, moved to the location, our surgeons hold me and told me: hurry up, extract the liver and two kidneys.

I turned into a robot trained to carry out its duty. Those police officers and my assistants put the body on the bed inside van already. The victim was a man in his 30s, unshaved with long hair and civilian clothes. The bullet gone through his right chest.

The nurses have prepared the body, two chief surgeons standing on my left observing my movement, I asked to apply anaesthesia, they said no need "We will apply if it is needed". It meant they will observe if the man is not moving and then they will do something. The man seems already dead anyway, so I started my insertion, the cut designed as upside-down "T" shape, to expose internal organs as wide and possible. My scalpel finds its way cutting his skin, blood could be seen, it implies that his heart was still pumping blood, he was alive! My chief surgeon whispered to me: hurry up! ...

It is not known how the organs were handled after extraction, or to what purpose they were put. Tohti reported that the two chief surgeons put the organs into a box and drove them away.

165. 1990 – Enver Tohti also gave an account of three teenage boys in 1990 with U-shaped scars consistent with single kidney extractions.

166. Tohti, in his oral evidence (in December 2018), produced a contemporary photograph[91] of a sign on the floor of an airport in Xinjiang saying, 'Special passenger, human organs transportation pass-way', implying this indicated the scale of present transplant activity in that area of China.

167. 2002 – In April 2002, Zhiyuan Wang received a phone call from a guard who had tortured a woman for a week and then been on guard while surgeons cut her open without anaesthetic for her organs as she shouted out, amongst other things, 'Falun Gong is good'.[92]

---

[91]   Ibid

[92]   Appendix 2A, Witness 30

168. June 2005 –as reported in An Update by Kilgour, Matas and Gutmann (2016), a specific lethal injection technique and field experiment was the subject of investigation by a researcher in Suijiatan:

> 'Through the entire process of a convict's death via lethal injection, the healthy person's vital signs were measured before and after the injection, the amount of poison residue in various organs afterwards, the prisoner's psychological changes when facing death ... this data will provide important help to organ transplantation after death by lethal injection and other aspects of human organ transplantation. Whether in China or abroad, this is cutting-edge research.'

The evidence as reported is supportive of forced organ extraction having taken place at scale under the leadership of Wang Lijun, who was Director of the Onsite Psychological Research Centre under the auspices of the Jinzhou Security Bureau.[93] (See also paragraph 172)

169. 2006 – A woman with the pseudonym 'Annie' told the Epoch Times newspaper[94] in March 2006: '…one of my family members was involved in the operation to harvest Falun Gong Practitioners' organs. This brought great pain to our family.' Annie's account described how her ex-husband had removed the corneas from 2,000 people between 2001 and 2003. These were Falun Gong practitioners, whose organs were removed after they had been 'executed' by injection. The organs were transported to other institutions as part of a commercial venture.[95]

170. 2006 – David Matas filed a 'Magnitsky Act'[96] submission in Canada, whereby individuals can be identified through a court process and thereafter sanctioned

---

[93]   Appendix 3, item 7 'An Update' p375.

[94]   The Epoch Times is a multi-language newspaper founded in 2000 by John Tang and a group of Chinese Americans associated with the Falun Gong spiritual movement.

[95]   Appendix 3, item 10, p7 of Bloody Harvest (Matas and Kilgour 2009). A detailed record of Annie's story is given on pp112 to 122. Kilgour himself interviewed Annie in 2003.

[96]   The first Magnitsky Act was introduced in the United States in 2012, intended to punish Russian officials responsible for the death of Magnitsky, a Russian lawyer who died in 2009 in highly suspicious circumstances in a Moscow prison after blowing the whistle about a massive fraud perpetrated by Russian tax officials. Its scope has been expanded to cover corrupt officials

for established corruption or human rights abuses. In his application he referred to articles in the Epoch Times: 'Shenyang Military Region Senior Physician Testifies to the Truth of Sujiatn Concentration Camp' (March 31, 2006); and on the Minghui website: 'Two Sources Testify Publicly about the CCP's Atrocities of Harvesting Organs from Living Falun Gong Practitioners' (April 22, 2006).[97]

171.   2008 – Unethical methods of organ extraction are also revealed in a case study, set out in the Update, of a combined heart-lung transplant carried out in May 2008. The donor was intubated by an endotracheal tube for ventilation of the lungs after being declared brain-dead. This suggests that the donor was breathing spontaneously prior to intubation. (See also paragraphs 173-174) This is inconsistent with international ethical practice; declaration of brain death requires apnoea and the repeated assessment of the potential donor over at least 48 hours by more than one physician. The authors of the case study reported 38 similar procedures.[98]

172.   2012 – Wang Lijun, an acolyte of Politburo member Bo Xilai, rose to be Director of Tieling City Security Bureau and then head of the Public Security Bureau in Jinzhou, where he hugely increased surveillance of Falun Gong practitioners, and set up the Onsite Psychological Research Centre. Wang's 'research' pioneered lethal injections for organ harvesting. His research centre may, thus, have been directly involved in an extensive programme of organ harvesting. In February 2012, after a power struggle in China involving Bo Xilai, Wang, then head of the Chongqing Public Security Bureau, is said to have tried to inform the US consulate in Chengdu about the harvesting of organs from Falun Gong practitioners. The US consulate surrendered Wang to the Chinese authorities. This was despite a letter from 100 US Representatives to the Secretary of State, Hillary Clinton, opposing the surrender – apparently no response was received to the letter.[99]

---

and human rights violators. Similar acts had been adopted in the EU, Canada, UK, Australia and many other European countries.

[97]   Appendix 2B, item 29, Magnitsky Act p41.
[98]   'An Update' *supra*, p371
[99]   *Ibid* pp374 to 376.

173. Dr Huige Li gave evidence of the four methods of live organ-harvesting practice in China.[100]

Incomplete execution by shooting: this is described by Enver Tohti (above) and in a report by Jiang Yanyong, a high-ranking military doctor from Beijing speaking to Hong Kong journalists in 2015. Li reported that in his interview, Jiang Yanyong said: the practice was 'relatively common'.

After lethal injection: Li described how the relatively lax Chinese laws defining death after lethal injection left loopholes which have been systematically exploited. Death can occur under the legal definition within tens of seconds of injection, and Li states that it can be assumed that all organ procurement after lethal injection happened on still-living bodies

Execution by organ explantation: Li referred to a paper published in 2003 describing the major points of heart removal. Li argued that the lack of criteria for brain death before 2003 meant that the donor could not be brain dead, and thus the fact that the beating heart was stopped with cold cardioplegia for extraction was the cause of death.

Organ harvesting under the pretext of brain death: Li provided evidence from Chinese scientific papers that after the 2003 enactment of brain death criteria in China, in many cases organ donor patients were described as having been endotracheally intubated *after* definition of brain death. This is not possible. Brain death is associated with the inability to breathe spontaneously (see paragraph 171 above). These patients cannot have met the criteria for brain death acceptable elsewhere. They were, therefore, alive at the time of organ donation, even if not conscious of it.

174. The Tribunal notes as important, Li's evidence about the removal of organs, by whatever means, without brain death having been formally established. If the donor was breathing spontaneously before the procedure, the donor must be considered to have been alive. The mode of death must then be related to the removal of the organs. A lethal injection before the commencement of organ extraction forces the pace. The organs must then be removed very quickly if they are to function well after transplantation. A donor heavily sedated (similar to an anaesthetic), ventilated and medically supported could have organs removed more carefully and with a better chance of organ preservation. The act of organ removal would still kill the donor.

---

[100]   Appendix 2A, Witness 37

Indirect Evidence of Forced Organ Harvesting

175. 'Indirect' evidence includes witness statements to the Tribunal from which incidents of forced organ harvesting could be inferred, or hearsay of other sorts allowing such inferences. Again this evidence is presented in chronological order based on the years the events referred to took place.

176. 1940 – China's first recorded case of using prisoners for medical purposes was in 1940, when three 'counter-revolutionaries' were killed on orders of Communist Party official Kang Sheng in order to produce cadavers for dissection. Documents dating from 1962 show that the CCP's Central Military Commission initiated a policy that all death row prisoners and serious offenders may be treated according to the needs of national and socialist development and can be dealt with according to the 'revolutionary protocol,' under which enemies of the state are deprived of all rights and utilized as state resources.[101]

177. 1960s-1980s – The COHRC report explains that China began to conduct experiments in organ transplantation in the 1960s. The first recorded instance of organ harvesting from a Chinese political prisoner during, or following, execution was in 1978. In 1984, multiple government bodies and ministries jointly promulgated a regulation allowing the bodies and organs of prisoners to be used at will by the State under certain conditions. China later started using organs from prisoners of conscience and minorities on a small scale.[102]

178. 2001 – In January 2001, Liu Yumei was told on arrest to give her name and address or all her organs would be harvested.[103]

179. 2002 – In May 2002, in Beijing Women's Labour Camp, Liu Huiqiong (aka Zeng Hui) was told by Division Chief Zhaofeng and Section Chief Li Shoufen, in presence of others, that Falun Gong practitioners are kept as spare goods.[104]

---

[101] Appendix 2A, Witness 36. See also paragraph 147 above
[102] Ibid
[103] Appendix 1A, Witness 14
[104] Appendix 1A, Witness 5

180. 2001-2005 – A prison doctor sympathetic to Falun Gong practitioners told Yu Xinhui secretly: *'Don't go against the Communist Party. Don't resist them. Whatever they tell you to do, just do it. Don't go against them forcefully. If you do, then when the time comes, you won't even know how you will have died. When it happens, where your heart, liver, spleen, and lungs will be taken, you won't even know either.' and 'Falun Gong practitioners, they all practice qigong. They often exercise their bodies, so their bodies are very good. So, think about it, those organs are of course very good also. So, do you think we'd rather pick you practitioners or those other prisoners? Those prisoners all abuse drugs or alcohol. Otherwise they still have many unhealthy habits. It might happen that, when you take their organs, they are damaged beyond repair. You practitioners' organs are the best.'*[105]

181. 2003 – Xuezhen Bao told of the disappearance of Falun Gong prisoners who had been medically tested but had refused to give their names. [106]

182. 2005 – Dr Jacob Lavee, former Chair of the Israel Society of Transplantation, had a patient in his department with a severe heart condition, who was continuously hospitalized for over one year. The patient was on the Israeli waiting list for heart transplantation throughout this time. He was then told by his medical insurance company that he could go to China in two weeks' time, where he would be scheduled to undergo heart transplantation on a specific date. When asked by Dr Lavee how such an operation could be scheduled ahead of time the patient responded that he had not bothered to inquire. The patient went to China and underwent the operation on the exact date, as promised. This would not be possible in countries relying on standard transplant practices.[107]

183. Pre 2006 – Edward McMillan-Scott gave an account of the imprisoned best friend of Cao Dong, whose body, lying in a morgue, was found to have holes where body parts had been removed.[108]

184. 2006 – In 2006, Yu Jing told the receptionist at the Zhongshan Hospital Building in Shanghai that a family member of one of her friends needed to

---

[105]   Appendix 1A, Witness 11
[106]   Appendix 1A, Witness 18
[107]   Appendix 2A, Witness 31
[108]   Appendix 2A, Witness 38

have an organ transplant and which department should he visit? A doctor, aged 70 or more, in a white robe, replied that it was very troublesome because it needs matching and many tests need to be done. Yu Jing said that *those are things to be done by you doctors'*, and asked what did the patient's family need to do? The doctor replied: *'money'*. She told him that money was not a problem. Then he said: *bring the patient here*. She replied: *It depends on what time you can do organ transplant surgery. The patient will come ahead of that time. But if it takes you three years, five years, eight years, 10 years before you get an organ, it wouldn't be good for the patient to come so much in advance.* The doctor said: *If it takes that long, the patient would be dead already. In our hospital, it takes only half a month for an organ transplant. ... the organs are all good organs from young people, just ask the patient to come ... we only need to pay the hospital – ¥400,000, maybe over ¥400,000. It would be safer if you have ¥500,000.* Then he asked where the patient was. She told him the patient was in Hebei. He said: *tell the patient to come quickly.* [109]

185.　2006 – George Karimi, in prison for matters not related to Falun Gong, gave an account of executions and of conversations about organ harvesting from executed prisoners, specifically about 'prisoners not needing organs after death'. He gave one account of a guard, who knew of or dealt with 24 or 25 Falun Gong prisoners being executed and only one being spared, and explained that the one spared was unwell – 'if sick, organs are of no use'.[110]

186.　2006 – In July, 2006, Dr Torsten Trey talked with two transplant doctors from China at the World Transplant Congress in Boston. One of the doctors worked in a research laboratory at the University of Hannover, Germany. He had been invited by two Chinese hospitals to return to China to open a transplant department. When asked how this transplant boom can be explained and where all the organs come from, the doctor replied: 'from Falun Gong practitioners'. The other transplant surgeon from the Tianjin transplant centre said, that they performed 2,000 liver transplants in 2005.[111]

---

[109]　Appendix 1A, Witness 20

[110]　Appendix 1A, Witness 4

[111]　https://chinatribunal.com/wp-content/uploads/2019/04/April_2019-DAFOH-Report-on-Forced-Organ-Harvesting-in-China.pdf

187. 2007 – Jintao Liu (Tony), imprisoned April to 14 May 2007 in a cell with about eight drug addicts, who were regularly induced to abuse Falun Gong practitioners. '*Those drug addicts were rostered on shifts to persecute me by the guards' order. The cell has surveillance camera installed, so the guards know everything happened inside. One day a drug addict inmate was beating my back and waist, another inmate came in from outside yelled at him: "don't injure his organs". I felt strange why these guys did not care about my well-being but cared about my organs. What's more, I knew the drug addict inmate came from outside was just said what the guards' let him say, because without guards' order nobody could came to the cell.* Doctors pushed plastic tubes through his nose into his stomach. They often pulled the tubes in and out several times, to torture him. Prisoner Zhang Guobing also urinated into the sticky fluid used to force-feed him. After two weeks, the guards realised that their torture methods hadn't changed his resolve, so they transferred him back to the Fourth Brigade where his persecution continued. They shoved his faeces into his mouth. Zhang Guobing ordered other inmates to strip him, and then forced a toilet brush handle into his anus. They pushed the handle so hard that he couldn't defecate.[112]

188. Before 2009 – A vice-president of a medical university reported to Yang Guang, a China expert who resides in Denmark, that before 2009 two hospitals of which he was in charge each conducted 2,000 to 3,000 organ transplants every year. '*[Having] a pool of living organ sources meant tissue matching took less than a month, sometimes as short as 48 hours …The 610 Office transported organ sources to the hospitals in prisoner transport vehicles. … We only get serial numbers [of the "organ sources"] and knew only that they were Falun Gong practitioners. Such cases accounted for 90% of transplants in the hospitals … All the serial numbers and data of organ transplants were reported to the supervising Chinese Communist Party Committee at the end of each year, and then were removed from our computers under the supervision of 610 Office personnel … Since 2000, the 610 Office started to supply us such kind of organs of Falun Gong practitioners. There were no names and addresses, just their gender, age, and a serial number.*'[113]

   [The real name and former workplaces of Yang's contact were verifiable by the authors of the Update online. Yang Guang was not called as a witness to the Tribunal because he became available too late for the evidence hearings;

---

112   Appendix 1A, Witness 6

113   https://endtransplantabuse.org/an-update-chapter-twelve-a-state-crime/#_edn2057

there is no known reason to doubt the account of what he says given on page 403 of the Update]

189. 2002-2012 – Yang was told in 2012 by someone who worked at the Ministry of Public Security, and was in charge of informant stations of a major city on the coast of mainland China, that as far as he knew, over the past decade at least 500,000 Falun Gong practitioners' organs were harvested for transplants in civilian hospitals in China.[114]

190. 2013 – Yukiharu Takahashi, a Japanese journalist, interviewed three beneficiaries of transplantations that had happened in China in 2013. In 2018 he contacted a mediating organisation that arranged transplants for Japanese patients in China. The terminology used by the Chinese changed from 'organs from death-row prisoners' to 'organs from Beijing', and this became a commonly used euphemism implying the source was death-row prisoners. The euphemism is consistent with the practice being one that could not be conducted openly. The change in terminology happened between 2010 and 2018, probably between 2015 and 2018. Prices paid by the recipients were US$200,000 for a kidney; US$300,000 for a liver. Recipients were all told there would be a waiting time of about two weeks (compared with several years for liver transplant in Japan). All three recipients went to a hospital in Tianjin; the recipient of the liver was told the donor had been in a traffic accident; the other two guessed or were told their kidneys came from death-row prisoners, one donor being said to be 37 years old.[115]

191. 2015 – Huige Li reported that in 2015, Jiang Yanyong, a famous high-ranking military doctor in Beijing, talked to Hong Kong journalists about the practice of organ harvesting from still-living bodies. His statement implies that this brutal practice was relatively common.[116]

192. 2016 – In 2016, a phone call was made to Jiabin Zhu, who was in charge of the 610 office, about the death of Yixi Gao. Jiabin Zhu said his organs were harvested. (name of witness, who was heard by Tribunal, withheld for security reasons).[117]

---

[114]   Ibid
[115]   Appendix 2A, Witness 43
[116]   Appendix 2A, Witness 37
[117]   Appendix 4, Item 32

193. 2017 – Gulbahar Jelilova, a Kazakh national forced to adopt Uyghur identification papers by PRC police was imprisoned with Uyghurs in Xinjiang. She heard from the women there that organ harvesting was taking place. Many women were taken from the cells (including from her cell) and they did not come back. She was taken away for interrogation lasting 24 hours but returned to the cell. Many other women never returned after being taken away for questioning.[118] She also gave evidence of how on the night of arrival at the No.3 prison, she was stripped naked for a medical examination that included giving blood sample and urine samples, before being placed in a cell. In less than one week, she, along with other prisoners, were taken, with black hoods over their heads, to an unknown place where they were examined, and had blood samples taken and underwent ultrasound tests. They were stripped naked at weekly examinations. Many other prisoners had medical examinations almost daily. On the 27 August 2018, before Jelilova was due to be released, she was taken to a big prison hospital for a check-up.

194. The Tribunal's conclusions on this category of evidence follow here. Before looking at them, the reader may wish to pause and consider what conclusions they themselves would reach on the evidence, bearing in mind that the Tribunal's decision-making for this particular category of evidence was on the basis of an imagined country, free of negative reputation of any kind. The reader may wish to perform similar exercises with each of the Tribunal's following conclusions.

195. The Tribunal found all witnesses who gave evidence on these categories to be believable and they found nothing to cause doubt about any one of them. None had any particular purpose to serve that the Tribunal could discern or imagine. The evidence was often distressing for the witnesses to give, and horrifying for all present to hear. In its overall and final assessment, the Tribunal has in mind in that none of the witnesses has been cross-examined in any adversarial way and that, accordingly, the Tribunal should approach all witnesses with caution before finding their evidence convincing; it has applied its usual discipline, explained above under paragraph 68 above', to assessment of written or video material.

There is some direct and indirect evidence of forced organ harvesting over several decades. The mechanisms by which it may be done are clearly

---

[118]   Appendix 1A, Witness 25

described. The 'industrial scale' of the practice claimed by some might lead to an expectation of much more evidence being publicly available than is, so far, the case. The Tribunal questioned why this should be.

196.   Doctors have spoken of the 'Do as you are told, or else' philosophy that maintains the CCP's control over much of Chinese life, and, in evidence, the Tribunal was told that this operates within hospitals too. The large number of military and police hospitals involved in transplantation is surprising and lends support to the arguments about the organisational structure, including the military structures, supporting expansion of transplantation services. Rapid extraction of organs from prisoners has clearly happened frequently.

197.   On the basis of the evidence, the Tribunal concludes with certainty that, over a period that began before the end of the 20th century, forced organ harvesting happened in more than one place in the PRC and on more than one occasion, and has continued since, as shown by a variety of evidence. This evidence is insufficient *in itself* for the Tribunal to reach any overall conclusions in regard to a pattern of conduct over time and geography.

198.   However, before leaving this evidence, it may be important for this Judgment to seen in the setting of the many other reports that have covered forced organ harvesting in China, reports that have never been challenged by the PRC. The various reports collectively can be seen as providing a consistent narrative that fits with the Tribunal's Judgment, which was formed only on the evidence it heard.

Reports that the Tribunal has dealt with in some detail (see paragraphs 19 and 20 above) mostly start their reporting of events at about the year 2000. However an earlier 1994 report of Human Rights Watch, for which the Tribunal heard no witness and on which it did not rely at the time of Judgment, may be thought now to provide information of background and 'setting' of particular interest, given the long history it lays out from the days of Chairman Mao onwards.

It was written to deal with the number of capital punishment executions and the human rights violations inherent in trials and executions, and in the use of the bodies of those executed for organ transplantations. At that time Falun Gong was favoured by the PRC and no question of harvesting organs from Falun Gong practitioners arises. However the report may be seen as of particular interest at this stage for what it suggests about:

the importance of forced organ harvesting from prisoners for economic reasons; its importance to party members; the culture in which at least some doctors were willing to work; the role of doctors in performing blood tests and the need of such tests for forced organ harvesting; the consistency of accounts of execution methods with what the Tribunal heard from at least two witnesses.

The heavily end noted report recorded, among many other things:

*China's organ transplantation program began during the 1960s, when a number of kidney transplant operations were conducted **with the help of foreign medical advisers**; the program was not publicly announced, however, until 1974. (emphasis added)*

By 1984, at least 98 hospitals around China had begun to carry out organ transplant operations, and a national coordinating body, the Organ Transplantation Registration Center, had been established in Wuhan. ... The vast majority of kidney transplant patients in China now receive expensive follow-up treatment involving CsA therapy. In addition to the drug's lifesaving benefits, widespread use of CsA unavoidably introduced a major new financial element into the organ transplantation process, for its high price created not only a need to cut costs in other areas, but also an incentive to provide organ transplants for high-paying foreign customers as a way of subsidizing wider domestic availability.

Chinese doctors participate in pre-execution medical tests, matching of donors with recipients and scheduling of operations ... Surgeons are commonly present at execution grounds to perform on-site removal of vital organ.

In August 1992, a recently-released Chinese prisoner informed another Hong Kong newspaper that: 'A team of doctors was always on hand at execution grounds in major cities such as Beijing, Shanghai and Guangzhou, and, once the prisoners had been shot, the doctors immediately dissected the bodies and removed the organs required.'

Medical personnel, who have been notified by the court in advance of the time and place of execution, are also present on the scene, and the moment death is announced they move swiftly to extract the organs. The government's 'Temporary Rules Concerning the Utilization of

Corpses or Organs from the Corpses of Executed Criminals' stresses in chilling detail the secretive nature of the organ harvesting process and the furtive role performed by medical personnel.

... the post-1983 criminal justice system in China [had] secret regulations permitting courts to pass death sentences on those found guilty of certain types of nonviolent dissidence. A top-secret Communist Party directive, issued in August 1983 on the eve of the first 'crackdown' campaign, however, listed 'seven categories' (qige fangmian) of criminal elements who were to form the main target of the crackdown and upon whom expedited death sentences could be passed. According to the directive, detainees of these seven types were all to be 'dealt resolute blows and given severe and prompt punishment ... Those requiring severe punishment must be sentenced heavily, and those who deserve to die must be executed.' The 'seventh' category comprises: 'Active counterrevolutionary elements who write counterrevolutionary slogans, flyers, liaison messages and anonymous letters.'

The involvement of Chinese doctors and other medical personnel in the process of removing executed prisoners' organs is necessarily extensive. Before the executions take place, medical workers perform blood tests to determine the prisoner's health and suitability as an organ donor. Hospitals are notified ahead of time of when the execution is to be held so they may arrange a donor-patient match and prepare to make the transplant. Medical personnel are also present at the execution ground, awaiting the moment of death so that they can immediately remove the organs and rush them back to the hospital to perform the operation.

The use of corpses or organs of executed criminals must be kept strictly secret, and attention must be paid to avoiding negative repercussions. [The removal of organs] should normally be carried out within the utilizing [medical] unit. Where it is genuinely necessary, with the permission of the people's court that is carrying out the death sentence, a surgical vehicle from the health department may be permitted to drive onto the execution grounds to remove the organs, but it is not permissible to use a vehicle bearing health department insignia or to wear white clothing. Guards must remain posted around the execution grounds while the operation for organ removal is going on.

Still more shocking is the revelation – made authoritatively in an official Chinese law textbook – that executions are sometimes deliberately botched so that the victims' bodies can be kept alive longer, thereby making organ transplantation procedures more viable. According to the official source, 'A very few localities, in order to be able to use particular organs from the criminals' bodies, even go so far as to deliberately avoid killing them completely when carrying out the death sentence, so as to preserve live tissue.' In other words, vivisection sometimes occurs.

Finally, when cranial injury would destroy coveted body parts, prisoners are sometimes unlawfully shot in parts of the body other than the head. A former Shanghai police official, interviewed by Asia Watch (now HRW/Asia) in 1990, reported witnessing the execution of a prisoner whose eyes were desired for transplant purposes: 'In order to preserve the eyes, the prisoner was shot in the heart. This is what happens. If they need the heart, the prisoner would be shot in the head instead.'

Government cadres, however, are reportedly given preferential status for organ procurement.

In the senior cadre wards of high-level hospitals, organ needs are recorded promptly. Instructions from the [Party] leadership say that medical departments should naturally expend every possible effort to meet the needs of loyal servants of the revolution, and so organs from condemned prisoners are first of all reserved for their use. Long before the prisoner is executed ... his or her health records, details of blood type and so forth will have been sent to the hospital, which then merely waits for the bullet being fired.[119]

Evidence of Medical Testing of Falun Gong Practitioners and Uyghurs

199. Blood testing is a pre-requisite for organ transplantation as donors need to be matched with recipients so that antibodies present in the recipient do not

---

[119] Human Rights Watch Reports August 1994 Vol. 6, No. 9 CHINA ORGAN PROCUREMENT AND JUDICIAL EXECUTION IN CHINA https://www.hrw.org/reports/1994/china1/china_948.htm#N_12_

interact with antigens present on the donor organs, leading to rejection. The only way for transplantation to succeed at scale is to have databases matching donor with recipient tissue types. [120]

200. The Tribunal heard several witnesses describe blood being taken from them when they were prisoners of the PRC for tests whose purpose was undefined. Many also described other tests, including ultrasound, radiographic and physical organ examinations. If they refused initially to take the tests or give blood samples, guards forced them to do so.[121]

201. Falun Gong practitioners in detention were 'systematically subjected to blood tests and organ examinations'. Other prisoners were not tested. Matas and Kilgour reported that the Falun Gong practitioners were never told either the reason for the tests or the test results. They argue that there is no rational health reason for such testing or organ examinations, mainly because the health of Falun Gong prisoners was otherwise disregarded by the authorities.[122]

202. Dr Trey, an expert witness, recalled having spoken to a Falun Gong practitioner who, during two years of detention, had blood tested 10 times, 'without having any health issues'. Trey raised the question '*Why would detained Falun Gong practitioners receive specific physical examinations (including X-rays, ultrasound, blood tests) while at the same time being subjected to brainwashing, labour work, torture or torture death?*' He postulated that the only rational explanation was that purpose was to a build up a systematic medical databank of potential living organ donors. [123]

203. Wang Xiaohua, interviewed in Montreal by Gutmann, explained how he was taken to a camp hospital for a 'physical' where he and others gave a urine sample, and had an ECG, an abdominal X-ray and an eye exam. No results were ever given to him or any others.[124]

---

[120]   Appendix 3, item 10, Bloody Harvest pp. *50 et seq*. Gutmann

[121]   Appendix 2B, item 47 www.dafoh.org/implausible-medical-examinations-Falun-Gong – forced-labour-camp-workers

[122]   Bloody Harvest, *supra*, (Matas & Kilgour, 2009, pp50-54); Individual witness evidence to them is given on pp51-54.

[123]   Appendix 3 Item 11 State organs; transplant abuse in China (eds Matas & Trey, 2017) pp21-22.

[124]   Appendix 3, Item 4 The Slaughter (Gutmann, 2014) pp 217-219.

204. The questions raised by Trey (paragraph 202 above) are appropriate, but the Tribunal has seen no specific independent evidence confirming what the tests were, what the resultant findings were and for what purpose they were used. As Gutmann points out some tests were obviously configured to detect the SARS virus.[125]

205. Lin Jie reported that while she was in Chongqing Yongchuan Women's Prison, at least 100 Falun Gong women were examined 'all over the body, very detailed. And they asked about our medical history'.

206. 2002 – Jing Tian, in 2002 in Shenyang Detention Centre, observed comprehensive physical tests and 'expensive' blood tests (eight tubes per prisoner).

207. 2003 Dai Ying, in 2003 in Shansui Labour Camp, recalls 180 Falun Gong practitioners were -x-rayed and had large blood samples taken, urine tests and 'probes', plus physical examination. The tests seem to have been performed on Falun Gong practitioners and Christians... but not other prisoners.[126]

208. 2000s – Interviews carried out by Jaya Gibson in the early 2000s reported that over 90% of the Tibetan Buddhists interviewed who had been imprisoned in the 1990s had undergone blood tests. The samples were large enough in size to be utilised for transfusion to others or blood banking for future use, as well as for medical tests.[127]

209. 2014 – Blood and other medical tests are discussed in the Update. Here again, it is stated that Falun Gong practitioners, Uyghurs, Tibetans and certain House Christian groups were frequently subjected to blood testing and medical examinations, while other groups were not. The authors quote as sources their own previous research and publications, but also numerous examples on www.minghui.org. They state:

> In April 2014, in Guizhou, Liaoning, Hunan, Hubei, Beijing and other locations, police entered practitioners' homes and forcibly took blood samples and cheek swabs. The policemen claimed to be following

---

[125]   Ibid, pp234-235
[126]   Ibid, p239
[127]   Ibid

orders from above. In one month, sixteen practitioners in the Dandong area of Liaoning Province had blood samples forcibly collected by police.[128] [129]

210. Testing of a Kazakh (identified as a Uyghur by ID documentation forced upon her) Gulbahar Jelilova has been set out in some detail at paragraph 193 above.[130]

211. No evidence of the purpose of this testing has been given by the authorities of the hospitals or prisons to those who gave evidence to the Tribunal; nor has any explanation of its purpose been given to other inquiries into forced organ harvesting.

212. Consistent with its duty set out under paragraph 64 above, the Tribunal has considered potentially beneficial uses of such tests, other than for tissue typing for potential transplantation. These include searching for infection (potentially transmissible to others), defining a baseline state of organ function at the onset of imprisonment, or searching for other disease. For such tests to be of any value, they would have had to be performed on everyone, not specific sub-populations, and action would have to be taken to treat or eliminate identified diseases or infections. No evidence has been heard or read by the Tribunal to support such explanations.

213. Furthermore, DNA testing, which might encompass a whole range of tests, from Human Leukocyte Antigen (HLA) tissue typing through various complexities of genome sequencing, allows of several explanations. These include tissue typing, as indicated, using HLA DNA coding rather than conventional serotypic analysis; building a DNA bank for identification and relationship purposes [security]; potential business development by having a genome profiling map of a very large population, which would allow R&D to develop in drugs and therapeutics, as well as be a resource to accelerate the development of efficient genotyping. Again, no evidence supporting such

---

[128] The Update, *supra* pp409-410. See also http://en.minghui.org/html/articles/2014/ 7/19/2101.html

[129] Dandong Police Claimed It Is a 'Task' to Forcibly Perform Blood Tests on Falun Gong Practitioners – Terrible Secret Lies Behind. The Epoch Times http://www.epochtimes.com/ gb/14/9/19/n4252384.html

[130] Appendix 1A, Witness 25.

possible explanations has been offered on any occasion by the PRC – even though they would be easy to prove if they were the underlying reality.

214. 2001-2002 – Liu Huiqiong (aka Zeng Hui; see also above paragraph 179) was detained for several years and subjected to medical tests on eight occasions but was told that the results were 'state secrets'. In September 2001, she and others were tested, and told that if they did not submit to tests they would be killed. In October 2001, she was told not to eat before medical tests that involved X-rays, blood tests, and examination of organs and private parts. These tests were carried out on 700 Falun Gong women in Divisions 1 to 7 and armed military police were present at hospitals to maintain order. The armed military police were reported to have the freedom to attack Falun Gong men and women. In mid-December 2001, an elderly female Falun Gong (also known as Falun Dafa) reportedly shouted, 'Falun Dafa is good' and was then dragged out, assaulted and locked in a basement. After being instructed not to eat or drink on a particular morning, 40 Falun Gong practitioners were subjected to medical testing in the presence of armed military police.[131]

215. Ethan Gutmann gave an account of eight extended interviews with Falun Gong practitioners in which evidence of testing for organ function emerged without any prompting or direct questioning;[132]

216. 2000 – Hong Chen was detained in 2000, and her blood was tested three times;[133]

217. 2001-2002 – Huang Guohua was tested three times for liver function; blood was drawn, and he was eventually told by the physician that the blood was very thin, like that of a 70-80 year old man;[134]

218. 2001-5 – Yu Xinhui was detained in Guangdong Sihui prison between 2001 and 2005, and subjected to physical check-ups and blood-tests. The prison personnel said tests were for the purpose of determining 'whether we had AIDS or any contagious diseases'. Between 2003 and 2005, he underwent three more so-called check-ups: blood pumping (taken to mean blood testing

---

[131]   Appendix 1A, Witness 5
[132]   Appendix 2B, item 35
[133]   Appendix 1A, Witness 7
[134]   Appendix 1A, Witness 10

– the amount of blood taken was enough to fill a tube); a urine test; he was asked if he had any history of heart, liver or kidney problems; and his eyes were examined. The prison doctors wore white uniforms. Military police stood watching throughout the check-ups. He had three chest X-rays with exactly the same procedure. A black rubber tube, as thick as a finger, was stuck into his mouth and all the way down to his stomach.[135]

219. Xuezhen Bao underwent tests including an ultrasound when the doctor said: 'This one is useless, it is a mess full of stones, everywhere she is useless'. They also attempted eye testing. [136]

220. Yin Liping said testing included ultrasound – violent forced testing. Five Falun Gong women had chest X-rays and the doctor said all their lungs were shining bright;[137]

221. 2005 – Li Lin Lin reported organ testing in the van, at the prison gates, of Falun Gong practitioners who had not renounced faith.[138]

222. 2005-2006 – Feng Hollis, detained in Beijing Haidian District Detention Centre, in Beijing Women's Forced Labour Camp and the Beijing Forced Labour Dispatch Centre gave an account of all Falun Gong women in the labour camps being subject to regular checks at three- to four-monthly intervals. These tests included blood pressure measurements, blood tests, chest X-ray, and ultrasound inspections of kidneys.[139]

223. 2002-2004 – On 8 May 2002, Yang Jinhua, 'on the way to be sent to No 2 Female Labour Camp in Shandong Province, was taken to a hospital for comprehensive physical tests.' Later she was tested physically several times at the clinic in the labour camp. At the end of September 2004, she was taken by bus, with many other inmates from the labour camp, to a 'courtyard'. After she had been fingerprinted, a woman in a white robe measured her blood pressure and listened to her heart with a stethoscope. She was asked to sit at a table and a woman asked her to extend her arms and then drew a large

---

[135]   Appendix 1A, Witness 11
[136]   Appendix 1A, Witness 18
[137]   Appendix 1A, Witness 17
[138]   Appendix 1A, Witness 15
[139]   Appendix 1A, Witness 2

tube of blood from her wrist. After these tests she was sent back on to the bus and returned to the labour camp.[140]

224. Lijuan Tang 'was forced to take irregular physical tests and blood tests'. She couldn't recall how many times she was tested while being held in the prison, but no less than five or six times. In addition, during examinations her abdomen was pressed and checked very carefully, and her corneas were also checked. Once, the prison authorities hired a doctor from an outside hospital to carry out eye checks. He made a very careful examination of her eyes. When thinking back, she believes these tests were preparing her as a target for live organ harvesting. 'If my sister had not called the prison very constantly, telling them that she would not let them get away if I were not to be released alive, I would have been probably dead.'[141]

225. The Tribunal must ask itself why a prison management system might test anyone in the ways described, when such testing was not required for the purposes of internment. The quantities of blood taken do not appear to have been sufficient to permit transfusion to others. The apparent limiting of testing to certain groups does not support an epidemiological approach, say for the control of infection, since the entire population of the prison would need to be tested for it to have value. Further, the assessment of internal organs by ultrasound could only be to determine how the organs looked structurally. It could be postulated that such examinations might have been done to assess the state of an organ before or after physical abuse, which, according to evidence, occurred frequently in the camps. However, the routine application of such tests as is described, is more consistent with a baseline assessment of organ status for other purposes, specifically potential organ donation.

226. On the basis of the above evidence the Tribunal concludes with certainty that the medical testing of groups including Falun Gong and Uyghurs was related in some way to those groups, because other prisoners were not tested. The nature of the testing is highly suggestive of methods used to assess organ function. The use of ultrasound examinations further suggests testing was focused on the condition of internal organs. No explanation has been given by the PRC for this testing of blood or otherwise.

---

[140]   Appendix 1A, Witness 21
[141]   Appendix 1A, Witness 24.

Evidence of Incarceration and Torture of Falun Gong Practitioners

227. As explained above, the Tribunal has approached evidence without regard to the PRC's general record of human rights violations. This approach might suggest that evidence of specific bad conduct, for example, torture of religious or ethnic groups, by the state should be disregarded altogether. However, given the disregard for human life implicit in a pattern of human rights violations by the PRC, the Tribunal has been mindful that there *may* be several PRC objectives in any forced organ harvesting that *may* be proved, for example:

- Making financial profit from the sale of organs;
- Allowing for the rapid development of transplant skills in order for the PRC to lead the world on this medical practice;
- Suppressing the practice of Falun Gong or those observing religions by letting it be known that practitioners may be arrested and 'disappeared';
- Persuading Falun Gong practitioners to renounce their beliefs by making them face organ harvesting consequences;
- Killing Falun Gong practitioners in order to remove them from the PRC and *thereby* reduce the risk of their encouraging others to take up Falun Gong;
- Dehumanising practitioners of Falun Gong to ensure perpetrators of torture would do all that was needed of them.

228. The Tribunal takes the view that understanding the scale and scope of imprisonment without any due process, followed by torture of those incarcerated is of *potential* significance for the Tribunal's Judgment for the following reasons:

- It provides a further context in which the treatment of Falun Gong practitioners as a group by the Chinese authorities may be viewed;
- It contributes to an overall understanding of the different sets of crimes that may have been inflicted on Falun Gong practitioners; and
- It reveals the allegedly widespread and systematic way in which such actions were undertaken.

229. Every witness who appeared before the Tribunal and who identified as a Falun Gong practitioner while in the PRC, and who had been either detained and/or arrested by law enforcement authorities in the PRC, and/or sentenced by a court in the PRC, for being a Falun Gong practitioner, stated that they had

been tortured while incarcerated. It would appear that these acts of torture occur(ed) all across the country.

230. In March 2006, a whistle-blower senior physician from Shenyang Military Region's Logistics Department told the Epoch Times that: 'Across China, there are at least 36 secret camps similar to the one in Sujiatun (concentration camp). Located in Jilin Province, the camp, codenamed 672-S is detaining more than 120,000 Falun Dafa practitioners, felons, and (political) dissidents.' The surgeon also spoke of 'the bulk transferring of 7,000 captives from Tianjin to Jilin province by a rail train by fully armed [military] and took place at night. All the captives were cuffed to handrails, like a line of de-feathered chickens.' [142]

231. According to the various witnesses, the torture took many forms. Physical punishment: being forced to adopt a particular physical posture for long periods of time, being hanged/suspended from a height using handcuffs, being stretched using cloth belts, being deprived sleep and food, prodded with electric batons, forced to do manual labour, denied access to the toilet or to bathing facilities, being forced to consume medication or drugs, being publicly humiliated (including by humiliating sexual violence). Psychological torture, for example, being made to write 'confessions' and/or 'undertakings' about Falun Gong activity and watching programmes that portrayed Falun Gong practitioners negatively, was also inflicted. Detailed accounts of such practices can be found in the various witness statements and oral evidence provided to the Tribunal.

232. In some instances, physical and psychological abuse was inflicted by cellmates of the detained person on the orders of the detention authorities.

233. Attempts to protest against arrests, and also against poor treatment, by way of hunger strikes, resulted in force-feeding by the detention authorities (see testimony of Dai Ying in paragraph 234 below).

234. As an example, the evidence of one witness, Dai Ying,[143] is set out in detail here. Dai Ying's evidence of her suffering is consistent with that of others:

---

[142]   Appendix 2B, item 29, Magnitsky Act, Paragraph 49
[143]   Appendix 1A, Witness 1

On 21 July, 1999, fellow practitioners and I went to the Shenzhen City appeals office to appeal to the government. Instead of finding help, the police arrested us. My husband was secretly detained ...

Dai Ying was not allowed to defend her husband, and Shenzhen City Juridical Bureau forced the retained lawyer, Ms. Xu, to void her contract and thus barred her from representing the husband in court.

They did not allow any appointed lawyers or family members to be in the courtroom for Dai Ying's husband's case; instead, they appointed a lawyer who pleaded guilty on his behalf at Futian District Court.

Dai's husband was sentenced to a four-year term at the end of February 2000. On 5 March, 2000 Dai went to Beijing to appeal. Police officers detained her, took her back to Shenzhen City, where she was held in Futian District Detention Centre:

Just because I wanted to help my husband ask the government for justice, I was deemed guilty and detained, awaiting my sentence to be passed.

In order to resist and protest the persecution, I went on a hunger strike. Three days later, police officers from the detention center began to force-feed me. Forced- feeding has become a means for guards to torture Falun Gong practitioners.

They carried me outside. Four or five guards held me down. They put a very rigid tube into my nose until I bled. When the tube did not reach my stomach, they forced my teeth open with a screwdriver. Then they put a bamboo barrel with a very sharp end into my mouth with a lot of force. My mouth hurt immediately. After that, they force-fed me with food or condensed salt water. I felt like choking. Food and blood came from my mouth and nose and went all over my clothes. After they finished the forced-feeding, I felt as if I had died. I was force-fed every two to three days. One time during the force-feeding, I held my teeth closed very tightly. Doctor Zhou from the detention center used a large screwdriver to force my mouth open. I lost two front teeth and my upper and lower front teeth became loose.

Practitioner Wang Xiaowen also lost two front teeth. I witnessed practitioner Ms. Xue Aimei being forced-fed with chilli oil and chilli

71

powder. After she returned to her cell, her nose and face were all bloody and she was covered with chilli oil and food. Because we hadn't committed any crimes and were being detained illegally, all of us refused to wear the detention center uniforms.

Dai Ying was forced to do hard manual labour daily making leather shoes her until fingers developed blisters and became deformed. These products were exported to the US, Europe, and other countries. She was forced to work from 7:30am to midnight, and sometimes until 1:00am without any breaks during the week or at weekends:

A cell was just a little over 30 square meters. There was a washroom, but there were over 30 people in the one cell. We had to sleep on our sides and often with our head next to another's feet.

Dai Ying was sentenced to a three-year term:

On March 8, 2001, I was transferred to Shaoguan Prison (currently Guangdong Province Women's Hospital) for further persecution. Because I refused to give up Falun Dafa, Political Instructor Luo Dai, Team Leader Zheng Zhue, Team Leader Cai Guangping, and Assistants Lin and Yang took turns talking to me daily. They used hard and soft tactics, threatened and cursed me, and attempted to brainwash me. They often forced me to watch TV programs defaming Dafa and Teacher. When I refused to give up Falun Dafa, they tortured me. They forced me to stand facing the wall, without moving or sitting down. They also deprived me of sleep. Besides talking to me, the only thing they could think of was to make me stand for a long time. Three days passed and I couldn't keep from falling down, but they woke me up and forced me to stand again. Then I fell again, stood up, fell again. Not until I couldn't stand up anymore did they allow me to sleep. Then they told me to stand again. This went on and on relentlessly. Occasionally, they allowed me to sleep for no more than two hours.

Dai Ying was generally watched by other prison inmates when she was eating, using the bathroom, and taking a shower. They monitored her closely. They always found fault with her, and swore at and humiliated her. They recorded what she said and reported it to the guards:

I didn't give up my belief. Therefore, the guards often shocked me with electric batons. They also threatened me, "If you are not 'transformed', you will be taken to the Great Northwest". The Great Northwest is located in the north-west of China. Not many people live there but there are concentration camps, where many of the detained have disappeared. After just one month of this inhuman torture I developed high blood pressure (before, my blood pressure was normal). It exceeded 220. I felt muddle-headed. Even so, they still forced me to do 14 hours of hard labor daily. When I didn't reach the quota, they didn't allow me to take a break. I made saddles and light chains to hang on Christmas trees. I was totally exhausted. Seeing that I didn't give up practicing Falun Gong, guard Lo said, "I have been treating you too nicely". She threatened to lock me up with a mental patient in solitary confinement and have that mental patient spray urine on me. She asked me to think about it for 15 minutes. After I told her that I didn't care, she gave up...

A few days later, at about 10:00pm, guard Li and three criminal inmates carried me to the basement. The inmates pressed me down and tied me so that I couldn't move. Guard Li was holding an electric baton and began to shock me. He shocked me at my acupuncture points and my sensitive parts. ... I was in terrible pain. I couldn't stand up. That time, they shocked me for between 30 and 40 minutes. The next morning, I could no longer see clearly. This was the result of being shocked for a long time. I demanded that team leader Zheng and guard Yang take me to Li City Hospital, which was outside the prison. The diagnosis was that the blood vessels and vision nerves at the bottom of my eyes were injured. I went blind in my left eye, and my vision was 0. The doctor said that it couldn't be healed, and I would lose my vision in that eye completely. In addition, it also would impact my right eye. My right eye was 0.1, and my left eye became 0.

Liu Cheng, a prisoner who participated in my persecution, said, "You are not treated the most inhumanly. Song Ping was tortured worse than you. What you suffered was only one tenth of what she suffered. When she was shocked, they poured water over her. Once she was wet all over her body, they shocked her with a few electric batons at the same time. She was shocked until she bounced off the wall then bounced back to the ground. Then she was shocked again. She was wounded all over. She could no longer eat. Then she was taken to the hospital.

After being shocked, I became blind. However, Guangdong Women's Hospital still forced me to do hard labour.

When my family came to visit, I had to be escorted by two guards. The meeting room is isolated from the outside with walls and windows. We can only communicate through the telephone. Behind me, there was a guard holding another phone to monitor my discussion. He recorded it at the same time.

We were not allowed to inform family members about the persecution we suffered. If we ever said even half a sentence about what was going on inside the jail, our phone would be cut off, and we would lose the chance of being visited ever again. Therefore, if a person was detained in the prison, he was forbidden to hear any outside news, nor could those outside find out what was going on inside. Only two months before my term was due to expire did they agree to have someone bail me out for medical reasons and let my family take me home.

Two months after she returned home, at 10:00 pm on February 27, 2003, police officer Wang Xiang from the 610 Office in Shenzhen City and more than 20 police officers broke into Dai's home:

They took my husband and me to Futian District Detention Center, where I met practitioner Ms. Wang Suqin, who was 67 years old. She told me that when police officers from the 610 Office in Shenzhen City interrogated her, they locked her in a small room. Although it was a very cold winter, they ran fans non-stop for two days and nights and deprived her of food and sleep. She told me that her son, Li Xiaoqiu, was also detained at Futian District Detention Center. Her daughter suffered from inhuman torture from the police officers in the 610 Office of Shenzhen City. Her daughter asked someone to pass a note to her [Wang], which said that she would never commit suicide. Even if [the authorities claimed that she had], she would have been tortured to death.

Because Dai Ying, after being home for only two months, was not 'transformed', she was again taken to a forced labour camp, for another two years. She was detained in the No3 Team in the No1 Ward of Sanshui Guangdong Province Women's Forced Labour Camp:

At Sanshui Forced Labor Camp, I was detained in a small cell. The windows and doors were covered so that people could not see what was going on inside. I was tortured by the head of the forced labor camp, Xie Tang; Divisional Manager Ge Chen; Team Leader Sun Tang Zhang; and guard Liu Ai. They didn't allow me to write letters to my family nor allow my family members to come and visit me. They tried to brainwash me, took turns talking to me, forced me to write my "understandings" daily, deprived me of sleep and forbid me from going to the bathroom. This kind of mental torture and brainwashing was the most painful. I had noticed that some practitioners became very sick after being forced to undergo brainwashing. Some could no longer walk. Over 30 practitioners suffered from high blood pressure. I also saw that a female practitioner was persecuted to the point of mental collapse. The guard didn't notify her family. Some were skin and bones from the torture. Some were transferred to other places where they were cruelly tortured. Every time practitioners were transferred; guards brought other people into their cells and closed the doors. The practitioners who were dying were wrapped in blankets and carried by guards and prisoners secretly downstairs. No one knows what happened to them.

They were forced to do hard labour sorting garbage:

The garbage came from Hong Kong. It stank. We had to take all plastic and metal from the garbage. This is the type of work no one else wants to do, but we were forced to do it. Everyone was assigned a quota. If we couldn't meet the quota, our [prison] term would be extended.

In April 2004, about 160 practitioners were locked up in one room. Many police officers and doctors from Foshan City People's Hospital gave us injections and performed medical exams. I asked team leader Sun, "How come you are only examining Falun Gong practitioners and not the other prisoners as well?" She said, "Even though they want injections, they will not receive them. This is the special care the government gives you guys." A few police officers brought in a practitioner who had fainted after being injected. After seeing this, all of us resisted and did not cooperate. I was not given an injection, but some practitioners were given injections. Seeing all of us resist it, they stopped giving injections.

Some days later, police officers took a few practitioners to the forced labour camp clinic. Doctors from Foshan City People's Hospital performed examinations, took blood for testing, did electrocardiograms, X-rays, and so on. The equipment to carry out these procedures was brought in by staff from Foshan City People's Hospital, some of it installed in luxury buses.

When the doctors were giving me an electrocardiogram, they appeared to have found a problem. One asked in detail whether I had a heart problem. I said, "I was persecuted for three years, and I suffered cruel punishment. My heart sometimes stopped beating." During this medical check-up, the doctors pressed and tested my kidneys. One asked me, "Do they hurt?" They took a lot of blood. When I asked the doctor why they took so much blood, the doctor said that it was needed to test for a number of things. In the end, every Falun Gong practitioner had been given a medical check-up and had his or her blood tested. Even those who had developed a mental disorder were not exempt.

Other, non-Falun Gong practitioner prisoners didn't have to go through this. At that time, I already knew that the medical check-ups were not for our health. After the exams, I discovered that some practitioners had disappeared; I didn't know where they went. The warden said, "If you don't give up Falun Gong, we transfer you to other places." I never heard from the practitioners who were transferred.

I understood the reason for these medical tests after I heard about the CCP harvesting organs from living Falun Gong practitioners. Then I understood the depth of their deceit.

Because of the long-term persecution at Sanshui Women's Forced Labour Camp, Dai Ying was on the brink of a mental breakdown. Her blood pressure was as high (250mm Hg). She often felt dizzy. Staff at the forced labour camp realised that her life was in danger and were afraid to take responsibility. On 30 September, 2004, they told her family to pick her up and bail her out for medical reasons.

A year later, on the evening of September 7, 2005, police from the 610 Office in Shenzhen City started another round of persecution. Dai Ying and her family were warned before the police officers arrived, so left home. The police searched for them citywide. They tried to track them down with electronic equipment and set up video cameras on the road and at the exits from Shenzhen City in an effort to locate them. After Dai Ying's family left home, they wandered around for nearly two months trying to get to Thailand. Once in Thailand they went to the UN Refugee Board:

> *We told them the truth about the persecution of Falun Gong in China and our experiences. With their help we escaped the CCP persecution and now live in Norway.*[144]

235. There are also accounts in the evidence of others which extensively detail the forms of torture practised.[145] Witnesses giving evidence at the Tribunal, and in other documents, reveal the gravity of the alleged torture practices and their consistency. Those of particular note include:

Feng Hollis (for her medical testing see paragraph 222 above)[146] – detained 1 March 2005-11 April 2005 Beijing Haidian District Detention Centre; 11 April 2005-25 April 2005 Beijing Forced Labour Dispatch Centre; 25 April 2005-1 September 2006 Beijing Women's Forced Labour Camp:

> *I was held in a detention centre, and later given two years forced labour in Beijing Women's Forced Labour Camp without any legal procedure.*

Feng Hollis described the torture she underwent in detention:

> *Forced to sit on a stool for over 20 hours a day with feet closed, rest hands on knee, back straight, eyes must open and not allowed to move without permission from drug addict inmates.*

> *Limited food each meal. Equal to one slice of bread.*

---

[144]   Appendix 1A, Witness 1

[145]   Li Lin Lin (Appendix 1A, Witness 15); Han Yu (Appendix 1A, Witness 16 – she was detained in 2015, her father and mother were detained in 2004); Yin Liping (Appendix 1A, Witness 17 – includes filmed rape); and Xuezhen Bao (Appendix 1A, Witness 18)

[146]   Appendix 1A, Witness 2

Limited water to drink, even in summer under 40 degree. Was given only 500ml a day.

Forced to watch videos slandering Falun Gong. Limited sleep. 2-4 hours a day.

Not allowed to wash hair, clothes and take shower. Was only allowed to do so after I went on hunger strike.

Forced to do hard labor.

Excerpts from her evidence include:

When I was held in my local detention centre, police officer Liu Dafeng ... took me to his office every evening after 10pm. Upon entering the office, he began swearing at me using very dirty and obscene language. When he had finished interrogating me, he told me to sign their paperwork to renounce Falun Gong. I refused every time.

Because I refused to sign his paper, one time he grabbed my coat and pushed me against the wall, and at the same time he kicked my legs.

Pressure, and brainwashing, to renounce Falun Gong continued at the detention centre and in the labour camp:

In June 2005, I was taken to the so-called Intensive Assault Unit. This unit was established specifically to deal with practitioners who refused to renounce their belief.

In the "Intensive Assault Unit" I was locked in an isolation cell. Three drug addicts monitored me; each being assigned an eight-hour shift. They recorded every detail of my daily activities, such as at what time I drank water, how much I drank, and when I used the toilet, and whether I was passing water or stool. If it was passing water then how much did I pass and what was the colour of the urine, yellow or clear. If I was passing stool, they recorded whether it was dry or liquid. What was my facial expression? Whether I was happy or not happy? What did I say? When I was in bed, did I lie flat or on my side and when I turned over? The purpose of this detailed record was used as a reference for finding a psychological breakthrough.

Feng Hollis reported that at the detention centre, she was told, on hearing her sentence, that if she thought she was innocent she would be able to appeal when she arrived at the labour camp, but this was never allowed. She supplied a copy of the verdict passed on her.

Zhang Yanhua[147] – detained more than once between 2001 and 2017:

Since 1999 when the persecution started, the prison is a place to torture and humiliate practitioners.

The purpose of torture is to force practitioners to give up the belief. The torture methods include hanging for a long time on the wrists, freeze, stand still for over 12 hours, sleep deprivation for 7 nights while tied up. I was once locked up in a room from 5am to midnight. The window on the door was covered with paper. A dozen inmates (non-practitioners) and 2 to 3 guards would surround me and defame Falun Gong, humiliate me and torture me. They said, "If you give up Falun Gong, and say it is not good, say you have been deceived, we will not treat you like this. We will let you sleep and rest."

The type of tortures in the police station include being tied up on the iron bench for 2 days and 1 night, the four limbs being tied and stretched for a long time, sleep deprivation.

The purpose was to have me sign a statement. The police said, "The statement is to say that you are guilty for distributing flyers and hanging up posters. You must sign quickly. If not, I will torture you."

In the detention centre, 'in order to force me to do labor, they stripped off my clothes and poured cold water on me. They asked other inmates to beat me. I said to the police, "the inmates beat me." The police said, "You don't work, you don't obey the rules, that's why they beat you." I said, "You are breaking the law." the police said, "Yes."

The tortures include freeze, being handcuffed in the back, and feet were also cuffed, sleep deprivation for 7 to 8 days, force feed while I

---

[147]   Appendix 1A, Witness 8

was on hunger strike, the food that was force fed to me contained large amount of salt.

Jiang Li[148] –

My father was abducted by police the third day after the Wenchuan Earthquake in 2008 when he was at home watching TV.

The police didn't present any ID or warrant. He was sent from Youxi Police Station to Jiangjin Detention Centre, then sentenced to Xishanping Labour Camp for a year, without having any legal documents. During his detention, my sister Jiang Hong once went to the National Security Bureau and inquired about my father's situation. Mu Chaoheng, a policeman from the National Security Bureau, said that he had the power and that he could persecute whomever he wanted to for as long as he desired ...

On January 27 2009, at 3.40pm, I myself, Jiang Hong, Jiang Hongbin, and my niece Jiang Guiyu went to Xishanping Labour Camp to visit Jiang Xiqing. ... Jiang's health was normal.

On January 28, 2009, Chongqing Xishanping Labour Camp called to notify us that Jiang Xiqing died of acute myocardial infraction at 2.40pm that afternoon. ... After several hours of negotiation, at 10.30pm on that day, [we] went to the mortuary. When Jiang Xiqing was pulled out from the freezer, his body was found to have many bruises on it, but it was still warm on his philtrum and his chest.

All members of our family felt father's body and it was warmer than the hand; my father's upper teeth were tightly biting his lower lip (the expression on his face was full of pain.) 'We asked for emergency rescue and were declined brutally.

Jiang Li's family members shouted loudly for help and called 110, but they were dragged away by force. Jiang Xiqing, still with obvious signs of life at that time, was pushed back into the freezer in the mortuary.

---

[148]   Appendix 1A, Witness 9

On February 8, 2009, Jiang Xiqing's body was forcibly cremated. The autopsy report delivered to Jiang's family was issued around 40 days after the autopsy. At a meeting with the family, the director of Prison and Detention Centre Supervision stated that 'Jiang Xiqing's organs were all extracted and made into specimens'.

Huang Guohua[149] – detained: Oct 31, 2000-Jan 30, 2001, Nov 20, 2002-Dec 16, 2003

No 1 Re-Education Through Labour Camp, Guangzhou City, Guangdong Province

One day in December 2002, ... in Haizhu District Detention Center, the '610' policeman wanted me to give up my belief in Falun Gong. I rejected their unreasonable request, as one cannot simply just give up their spiritual beliefs. The '610' policeman was very angry. They moved me to another room and locked me on the "death bed" or "dead person's bed". I was locked there for more than 12 hours. After that, the policeman locked my four limbs with a heavy chain that was nailed to the floor for more than 7 days. I wasn't allowed to go to the bathroom and had to release myself right where I was cuffed.

On 31 December 2002, '610' policeman transferred me into Guanzhou Forced Labor Camp, the Second brigade. That policeman Bi Dejun asked me to write a letter of guarantee to give up Falun Gong, of course I rejected him. At this time, three people who were known to be particularly vicious, appeared. Their names are Wang Feng, Cui Yucai, and Jiang Yong. They were all black-handed drug dealers, who used drugs.

They deported me to a remote room. At the first, they're punched and kicked me, hit my abdomen with their knees, and hit my back with their elbows. Then they twisted my arm and pressed my head on the concrete floor. A person jumped up and used his weight to smash my head with his foot. It felt like my head will be crushed at any time. They had already taken off my shoes earlier. The other torturer jumped and stomped on my fingers and toes. It felt like my fingers and toes were crushed. The last torturer fiercely hit my back with his fists. I don't know how long they beat me, they only stopping once they've become exhausted and sat on the ground.

---

149   Appendix 1A, Witness 10

After that, I was held alone for more than six months in a room with no sunlight. Eight people were on duty for 24 hours, guarding me. They also recorded down all my words and deeds–and even my behaviour after sleeping was recorded to try and decipher my thoughts. Every day they forced me to watch a lot of videos that slandered Falun Gong to mentally break me. This kind of mental and spiritual torture was crueller than any physical torture I had suffered.

Six months later, the policeman released me out from that small dark room. However, the policeman forced me to kneel down to them and say "Thank you for saving my life" every morning, until I was released out of labour camp. If I did not smile and say "Thank you for saving me life" to the policeman, they would force me to watch more videotapes that slandered Falun Gong.

Huang also gave an account of the death of his pregnant wife, said to be suicide, but considered otherwise by the witness.

Lijuan Tang (see paragraph 224 for medical testing)[150] – detained April 4, 2008 to October 25, 2011 Guangdong Women's Prison

I was detained illegally by the Chinese Communist Party ... for 3 years and a half, and I had been tortured by all kinds of brutal methods of torturing. The "reason" for their torturing me was that I would not abjure my belief.

Methods of torturing I have experienced include the following:

Not allowed to eat they said food was for criminals only

Not allowed to go to the toilet: I had to urinate sometimes in my pants. Pants became dry due to my body heat. I was not allowed to take any shower or wash. As it is tropical climate in Guangdong, my body stank as a result. Then the police directed inmates to find fault with me

Not allowed to sleep: once I was not allowed to sleep for almost 20 days. When my eyes closed, they used a nib to prick my body and

---

[150]   Appendix 1A, Witness 24

my legs. The pricking caused red blood dots which festered, and flesh stuck with pants.

Forced to take drugs: they claimed these were antihypertensive agents. I had no idea whether they were true or not; my health just went from bad to worse, and my weight dropped from over 70kg to less than 50kg.

Humiliation: there was no dignity at all when I was detained illegally. They slandered Falun Gong and made up lies about Falun Gong. I was forced to admit that I was a criminal. They beat me and scolded me at their will. They even took off all my clothes to search my body. Words of humiliation were seen everywhere.

236. Witnesses repeatedly recounted medical testing being performed on them, and not on any other group of detainees or prisoners. The tests included: electrocardiograms, X-rays, blood testing, saliva and urine testing, and kidney ultrasonic wave checks.

237. None of the allegations of torture could be independently verified by a witness who had observed and could verify the account of the person giving evidence of having been tortured. However, the *detail* that some witnesses were able to provide should be noted – see, for example, the evidence of Yang Jinhua[151] who was detained many times in the period 1999-2006. She detailed nine methods of torture, including diagonal handcuffing, lashing, 'stewing the eagle' (i.e. no sleep, food, use of toilet for days, forced feeding etc).

238. The similarities of the testimonies from witnesses from different parts of China, and the similar patterns of torture that were allegedly inflicted are striking.

239. Physical abuse, by way of being beaten, was also alleged by non-Falun Gong witnesses who appeared before the Tribunal, and is dealt with, so far as Uyghurs specifically are concerned, below (paragraphs 241 to 261).

240. On the basis of the above evidence the Tribunal concludes with certainty that acts of torture have been inflicted on persons detained by the Chinese

---

[151]   Appendix 1A, Witness 21

authorities for their practice of, support for and defence of Falun Gong and for no other reason. In other countries the practice of Falun Gong would not be considered or constitute a criminal offence. The Tribunal is certain that such acts of torture have taken place at many different sites in China over a long period of time and that acts of forced labour are or have been particularly harsh and brutal. Acts of torture generally reveal an overall consistent attitude and approach of the PRC towards practitioners of Falun Gong that is systematic in nature and designed to punish, ostracise, humiliate, dehumanise, demean and demonise these practitioners into renouncing and abandoning their practice of Falun Gong.

Evidence of incarceration of Uyghurs

241. In 1949 the CCP took control over the Xinjiang Uyghur Autonomous Region, a region located in the Northwest, sharing a border with Kazakhstan, Kyrgyzstan, Tajikistan, and Pakistan. As a result, the population balance, which was once predominantly Muslim, shifted with the resettlement of Han Chinese making the Muslim populations the minority in the region.[152]

242. The Muslim minorities, namely the Uyghurs, the Kazakhs and the Uzbeks, have become the focus of a CCP crackdown in the region. The CCP has placed restrictions on the daily lives of the Uyghurs. For example, there are bans on fasting during Ramadan, and prohibition of long beards and wearing veils in public.[153] In Xinjiang, religious activities can only take place in registered venues, while practice in government offices, public schools, businesses and 'other places' is prohibited.[154]

243. These actions, along with the restrictions on other religions and their adherents, for example, Tibetan Buddhists, House Christians, and Falun Gong practitioners are part and parcel of the CCP's policy of *sinicization*, whereby the government interferes with religious and cultural activities so that traditions and doctrines conform to CCP objectives.[155] A pivotal moment

---

[152]   Appendix 2A, Witness 33, Sarah Cook, 'The Battle for China's Spirit' Freedom House Special Report, February 2017 pp 68-69. For another detailed history of the Uyghurs, see Ethan Gutmann, The Slaughter, *supra*, pp 9-30

[153]   Sarah Cook, *supra*, 2017 p66

[154]   Ibid pp71-72

[155]   Ibid p17

in the region occurred in 1996 when the CCP launched 'strike hard' campaigns to stop what they said were illegal religious activities.[156]

244. The Uyghurs not only face religious repression but ethnic discrimination. It is reported that Chinese authorities continue 'to abuse the entire Uyghur population of Xinjiang under the guise of "stability maintenance" or "counterterrorism"'.[157]

245. The CCP has introduced 're-education camps' in order to give 'patriotic re-education'.[158] Uyghur and Kazakh survivors of the camps gave evidence to the Tribunal that they were asked to sing 'red' songs (hailing President Xi) and were taught and examined on Mandarin.[159] One survivor testified that food rations were dependent on speaking mandarin and no other language.[160] The camps are known as *Laogai* (reform through labour) where, as the Tribunal heard from various witnesses, multiple forms of torture and murders of political prisoners take place.[161]

246. It is believed that there are 'in the hundreds of thousands, and possibly millions' of Uyghurs in prison. The overflow from these prisons has resulted in the transfer of Uyghurs throughout the PRC according to PRC police officers, speaking anonymously.[162]

---

[156] Appendix 3, Item 60, Human Rights Watch, 'Eradicating Ideological Viruses: China's Campaign of Repression against Xinjiang's Muslims' 2018, p11-25, https://www.hrw.org/sites/default/files/report_pdf/china0918_web.pdf

[157] Appendix 3, Item 16, A Report of the Conservative Party Human Rights Commission, p41, June 2016, http://www.conservativehumanrights.com/reports/submissions/CPHRC_China_Human_Rights_Report_Final.pdf

[158] Sarah Cook, supra, 'The Battle for China's Spirit' Freedom House Special Report, February 2017, p17

[159] Appendix 1A Witness 19, evidence of Omir Bekali; Appendix 1A, Witness 25, evidence of Gulbahar Jelilova; Appendix 1A, Witness 27, evidence of Mihrigul Tursen,

[160] Gulbahar Jelilova, *supra*.

[161] Sarah Cook, *supra*, 'The Battle for China's Spirit' Freedom House Special Report, February 2017 p. 18. See also Ethan Gutmann, The Slaughter, *supra*, p143

[162] Appendix 3, item 64, Radio Free Asia, 'Xinjiang Authorities Secretly Transferring Uyghur Detainees to Jails Throughout China' October 2, 2018, https://www.rfa.org/english/news/uyghur/transfer-10022018171100.html

247. In his book The Slaughter, Gutmann notes that the Uyghurs were the first group targeted for their organs, beginning in the 1960s.[163] He further states,

> *Xinjiang has long served as the [CCP's] illicit laboratory ... at some point during the last decade, the Communist Party authorized the creation in the Tarim Desert of another grand experiment – the world's largest labour camp, roughly estimated to hold fifty thousand Uyghurs, religious prisoners, and hardcore criminals. In between these two ventures, the first organ harvesting of political prisoners was implemented. And again, Xinjiang was ground zero.*'[164]

248. Gutmann gave evidence to the Tribunal in December 2018 that 'over the last 18 months, literally every Uyghur man, woman, and child – about 15 million people – have been blood- and DNA-tested, and that blood testing is compatible with tissue matching'. (While not doubting the sincerity of Gutmann's views on this topic the Tribunal has insufficient evidence to reach the strong conclusion he ultimately reaches).[165] Enver Tohti corroborated this in his statement to the Tribunal, where he detailed news in June 2016 that the CCP gave Uyghur people free national health examinations.[166] He suspects that 'CCP is building their national database for organ trade' and the number of samples collected has 'exceeded 17 million.' (This is one example of where the Tribunal felt caution was necessary and it was unable to conclude that compatibility with tissue testing was necessarily conclusive of it, or that Tohti's honest suspicion could be of much evidential value).

249. Dolkun Isa,[167] the World Uyghur Congress President addressed a roundtable

---

[163] Ethan Gutmann, *supra*, The Slaughter, p14

[164] Ibid p14. Gutmann also testified before the US Committee on Foreign Affairs Joint Hearing in 2016, 'In 1997, following the Ghulja massacre, a handful of political prisoners, Uyghur activists were harvested for a handful of aging Chinese Communist Party cadres. Now, perhaps those organs were simply prizes seized in the fog of war. Perhaps the harvesting of prisoners of conscience could have ended there.'

[165] Appendix 2A, Witness 35, Ethan Gutmann.

[166] Appendix 3 Item 62. This was reported by Radio Free Asia in an article provided as reading material to the Tribunal, Radio Free Asia, 'Uyghurs Forced to Undergo Medical Exams, DNA Sampling' May 19, 2017, https://www.rfa.org/english/news/uyghur/dna-05192017144424.html

[167] Appendix 2A, Witness 52

in the UK Parliament in 2017: *'On the one hand, collecting blood samples allows the Chinese government to establish a genetic database of the Uyghur people to further monitor, control and repress them. This genetic information also facilitates organ harvesting, making it easier to compare blood types and compatibility of potential Uyghur victims.'*[168] Dolkun Isa testified before the Tribunal that he received communications within China from Uyghurs that organ harvesting is taking place. He also stated that there are injections and unknown medications given to the Uyghurs in detention.

250. Edward McMillan-Scott stated before the Tribunal in December 2018[169] that:

> *In 2018, credible reports that some 1,000 new camps have been constructed to accommodate Uyghur dissidents ... The significance of this is that there is testimony available that the Uyghur themselves have been eviscerated and their organs taken for transplant, again most of them neither smoke nor drink and this is seen as a premium market for the organ transplant trade, as with FG.*

251. The Tribunal heard live evidence from seven Uyghur survivors.

252. Dr Enver Tohti (see above) gave evidence, consistent with other Uyghur survivors who gave evidence to the Tribunal, that their heads were shaved in detention.[170]

253. One Uyghur witness said that when family members came to see the body of a deceased relative, they were not allowed to see the entire body but only the head. In the Uyghur tradition, the burial custom would dictate that the body be cleaned in order for the burial to take place. This was denied to family members and they were only allowed to see the face, which indicated to them that organ harvesting had probably taken place and that was why the remainder of the body could not be seen.

---

[168] Appendix 3, item43, World Uyghur Congress, 'WUC President Speaks on Organ Harvesting at Roundtable in UK Parliament' December 14, 2017, https://www.uyghurcongress.org/en/wuc-president-speaks-on-organ-harvesting-and-uyghurs-at-hearing-in-the-uk-parliament/

[169] Appendix 2A, Witness 38

[170] Appendix 1A, Witness 13

254. Omir Bekali,[171] who is a Uyghur, but a Kazakh citizen, stated that at the police station he had blood samples taken and was given a full body check and an ultrasound on his back and chest. In evidence, he said that it felt like the tests lasted about 2 hours. He was given another full body examination at a hospital, before being tortured and interrogated. He said that the medical examination was the same as before except, he had a black hood over his head. He stated: 'I was terrified that they might open me alive to remove some of my organs to sell them.' He also said that during his imprisonment 'my ankles were shackled together and then one ankle was chained to the bed. I was to spend every day and night … eating, sleeping and carrying out my ablutions on the bed with the occasional wash by the young guards. And I remember that day vividly because they now used a metre of chain attached to my upper arm and ankle to bring me into a crouching position. Mr Bekali stated he suffers from post-traumatic disorder and cannot sleep properly. He was barely given food to eat. He was not allowed to visit with his family until he was able to speak Mandarin.

255. Gulbahar Jelilova,[172] in addition to evidence about medical testing (paragraph xx above), explained how women were treated generally. This included being placed in overcrowded and dirty cells where the women took turns to sleep as there was not enough space for everyone to lie down. They were barely given food to eat. They were given showers once a week with one bar of soap, which resulted in body sores for the women. She stated that they were given pills that caused disorientation and stopped their menstrual cycles. She said she witnessed many women having mental breakdowns as a result of the conditions in the prison.

256. Mihrigul Tursen[173] stated that while she was in detention her head was shaved and she was interrogated for days and nights without sleep. She was physically examined and then locked up in a mental facility because of her seizures. Although she was medically paroled, she returned to detention a year later where she was taken to the hospital, stripped naked, and put under a 'computerized machine.' Mihrigul Tursen stated that during her detention she was put in a cell with 60 people and the women in her cell would have to take turns to sleep. She was chained by her wrists and ankles. During her

---

[171]   Appendix 1A, Witness 19
[172]   Appendix 1A, Witness 25
[173]   Appendix 1A, Witness 27

time in the cell the women would be ordered to wake up at 5am each morning and fold their blankets in a particular way, otherwise they would be taken from them. She stated that they were given unknown pills which reduced 'cognition level' and the women were given a white liquid which stopped their menstrual cycles. *'As if my daily life in the cell was not horrific enough, I was taken to a special room with an electric chair, known as the Tiger Chair. ... I was placed in a high chair that clicked to lock my arms and legs in place and tightened when they press a button. The authorities put a helmet-like thing on my head. Each time I was electrocuted, my whole body would shake violently, and I could feel the pain in my veins.'* Tursen stated that she witnessed the death of many of her cellmates during her time in detention. Some women died because of the white liquid they were given to stop their menstrual cycles. She testified of nine deaths she witnessed that were as a result of starvation, torture, and denial of medical treatment.

257. Abduweli Ayup[174] gave evidence that during his imprisonment he was forced to clean faeces out of toilets. He also described a torture method in a 'Tiger Chair' to which his ankles, wrists, and neck were secured by chains. The police would beat and threaten him to make him admit to committing the crimes he was accused of. Ayup stated he never admitted to anything and that he was stripped of his clothing and thrown into a cell where he was then raped by 20 criminals.

258. All Uyghur witnesses who provided statements to the Tribunal, with the exception of Dr Tohti, were detained and no one in their families was notified of any legal proceedings. These Uyghur witnesses were not formally charged with crimes and not provided any due process rights, which Clive Ansley, in his evidence regarding the Chinese criminal system, says is standard practice.

259. Through great efforts, the family members of these Uyghur survivors were able to locate them.[175] In some instances, such as that of Dolkun Isa, family members died in prison, with no further contact with the outside world.

260. Further detail of the above and similar events may be found in the witness statements and pre-reading material on the website of the Tribunal.

---

[174]   Appendix 1A, Witness 3.

[175]   Ethan Gutmann, The Slaughter, *supra*, p282. Gutmann believes that enforced disappearances of Tibetans, Uyghurs continued into 2014

261. On the basis of the above evidence the Tribunal concludes with certainty that acts of torture have been inflicted on Uyghurs as well as others, as set out above. Acts of torture generally reveal an overall consistent attitude and approach of the PRC towards Uyghurs, which is systematic in nature and designed to punish, ostracise, humiliate, dehumanise and demean them. It is clear that Uyghurs have been routinely forced to undergo regular medical testing.

Evidence about Christians, Tibetans and Foreign Nationals

262. Aside from members of the Uyghur and Falun Gong practitioner communities, evidence was presented to the Tribunal regarding other groups that *could* also be victims of organ harvesting in the PRC.

263. According to Freedom House, persecution against Protestant Christians and Tibetan Buddhists has increased.[176] The Freedom House report indicates that 'numbers of religious prisoners across China – Christians, Tibetan Buddhists – have over the past decade been a key source of forced labour while in custody. They were forced to manufacture products for both domestic consumption and foreign export under oppressive, unsanitary conditions.'[177] The use of forced labour in camps was further corroborated by almost all Uyghurs and Falun Gong survivors who gave evidence to the Tribunal.

264. In The Slaughter, Ethan Gutmann makes reference to several different minority groups outside of Falun Gong practitioners and Uyghurs that would be potential sources for organ harvesting.

265. Gutmann states that after the Tibetan uprising of 2008, many prisoners were shifted to Sichuan, a place of much organ harvesting according to Matas and Kilgour, and Qinghai Province. In addition, construction of modern hospitals within Tibet increased dramatically.

266. Gutmann estimates that, in August 2008, 700 to 1,000 monks were sent to military detention centres, the most prominent based in Golmund, close to the First Affiliated Hospital of Qinhai University. Hundreds have not returned.

---

[176]   Freedom House Report, *supra*, p2 and p21.
[177]   Ibid.

He concludes 'the ongoing Tibetan policy of dialogue with China appears not to have inhibited the harvesting of Tibetan prisoners of conscience.'[178] While not in any way doubting Gutmann's honesty and reliability as a witness of factual matters –and as explained above – the Tribunal has not felt able always to reach the strong *opinions* reached by Gutmann. It is true that he has had very wide experience of many kinds but he cannot be treated as an expert on matters the Tribunal has to decide on the basis of evidence presented – nothing else.

267. Further, Gutmann detailed a small investigation that was done by Jay Gibson, a colleague of his. Gibson interviewed about forty Tibetans who had suffered incarceration in China since the 1990s. 'The one consistency: blood testing often in large enough samples (350ml) that it may have been actual blood banking, particularly in the notorious Gusta Detention Centre in Lhasa. Only one out of ten prisoners had never been tested.' Gibson reported to Gutmann more narratives which conformed to 'the organ-harvesting physical examination pattern'.[179] The Tribunal treats with caution the conclusion of Gibson/Gutmann about conformity because of the levels of hearsay involved.

268. Gutmann submitted an additional statement to the Tribunal raising the issue of whether the persecution of Falun Gong practitioners is an isolated event. He states, 'the discovery that "Eastern Lightning" House Christians were also being tested for their organs emerged organically [without prompting of any kind] from interviews…'[180]

269. Dr Torsten Trey submitted a 2019 report to the Tribunal which specified four religious groups: Falun Gong practitioners, Christians, Uyghur Muslims, and Tibetan Buddhists. When the Tribunal asked Dr Trey about possible organ harvesting from Christians, he stated that there is not enough data available to determine the issue. With regard to Tibetans, Trey stated that organs procured from Tibetans would need to be 'transported across country'.[181]

---

[178]   The Slaughter, *supra* pp244-246

[179]   Ibid pp242-244

[180]   Ibid p239. See also Ethan Gutmann's Statement to the Tribunal Appendix 2A, Witness 35.

[181]   Appendix 2A, Witness 47 Doctors Against Forced Organ Harvesting, 'Report on Forced Organ Harvesting in China' January 31, 2019, p30

270. Gutmann countered this statement in his second appearance before the Tribunal and stated that there is enough data to indicate that Christians are a source of organs.[182]

271. In a Human Rights Without Frontiers Report titled Tortured to Death, the authors state that the CCP has labelled the Church of Almighty God 'xie jiao' (an evil cult).[183] This report includes several accounts from family members and the death of loved ones who died in Chinese prisons. All the accounts are consistent with the pattern of torture and abuse the Tribunal heard from Falun Gong and Uyghur victims and survivors. This torture and abuse include, sexual violence,[184] beatings with objects,[185] torture with the Tiger Chair,[186] and forced starvation.[187]

272. There are three instances within the report that indicate a possibility of organ removal. In the first, the witness states that the deceased had died of heart problems shortly after detention (although there was no history of a heart condition). The family say that when they were able to inspect the remains 'one long cut had been made extending from her neck to her stomach'. The policy officer informed the family that the 'body had been dissected – her brain, heart, liver, and lungs had been removed'.[188]

273. In another account the family noted that 'her abdomen was misshapen, there was a long scar that had been sewn up across it.'[189] The family suspected this was the result of organ harvesting.

274. In the final account, a mother was given permission to visit her daughter who was in a coma. The mother noted a '3 centimetre long scar above her right

---

182   Appendix 2A, Witness 49 Ethan Gutmann, evidence to the Tribunal, April 2019

183   Tortured To Death, published by Human Rights Without Frontiers and Bitter Winter in Belgium, (2018). p8

184   Ibid p28.

185   Ibid pp 10, 19, 26, 30, 55

186   Ibid pp 14, 56

187   Ibid pp 30, 44, 48, 54

188   Ibid p 24

189   Ibid p 37

ear.' The doctor stated the scar was 'from sleeping'. The official cause of death given by the hospital was 'brainstem bleeding'.[190]

275. In addition, the issues concerning a lack of due process arise in these accounts. Members of the Church of Almighty God were arrested for possession of religious material or proselytizing. In all these accounts, no person arrested was given any due process to determine their guilt or innocence and the families had no way of appealing decisions, or finding out more information when their loved ones had died. Furthermore, all victims in these accounts died from various medical reasons that were not present when they were taken into custody.

276. In addition to possible organ harvesting from adherents of different ethnic and religious groups, the Tribunal was made aware that foreign nationals could be subjected to the practice. The Tribunal received a witness statement from a Swedish national. He stated that he had been arrested in China in 2003 for allegedly counterfeiting money. In prison he observed there were other foreign nationals, from places like Taiwan and Sierra Leone. The witness described how torture was rampant in the prison and in many cases prisoners were directed to torture and kill certain other prisoners[191]

277. Further details of the above and similar events may be found in the witness statements and pre-reading material on the website of the Tribunal.

278. On the basis of the above evidence the Tribunal concludes with certainty that identifiable groups other than Falun Gong practitioners and Uyghurs – for example Protestant Christians and Tibetan Buddhists – have been incarcerated and tortured in similar ways to Falun Gong practitioners and Uyghurs.

Evidence of Rape and Other Sexual Violence

279. The Tribunal heard from a significant number of witnesses at its two hearings detailing evidence of rape and sexual violence against detainees in the PRC's prison system.

---

[190]   Ibid p 53
[191]   Appendix 1A, Witness 4

280. Dai Ying (see also paragraph 234 above on torture generally), said that while detained in detention guards stripped over 20 female practitioners and pushed a naked female Falun Gong practitioner out of her cell to show her to male prisoners, just to humiliate her.[192]

281. Liu Huiqiong, (see also paragraph 214 on torture generally), also known as Zeng Hui, said that in a medical examination, she was forced to have her private parts examined in 'an insulting way'. On 5 March 2001 she was detained and a police officer started to unbutton her clothes. 'He humiliated me and said "don't think about going back to your cell. I will sleep with you for sure."'[193]

282. Jintao Liu (Tony), (also in paragraph 187 above), said that in November 2007 while being subjected to torture by prison guards and other inmates, he had a toilet brush handle forced into his anus so hard he couldn't defecate.[194]

283. Zhang Yanhua, (also at paragraph 235 above) was asked whether there was a reason she had been tortured. She replied: 'The prison is a place to torture and humiliate practitioners.' The Tribunal believes that in this case and in other witness statements 'humiliation' is a euphemism for rape or sexual violence.[195]

284. Li Lin Lin, (see also footnote 145 above) described as a housewife, says that while in detention she was forced to take contraceptives.[196]

285. Yin Liping, (see also paragraph 220 above on medical testing and paragraph 235 on torture generally) said that on the 19 April 2001 she was incarcerated in the Masanjia Labour Camp. There, she said she was locked up with more than 40 men of unknown identity and was raped by these men, one of whom video-recorded her ordeal.[197]

286. Xuezhen Bao (see also paragraphs 181 and 219 on indirect evidence of forced organ harvesting and medical testing) says she witnessed the treatment of

---

[192] Appendix 1A, Witness 1
[193] Appendix 1A, Witness 5
[194] Appendix 1A, Witness 6.
[195] Appendix 1A, Witness 8.
[196] Appendix 1A, Witness 15.
[197] Appendix 1A, Witness 17.

a Falun Gong practitioner who had a physical examination that was used to 'cheat her and aborted her baby'. She said this woman was 'cheated and coerced many times'.[198] This was understood by the Tribunal as an understatement of something far worse.

287. The COHRC (China Organ Harvest Research Centre) report of the 28 November 2018 set out a list of atrocities perpetrated against Falun Gong practitioners by the PRC, including rape, gang rape and sexual torture. [199]

288. The Human Rights Law Foundation also listed such acts, including rape and sexual assault. In the same document Gao Zhisheng, a well-known lawyer said he witnessed 'immoral acts that shocked my soul; the most [being] ... lewd yet routine practice of attacking women's genitals by 610 staff and police. Almost every women's genitals and breasts have been sexually assaulted ... almost all [prisoners] ... be they male or female were stripped naked before torture.'[200]

289. In his evidence Edward McMillan-Scott claimed that Falun Gong prisoners were subjected to 'progressively brutal treatments involving electric prods ... always including the genitals'.[201]

290. On the basis of the evidence above the Tribunal concludes with certainty that the PRC has orchestrated within its penal system the endemic perpetration of rape and other acts of sexual violence and humiliation against male and female prisoners including Falun Gong practitioners. Specifically, the use of electric batons on the genitals of both men and women is prevalent

Evidence of Public Statements by the PRC about Falun Gong

291. In 1999 Jiang Zemin described Falun Gong as 'something unprecedented in the country since its founding 50 years ago'. In addition, on 7 June 1999, Jiang issued an unequivocal order to 'disintegrate' Falun Gong practitioners.[202]

---

[198]   Appendix 1A, Witness 18.

[199]   Appendix 2A, Witness 36.

[200]   Appendix 2A, Witness 40 See also http://hrlf.net/wp-content/uploads/2014/08/Spain-Jiang-Zemin-Amicus-Curiae-Brief-.pdf p11.

[201]   Appendix 2A, Witness 38.

[202]   Appendix 2B, item 33, Freedom House Report p112

292.   Further, in the same 7 June 1999 order, Jiang issued the following instructions: 'all CCP central departments, all ministries, all provinces and all cities must co-operate with the 610 Offices very closely'.[203]

293.   In July 1999, Wen Shizeng issued instructions 'to follow orders of Jiang's Central Committee of the Chinese Communist Party (CCCCP) to eliminate Falun Gong'[204]

294.   In 1999 Jiang Zemin also issued instructions through the CCCCP launching a douzheng (violent suppression) and zhuanhua (forced conversion).[205]

295.   On 20 July 1999 the CCP Central Committee's Notice of Forbidding CCP Members to Practice Falun Gong stated that: 'the transformation task for CCP members who practice Falun Gong must be accomplished'.[206]

296.   On 24 August 1999 Xinhua News Agency published the following notice from the Office of the CCP Central Committee: 'to better accomplish the mission of transforming the majority of the Falun Gong practitioners ... if they do not hold the "correct opinion"'[207]

297.   In early Sept 1999 Luo Gan (head of the 610 office) said: 'Whoever is found to be practising Falun Gong should be secretly arrested and sentenced to a life sentence until death.'[208]

298.   In early September 1999 Jiang Zemin issued a directive as follows: 'Beating them to death is nothing. If they are disabled from the beating, it counts as injuring themselves. If they die, it counts as suicide!'[209]

299.   In October 1999 Ding Shifa also issued instructions to 'diligently[210] participate in the Falun Gong douzheng with full political enthusiasm and prevail'.

---

[203]   Appendix 2B, item 36, Medical Genocide p9

[204]   Appendix 2B, item 40 (F), Campaign against FG p7

[205]   Appendix 2B, item 40 (G), Jiang Zemin liable for Torture p6

[206]   Ibid

[207]   Ibid p10

[208]   Appendix 2B, ibid

[209]   Appendix 2B, item 36 Medical Genocide p11, See also paragraph 147 above.

[210]   Appendix 2B, item 40(F), Campaign against FG p5, pp.7-8.

300. On 30 November 1999 Li Lanqing announced Jiang's directive about Falun Gong practitioners as follows: to 'ruin their reputations, break them financially, and destroy them physically'.[211]

301. In 1999 Luo Gan promoted the so called 'Masanjia experience' – a brainwashing programme introduced to persuade or force Falun Gong practitioners to renounce their faith; write repentance letters; give up all Falun Gong materials and literature; and denounce other practitioners and the founder of the faith.[212]

302. In Sept 2000, Jiang Zemin said, in a CBS interview: 'after careful deliberations, we concluded that Falun Gong is an evil cult'.[213]

303. In January 2001 Huang Jiefu told the Yangcheng Evening News that there was a 'struggle against Falun Gong [because it is] a serious political campaign. We have no mercy towards the few active members.'[214]

304. On 13 Feb 2001 a meeting was held at the Bureau of Justice in Chonquing at which lawyers were ordered to 'recognise fully the importance of the persecution of Falun Gong (the religion and its adherents)'.[215]

305. In February 2001 Huang Jiefu said: 'Opposing Falun Gong is a grave political struggle. We must not be soft-hearted when dealing with a little group of hardcore reactionaries.'[216]

306. In March 2002, there were Directives from 610 Office as follows: 'Firstly, eradicating Falun Gong is an arduous political task; do not be afraid of bloodshed and deaths; Secondly, tightly conceal the deaths and prevent leaking of information, which could lead to negative international impact; Thirdly, all levels of prosecution and judiciary branches of the government should not conduct investigations into the deaths or injuries of Falun Gong practitioners. Everyone should give way to the big picture.'

---

[211]   Appendix 2B, item 36, Medical Genocide p10

[212]   Appendix 2B, item 40(D), Brainwashing p77

[213]   Appendix 2B, item 40(B), Role of Jiang Zemin p8

[214]   Appendix 2B Magnitsky Act p4

[215]   Appendix 2B, item 40(F), Campaign against FG p5

[216]   Appendix 2B, item 36, Medical Genocide p18

307. In 2009, a book was published, entitled Prevention Of Cults In The New Era.[217] The following quote is extracted from it:

> *Falun Gong and similar evil religions are like viruses corroding the organism of humanity, warping the souls of believers, destroying social order, disrupting economic development, and have become a public nuisance to mankind and a cancer on society. ... Launching a deep douzheng against Falun Gong and other evil religious organisations is a duty shared by the whole Party, the whole country and the whole society.*[218]

308. There has been promulgation of *douzheng* by various party officials including Jiang Zemin, Li Lanqing, Wang Maolin (Leadership Team). Wang Maolin, in his book Falun Gong and Evil Cults, speaks of 'the importance and necessity of *douzheng* against Falun Gong'.[219]

309. Furthermore, China's official position towards Falun Gong practitioners is reflected in a document produced by ETAC at the Tribunal's request.[220] In October 2015 the PRC provided advanced responses to a List of Issues in to be dealt with by The UN Committee Against Torture on 17 and 18 November 2015. The PRC maintained complete compliance with the provision of the Convention against Torture but at paragraph 24 said:

> *The so-called "harvesting of organs of Falun Gong practitioners" is a rumour entirely fabricated by Falun Gong. On the contrary, it is precisely these preposterous and evil tales fabricated by Falun Gong that are exerting mind control on [Falun Gong practitioners] and causing a large number of fanatical followers to commit self-mutilations and suicide.*

Many of the other responses by the PRC are completely at odds with evidence received by the Tribunal.[221]

---

[217] Published by Zhejiang Province Anti-Cult Association (Internal Circulation) 2009. See Appendix 2B, Item 34 footnote 31

[218] Appendix 2B, item 34, Profiles of Chinese Transplant Surgeons paragraph 23, Summary of Evidence.

[219] Appendix 2B, item 40 (F), Campaign against FG p.7.

[220] Appendix 4, item 17

[221] https://www.hrichina.org/en/excerpts-chinas-responses-committee-against-tortures-list-issues

310. On the basis of the above evidence the Tribunal concludes with certainty that the PRC and its leaders have actively incited the persecution, imprisonment, murder, torture and humiliation of Falun Gong practitioners with the sole purpose of eliminating the practice of and belief in the value of Falun Gong.

Evidence from Telephone Calls to Hospitals and PRC and CCP Officials

Evidence of Investigations by WOIPFG (the World Organization to Investigate the Persecution of Falun Gong)

311. WOIPFG, as noted at paragraph 48 above, conducted a wide-ranging investigation of the PRC lasting nearly14 years, commencing in March 2006 and recording over 2,000 telephone calls to members of the standing Committee of the Politburo, other officials including at the 610 office, police, military hospitals, doctors and other staff in hospitals and transplant brokers. (see chapter 2 of their report The Final Harvest see http://www.upholdjustice. org/node/284).[222]

312. Telephone calls were always made on the basis of the investigator practising deception on the person called, pretending either to be someone with a need (for her or himself or another) of an organ or to be someone with official position. The objective was to establish whether the person receiving the call would reveal whether the source of any organ was a prisoner, in particular a Falun Gong prisoner, and/or whether the PRC itself was complicit in any forced organ harvesting of Falun Gong practitioners.[223]

---

[222]   Appendix 2A Witness 30 Dr Zhyiyuan Wang, 'Submission of World Organization to Investigate the Persecution of Falun Gong (WOIPFG),'

[223]   A measure of ambiguity exists in the papers about whether Matas and Kilgour commissioned the making of some phone calls independently of WOIPFG (see, eg, Torsten Trey who explained: 'In July 2006 David Kilgour and David Matas completed a two-months investigation and published their first investigative report alleging that organs were harvested from detained Falun Gong practitioners. In 14 recorded phone calls doctors in Chinese hospitals admitted to various degrees that they use "fresh organs" from Falun Gong practitioners for their transplants'. https:// chinatribunal.com/wp-content/uploads/2019/04/April_2019-DAFOH-Report-on-Forced-Organ-Harvesting-in-China.pdf Paragraph 2.3.)

    Matas and Kilgour have clarified as follows:

313. On one view the WOIPFG investigation overall deals conclusively with nearly all of the issues being considered by the Tribunal.

Approach by the Tribunal to the Work of WOIPFG

314. The findings of a body such as WOIPFG, that has a clear 'activist' purpose, may be subject to comment and criticism from some, fair or otherwise. In a recent report Matthew Robertson quotes Graham Fletcher, formerly the First Assistant Secretary in Australia's North Asia Division, as recorded in Hansard on the 8 June, 2108: '*I've looked at the reports as well, and often it's someone ringing from overseas. Who are they really speaking to? It's not the kind of evidence you'd put into a courtroom*'.[224]

315. In a similar vein Clause 2.36 of the 2018 Australian Parliamentary Sub-Committee Report, Compassion not Commerce, noted:

'The Coalition to Investigate the Persecution of the Falun Gong in China (CIPFG) asked [us] Matas and Kilgour by letter on May 24th, 2006 to undertake an investigation into forced organ harvesting of FG practitioners in China. We were first asked informally and so began work before that date. Some of the recordings used were from WOIPFG's previous work. These were calls that were useable, according to our methodological standards. The dates of all the calls we used are set out in Bloody Harvest. Some of the call excerpts published in *Bloody Harvest* were dated March 14 to 16, 2006. These would have been calls we drew from WOIPFG's previous work. We had independent translators translate the audios of the WOIPFG calls we chose to use. Through a personal contact we also contacted volunteers to conduct additional telephone investigations for our research. We gave the directions to the callers for who to call and for the method of the call via interpreters. (that they were to be recorded from pick up to put down) These calls were conducted in 2006 including a call to Dr Lu Guo Ping (see paragraph 425 below (Response of ETAC to Compassion Not Commerce 2.36)); through discussion it has become apparent that the caller who made this particular call was volunteering for both David Matas/David Kilgour and WOIPFG at the same time. David Matas and David Kilgour were unaware of this at the time. They had not approached WOIPFG at any time to conduct calls for them. The caller had previously (and still does) volunteer for WOIPFG so provided the audio of the Lu Guoping call to WOIPFG who translated the call for their own report. David Matas and David Kilgour had their own translation done of the audio at the time. Due to the fact that this caller was also volunteering for WOIPFG at the time, David Matas and David Kilgour have now agreed that this particular call could be considered joint research.'

[224] Australian parliamentary Hansard, June 8, 2018. For the Tribunal's provisional assessment of Mr Fletcher, now Australia's ambassador to the PRC, see paragraph 425 below and footnote 303.

The Submission of Doctors Against Forced Organ Harvesting highlighted transcripts of purported telephone conversations between Bloody Harvest researchers posing as prospective patients and staff at Chinese hospitals. In these alleged transcripts, the hospital staff appear to indicate that organs sourced from imprisoned Falun Dafa practitioners are available for transplantation. However, it is not possible to evaluate or confirm the authenticity of this material.

316. It is hard to know precisely what the Australian Sub-Committee meant by 'authenticity' in this context. The Tribunal found no difficulty with evaluation or confirmation, starting as it did from a position of complete neutrality as to overall outcome.

317. In a forthcoming publication, Authentication and Analysis of Purported Undercover Telephone Calls Made to Hospitals in China on the Topic of Organ Trafficking,[225] Matthew Robertson, who is associated with Falun Gong but recognised by the Tribunal as an expert on certain matters, observed of WOIPFG:

Its approach to research and information gathering often overlaps with human rights advocacy and/or religiously inspired moral persuasion. WOIPFG clearly states that the goal of its work is to gather the evidence required to bring to justice the perpetrators of alleged crimes against humanity against Falun Gong practitioners. All this means that on a fundamental level WOIPFG does not understand its role to be as an objective gatherer of scientific information, but rather an investigator searching for evidence of crimes in order to expose them. This adversarial orientation inevitably has downstream effects on how information has been gathered, stored, and presented to the public.

---

[225]   See report at https://chinatribunal.com/wp-content/uploads/2020/02/Authentication-and-Analysis-of-Purported-Undercover-Telephone-Calls-Made-to-Hospitals-in-China-on-the-Topic-of-Organ-Trafficking_MatthewRobertson_VOCWorkingPaper.pdf
    Matthew Robertson, China Studies Research Fellow, Victims of Communism Memorial Foundation: 'Authentication and Analysis of Purported Undercover Telephone Calls Made to Hospitals in China on the Topic of Organ Trafficking' prepared for Victims of Communism (VOC). Robertson does not single out Matas and Kilgour telephone calls from those of WOIPFG and it is clear that at least on some occasions there was common use of the same investigators. The Tribunal assesses all telephone calls of which it has evidence.

In this passage Robertson appears to have doubt about WOIPFG's ability to be objective, without giving a reason. As observed at paragraph 52 above, there is 'no presumption of disbelief in what people say about facts'; the need for caution arises only wherever there is a reason for doubting some piece of evidence (a 'reasonable doubt')' even though there should only ever be limited reliance [by Tribunal members] on *expert witness opinions* on final issues.[226] The characterisation by Robertson of WOIPFG as a body *seek[ing] to bring to justice the perpetrators of alleged crimes against humanity against Falun Gong practitioner* might lead readers to ask whether they should doubt the factual accuracy of anything, or everything, that Jewish 'Nazi hunters' have ever recounted, simply because they are Jewish? The Tribunal thinks

---

[226]   In a further recent report, 'Organ Procurement and Extrajudicial Execution in China: A Review of the Evidence' Matthew P Robertson, China Studies Research Fellow, Victims of Communism Memorial Foundation January 1, 2020, Robertson appears to recognise this distinction at footnote 37: 'Our inclusion and discussion of WOIPFG data in this report by itself indicates some level of confidence in their research, but additional qualification is appropriate. WOIPFG's *raw collection and documentation efforts* — **which have been thorough and vast** — should be distinguished from both their *analytical process* as well as their *presentation style*. In the first category, raw collection, we have no reason to doubt the reliability of their work as a whole. We have obtained 25 gigabytes of hospital website archives, pdf and png files of medical papers, doctor biographies, video files, and much more, which WOIPFG researchers collected by going to the websites of hospitals one by one, taking screenshots, logging archives, and inputting data. In almost all of the numerous cases we have checked, these corresponded to the publicly available data. We have found a number of instances in which the original source says something slightly different to what WOIPFG says it says, or where WOIPFG's interpretation may be construed as imprecise or perhaps overly emphatic (counting all beds in one hospital's hepatobiliary surgery department as transplant beds, and counting dialysis beds in a renal department as transplant beds, for example), but these cases appear to be on the margins. Occasional mistakes and conflations may be expected when dealing with tens of thousands of complex data points. We have interviewed WOIPFG researchers and investigators at length about their procedures, which, with the exception of their undercover telephone calls, are based on accessing publicly available data. Forming a judgement on WOIPFG's reliability in gathering publicly available data should be sharply distinguished from judgements about their analysis or style of presentation. In some instances, it appears that the failure to make this distinction has led to their work being disregarded, to the detriment of advancing knowledge on this issue. **We are pleased to make use of the remarkable body of primary data they have collected, much of which is no longer available**, while submitting it to our own process of analysis.' [emphasis added]

The Tribunal reads this passage as fulsome endorsement by someone taking a fine academic approach to the integrity of WOIPFG's work; an endorsement that accords with the Tribunal's own assessment, as set out at paragraph 340 below

the characterisation unhelpful and maintains its 'juror' approach. Individuals giving accounts of facts should be credited unless there is reason to doubt; not otherwise.

318. Finally, it should also be noted, the Australian Sub-Committee's approach – or even Robertson's report – may suggest there could be a possible cause for *reasoned* doubt simply because of the human wickedness revealed in what people may recount. Many events can be described as unbelievable that are not at all unbelievable, but simply things listeners or readers would prefer not to have to believe – against which they may resist out of a determination to see humans, and nation states that represent humans, as other than they are. The Holocaust does not stand alone as an example of recent state-sponsored human wickedness – the massacres in Indonesia in 1965, the killings by the Khmer Rouge and the butchery in Rwanda of the Tutsis are but three others that may be described as 'unbelievable' when they are only too believable and indeed established facts.[227]

Robertson's Report

319. In his report Robertson sets out the significant lengths to which he went in verifying that the phone calls were indeed made and that the recipients of the calls were genuine as WOIPFG explained. This verification included;

- cross referencing call logs and dialling hospitals,
- calling surgeons to match phone numbers,

---

[227] We may not want to have to believe things but that does not generate a reason to doubt them when they are described. The Pole Jan Karski encountered unreasoned doubt from US Supreme Court Justice Felix Frankfurter– himself a Jewish friend and adviser of President Roosevelt – in 1943 when Karski's face to face account of his own first-hand experiences of Polish Ghettos and death camps was met with: 'I am unable to believe you', Frankfurter explaining that he did not say Karski was lying just that he was unable to believe him. Why not? No reason given, and the disbelief came at what cost? See 'Karski, How One Man tried to Stop the Holocaust by Wood and Jankoswski, John Wiley and Sons 1994, p188. And on the issue of what humans do to each other without resistance, public executions that included disembowelling drew huge crowds in London until three centuries ago, public hangings in Central London only stopped in 1868 because the crowds of baying onlookers were too large to handle. Accounts of these events are undoubted facts. Would accounts of public tolerance of, and amusement by, public quartering of humans still alive otherwise be believed? It may be thought that to disbelieve without reason a human account of something factual comes at risk.

- observing calls made by WOIPFG investigators,
- reviewing calls recorded by telephone companies and comparing them for length of calls and,
- logging into investigators secure portals.

320. Although Robertson explains that the record keeping and data management of some of WOIPFGs work has been less than methodical, he was able to match a number of calls from a 'convenience sample' to records held. More important *no error was identified.*

321. Robertson states: 'We believe we have taken every reasonable and feasible precaution to establish the veracity of the telephone calls provided by WOIPFG.'

322. The veracity of the telephone calls is, of course, for the Tribunal members to decide – they will not, as explained, accept expert opinion on 'final' issues. The Tribunal does nevertheless note and apply in its final decision-making the factual account given by Robertson in his report that clearly supports the integrity of WOIPFG's investigation.

323. Robertson has undertaken extensive research relating to Falun Gong and so might justify the same caution he posits the Tribunal should feel for WOIPFG generally. The Tribunal has considered his evidence in exactly the same way as it has considered evidence of any who have shown particular interest in Falun Gong practitioners' suffering, whether or not themselves Falun Gong practitioners.[228] *If* any caution is necessary – the Tribunal repeats the negative contained in paragraph 52 and 317 above – then it must apply to all who came to the Tribunal with evidence in support of the allegations against the PRC and a record of giving some support for Falun Gong. The Tribunal approached the evidence about WOIPFG and Robertson's evidence – without any *presumption* or *assumption* of doubt – in the regular way of decision-making by jurors.

---

[228] Some witnesses at the Tribunal did say whether they were Falun Gong practitioners; others did not. The Tribunal accepts this to be a matter of personal choice. Recorded in the judgment where thought relevant or of interest.

The Tribunal's Approach to WOIPFG

324. The Tribunal approached the evidence provided by WOIPFG first, by asking whether Dr Wang, the witness who provided evidence of WOIPFG's work, was an honest and reliable witness and second, by asking whether WOIPFG was a body of integrity conducting research in the way shown by evidence. As to integrity it needs to be noted that where phone calls were made to hospitals it was not possible to check by scientific means whether the voice of the person answering was the voice of the same person recorded elsewhere.[229] A similar consideration arises with telephone calls to PRC or CCP officials. The integrity issue may include whether in these circumstances the researchers might have been simply putting on a show and calling others in their activist group with the aim of deceiving their audience (as urged, without supporting evidence of any kind, by Graham Fletcher of the Australian government – see paragraph 314 above). In addition, there exists the possibility that western understanding of answers given by Chinese officials could be 'lost in translation', literally or in an interpretive sense. To that end, three academics were asked to provide comment on the content of 30 phone calls (see additional submissions). None of them made comment that would suggest any misinterpretation.[230] Between delivery of the Summary Judgment on 17 June 2019 and printing of this full Judgment there were further tests performed

---

[229] Consideration was given by Matthew Robertson to proving identity of voices on tape recordings recording of known individuals in the very few cases where the person called might have been recorded already elsewhere or where the person could be contacted by telephone independently to make a recording of her/his voice for comparison. It became clear that the quality of recordings of the voices made such an exercise impossible

[230] See: Phone call content verification report (for WOIPFG Investigation Calls) Appendix 2B, item 42. Terms of reference were as follows: Three academics were approached (not FG practitioners or Uyghurs) to provide comments on the content of 30 phone calls from the WOIPFG submission to the China Tribunal. A link to the audio and a spreadsheet with two columns were provided (see pdf documents). The written transcripts and WOIPFG reports were not provided, phone call recipient names were not provided.

Commentators did not see the comments from other commentators

Instructions to academics/commentators:

'One particular submission the Tribunal received is from an organisation that has made investigative phone calls to Chinese doctors and officials regarding forced organ harvesting. In total there are 30 phone calls with most calls being 2-6 mins long. The Tribunal has requested that a few native Chinese speakers listen to the calls (or a portion) and comment on what is happening in the call and the outcome of the call. The responses in some calls are ambiguous when translated into English, whilst others seem quite clear. It is not necessary to actually

on a sample of five telephone calls as recorded by WOIPFG in its report The Final Harvest (The Final Harvest, one of many WOIPFG reports, had not been referred to specifically in evidence hearings). The five calls were listened to by independent translators who checked original translations and, where they considered appropriate, provided some fresh translations. Two of the calls summarised in paragraph 336, were among the five. No significant error in the original translations was identified in any of the five calls.[231] See Appendix 4, item 34.

325. The Tribunal concluded first, that Dr Wang was an honest witness and second, that the investigation was one of integrity and that there was absolutely no reason, and no evidence of any kind, to doubt that investigators of WOIPFG were calling, or seeking to call, the people they said they were calling.

326. In the absence of *either* of these conclusions by the Tribunal, the telephone call evidence would have been accorded no significance.

327. These two conclusions do not, of course, by themselves determine the value of telephone calls that were expressly designed to deceive those called into saying things against their own, or a hospital's, or the PRC's interest.

---

translate the call into English as this has already been done unless you want to highlight any particular part of the call.

There is no need for a translation, more your comment on what is happening in the calls and the outcome of the calls. If you do wish to highlight and comment on a particular part of a call in your notes that would also be helpful.

The calls are by investigators who called into China pretending to be someone else so as to capture information about organ harvesting. In some cases they are pretending to be someone in need of an organ, or who has a family member in need of an organ. In other cases they pretend to be someone from an official office.'

See report at https://chinatribunal.com/wp-content/uploads/2020/02/Phone-call-content-verification-report.pdf; and https://chinatribunal.com/wp-content/uploads/2020/02/PhoneCallsVerification_AcademicCommentators_15May.pdf

[231] One of these two calls was capable of being subject to a technical voice recognition process by an expert who reached the conclusion that *'the voice in the questioned telephone call is very similar to and consistent with that of Bai Shuzhong in respect of the parameters examined; I have found no differences that would indicate that the voice in the call is not his.'* *(See the report by Prof. French* https://chinatribunal.com/wp-content/uploads/2020/02/Report-on-Forensic-Examinations-of-Recordings_Prof-French_A.pdf)

How the Tribunal Approached what was Said in Telephone Calls

328. The Tribunal has had the following considerations in mind it is approach to phone calls made with the purpose of deceiving those called:

    a.   A percentage of calls to medics, hospitals etc were met by denials, outraged responses etc ….;

    b.   Where someone is confronted with no prior warning by a proposition that is surprising or outrageous, she or he may not necessarily give the best or most accurate or honest response because of the surprise;

    c.   Hospitals seeking transplantation business may not tell the truth – and may indeed lie – about their capacity, including about their ready access to organs from young Falun Gong practitioners for business reasons;

    d.   Political or similar leaders confronted by people on the phone who seem to hold official office may answer according to what they assume is wanted by way of an answer;

    e.   Answers such as 'yeah, yeah, yeah' to difficult questions about access to Falun Gong organs need not necessarily be the same as a clear 'yes' and should be approached cautiously for what they signify;

    f.   Answers given to callers who were practicing deception could best be evaluated by hearing from the person who gave the answer; none of the people called by WOIPFG was a witness or even known to be available as a witness for the Tribunal to hear.

329. On the other hand,

    a.   Answers amounting to statements against the interest of the person speaking – such as acknowledged engagement in practices whereby Falun Gong prisoners were killed for their organs to be harvested – may be more likely to be right than otherwise. Why admit something adverse to yourself, it is often argued?

    b.   Being asked specifically about provision of Falun Gong practitioner organs must have focused the minds of those questioned and would be likely to elicit answers genuinely related to Falun Gong practitioners;

    c.   Patterns of broadly similar answers and reactions by people from different sectors of the hospital/medical section of the PRC, in different places, and over time may lend support to the proposition that one or more of the individual answers may be true in substance, and a mere pattern of broadly similar answers about matter arguably contrary to self-interest may generate a reliable *general* conclusion;

d. Answers by PRC or CCP officials that would be revealing, if true, of PRC or CCP involvement in forced organ harvesting might reflect the impunity felt by those officials operating in a powerful state machine (depending, of course, on the view any individual assessing the evidence held of the power of the state machine). This was certainly the case, it would appear, in the call made to Zhu Jiabin of Mudanjiang City's 610 office. (Appendix 2B item 30. WOIPFG list of calls Appendix 11 – Evidence 15).

330. Those reviewing the material provided by WOIPFG – summarised below and available in full on the Tribunal website and the internet – may reach conclusions stronger than that of the Tribunal, set out at paragraph 340 See report at https://chinatribunal.com/wp-content/uploads/2020/02/Phone-call-content-verification-report.pdf; and https://chinatribunal.com/wp-content/uploads/2020/02/PhoneCallsVerification_AcademicCommentators_15May.pdf below, a conclusion that is in accordance with the cautious approach taken by the Tribunal in respect of all other areas of evidence.

History of Some Calls

331. Following media reports that Falun Gong practitioners were being killed for their organs, which surfaced in March 2006, WOIPFG initially commissioned two mandarin speaking investigators, 'M' and 'N', who began making calls to a number of hospitals and transplant doctors together with other CCP officials.

332. The majority of the calls followed a similar pattern, with M or N asking to be put through to the transplant department and seeking general information. M or N was then usually handed on to a doctor, but on occasion to a prison or court official.

333. M made 80 calls to different hospitals and of these 10 admitted they used Falun Gong practitioners (FGP), 5 said they could procure the same, 14 said they used live organs and 10 said the source of the organs was a secret. No information is available with regard to the remaining calls.

334.   N made calls to almost 40 hospitals, of which 5 admitted using FGP organs. In addition, N made calls to 40 detention centres of which 4 admitted using FGP organs.

335.   The calls listed were recorded and translated by a certified translator with the Government of Ontario, Mr CY. The original recordings are also available.

336.   Excerpts and a précis of some of those calls are set out below. The excerpts and the calls themselves are not included in full, but complete transcripts are available at https://chinatribunal.com.

On the 22 May, 2006, in a call made to Dr Lu Guoping of Nanning City Minzu Hospital, the doctor appears to make a direct and incontrovertible admission that that organs from FGP are used:
Q: It is said that the organs from FGP are relatively healthy and better. Do they use this kind as well?'
A: Right, right, right. Usually the healthy ones are chosen.'
Q: What I mean is that the organs from FGP are better. Do they use this kind as well?'
A: Right, right, right.

Remarkably, Phoenix TV subsequently produced a PRC response to a transcript of the call which had been made public. In it, Lu Guoping acknowledges receiving the call but appears to challenge his recorded answers as follows:

'I told her I was not involved in the surgical operations and I had no idea where the organ came from. She asked me whether these organs came from prisons. I replied no to her in clear cut terms.' Dr Lu goes on to refute various parts of the transcript and states that it has been 'distorted or mutilated'. What appears to be clear is that Dr Lu, who knew of the transcript but may not have been aware of the tape recording, was a participant in the call and therefore is the author of the words in the transcript, contrary to his subsequent denials.

On the 8 June, 2006, M calls the Mishan City Detention Centre and speaks to Mr Li, who directly acknowledges the availability of FGP 'suppliers':
M: How many FG suppliers do you have?

Li: Quite a few.

M: Are they male or female?

Li: Male.

M: … how many do you have?

Li: Seven, eight, we have at least five, six now.

On the 15 March, 2006, N speaks to Director Song at the Oriental Transplant Centre, Tianjin City who confirms that the source of kidneys is alive.

N: 'Her doctor told her that the kidney is quite good because he (the supplier) practices … FG.'

Song: 'Of course. We have all these who breathe and with heartbeat.'

[This call was tested as to translation (see Appendix 4, item 34)]

On the 16 March, 2006, M calls the Shanghai Zhongshan Hospital Organ transplant and speaks to an unidentified doctor who acknowledges the source of the organs as being from FG.

M: 'Is there are a source of organs that come from FG?'

Doctor: 'All of ours are that type.'

On 16 March, 2006, M calls the Quanfoshan City Liver Transplant Hospital, Shangdong province and speaks to an unidentified doctor who confirms the source of organs as being FG.

M: The supply of liver …. the ones from FG, I want to ask if you have those types?

Doctor: It is OK if you come here.

M: 'So that means you have them?'

Doctor: In April there will be more of these kind of suppliers… now, gradually we have more and more.

On the 16 March, 2006, M speaks to Dr Dai at the Shanghai Jiatong University Hospital who confirms that the source of organs are all alive, states a number of 400-500 cases that 'we' have and a price at RMB 150-200,000.

M: 'We want fresh alive ones.

Dr Dai: They are all alive, all alive.

On 14 March, 2006, M speaks to Dr Wang at the Zhenzhou Medical University Organ Transplant Centre who confirms that FGP are the source of organs.

M: That is the kind that practices this type of FG.
Dr Wang: For this could you rest assured.

On 30 March, 2006, N speaks to an unidentified official at the Tongji Hospital who confirms that the organ suppliers are alive.
N: We hope the kidney suppliers are alive… using living bodies from prisoners who practice FG. Is that possible?
Official: It's not a problem.'

On 11 April, 2006, an investigator speaks to Dr Wang at the No 1 Hospital University of Xian who confirms that the organ source is both live and from FG.
Investigator: There are some labour camps that jail FGP and then the organs are removed from their live bodies…
Dr Wang: Yes, yes. What we care is the quality…

On 12 April, 2006, N speaks to Dr Zhu of the General Hospital of Guangzhou Military Region who states that they have, albeit limited, a supply of kidneys from FG.
Zhu: 'We have very few kidneys from FG.'
N: But you still have some?
Zhu: It is not hard for blood type B.

On 26 April, 2006, an investigator (unclear if this is N or M) speaks to Chief Physician Xu at the Air Force Hospital at Chendu, who unequivocally confirms the source of organs as being FG.
Investigator: It should be from the young and healthy who practice FG.
Xu: No problem.

On 23 May, 2006, N speaks to an unidentified official of the Jianzhou Intermediate People's court who is explicit in referring to the availability of organs from young FGP.
N: …we always (got) kidneys from young and healthy people who practice FG … I wonder if you still have such organs in your court right now.'
Official: …it is you who will come here to get them.

On 13 September, 2006, Bo Xilai, then minister of Commerce accompanied the Chinese Premier, Wen Jiabao, on a visit to Hamburg. An investigator who claimed to be the First Secretary at the Chinese Embassy in Germany phoned Bo Xilai and asked him to identify who gave the order for live organ harvesting of FGP. Bo Xilai confirms that it is the Premier.

First Secretary: '… that is to say, regarding the matter of live organ harvesting of FGP, was that your order or Jiang Zemin's order?'

Bo: President Jiang's.[232]

On 25 October, 2006, an investigator speaks to an unidentified doctor at the Shanghai Ruinjin Hospital who confirms the use of FGP as a source of organs, and that the practice is widespread in other hospitals.

Investigator: '… he refers to that kind from FG, right? Do use this kind as well?

Doctor: Yes.

Investigator: Wow, you use that kind as well?

Doctor: Every hospital is the same.

Investigator: …it is because FG kind is much healthier, right?

Doctor: Correct.

On the 14th November, 2006, M speaks to an unidentified doctor at the No 1Hospital affiliated to Mongolia Medical College who confirms FG as an organ source.

M: That type, the FG type is better…

Doctor: I know, I know.

Investigator: Right. That kind that practices FG, they are very healthy.

Doctor: I know, I know.

On 8 August, 2007, Zeng Quinhong attended the 60th Anniversary Celebration of Inner Mongolia Autonomous Region. A WOIPFG investigator was able to reach him at his hotel room. During the phone conversation, Zeng did not deny the statement that 'Military armies participated in live organ harvesting from detained Falun Gong practitioners.' (The Final Harvest 2.6)

On 26 September, 2008, Wei Jianrong admits that organ harvesting 'started a long time ago'. (The Final Harvest 3.2-no transcript.)

In November 2008, Zhou Benshun, the then Secretary-General of Central PLAC, accompanied Zhou Yongkang, the director of Central PLAC, on a

---

[232]   Appendix 2B, item 30 Appendix 2.

visit to Australia. A WOIPFG investigator disguising himself as Yang Hui, Head of the Second Department of PLA General Staff Headquarter, tried to collect testimony from Zhou Benshun. Zhou admitted, 'Such things as live organ harvesting from Falun Gong practitioners in our country – it does exist in our country.' (The Final Harvest 3.1)

On 17 April, 2012, an investigator questions Li Changchun (a Politburo member)
Investigator: we should use Bo Xilai's in murdering and removing organs from FG practitioners to convict Bo.
Li: 'Zhou Yongkang is in charge of this specifically. He knows it. (The Final harvest 2.3)

On 13 September, 2012, Tang Junjie (former deputy secretary of PLAC in Liaoning province) was asked

'What directions or commands did Bo Xilai give regarding removing organs from FG practitioners.'
Tang: 'I was asked to take care of that task. (The Final Harvest 3.3)'

[This call was tested as to translation (see Appendix 4, item 34) and voice recognition See https://chinatribunal.com/wp-content/uploads/2020/02/Report-on-Forensic-Examinations-of-Recordings_Prof-French_A.pdf)

On the 30 September, 2014, Bai Shuzhong, minister of health for the People's Liberation Army admitted that Jiang Zemin gave direct orders to extract Falun Gong organs.
Investigator: When you were head … regarding taking organs from the detained FG people, was it an order from Wang Ke …'
Bai: Back then, it was Chairman Jiang.
Investigator: We also obtained some intelligence…..the Joint Logistics Department had detained a number of FG people as live donors, is that true?'
Bai: '… after Chairman Jiang issued the order, we all did a lot of work against the Falun Gong practitioners' (The Final Harvest 1.1)

On 15 June, 2015, an investigator called Zhang Dejiang while he was on a trip to India.
Investigator: Comrade Jiang Zemin wanted to know if Zhou Yongkang had confessed the fact the Jiang Zemin made the decision of live organ harvesting….
Zhang: Can we talk after I am back in China? Okay?. (The Final Harvest, 2.2)

On 24 June, 2015, a call was placed with Zhang Gaoli a member of the Politburo Standing Committee. The investigator, posing as a secretary (Liu) at Jiang Zemin's office, states that he is calling on behalf of Jiang Zemin who is concerned at court action that is being brought at the Supreme Procuratorate and Zemin's accountability for ordering the removal of organs from 'millions' of FGP. Liu seeks Zhang's assurance that that the matter will be repressed at a Politburo meeting, to which Zhang agrees.

Liu: You know the responsibility of live organ harvesting from several million FGP is enormous. You know that right. You understand … You need to take care of that.'

Zhang: Tell president Jiang not to worry.

On 26 June, 2015, a call was placed to Chen Yongfeng at the Liver Transplantation Department of Zhengzhou People's Hospital in which Chen initially states that he has carried out one procedure that day and they had a donor with a cerebral haemorrhage who was three days older than 16 with a liver of more than 700 but less than 800gms which was harvested at 9 o'clock. He confirms that the waiting time for a procedure is one week.

Investigator: … roughly how long is the waiting time?

Chen: Usually about a week.

On 21 June, 2016, an investigator collecting evidence on the alleged murder and forced organ harvesting of the organs of Gao Yixi, calls the Head of the 610 Office in Mudanjiang City. The transcript provides an explicit and frank admission that Zhu Jiabin of the 610 Office is a perpetrator of murder and organ harvesting and that he does so with impunity.

Investigator: You carved out his organs and you think you can get away with it?

Zhu: Sold them!'… After slaughtering and opening up the belly, you just carve out the organs and sell them I only know to sell organs for money after organ harvesting. That is my principle… If you had guts to stand in front of me now I would live organ harvest you … My name is 'the butcher'… I am called the butcher specialising in live organ harvesting … Its nothing, just like slaughtering pigs. You come over to shave their hair first and then split open the belly. I would carve out whatever I need. After scooping the organs out, I would sell them.'

On 26 May, 2017, an investigator calls Director Wang at Yasntai Yuhuangdong Hospital and Dr Wang confirms that the waiting time for a kidney is two weeks or less. He has a detailed discussion regarding the price, the terms of the payment, who receives the money and that the donors are young.

Wang: … yes, including the physical examination, it will be within half a month, within two weeks. … The complete package is, the whole thing will cost over 500,000 yuan.

Investigator: So how much is your portion?

Wang: 400,000 yuan.

Investigator: So you can still find that kind from the prison?

Wang: You need to find the ones under 30 years old.

On the 10 June, 2017, a further call was placed to Dr Wang in which he confirms that kidneys are available at 10 days' notice and that the source is a very young person. He also confirms that the hospital has carried out hundreds of procedures every year and that it circumvents the official Red Cross 'network' and has its own channels to source organs. He also confirms the price as less than 500,000 yuan, but more than 400,000.

On an unspecified date an investigator calls Chen Qiang, a kidney broker at the PLA (People's Liberation Army) No 37 in Beijing, During the call Chen confirms that his boss will show information positively identifying FG as the source of organs. Falun Gong prisoners were imprisoned around the time of 2003 without records of their names and were therefore accorded codes.

Chen: How to positively identify FGP, well when the time comes… our boss will have people show you information. … There were tons of FGP on file around 2003 … If they could not find out the real name, they just left code numbers, you know … such an operation is like a supply chain, you know.

On an unspecified date a call was placed to a policeman at the Intermediate People's court of Jinzhou in which the investigator seeks confirmation that kidney donors are young and healthy and practice FG. The responses are tentative but do not disclaim the request.

Investigator: We have been obtaining kidney donors from courts and detention centres, from those donors who are young and healthy and practice FG. Now there are fewer such donors.

Policeman: Mmm, mmm.

Investigator: So, I don't know if your court is still able to provide such donors.

Policeman: That depends on your situation … we might be able to provide it.

A graphic call was made to a police officer from Jinzhou City – the date of the call is unspecified, but it refers to events that took place on 9 April, 2002. In it the officer describes, as a witness, the torture of a woman who was then killed by means of the extraction of her organs without anaesthetic. Her heart and then her kidneys were removed. 'When the knife touched her chest she shouted 'Falun Gong is good.' … her heart was carved out first and then her kidneys. When her cardiac vessels were cut by the scissors she started twitching. It was extremely horrible.' (See also paragraph 167.)

The Tribunal's Approach to the Evidence of Telephone Calls

337. The volume of what are effectively admissions from medical staff – in many cases the direct acknowledgement and admission of the practice of organ harvesting from live donors (mostly Falun Gong) by these parties – the verification work undertaken by Matthew Robertson and the honesty (as found) of Dr Wang leaves the Tribunal in no doubt that Mr Fletcher is quite wrong in his cursory dismissal of this very important body of evidence.

338. The Tribunal concludes that the calls were made and that they add significant weight to the Tribunal's judgment.

339. There is powerful evidence of responsibility for forced organ harvesting from those who were agents of the state, significantly as recently as 2014. The PRC has been given a chance, through the hearings at the Tribunal and by material posted on the Tribunal website, to challenge the accuracy of these calls. No challenge has been made to the Tribunal, publicly or otherwise. The Tribunal has no reason to doubt the accuracy of recordings of calls with those who were agents of the state.

Conclusions about the Evidence of Telephone Calls

340. On the basis of all evidence, the Tribunal concludes, with certainty, that telephone calls were made to hospitals and individual medical staff including senior surgeons and that the translations of the recorded calls are accurate. The Tribunal further concludes, with certainty, that the hospitals telephoned were offering organs for sale, that those organs were from people who were alive at the time of the calls and that those organs were available to the callers on short notice.

341. The Tribunal is also certain that responsibility for forced organ harvesting by the PRC itself is also demonstrated through things said by those who were agents of the state. The Tribunal has no reason to doubt the accuracy of these recordings. The PRC has been given a chance, through the hearings at the Tribunal, and material posted on the Tribunal website, to challenge the accuracy of these calls. No challenge has been made to the Tribunal publicly or otherwise.

The Scale of Transplant Activity in China

342. There are constraints on the total number of organ transplants that any country can perform. These constraints comprise:

- The number of potential (and eligible) donors;
- The number of organs or parts of organs obtained at each organ donation procedure;
- The number of organs extracted which actually are transplanted into recipients. Some extracted organs may prove unsuitable and be 'wasted';
- The resources and facilities available to perform transplantation;[233]
- Staff (medical, surgical, anaesthetic, nursing, technical, laboratory, administrative, data management, co-ordination experts and many others);
- Hospitals, and within them, beds dedicated to transplant patients;
- The organisational infrastructure to match donor with recipient. This means adequate and accurate tissue typing, accessible and accurate databases, and transportation arrangements for donor organ and recipient;
- Appropriate equipment for post-transplant organ function monitoring;
- Adequate supply of effective anti-rejection therapies.

343. Organs should only be transplanted from:

- Voluntary live donors in the context of a single kidney, a part of a liver or a lobe of lung.
- Confirmed brain-dead (against established criteria) donors, or post-circulatory death donors, in the context of whole organs (lung, heart, whole liver, small bowel, pancreas, both kidneys and corneas)

---

[233]   Textbook of Organ Transplantation Editor(s): Allan D. Kirk MD, PhD, FACS, Stuart J. Knechtle MD, Christian P. Larsen MD, DPhil, Joren C. Madsen MD, DPhil, Thomas C. Pearson MD, Steven A. Webber MBChB, MRCP Copyright © 2014 John Wiley & Sons Ltd

344. International transplant authorities expect transparency and completeness of data collection in relation to all the above, in accordance with The Declaration of Istanbul.[234]

345. China has, in effect, regarded such data as a state secret. There is no transparency, and there are grave doubts over all official data, including some of the most recent.[235]

346. It is important to note that the reporting of transplantation activity can be confusing. For example, the *total* number of transplants is a complex statistic, itself comprising individual organs from a variable number of donors. It may include both live and deceased donors, and the recipient may receive more than one organ (eg heart and lungs). In an ideal world, it would be better to subdivide transplantation activity by organ transplanted and by donor source and type. However, the figure that is often used to indicate the *scale* of transplantation in a particular country, related to the population, is a number *per* million. Once again, no such official data are available from China.

347. There is no doubt that interpreting the available information from China over the last 20 years is challenging, largely because of the lack of transparency. It is useful therefore to report transplant rates in a well-regulated country, such as the UK, with established and transparent data reporting. In the financial year 2018-19, when the UK population was just under 68 million, according to data available from NHS Blood and Transfusion[236] there were 6,077 people on the transplant waiting list, 4,990 transplants, of which 1,600 were from deceased donors, 46% of whom had been on an opt-in donor register (the remainder being consented by the donor's family, who were approached after death was declared inevitable). 'Live' donors donated 1,017 kidneys and 22

---

[234] The Declaration of Istanbul was created at the Istanbul Summit on Organ Trafficking and Transplant Tourism held from 30 April to 1 May 2008 in Istanbul, Turkey. Clause 6 of the 'Principle of The Declaration of Istanbul' reads 'Designated authorities in each jurisdiction should oversee and be accountable for organ donation, allocation and transplantation practices to ensure standardization, traceability, transparency, quality, safety, fairness and public trust.' See further https://declarationofistanbul.org/

[235] Appendix 2B, item 44 'Analysis of official deceased organ donation data casts doubt on credibility of China's organ transplant reform' Matthew P. Robertson, Raymond L. Hinde, Jacob Lavee; January 26, 2019

[236] https://www.odt.nhs.uk/statistics-and-reports/annual-activity-report/

segments of liver. Thus, there were 2,639 donors of solid organs in that year from whom an average of 3.2 organs were retrieved per donor. Rounding these figures for simplicity, 2,700 donors resulted in 5,000 actual transplants.

The data also shows that in 2018-19 there were 14.6 donors per million of population in the UK. On a similar basis, and if it had a system of equivalent efficiency, China's population of almost 1.4 billion could be expected to generate 20,440 donors per year and thus approximately 38,000 transplants per year.

348.   In the absence of validated, externally auditable and complete data from the Chinese state, it is necessary to relate different sources of data to deduce what are the real data for transplant activity in China. 'Triangulating' data from other, multiple and different, sources is both rational and indeed the only way to approach the numerical data. This was the approach adopted by Kilgour, Gutmann and Matas.[237] The Tribunal has relied on their very detailed and well referenced research in this area and is of the opinion it is correct so to do. The weight of evidence they have collated from a wide range of sources is convincing in terms both of scale and consistency.

349.   Organ transplantation activity has grown rapidly in China since the turn of the century, supported by official policy.[238] In order to describe that rise in activity, the Tribunal must summarise the evidence for such growth in a number of areas.

The Number of Hospitals Undertaking Transplantation

350.   There was no government approval system in China for transplant hospitals until 1 July 2007, when in response to criticisms of the source of organs for transplantation and in order 'to rectify and regulate' the market, hospitals were required to obtain a permit to function as a transplant centre.[239] One thousand hospitals applied but only 146 received permits. Some hospitals only had limited permits. It is reported that up to 566 other hospitals without permits continued to perform transplants[240]. This total of 712 hospitals

---

[237]   Appendix 3, item 7 Bloody Harvest/The Slaughter; an Update, June 2016, p11

[238]   Ibid, Chapter 3 pp19 *et seq.*

[239]   Update, *supra*, p316

[240]   Ibid

performing transplants is in contrast, and in contradiction, to the comments of Wang Haibo in paragraph 425 below (Compassion Not Commerce 2.48).

351. Although the *official* number of transplant centres in China is upwards of 146, it has been stated by several authors that there are many more hospitals either performing or claiming to perform, organ transplantation.[241] These various indications and estimates, and the explanation for any differences, appear on pages 16-19 of the Update.[242]

352. As well as numbers of hospitals, it is also necessary to look at the number of beds within hospitals available for transplant patients and at the number of staff with transplant training dedicated to such care. A hospital claiming to do transplants may only have done one operation or have one dedicated bed.

353. The Tribunal has considered whether individual hospitals might have had reason to inflate or deflate their reported activity. It may be in the interests of the hospital to exaggerate experience for commercial reasons as part of a marketing exercise, or to please higher authorities with a policy of expanding transplantation.

The Rapid Expansion of Transplant Facilities

354. Following a change in PRC policy on 23 March 2012,[243] there was a huge expansion in hospitals apparently devoted to making transplantation a key part of their growth strategies. Many medical facilities, including hospitals, are run and staffed by military and police authorities, and both were required to be commercially viable and this too may have been a stimulus for expansion. The rate and scale of expansion are relevant because of an apparent mismatch between the availability of *voluntary* donors and the rapid growth in the number of transplants performed.

The Number of Transplants Performed

355. The Global Observatory on Donation and Transplantation publishes transplant numbers from official sources for countries around the world. Their data

---

[241]   Ibid p316
[242]   Ibid, pp16-19
[243]   Slaughter, *supra*, p263.

indicates that between 2004 and 2014 there was a steady worldwide growth in transplants of 2-3% per annum.[244]

356. Prior to this period, transplant numbers in China were reported to have increased from under 4,000 per annum in 1999 to 12,000 per annum in 2004 – an increase of 300% over five years.[245] But from 2004 to 2014, the official Chinese annual transplant volume (as reported in a number of sources) showed no further increase and remained about 10,000 per annum; a remarkably consistent figure given the simultaneous massive growth in transplant facilities, staff and infrastructural investment. In the absence of any publicly available hospital- or regional-level data from China, researchers have had to acquire relevant data in different ways.

357. The extensive investigations set out in the Update reveal that individual hospitals were reporting – on their websites, in newsletters, media reports, scientific papers *and* during a series of phone calls made by various investigators – significantly higher numbers of transplants than could possibly fit with any official figures. In addition, reported activity of individual surgeons also aggregates to more than the official figures published by the PRC.

358. When, in July 2007, the PRC's then Ministry of Health issued transplant permits to 146 hospitals (see paragraph 350 above), a prerequisite for receiving a permit was a minimum bed capacity. To qualify, hospitals needed 15 beds dedicated to liver transplants and 10 intensive care unit (ICU) beds. For kidney transplants it was also 15 and 10 respectively.

359. Based on these figures the Update provides an estimate of the total number of transplants in the PRC in any one year during that period. Assuming the 146 approved hospitals each had the minimum beds required for both liver and kidney transplants, the Update authors calculated a minimum of 5,775 beds in the PRC. They then assumed 100% bed utilisation and 12 transplantation procedures per bed per annum. The result is 69,300 transplant procedures per annum (5775 x 12). And, as explained above (paragraph 351above), the 2007 figure of 146 approved hospitals is probably a major understatement of the true number of hospitals, licensed or not, performing transplant operations.

---

[244] http://www.transplant-observatory.org/

[245] Appendix 2B, item 47 Doctors Against Forced Organ Harvesting 2019 report. (page 8)

360. Between 2010 and 2012, the People's Liberation Army No 309 Hospital transplant centre increased its number of beds dedicated to transplant patients from 316 to 393 (although at some point its website referred to only 330 beds). Nonetheless, even 316 beds and 12 procedures a year per bed would result in 5,767 transplants per annum on the same assumptions as above.

361. By 2011, the Southwest Hospital had expanded to 200 beds for transplant patients and the Xijing Hospital to 110 beds. A clear picture of the scale and professionalism of the Southwest Hospital and of the claims made by surgeons about the number of transplant operations they performed is shown in its own publicity material.[246]

362. It is not unreasonable to suggest, on the assumptions made, that a handful of hospitals could account for more than the approximately 10,000 transplants officially acknowledged by the PRC in 2016.

363. According to the Update, during this era individual hospitals reported performing more transplants than claimed by the PRC for the country as a whole. The range of evidence relating to individual hospital activity is too extensive to be included in the text of this Judgment, and the reader is referred to pages 14-279 of the Update. However, included below is a small sample of the evidence of hospital activity:

- In March 2013, transplant surgeon Huang Jiefu (currently chairman of the China National Organ Donation and Transplantation Committee – and frequent spokesperson for the Chinese transplant community) told the Guangzhou daily: 'Last year (2012) I did over 500 liver transplants.'[247]
- On 14 March 2013, the Guanzhou daily reported that the First Affiliated Hospital of Sun Yat-Sen University had carried out 19 transplants in one day.[248]
- On or around the 31 January 2013, the Quzhoo Evening News reported that Zheng Shusen had performed a total of 1,104 liver transplants (over

---

[246] https://chinatribunal.com/wp-content/uploads/2020/02/WOIPFG_files_Southwest_GoogleTranslation.pdf – translated by Google Translate. The original is at https://chinatribunal.com/wp-content/uploads/2020/02/WOIPFG-files-Southwest-original.pdf

[247] Appendix 2A, Witness 29 Magnitsky Act https://chinatribunal.com/wp-content/uploads/2019/06/MagnitskySubmission_OfficialsSurgeons_Final.pdf paragraph 42

[248] Appendix 2A, Witness 30, Evidence 7(3)

what period is not clear), but by September 2015 the number had risen to 1,400 and by February 2016, to nearly 2,000.[249] (So during the five months between the latter two dates, 600 transplants were carried out by this one surgeon, representing approximately 6% of the total official number of 10,000 transplants carried out in China for 2015-16.)[250]

- The People's Liberation Army Hospital No 309 employs several leading doctors who claim to have carried out in excess of 5,000 procedures between them.[251]
- Liu Dong of Guandong No 2 Provincial People's Hospital claims to have performed over 2,000 liver and kidney transplants.[252]
- In September 2013, Zhu Jiye, Director of the Organ Transplant Institute of Peking University issued a statement: 'Our hospital conducted 4,000 liver and kidney transplants within a particular year'. (This represents 33% of the total peak of 12,000 transplants acknowledged by the state authorities in that year.)[253]

364. The number of licensed, and unlicensed, hospitals performing transplant operations, together with the prolific work of a small number of surgeons, leads to the conclusion that a very large number of transplants were, and are, carried out in the PRC each year. Kilgour, Matas and Gutmann's assertion in the Update of upwards of 60,000 and as many as 90,000 transplant operations per annum seems reasonable; this would be between approximately six to nine times the official figure claimed by the PRC. However, the exact number is not, and is unlikely to be, verifiable.

365. The director of the China Organ Transplant Response System (COTRS), Wang Haibo, suggested, in an interview in February 2017, that estimates in the order of 60,000 to 100,000 transplants per year were 'ridiculous', and 'more than the rest of the world put together'.[254] He argued that it was up to external investigators to 'prove' the numbers and not up to the PRC to prove

[249]   Appendix 2A, Witness 34 Profiles of Chinese Transplant Surgeons https://chinatribunal.com/wp-content/uploads/2019/06/12_SurgeonProfileOne_ZhengShusen.pdf p4

[250]   See Appendix 2B, item 44, Robertson *et al* pre print https://osf.io/preprints/socarxiv/zxgec/ p18

[251]   Bloody Harvest/The Slaughter an update, *supra.* p291

[252]   Ibid, p270

[253]   Ibid, p90

[254]   Appendix 4, item 10 https://www.youtube.com/watch?v=flhSY0evT0o

the veracity of its transplant figures. He made his argument on the basis that there were only 169 hospitals doing transplants in the PRC compared with 300 hospitals (his number) performing transplants in the US. On that basis, he said, the US should be performing 120,000 transplants a year. – which it is not. Wang's assertion would be correct, of course, if the USA were forcibly extracting organs, in which case 120,000 per annum would be perfectly plausible – but it is not.

Donor Numbers and Origin

366.   In the early days of transplantation in China, organs were thought, and said, to be obtained solely from executed prisoners.[255] The numbers of donors at that time could only be derived from the number of transplants reported, which should have been limited to the number of executed prisoners whose organs were useable for transplantation (there is some evidence that prisoners awaiting death by execution might often have organs affected by lifestyles of drug and alcohol abuse, or by general ill health, which reduced their viability for transplantation). Over time, international pressure appears to have resulted in a reduction in the use of organs from death-row prisoners, but the number of transplants continued to rise.[256]

367.   China did not have a deceased organ donation system in the conventional sense until 2010 and this existed only as a pilot programme until 2014. During this period, the number of kidney transplants and liver transplants performed continued to grow, rising from 66 in 2010 to 7,081 in 2015, according to figures extracted from the COTRS 2017 data.[257] There is no satisfactory official explanation of where the donor organs came from since the voluntary donation system was only at a pilot stage for much of that period.

368.   In September 2013, a formal voluntary donation scheme was established under the governance of COTRS.[258] By 2017, the declared number of registered donors in the PRC was 375,000.

---

[255]   Appendix 2B, item 31, The Impact of Use of Organs, J Lavee p2. See also Appendix 1A, Witness 26

[256]   https://duihua.org/china-executed-2400-people-in-2013-dui-hua-2/ and Robertson *supra*, at paragraphs 5&6

[257]   Robertson, *supra*, page 18

[258]   Chin Med J (Engl). 2016 Aug 20; 129(16): 1891–1893

369. In any country, for every 1,000 registered donors there will, in any one year, be a number – call it x – who will die and whose organs will be useable for transplantation – known as 'eligible donors'. The ratio, or conversion rate, of registered donors to eligible donors in any year ie the ratio of 1,000 to x in the hypothetical example – is likely to be reasonably standard across many countries, there being no reason for wildly atypical ratios.

Yet, in 2017, the 375,000 donors in the PRC resulted in 5,146 eligible donors (See Appendix 2B, item 44 (Robertson et al -Analysis of Official Deceased Organ Donation p7)) (ie at least 5,146 transplants, see paragraph 341). This is a conversion rate of 1.4% – 140 times greater than that of the US where, in the same year, 140 million registered donors resulted in 10,824 transplants – a conversion rate of 0.008%.

370. Doctors Against Forced Organ Harvesting (DAFOH), a voluntary cross-border network of medical professionals, monitored the register of voluntary organ donors in the PRC for 18 months from 2014-2016. In the course of its monitoring, DAFOH discovered a significant discrepancy between voluntary organ donor numbers and organ transplant volumes[259].

371. DAFOH discovered that 25,000 registered organ donors were added to the organ donor registry on a single day in December 2015. Such a sudden large increase seems to the Tribunal to be implausible. The sharp increase in numbers suggests data manipulation. DAFOH has provided a chart that demonstrates the anomalous rise in the organ donor numbers in the registry[260].

372. The mismatch between the number of transplants performed each year in the PRC and the number of registered donors is substantial. There are more transplants than could possibly come from the pool of registered donors. Clearly some transplants (of one kidney or a lobe of liver, for example) may have used live donors, but the mismatch in numbers cannot possibly be explained by this factor alone. Given that the PRC asserts that it no longer

---

[259]   Appendix 2B, Item 47 https://chinatribunal.com/wp-content/uploads/2019/04/April_2019-DAFOH-Report-on-Forced-Organ-Harvesting-in-China.pdf pp17-21, Doctors Against Forced Organ Harvesting

[260]   Appendix 2A, Canada Magnitsky Act Submission, paragraph 64,
DAFOH's Chart: https://dafoh.org/wp-content/uploads/Registered-organ-donors-in-China-2015-2016.jpg.

uses the organs of executed prisoners for transplants, the very substantial mismatch is wholly unexplained and demands justification.

Important issues are therefore raised:

373. Are official transplant numbers in China credible, audited and traceable back to individual hospitals as they are in the rest of the world? The Tribunal can find no evidence of this in the public domain.

374. Are the transplant numbers estimated in the Update as a result of triangulating data from individual hospitals and other sources credible, audited and traceable? The calls have been recorded, the website pages stored, and the papers published. The authors have chosen not to define *absolute* numbers, but to describe a range of potential numbers from conservative to more 'generous' upper limits, in order to take into account a degree of over- or under-reporting. The Tribunal finds this approach rational; the evidence and analysis is viewable in the Update.

375. China is a large country of around 1.4 billion inhabitants. It has a declared policy of expanding transplantation – a policy of potential public good.[261] Given that policy, together with the expansion of transplant facilities in number and size and the evidence that non-licensed hospitals are also performing transplants, it would be expected that transplant numbers would be large and rising.

376. These data once again lead to the question, where do the donor organs come from? Ethical transplant practice requires an open and honest audit trail of donor origin, not only for general statistics and system management, but also to ensure that any issues which arise relating to a transplanted organ (for example, malignancy) may be studied and prevented in the future. Evidence suggests that no such audit trail exists in China for the vast majority of transplants.

Short Waiting Times for Transplantation

377. Transplantation is not like elective surgery. One cannot 'book' most transplants unless the organ is coming from a live donor. With transplantation

---

[261]   Since 2000 China has prioritized organ transplantation in its national strategy See Appendix 2A, Witness 36 (China organ Harvest Research Centre report Nov 28 2108, p3

from deceased donors, the transplant can only go ahead when the team managing the recipient are made aware of a suitable donor. Patients have to wait. When a patient is put on the waiting list in the UK, they are likely to receive information indicating an estimate of how long they might wait, based on data shown publicly on the NHSBT website. The waiting times can only be estimates. Several hundred people die waiting each year. By contrast, many of the waiting times for transplantation reported from China to the Tribunal have been incredibly short.

378.	Even in countries with long-established and well publicised transplant programmes, there are always more people needing a transplant than available donors. With voluntary donation systems, where organs come from people who die having previously given consent for their organs to be transplanted at death or whose relatives give consent when death is inevitable, the mismatch between supply and demand generates waiting lists. The waiting lists are usually stored electronically and include relevant data of demographics, organ size, ABO blood type and tissue typing. Similar data are stored relating to voluntary donors, and this enables matching of donor to recipient after the death of a registered donor.

379.	In general terms, waiting times for organs can be months or years. For example, the average waiting time for a liver transplant in the UK is 135 days for adults, while for children it is 73 days.[262] For kidneys, the average wait is 2.5 to 3 years.[263] For hearts, the wait is described as months or years[264] and for lungs the wait is even longer.[265]

380.	The Tribunal has been presented with evidence of waiting times in the PRC that are much shorter than is usual in the rest of the world. Telephone call evidence reveals[266] that in the PRC waiting times as short as a few days are being offered to potential recipients willing to pay for organs. Dr Lavee's account of a patient being offered a transplant within two weeks is dealt with above in paragraph 23 and in more detail in Oral evidence on 8th December

---

[262]	https://www.nhs.uk/conditions/liver-transplant/waiting-list/

[263]	https://www.nhs.uk/conditions/kidney-transplant/waiting-list/

[264]	https://www.nhs.uk/conditions/heart-transplant/waiting-list/

[265]	https://www.thelancet.com/pdfs/journals/lanres/PIIS2213-2600(18)30380-1.pdf

[266]	See generally Appendix 2A, Witness 29 and Witness 30

2018.[267] Journalist Yukiharu Takahashi's account of organs being available on two weeks' notice is dealt with in paragraph 190.[268]

381. Another account comes from a witness who visited the Tianjin First Central Hospital in 2001, and was told by a nurse that organs were generally available in two weeks[269]. Further examples include evidence from WOIPFG (World Organization to Investigate the Persecution of Falun Gong) of interviews revealing short waiting times, including, as a particular example, a conversation with Wang Jianli of the Beijing Armed Police General Hospital indicating that 'a surgery can be arranged within one or two weeks'.[270]

382. Such waiting times are not compatible with conventional transplant practice and cannot be explained by good fortune. Predetermining the availability of an organ for transplant is impossible in any system depending on voluntary organ donation. Such short-time availability could only occur if there was a bank of potential living donors who could be sacrificed to order. If a single kidney, part of a liver or lung were to be used for transplantation then the death of the donor is not inevitable or planned. For a heart, a whole liver, lungs etc to be transplanted the donor must die.

Evidence Relating to Huang Jiefu

383. There have been many PRC doctors who have been involved in transplantation surgery. If the suggestions about forced organ harvesting from prisoners (whether or not prisoners of conscience) are correct then the mindsets in those doctors may be hard for citizens – including doctors – of other countries to understand. One doctor who features prominently in the material considered by the Tribunal is Huang Jiefu. He cannot stand for – or as in any way representative of – all doctors involved in transplant operations in the PRC. However, some detail of his double involvement – in surgery *and* in suppression of Falun Gong practitioners – provides a shaft of light that the Tribunal found illuminating, as a part of the background.

---

[267]   Appendix 2A, 31
[268]   Appendix 2A, Witness 43
[269]   Appendix 2A, Witness 30 Evidence 18
[270]   Appendix 2A, Witness 30 Evidence 19

384. Huang Jiefu's relevant history is covered in a Canadian Magnitsky Act[271] Submission by ETAC of March 2018.[272] 'Magnitsky' statutes, first used in the United States, exist in several countries and allow for financial sanctioning of human rights abusers from other countries. The Canadian government has not yet accepted the Canadian Submission but the Tribunal sees no reason to doubt its accuracy. It shows Huang to have been a pioneer of organ transplant techniques in the PRC since 1993. However he is said by some to be more than just a doctor. In 1999, he was reported to have led the party committee in the Sun Yat-sen University studying anti-Falun Gong literature. In May 2001, he was recorded as saying 'the struggle against Falun Gong is a serious political campaign. We must have no mercy towards the few active members.'

385. In September 2005, Huang ordered two spare livers of the required blood type from Guangzhou and Chongqing to do a demonstration transplantation operation in Xinjiang province.[273] The inference drawn by some, is that two people were killed to order so that 'back up' livers –which were never used –were available for his demonstration.[274]

---

[271]   The first Magnitsky Act was introduced in the United States in 2012. Its scope has been expanded to cover corrupt officials and human rights violators. Similar acts had been adopted in the EU, Canada, UK, Australia and many other European countries. See footnote 96

[272]   Appendix 2B, item 29 Magnitsky Act pp29-47.

[273]   Bloody Harvest/The Slaughter: An Update, p271 https://endtransplantabuse. org/wp-content/uploads/2017/05/Bloody_Harvest-The_Slaughter-2016-Update-V3-and-Addendum-20170430.pdf

[274]   Matthew Robertson in 'Organ Procurement and Extrajudicial Execution in China: A Review of the Evidence' – see footnote 226 below – explained that on his trip to Xinjiang Huang Jiefu travelled with Luo Gan, the Communist Party's security chief at the time; they were there for the 50th anniversary of the regime's annexation of the northwest border region. The two additional 'back-up' livers were obtained within 24 hours, after making a telephone call to the Third Military Medical University's First Affiliated Hospital in Chongqing. This extraordinary sequence of events — inconceivable in any Western medical context — is documented in four official Chinese publications. See: Sun, "25小时两例肝移植手术创纪录 [A Record Two Liver Transplant Surgeries in 25 Hours]."; Pan and Ye, "我国首例自体肝移植手术在新疆获得成功 [China's First Autologous Liver Transplant Is Successful in Xinjiang]."; "中国人体器官买卖的黑幕 [China's Organ Trade Secret]."; Xue, "卫生部副部长主刀, 我国首例自体肝移植手术在新疆获得成功 [With Deputy Health Minister Wielding the Knife, China's First Autologous Liver Surgery in Successful in Xinjiang]."

386. Huang claimed personally to have performed 500 liver transplant operations in the year 2012.[275]

387. In 2012, the Lancet medical journal published an article of which Huang was the first author, that said, *'China is the only country in the world that systematically uses organs from executed prisoners. ... About 10,000 transplant operations are performed each year in China, among which 65 per cent are organs from cadavers, and 90 per cent of which are executed prisoners.'*[276]

388. In the face of mounting pressure against questionable organ transplant practices in China, at the end of 2014 Huang announced that China would only use voluntary donations for organ transplants.[277]

389. In a revealing interview in 2015, Huang explained that Zhou Yongkang was the 'big tiger' and that it was 'clear where executed prisoners' organs came from'; Zhou Yongkang was the head of the central group dealing with Falun Gong issues and at centre of persecution of Falun Gong practitioners.

Veracity of Official Chinese Transplant Data

390. From the 1 September 2013, COTRS (China Organ Transplant Response System) was mandated by the Chinese National Organ Donation and Transplantation Committee to record data on allocation of all organs, no matter what the source, and to create relevant organ registries[278].

391. The PRC has asserted that from the 1 January 2015 all organ donations were sourced from voluntary donors. Huang Jiefu stated in public on 11 March 2015 that ending the use of death penalty prisoners for transplantation and establishing a comprehensive and transparent voluntary organ donation

---

[275] An Update, p324 https://endtransplantabuse.org/wp-content/uploads/2017/05/Bloody_Harvest-The_Slaughter-2016-Update-V3-and-Addendum-20170430.pdf

[276] Huang, Jiefu et al., 'A pilot programme of organ donation after cardiac death in China' *The Lancet*, Vol.379, Issue 9818 (2012), pp 862-865. http://www.thelancet.com/journals/lancet/article/PIIS0140-6736(11)61086-6/abstract

[277] See http://www.chinadaily.com.cn/china/2014-12/04/content_19025683.htm

[278] Chin Med J (Engl). 2016 Aug 20; 129(16): 1891–189

system amounted to 'saying farewell to the undignified past, we are starting a new hopeful chapter in the organ transplantation cause'.[279]

392. In 2017 the PRC said it had approximately 375,000 registered organ donors, which in the same year yielded 5,146 'eligible' organ donors (see also paragraph 369).

393. In addition, the Red Cross of China manages the China Organ Donation Administrative Centre which also publishes transplant data. These data come from the same source as COTRS data accumulated from local Red Cross branches. Therefore, the data published by the Central Red Cross and COTRS should be identical. The integrity of these data depends on such cross-correlation.

394. According to COTRS data (which was welcomed internationally) between 2010 to 2016 annual deceased voluntary donors went from 34 to 4,080, an increase of 12,000%; kidneys and livers transplanted went from 63 in 2010 to 10,481 in 2016, an increase of 16,636%.[280]

395. These data sets were analysed by Robertson *et al* in a paper published in January 2019.[281] Using a forensic statistical approach, the two central level datasets (Red Cross and COTRS) were assessed for evidence of manipulation. Features that would indicate that the data had been generated artificially by human manipulation included:

The COTRS data of the year-on-year increases of registered donors conformed to a simple quadratic equation, and this was mirrored by the Central Red Cross data, 'albeit imperfectly'. To quote Robertson *et al*: 'Contradictory, implausible, or anomalous data artefacts were found in five provincial datasets, suggesting that these data may have been manipulated to enforce conformity with central quotas.'

The 2017 and 2018 data from COTRS, when plotted against a simple quadratic equation, showed a remarkable, near perfect fit. The real-life likelihood of that being due to chance is remote, given the underlying contributors to the data; unpredictable patterns of death, transport issues, recipient matching, evolution of the system and several other factors.

---

[279]   http://www.china.org.cn/china/NPC_CPPCC_2015/2015-03/11/content_35021442.htm

[280]   Appendix 2A, Witness 44

[281]   Appendix 2B, item 44

Further, Robertson *et al* compared the COTRS data to those from 50 other countries and found no such fit with the same quadratic equation[282].

The authors suggested that their findings strongly implied that the official Chinese transplant data from COTRS had been manipulated by human hand to fit with the quadratic equation.

396.   The statistical arguments presented in the paper were so important and yet highly technical that the Tribunal felt it necessary to seek independent review of the Robertson *et al* paper, asking both about the appropriateness of the methods used and for comments on the likelihood of such a close fit to a simple quadratic equation.

397.   Professor Sir David Spiegelhalter FRS agreed that the methodology utilised by Robertson *et al* was appropriate. Spiegelhalter re-ran the regression analysis, and his results conformed exactly to those of Robertson *et al*. He also indicated that the chances of such a fit of data to a simple quadratic equation were 'remote'.[283]

398.   It is, therefore, reasonable to assume that some or all of the data provided by both COTRS and the Red Cross has been falsified.

399.   While the reasons for such data manipulation are not immediately obvious, the implications of such falsification are significant. Considerable effort has been expended by many international organisations to support the move to a voluntary donation system in the PRC after the announcement of a 'cessation' of the use of organs from executed prisoners. False data undermine trust at all levels – transplantation must be an open and ethical process to maintain that trust.

400.   The Tribunal is convinced by the arguments of Robertson *et al*, supported by the critical review of Spiegelhalter, that the COTRS data cannot be relied upon.

---

[282]   The authors used "*R-squared*" a statistical measure of how close the data are to the fitted regression line. See Appendix 2A, Witness 44 for further explanation by Dr Hinde in his oral testimony at p127. This approach was supported by Prof Spiegelhalter in paragraph 5 of his written submission to the Tribunal

[283]   Appendix 2B, item 44 Prof Spiegelhalter's written evidence to the Tribunal

401. If the activity data can be manipulated in such a way, what can be accepted from data provided by the PRC authorities? In consequence of Spiegelhalter's independent verification of Robertson *et al*'s approach, the Tribunal considers it rational to accept more readily the evidence accumulated by various other means by Matas, Kilgour and Gutmann in their separate, and now updated, books.

402. The Tribunal is satisfied that, in most countries, waiting times for organs of all kinds for transplantation is at best months and often years. Waiting times in the PRC are as little as two weeks. The gulf in waiting times between those in other countries and those in the PRC is unexplained. Similarly unexplained is the massive growth of physical infrastructure – hospitals and dedicated hospital facilities – providing transplantation services, together with commensurate growth in numbers of personnel working in transplantations. This infrastructure development often started before the institution of any voluntary donor scheme in the PRC.

403. The Tribunal is convinced that official Chinese transplantation statistics have been falsified. The Tribunal, thus, disregards PRC 'data' and concludes that, at the time of the most recent estimates, very large numbers of transplant operations have been carried out in the PRC. The Tribunal assesses as credible numbers of operations being between 60,000 and 90,000 per annum. This, when compared to the number of eligible donors on the PRC's own figures in 2017 of 5,146, leaves an incomprehensible gap. To achieve the numbers of transplantations performed – before and since the year of most recent estimate – there must have existed another source or other sources of tissue-typed organs; this in turn shows that there must have existed a body of donors unidentified in PRC material.

Evidence and Arguments Favourable to the PRC

404. There has been little evidence available or provided to the tribunal that is favourable to the PRC. Simple denials over the years by the PRC do not assist.

Doctors and an Academic Speaking Favourably of the PRC

405. Three doctors and an academic have spoken favourably of PRC transplantation practices. These are:

Professor Jeremy Chapman
Professor Philip O'Connell
Professor Francis Delmonico

Campbell Fraser PhD (Griffiths University Senior Lecturer in Business and Asian Studies. Publicly describes Falun Gong as a 'cult')

406. At least two, Delmonico[284] and Chapman[285], have visited the PRC as a guest of the PRC and found nothing amiss.

407. However, none of the doctors or Fraser has provided any evidence – in the form of records they have reviewed or patients to whom they have spoken – to justify or properly to explain their support for the PRC's historic or present transplantation practices.

408. All of the doctors and Fraser were invited to participate in the Tribunal's proceedings – their participation would have greatly assisted the Tribunal in its work. They all declined the invitations.

409. Further, although each did contribute in person to a recent report by an Australian Government committee (see paragraph 425 *et seq.* below), a review of their contributions by ETAC, at the request of the Tribunal, reveals that they produced no hard evidence to support what they said and could be criticised for their methodology or their experience in transplant surgery.[286] Although the Tribunal is cautious about accepting criticism coming from ETAC (because ETAC created the Tribunal and has members clearly of firm views about forced organ harvesting) the Tribunal finds force in the criticism they make. Given the Tribunal's overall approach to analysing *evidence*, as the doctors' and Fraser's various assertions are revealed by the ETAC commentary, and in other ways, as having no evidential support, and as all declined to engage with the Tribunal in a way that might have helped, the

---

[284]   https://tpm-dti.com/dti-foundation-visits-china/

[285]   https://www.theepochtimes.com/international-transplant-leaders-failed-to-disclose-connection-to-china-research_2140130.html

[286]   https://endtransplantabuse.org/australian-parliamentary-report-compassion-not-commerce-an-inquiry-into-human-organ-trafficking-and-organ-transplant-tourism/ Appendix 4. Item 28 https://chinatribunal.com/submissions/response_-compassionnotcommerce_austgovtreport_rogers_matas_hughes/

Tribunal is unable to find anything actually favourable to the PRC in the various things they have said.

410.   The Tribunal has also sought comment from TTS (The Transplantation Society), an international body of transplant surgeons. Its response was that it had no reason to disbelieve the PRC official pronouncements on its organ transplant practices – pronouncements that, the society said, were not its function to investigate or verify. The Tribunal finds this position to be contrary to that stated on the TTS website, where its policy and ethics objectives include: to *'provide global leadership in the practice of human transplantation'* and to *'promote ethical standards for clinical care and scientific investigation'*.

411.   Representatives of both The Transplantation Society and the World Health Organisation have spoken out in support of recent changes in human transplant systems in the PRC, particularly the development of the COTRS (China Organ Transplant Response System, see above) and the voluntary donor scheme. They argue that changes are being made and external criticism is not warranted. They have supported a transition for the sourcing of organs from death-row prisoners and suggested that executed prisoners are no longer used. They appear to believe the official Chinese figures to justify this support (see above for criticism of these figures).

412.   The Tribunal notes that the World Health Organisation is a specialised agency of the UN concerned with global public health. It operates in a multilateral stakeholder environment and may well be susceptible to political realities. Its statements on this issue have largely depended on information provided by TTS.

413.   The optimism of TTS and the WHO that the PRC's unethical practices have ceased is not supported by the evidence presented to this Tribunal, in particular evidence of the mismatch between numbers of voluntary donors and numbers of transplant operations. Taking into account the absolute lack of credibility of the PRC's official transplant statistics, as revealed by Robertson *et al*[287], it is very difficult to support the position of these two authorities, which both make strong claims for the need for ethical practice in medicine. For example, in May 2010, at the 63rd World Health Assembly,

---

[287]   Appendix 2B, item 44 https://osf.io/preprints/socarxiv/zxgec/

the WHO adopted WHA63.22 on Human Tissue and Transplantation, which condemned the purchasing of body parts and called for transparent and ethical systems in organ donation centres.

Government Committees Failing to Find the Allegations Proved

414. No official government body has, to date, pronounced on the criminality of PRC organ transplant practices.

415. Some governments have acknowledged the grave nature of the allegations against the PRC and have considered the substantial body of available evidence with some serious intent. Others, however, including the UK government, have sought to dismiss the allegations without making a judgment based on consideration of known facts and evidence. None of the reports of governments has been backed by the quantity or variety of evidence considered by this Tribunal, and doubts as to whether forced organ harvesting has occurred are expressed by them without the support of any analysis of evidence or explanation of doubts that can be tested or valued.

416. Before turning to opinions expressed by the UK and Australian governments, the Tribunal notes three things. First, committees of Congress in the US will have intelligence as good as any other country about the PRC. Second, no national body – knowing, as the US, UK, Australia do, of the Tribunal's work – has approached the Tribunal to suggest that intelligence has played a part in their assessments of the accuracy, or otherwise, of the allegations about forced organ harvesting made over a long period of time (see also paragraphs 66 above and 420 and 433 below on the subject of information coming from national intelligence operations). Third, the US has been less willing to dismiss the allegations than have the UK and Australia. House resolution 343 of the 114th Congress (2015-2016) recorded its position thus:

> *Expressing concern regarding persistent and credible reports of systematic, state-sanctioned organ harvesting from non-consenting prisoners of conscience in the People's Republic of China, including from large numbers of Falun Gong practitioners and members of other religious and ethnic minority groups*

and went so far as to resolve that the House:

condemns the practice of state-sanctioned forced organ harvesting in the People's Republic of China;

calls on the Government of the People's Republic of China and Communist Party of China to immediately end the practice of organ harvesting from all prisoners of conscience;

demands an immediate end to the 17-year persecution of the Falun Gong spiritual practice by the Government of the People's Republic of China and the Communist Party of China, and the immediate release of all Falun Gong practitioners and other prisoners of conscience; and...

calls on the United States Department of State to conduct a more detailed analysis on state-sanctioned organ harvesting from non-consenting prisoners of conscience in the annual Human Rights Report, and report annually to Congress on the implementation of section 232 of the Department of State Authorization Act, Fiscal Year 2003 (8 U.S.C. 1182f), barring provision of visas to Chinese and other nationals engaged in coerced organ or bodily tissue transplantation.'

The UK Government

417. The UK government has regularly taken a different line from that of the US, as revealed by the following extracts from answers to questions in the House of Commons and the House of Lords, presented in reverse order of date (and with underscores for emphasis added):[288]

18 Mar 2019 | HL14259 Lord Ahmad of Wimbledon | Foreign and Commonwealth Office

...The British government fully supports the Declaration of Istanbul (May 2008), which encourages all countries to draw up legal and professional frameworks to govern organ donation and transplantation activities. As the Minister for Europe and the Americas said in a Westminster Hall debate in

---

[288]   https://researchbriefings.parliament.uk/ResearchBriefing/Summary/CDP-2019-0069

October 2016: "Although I do not doubt the need to maintain close scrutiny of organ transplant practices in China, <u>we believe that the evidence base is not sufficiently strong to substantiate claims about the systematic harvesting of organs from minority groups. Indeed, based on all the evidence available to us, we cannot conclude that this practice of 'organ harvesting' is definitely happening in China."</u> ... The World Health Organisation (WHO) collates global data on organ donations and works with China. The WHO view is that China is implementing an ethical, voluntary organ transplant system in accordance with international standards, although the WHO does have concerns about overall transparency. ... We have not discussed the role of Dr Jiefu Huang (sic) with the WHO. We will continue to review any new evidence that is presented to us.

25 Feb 2019 | 796 c2 Baroness Goldie

At the moment, <u>our analysis</u> remains that the evidence available is not sufficiently strong to substantiate claims that state-sanctioned, systematic organ harvesting is happening in China ...the World Health Organization's view is that China is implementing an ethical voluntary organ transplant system, in accordance with international standards, although it does have concerns about overall transparency.

25 Feb 2019 | HL13634 Lord Ahmad of Wimbledon | Foreign and Commonwealth Office

We have serious concerns about the human rights situation in Xinjiang and reports of the Chinese government's deepening crackdown; ... We are aware of media reports that some Uyghurs may have been subject to unwanted DNA tests. More broadly, we are aware of reports that allege a process of involuntary organ removal is taking place in China and that minority and religious groups are being specifically targeted. My officials attended the final day of the recent tribunal into organ harvesting allegations, chaired by Sir Geoffrey Nice, QC. We are aware of the preliminary findings and await the final outcome of the tribunal in spring with interest. <u>With the evidence currently available we cannot substantiate the claims that state-sanctioned organ harvesting is happening in China.</u>

21 Dec 2018 | HL12218 Lord Ahmad of Wimbledon | Foreign and Commonwealth Office

We are aware of reports that allege that a process of involuntary organ removal may be taking place in China. ... The WHO view is that China is implementing an ethical, voluntary organ transplant system in accordance with international standards, although the WHO does have concerns about overall transparency. We will continue to review available evidence on this issue, including the preliminary findings of the Independent Tribunal into Forced Organ Harvesting.

14 Nov 2018 | 188826 Mark Field | Foreign and Commonwealth Office

We are aware of reports that allege that a process of involuntary organ removal may be taking place in China, including suggestions that minority and religious groups are being specifically targeted. The British government fully supports the Declaration of Istanbul (May 2008), which encourages all countries to draw up legal and professional frameworks to govern organ donation and transplantation activities. Reports by authors such as Kilgour, Gutmann and Matas are important sources of information about China's organ transplant system. They rightly question the lack of transparency in China's organ transplant system, whilst acknowledging that it is very difficult to identify the source of those organs and verify the number of organ transplants conducted in China. However, we do not agree with the claims of systematic organ harvesting of prisoners of conscience, assessing that the evidence they present does not substantiate such a claim. The World Health Organisation (WHO) collates global data on organ donations and works with China. The WHO view is that China is implementing an ethical, voluntary organ transplant system in accordance with international standards, although the WHO does have concerns about overall transparency. We continue to review available evidence on this issue.

08 Nov 2018 | HL11100 Lord Ahmad of Wimbledon | Foreign and Commonwealth Office

We are aware of reports that allege ... the UK government fully supports the Declaration of Istanbul ... As the Foreign and Commonwealth Office Minister for Europe and the Americas, Sir Alan Duncan, stated in a Westminster Hall debate in October 2016: "Although I do not doubt the need to maintain close scrutiny of organ transplant practices in China, we believe that the evidence base is not sufficiently strong to substantiate claims about the systematic harvesting of organs from minority groups. Indeed, based on all the evidence available to us, we cannot conclude that this practice of 'organ harvesting' is definitely happening in China." ... The WHO view is that China is implementing an ethical, voluntary organ transplant system in accordance with international standards, although the WHO does have concerns about overall transparency. We continue to review any new evidence that is presented to us.

06 Nov 2018 | 185605 Mark Field | Foreign and Commonwealth Office

We consider the Kilgour, Gutmann and Matas reports to be important sources of information about China's organ transplant system. These reports rightly question the lack of transparency in China's organ transplant system, whilst acknowledging that it is very difficult to identify the source of those organs and verify the number of organ transplants conducted in China. <u>We do not agree with the claims of systematic organ harvesting of prisoners of conscience, assessing that the evidence they present does not substantiate such a claim.</u> ... The WHO view is that China is implementing an ethical, voluntary organ transplant system in accordance with international standards. ... We continue to review any new evidence that is presented to us.

05 Nov 2018 | 185636 Mark Field | Foreign and Commonwealth Office

We have serious concerns about the human rights situation in Xinjiang and reports of the Chinese government's deepening crackdown, including credible reports of re-education camps and widespread surveillance and restrictions targeted at ethnic minorities. We are aware of media reports that some Uyghurs may have been subject to unwanted DNA tests. The UK supports the statement of 26 October by the European External Action Service highlighting concerns about Xinjiang. I raised our concerns about Xinjiang with Vice-Minister Guo Yezhou during my visit to China on 22 July 2018. The Foreign Secretary, Rt Hon Jeremy Hunt MP, also raised our concerns about the region with Chinese State Councillor and Foreign Minister Wang Yi during his visit to China on 30 July 2018. The UK raised our concerns about Xinjiang in our Item 4 statement at the September UN Human Rights Council.

01 Nov 2018 | 185002 Mark Field | Foreign and Commonwealth Office

Similar to later entries

29 Oct 2018 | 183334 Matt Hancock | Department of Health and Social Care

The Human Tissue Act 2004 prohibits commercial dealings in human material for transplantation and makes it an offence to traffic organs. Clinical advice to United Kingdom patients is not to travel to less well-regulated countries to seek an organ transplant. It is thought that very few patients in the UK choose to do so but data on those who do is not available. The government has welcomed China's move to stop using organs harvested from executed prisoners from January 2015. The government continues to monitor the degree of implementation of this commitment and encourages China to make further progress in bringing transparency to their organ transplant process.

22 Oct 2018 | 180659 Mark Field | Foreign and Commonwealth Office
Similar to later entries. Ends: *'Indeed, based on all the evidence available to us, we cannot conclude that this practice of "organ harvesting" is definitely happening in China.'*

12 Sep 2018 | 170313 Mark Field | Foreign and Commonwealth Office
Similar to later entries

Contributions to House of Commons debates, one before and one after the interim judgment of this Tribunal, were delivered by two MPs:

4 March 2019, Fiona Bruce MP
That this House notes with concern, allegations of forced organ harvesting in China and associated reports of suppression, persecution, torture and mass arbitrary imprisonment faced by religious and ethnic minority groups including Tibetans, Christians, Uyghurs, and practitioners of the traditional Chinese meditation, Falun Gong, that includes allegations of forced live organ extraction; acknowledges the interim judgement of the ongoing China Tribunal, chaired by Sir Geoffrey Nice QC, that such reports are beyond reasonable doubt, that in China forced organ harvesting from prisoners of conscience has been practised for a substantial period of time involving a very substantial number of victims; notes that Italy, Spain, Israel and Taiwan have introduced legislation banning their citizens from participating in organ tourism, and the Canadian Senate and Parliament have also approved similar legislation; urges the UK government to prohibit UK citizens from travelling to China for the purpose of receiving organ transplants; and calls on the UK government to give urgent consideration to other measures it could take to hold China to account for this alleged practice and to condemn it in the highest possible terms.

12 December 2017, Jim Shannon MP
That this House calls on the government of the United Kingdom of Great Britain and Northern Ireland to condemn the persecution of Falun Gong and the crime of harvesting organs from Falun Gong practitioners and other prisoners of conscience in China.

418. The UK government's repeated – if somewhat formulaic – answers express firmly the view that the evidence available is insufficient to prove that forced organ harvesting has been, or is, taking place, although the government does acknowledge that the PRC certainly used to harvest organs from capital punishment prisoners. The Tribunal assumed that the government could not take the positions it has done without having made a careful analysis of the available material – and indeed on 25 February 2019 (see above) Baroness Goldie stated: 'At the moment, our analysis …' and on 6 and 14 November 2018, Foreign Office minister Mark Field referred to 'assessing'.

419. With this in mind Counsel to the Tribunal wrote to Mark Field requesting provision of the analysis or assessment that must exist, and invited him to attend the April hearings of the Tribunal and to be a witness – he was offered to the opportunity to be the very last witness – in order to review all the evidence available to the Tribunal and to comment on it. A representative of the Foreign Office attended for a part of the last day of hearings, but did not offer to contribute in any way to the evidence or analysis available to the Tribunal, or to speak. No analysis of the kind that certainly *should* exist has been provided, and the answers to questions in both Houses of Parliament do nothing to explain the government's position apart from its placing some reliance on the WHO.

420. The Tribunal is left in the position of having to doubt whether any rigorous analysis of the material available on forced organ harvesting exists; if it did exist there can have been no good reason not to provide it to the Tribunal unless it contained intelligence material. As explained above, that seems improbable. Before the April Tribunal hearings there was an exchange of emails, following a Westminster Hall debate at which Field's position was unaltered. Immediately after the hearings there was an exchange of emails referred to in Paragraph 24 (footnote 39) above, which in no way supported any assumption that the government had done a proper analysis; if anything the reverse.

421. Although UK government statements may be superficially in favour of the PRC in respect of its organ harvesting practices, the Tribunal is left convinced that those statements are of no value to its work: they are not evidence; they identify no evidence; and they provide nothing by way of analysis.

The Government of Australia

422. The government of Australia published a report, in November 2018, of the Australia House of Representatives Joint Standing Committee on Foreign Affairs, Defence and Trade, Human Rights Sub-Committee (the Sub-Committee) titled Compassion, Not Commerce: An Inquiry Into Human Organ Trafficking And Organ Transplant Tourism.[289] This is the most recent of reports by any government into the allegations of forced organ harvesting and needs special and specific attention as it contains the nearest to a statement of position by PRC. In view of the PRC's failure to engage with the Tribunal or to counter any of the evidence, the Tribunal felt it important to give maximum attention to such defence as the PRC may have given to the Australian Sub-Committee.

423. In its conclusions, Compassion, Not Commerce was agnostic on the issue being dealt with by this Tribunal – see paragraph 425 below (Compassion not Commerce 2.81). It may be worth noting that the report had a very broad human rights focus. This may have allowed the forced organ harvesting issue to be 'diluted' to some extent within more general concerns about organ trafficking and transplant tourism.

424. The Tribunal asked ETAC to provide a response to the parts of the report that were of relevance to the tasks of the Tribunal. The Tribunal recognised that there might be comment on its turning to ETAC for this response.[290] However

---

[289] https://chinatribunal.com/wp-content/uploads/2020/02/CompassionNotCommerce_AnInquiryintoHumanOrganTraffickingOrganTransplantTourism_HumanRightsSub-Committee_AustralianGovttReport.pdf

[290] Since delivery of the Summary Judgment on 17 June 2019 there has been some criticism of the Tribunal having been created by ETAC. The criticism, for whatever purpose made, fails to understand the realities of the world where government and international bodies fail to do all the tasks that might be expected of them and, more generally, how allegations of crime are normally investigated and judged. Who else apart from a body like ETAC will act to establish a People's Tribunal when one is required? Maybe dispassionate NGO's – themselves often seen nowadays as part of the globalised establishment and thus subject to political agendas and pressures. Who could ever be expected to seek a resolution to the unanswered question dealt with by the Tribunal, but an organisation concerned about the question? Who chased Nazis for crimes against the Jews but Jewish organisations? Who, in a regular national criminal prosecution, perform inquiries and analyses of evidence but the very prosecution authority that is pursuing the allegation? So, the

ETAC is, without doubt, the body with best access to information and rationale for its inclusion experts in the area of interest and, notwithstanding the need to maintain separation and distance from ETAC, there was no reason to doubt the integrity of their work. Integrity, it should be noted, is not to be equated with accuracy of any conclusions ETAC reached. The Tribunal made its decisions on the basis of all evidence received, not on the basis of any ETAC conclusions (see above paragraphs 70 and 73).

425. ETAC's full response is available at https://chinatribunal.com[291] It is presented exactly as first provided to the Tribunal, there having been no to-and-fro of questions for clarification. Its authors are Susie Hughes (Executive Director of ETAC), David Matas and Wendy Rogers. Extracts from the Compassion Not Commerce report and from ETAC's responses that the Tribunal found of value are set out below, by reference to paragraph numbers of the report, but, to avoid confusion, without the report's footnotes, which the Tribunal has considered and can be found in the full report. Comments by the Tribunal are made by way of footnotes to this Judgment and a general review of the report and ETAC's responses is given in paragraphs 427-433.

Compassion Not Commerce, 2.11
Professor Jeremy Chapman AC, noted renal physician and Past-President of the Transplantation Society, told the Sub-Committee: ...countries where commercial transplantation is occurring [include] Egypt, Turkey, Pakistan, possibly Lebanon, India, Sri Lanka, possibly Singapore, Cambodia, Vietnam, Laos, China, Mexico and Venezuela ... they are mostly typified by having high inequality scores, by having low economic human development indicators and by having a large source of impoverished individuals on whom to prey for donors.

ETAC response
In our view, the nature of organ procurement in China is unique in that it involves State-sanctioned, large-scale killing of prisoners of conscience for their organs. We are not aware of commercial transplantation involving the systematic murder of individuals for their organs occurring in any country

---

criticism is misplaced. The Tribunal has preserved arm's length relations with ETAC and been alive to the need for caution in assessing any materials coming directly from ETAC; in this case, and for good reason, at the specific request of the Tribunal

[291]   Appendix 4, item 28

other than China. There is likely to also be a black market in commercial transplantations with live donors (kidneys) in China but we do not have information on that as it is a separate issue to the killing of prisoners of conscience for their organs. We note that in Prof Chapman's full testimony of 9 May 2017 to the Senate Inquiry, he states that his information about commercial transplantations was obtained at the 2017 meeting at the Pontifical Academy of the Sciences (PAS) on global organ trafficking. Huang Jiefu and Wang Haibo represented China at that meeting. At the time, ETAC contacted the PAS with concerns regarding the potential lack of transparency about China given Huang's longstanding involvement in transplantation in China and his own history of ordering spare livers (Rogers et al 2017) and requested that additional speakers be permitted. These concerns were dismissed, and the request denied (correspondence available on request).

Compassion Not Commerce, 2.16
The majority of countries in which organ trafficking is a growing problem appear to lack a properly established deceased organ donor system. (Dr) Campbell Fraser noted ......that one of the best methods to combat organ trafficking and transplant tourism is to develop [deceased organ donation systems].

ETAC response
.... most references to organ trafficking refer to black market sales from living vendors ... ... China lacked a deceased organ donation system of any sort until 2010 and had only a pilot program[me] until the end of 2014. ...... Since 2015, Chinese claims about voluntary donations are unverifiable and research suggests that the figures publicly quoted about donation rates are at least in part fabricated (Robertson et al 2019), indicating that China continues to lack a properly established deceased donation scheme ...... (Dr) Fraser has been referred to in Chinese State media, western media and in academic forums as an international human organ trade expert. He appears however, to have published only one paper concerning organ trafficking in his academic career, despite his claim to have been researching this topic since 2008. His sole published paper focuses on the role of social media in labour and human organ trading. In the abstract, the author refers to interviews with victims in 17 countries, but the list of countries is not provided, the methods are described in scanty detail (for example, there is no information as to how he contacted interviewees, or on his use of interpreters), and details of the necessary Australian human research ethics approval for this kind of

research are not provided. Given these omissions in his sole published paper, and the lack of other peer-reviewed and published accounts of his research, we have reservations about the extent and depth of (Dr) Fraser's claimed expertise.[292]

Compassion Not Commerce, 2.27
Other witnesses and submitters, such as Professor Chapman, (Dr) Campbell Fraser, and Dr Dominique Martin disputed these allegations as overstated and unsupported by the evidence available. The Sub-Committee also received evidence suggesting that China has undertaken a degree of reform towards the elimination of the use of the organs of executed prisoners. These matters are of ongoing debate amongst the international human rights community.

ETAC response
We note that the evidence referred to in footnote 49 [to paragraph 2.27] is a journal article authored by Huang Jiefu that contains assertions and proclamations of change, rather than evidence of ethical practice.

Compassion Not Commerce, 2.30
Professor Chapman disagreed that transplant infrastructure utilisation is a viable indicator, arguing that "you cannot invoke the same number of transplants as you would in an American hospital," based on transplant infrastructure alone. Professor Chapman also cited research and reporting from The Washington Post, which found that data compiled by healthcare information firm Quintiles IMS indicates that Chinese market demand for immunosuppressant drugs roughly reflects official transplant statistics.

ETAC Response
Prof Chapman claims that The Update erred in its estimates of transplant volumes as typically, in China, transplant recipient patients spend far longer in hospital than similar patients would in the USA or Australia. Prof Rogers clarified this statement in email correspondence with Prof Chapman as per her December 2018 witness statement to the Tribunal ("In that statement [13 June 2017] he [Chapman] says that the figure of 60,000-100,000 transplants per year (based on the research summarised in the Update) is a 'concoction'. On page 2 Prof Chapman provides details about the lengths of time that

---

[292]   see https://experts.griffith.edu.au/7759-campbell-fraser https://experts.griffith.edu.au/7759-campbell-fraser/publications

Chinese transplant patients spend in hospital, based upon which he concludes that if there were 60,000-100,000 transplants per year in China, there would need to be 30-40 times the amount of transplant infrastructure that there is in the US. His reasoning is hard to follow. I therefore sought clarification by email and was told that in China, patients stay in hospital for much longer than in the US or Australia – weeks compared to 4-6 days (Chapman, personal communication 6/6/2018, copy provided)[293]. This response indicates that Prof Chapman had failed to engage with the methodology in the Update and seemed unaware that in calculating the figure of 60,000-100,000 transplants per year, the authors allowed for a 4 week stay per person per transplant.").

I note here that Prof Chapman focuses on bed numbers and length of hospital admissions and does not acknowledge any of the other triangulating sources of information used in The Update. Specifically, where available, The Update used individual hospital posted figures [examples given[294]]. Prof Chapman also cites a Washington Post article that claims to prove that transplant volumes in China are far below the estimates in The Update and more aligned to official statements of transplant numbers, inter alia casting doubt on accounts of organ sourcing from murdered prisoners of conscience. The Washington Post article makes the claim that immunosuppressant drug sales data provided by the American medical data company Quintiles IMS supports the Chinese government's claims of transplant volumes. A number of academics raised concerns about relying solely upon the IMS data because of significant inaccuracies leading to unreliable conclusions. For example, using IMS data as an indicator of volume underestimates actual volume of transplants as the data take no account of either local production of immunosuppressant drugs sold in unofficial Chinese pharmacies or the low (by international standards) sales price of immunosuppressants in China. To illustrate the extent of these concerns, using the same method of estimating transplant volumes from immunosuppressant sales yields the clearly false conclusion that the number of transplants in Japan surpassed the number in China for several years. This letter and a full rebuttal of the Washington Post article are available on the ETAC website. In addition, David Matas presented an analysis of flaws in using IMS data to estimate transplant numbers at the

---

[293]   https://chinatribunal.com/wp-content/uploads/2020/03/InvitationsCorrespondence_withIndex_2020.pdf

[294]   Page 26 of The Update referencing endnote 52; page 63 referencing endnote 265; page 79 referencing endnotes 352 to 354; page 175 referencing endnote 855; and page 295 referencing endnote 1538

2016 TTS conference in Hong Kong in which he argues "It is frivolous to reject such a wide array of consistent cross-checked data [in The Update] by reliance on figures for share of global demand for anti-rejection drugs which in other countries produce nonsense figures for transplant volumes" (Matas 2016, https://endtransplantabuse.org/transplant-volumes-and-anti-rejection-drugs-by-david-matas-tts-madrid-2018/*).*

Compassion Not Commerce, 2.31
Dr Dominique Martin, Co-Chair of the Declaration of Istanbul Custodian Group, also doubted the validity of the use of transplant infrastructure as a basis for estimation, asserting: The methodology by which these large estimates have been derived simply does not add up. It is really a gross overestimate of any kind of transplant activity that has been taking place in China ...

ETAC response
Unfortunately, Dr Martin does not explain which aspects of the methodology of The Update she finds problematic. Here we note that The Update examined multiple data sources including:

Number of hospitals performing transplants (approved national military, civilian and regional; other types of transplant centres)

Number of transplant beds per hospital

Occupancy rates of transplant beds (individual hospital data, where available, plus estimates based on Chinese hospitalization times)

Building programmes for new transplant centres

Numbers of transplants per year per team/unit/centre/hospital (from multiple sources, e.g. hospital data including newsletters, reports by staff in the media etc)

Numbers of clinical transplant staff

Training capacity of teams/units/centres/hospitals

Research activities of transplant teams/units/centres/hospitals

Evidence of copious supply of organs (e.g. multiple transplants for the same patient; multiple simultaneous transplants; spare livers as back up for operation; short waiting times)

Growth in capacity for domestic production of immunosuppressive drugs

In the absence of further clarification from Dr Martin, we do not know which of these data sources she includes as "transplant infrastructure", whether she is aware of the full range of data sources underpinning the estimate of 60,000-100,000 transplants per year, or where she finds errors that she thinks result in a "gross overestimate" in The Update.[295]

Compassion Not Commerce, 2.36

The Submission of Doctors Against Forced Organ Harvesting highlighted transcripts of purported telephone conversations between Bloody Harvest researchers posing as prospective patients and staff at Chinese hospitals. In these alleged transcripts, the hospital staff appear to indicate that organs sourced from imprisoned Falun Dafa practitioners are available for transplantation. However, it is not possible to evaluate or confirm the authenticity of this material.

ETAC response

The DAFOH report only included two calls from 2006. Since that time there have been many more investigative calls, some of which have been submitted to the Tribunal by WOIPFG. The Subcommittee did not receive a submission from WOIPFG so have not seen these calls or questioned Dr Wang on them. Matthew Robertson is currently compiling a report for VOC evaluating the authenticity of the WOIPFG calls which we hope will be available before the Tribunal issues its final report.[296] *ETAC notes that the calls not only contain information on the source of the organs but also the short waiting times and payments made for organs.*

---

[295]   The Tribunal was struck, yet again, how those arguing against the propositions advanced over the years by ETAC and others, do so by unparticularised denials. The Tribunal would have liked to be able to 'weigh' the value of Dr Martin's observation but, in light of the ETAC response, cannot do so

[296]   Appendix 2B, item 44 – awaiting publication

The second call referred to in the DAFOH report was from the investigation Bloody Harvest (2006) with Dr Lu (Lu Guo Ping). After the report came out, Phoenix Television aired a documentary where Dr Lu was filmed talking about the recorded call. Lu Guo Ping acknowledges that he received the call and that he said what the transcript said he said, except for the part about Falun Gong. There is no indication in the Phoenix documentary that there is a recording. All the documentary suggests exists is a transcript. The documentary implies that David Matas and David Kilgour fiddled with the transcript. However, the fact that there is a recording means that the authors would have had seamlessly interwoven, in Dr Lu's own voice, the words that he admits having said and the words he denies having said. In 2006 this would not have been technically possible (we don't know if it's possible today). Moreover, the documentary states that all the calls in the Bloody Harvest investigation can be explained in this way. They could have said that the recorded responders were only saying that Falun Gong organs were available in order to promote the 'sale' and that these rogue promoters are being disciplined. (A common Communist form of deflection.) The fact this did not happen, in combination with the implausible alternative explanation given, supports the conclusion that the recipients of the calls (including Dr Lu) were originally answering truthfully. (The statements by Dr Lu in the Phoenix Television documentary can be viewed in the film Human Harvest.)[297]

Compassion Not Commerce, 2.41

(Dr) Fraser asserted his view that the apparent blood testing of imprisoned Falun Dafa practitioners may have been to support the detection of

---

[297] Appendix 3, item 46 Human Harvest. The Tribunal adopts with qualification the ETAC comment. The Tribunal heard a great deal of evidence about telephone calls. Phone calls were made by Dr. Wang (Appendix 2A, Witness 30 and Appendix 2A, Witness 42), Huang Wanqing (Appendix 1A, Witness 12), Xuezhen Bao (Appendix 1A, Witness 18), Yu Ming (Appendix 1A, Witness 22) and David Matas and David Kilgour in Bloody Harvest, *supra*, pp80-93. –

For call verifications see Appendix 4, item 32. It reached the conclusion at paragraphs340-341 above and paragraphs 455-456 below in its Conclusions about phone calls on a quantity and quality of evidence greater than, and different from, that heard by the Sub-Committee and has given careful consideration of the Sub-Committee's observation. The evidence about Lu Guo Ping is overwhelming as to dishonesty so far as he – admittedly only one individual – is concerned. The suggestion that Matas and Kilgour may have been party to the probably impossible task of corrupting the recording is rejected completely, not least because of the integrity the Tribunal found in these witnesses, an integrity that no other body – the Australian Sub-Committee or any other – has been willing to challenge in any articulated way.

communicable diseases, rather than for tissue typing to support organ matching for transplantation purposes. (Dr) Fraser stated: I asked [Falun Dafa practitioners], 'How much blood did you have removed?' they said they had two 10-millilitre vials of blood taken. I have consulted with my clinical colleagues, and we do not believe that two vials of blood is anything like what is required for testing for tissue typing, blood grouping and all the other tests that are required.

ETAC response

Prof Rogers provided evidence to the Senate Inquiry (13 June 2018) regarding the purpose and volume of blood taken from practitioners of Falun Gong while in detention. Contra (Dr) Fraser's assertions:

It is highly unlikely that blood was taken for the purpose of detecting communicable diseases as only FG practitioners were blood tested. If the blood testing were for infection control purposes, all prisoners would need to be tested in order for the programme to be effective. Multiple testimonies (eg in Gutmann's The Slaughter) independently and consistently report that FG practitioners were the only prisoners who were blood tested.

The assertion that the amount of blood taken is insufficient for tissue typing and other blood tests associated with organ transplant is incorrect. Prof Rogers verified this point with two separate transplant professionals, according to whom initial tests for tissue typing can be done on less than 10ml of blood (private communication, Australian transplant anesthetist and Israeli cardiac transplant surgeon). Once prisoners have been blood and tissue typed, this information can be stored and used for reverse matching to potential recipients, at which point, further testing for cross matching between individuals may be required. Thus, after initial testing for blood group, HLA antigens, infectious diseases etc, prisoners may then have been subject to further and multiple tests for specific cross-matching to potential recipients at later points in time.

We also note that during interviews that (Dr) Fraser conducted with Falun Gong practitioners in Sydney, several of the people he interviewed described organ scanning in conjunction with blood tests, but (Dr) Fraser failed to mention this relevant evidence in his 13 June statement.

Compassion Not Commerce, 2.44

In 2007, Dr Huang Jiefu, director of the China Organ Donation and Transplant Committee and then Vice-Minister of Health of the People's Republic of China, confirmed that the organs of executed prisoners were being used in organ transplants, but maintained that this was occurring on a *voluntary basis, saying ... most of the cadaveric organs come from executed prisoners. It should be clarified that, at present, the only prisoners who are subject to capital punishment in the PRC are convicted criminals. In addition, the relevant governmental authorities require that prisoners or their family provide informed consent for donation of organs after execution.*

ETAC response

... the 1984 law permitting removal of organs from executed prisoners remains on the books and does not require consent. Huang Jiefu uses the word "ban" quite freely. Mostly when he says something is banned, he is referring to Communist Party policy and not law. Even the law cannot be enforced against the Party. Claims of enforcement of law or policy are not independently verifiable.[298]

Compassion Not Commerce, 2.46

In December 2014, Dr Huang reportedly announced China would cease the use of organs sourced from executed prisoners from 1 January 2015. Dr Huang claimed this measure followed the establishment of a national digital organ matching and allocation system, the China Organ Transplant Response System (COTRS), in September 2013, as well as other initiatives to encourage voluntary deceased donation.

ETAC response

As noted above, there are many announcements of reform and claims about the move to a 100% volunteer donor system. However, these are impossible to verify in the absence of independent inspection of the claimed reforms, including access to the electronic system mentioned above. The existence of a national organ matching and allocation system (COTRS) does not provide any evidence about the source of the organs that are matched and allocated in that system. It is entirely possible that organs harvested from prisoners of conscience are entered into the system, alongside any organs procured from patients dying in hospitals who become donors. As per the testimony of Dr Shapiro (China

---

[298] The Tribunal was struck by the way that the features in Huang Jiefu's history that make him a witness to treat cautiously seem to have been completely overlooked by the Sub-Committee (see pages 51, 53 and 167 of the report). His publicly displayed ability to have two livers viable for transplantation but disposable as waste at his will, coupled with his public hostility to Falun Gong practitioners would ring alarm bells of concern as to credibility in any regular evidence-assessing body; but not, it seems, in the Australian Sub-Committee.

Tribunal, April hearing), there is no transparency about the source of organs, and even those who openly praise the alleged Chinese reforms are not willing to guarantee that all organs are procured from volunteers (testimony of Dr Shapiro, referring to his communication with Frances Delmonico).

Compassion Not Commerce, 2.47
(Dr) Campbell Fraser, Professor Philip O'Connell and Dr Dominique Martin all advised the Sub-Committee that to the best of their knowledge it would appear China is transitioning away from the use of the organs of executed prisoners. (Dr) Fraser observed: [China is] clearly moving towards an ethical, deceased donation model. There are still some isolated cases of executed prisoners' organs being used, but there is no evidence whatsoever that any of those organs are coming from prisoners of conscience.

ETAC response
Drs Fraser, O'Connell and Martin receive their information from Chinese organ transplantation specialists (notably Huang Jiefu and Wang Haibo) and (in the cases of Fraser and O'Connell) from visits to China as guests of the Chinese government. They have no information or evidence that is obtained independently or firsthand (rather than curated by and filtered through their Chinese hosts).[299] There may be a nascent scheme for obtaining organs from deceased patients, but the existence of such a scheme does not preclude the ongoing harvesting of organs from prisoners of conscience. Both sources of organs may be operating simultaneously, or each may be dominant in particular areas of China. Without accurate information we cannot know with any certainty. (Dr) Fraser has at no time presented research evidence in the public domain to support the assertions he makes here and elsewhere. We believe that China probably has a 'hybrid' system in place that incorporates several sources: (i) a small number of voluntary donations (secured at least in part through financial incentives to the family) (ii) criminal prisoners subject to the death penalty who have been redefined as 'citizens'; and (iii) and a large number of prisoners of conscience, primarily FG practitioners. It is our concern that Uyghurs are beginning to replace Falun Gong as sources of organs as the Falun Gong organ

---

[299]   The Tribunal accepts these comments as accurate and that they reduce, probably to nil, the value of Huang's and Wang's related accounts and the 'curated' and 'filtered' evidence. The Tribunal expresses no firm adoption of the remaining part of this comment by ETAC for which it has neither hard evidence nor any material to contradict the views of the authors of the response.

bank depletes. The Falun Gong population in indefinite arbitrary detention has been relatively stable since the early 2000s but is depleting secondary to widescale organ harvesting. We note that in the early years of transplantation in China, Uyghurs were not a viable source of organs nationwide because of the absence of a national organ distribution system. This is now in place, in partial evidence of which we have a photo of the VIP lane sign in the Kashgar Airport of Xinjiang giving priority to flights exporting organs from that area. The airport is near to Xinjiang mass arbitrary detention centres.

Compassion Not Commerce, 2.48

Professor O'Connell observed that China was moving away from the use of executed prisoners' organs in favour of deceased donation, "albeit with issues that we would say would be inappropriate in Australia and, I think, from a global ethical perspective are not appropriate." Dr Martin elaborated on these ethical concerns: "[China is] now offering financial incentives to families to agree to donation after death, which of course is preferable to executing people to take their organs but is not something that much of the international community would endorse".

ETAC response

As per our previous response, claims of reform made by these speakers simply repeat and amplify claims made by Chinese officials, and have not been independently verified by the speakers or anyone else. Frances Delmonico (past president of TTS) has stated under oath that it is not possible to access the military hospitals in China to ascertain sources of organs used in those facilities and was unable to offer assurances of ethical organ procurement to Dr Shapiro.

At the 2017 Pontifical Summit, Haibo Wang (sic) stressed the sheer impossibility of trying to fully control China's transplant activity since there are one million medical centres and three million licensed doctors operating in the country (as reported by New York Times Europe: Sparks Fly as Vatican Conference Challenges China on Organs. AP, Feb 7, 2017 https://www.scmp.com/news/china/policies-politics/article/2069050/ sparks-fly-vatican-conference-challenges-china-over

Further, in (Dr) Fraser's later testimony to the Senate Inquiry, he retreated somewhat from his earlier apparent certainty, stating:

'We are not in any way trying to say that our group has eradicated the problem of organ trafficking in China. We're also not saying that there are not prisoners of conscience in detention in China. We're not saying that at all. We accept a number of the testimonies that individuals have given about

certain human rights issues in China, and we're not trying to escape from that. We're also perfectly aware of the way the Chinese government will present facts. Some will call that propaganda. We have spent a lot of time trying to understand that there's going to be that element but, within that, we try and really hone down into what is really happening. We'll certainly never be able to know exactly everything that happens in China' (Fraser, 8 June 2018).

However, (Dr) Fraser provides no details as to how he and others 'try and really hone down into what is really happening' given that their only access to Chinese hospitals, transplant centres, medical personnel and transplant recipients is managed by their hosts and all communication is via interpreters or to those who speak English.

Regarding financial incentives to families of alleged voluntary donors, we refer the Tribunal to a report by DAFOH on this topic, which points out that such payments clearly violate principle 5 of the WHO Guiding Principles on organ transplantation and may also be in breach of Principles 6-8 (https:// dafoh.org/public-organ-donation-system-china-largely-depends-monetary-incentives-families-deceased-relatives/)

Compassion Not Commerce, 2.52

At the Pontifical Academy Summit (PAS) which was held by Holy See's Pontifical Academy of Sciences in 2016, Professor Huang [Huang Jiefu], professor and chairman of the China National Organ Donation and Transplantation Committee, presented data on China's new policy on prohibiting the use of organs from executed prisoners. According to a Xinhau news report, Professor Huang stated that: The total number of deceased donor liver and kidney transplant between 2010 and 2016 were 27,600 and China's Ministry of Health has submitted the detailed statistics to the Geneva-based World Health Organization (WHO) for public release. From the beginning of 2015, China imposed a total ban on the use of executed prisoners' organs for transplantation, Huang said, describing the process as "an arduous journey." "Rome is not built in one day, the same as for the forbidden city", he added. According to Huang, hundreds of foreigners used to come to China every year for transplant tourism before the Chinese government banned the practice in 2009. From 2007 to 2016, the Chinese authorities formed joint task forces and cracked down on 32 illegal intermediaries, investigated 18 medical institutions, prosecuted, convicted and imprisoned 174 people including 50 medical personnel, and eradicated 14 black market dens, Huang said, referring to the "Zero Tolerance" action to behaviours violating organ transplantation regulations and laws.

ETAC response

As per our response to 2.44 above, there is no way of independently verifying these claims, and both the legal status and practical reach of the "new policy" are unknown. There is, however, ongoing evidence of foreigners travelling to China for transplants (TV Chosun's Korean Documentary) indicating that the claimed ban on organ tourism has not been successful in eliminating this practice. China has not released for public scrutiny detailed statistics on donations and transplantations, contradicting Huang Jiefu's statement above. In addition, there is recent evidence that Chinese nationals are still receiving organs within extraordinarily short waiting times and Chinese transplant recipients have been recorded saying that the wait time depends on how much money you pay. Whilst we believe that international transplant tourism continues to China, large quantities of organs, probably the majority, are being provided to mainland Chinese.[300]

Compassion Not Commerce, 2.55

Citing data collated by participants of the Pontifical Academy of Sciences Summit on Organ Trafficking, however Professor Chapman observed however that the number of transplants being performed in China for foreigners has "collapsed" in recent years.

ETAC response

We agree that the number of foreigners receiving transplants in China may have decreased significantly since the mid-2000s when many hospitals openly advertised for international recipients. However, there are significant challenges in collecting data on recipients of extra-territorial transplants. In Australia and many other countries, there is no mandatory reporting of extra-territorial transplants, and no way for doctors who take up the ongoing care of patients who receive off-shore transplants of knowing the circumstances in which the transplant was received. In addition, given the illegality of organ sales to foreigners in all jurisdictions, there is a strong incentive for recipients to conceal the origin of their transplant to the extent possible. For these reasons, we believe it is impossible to know with any certainty how many foreigners continue to obtain transplants in China, especially as this is likely to be the only country where full liver transplants are available. ... ...Without seeing the data upon which Prof Chapman makes this assertion,

---

[300] The Tribunal accepts this comment and finds support from evidence it has heard in: Appendix 2B item 54 and Appendix 2A Witness 44

we are unable to provide further detail. The presentation at the Pontifical Summit on organ trafficking in China was made by Huang Jiefu and Haibo Wang (sic), and has been criticised for lack of detail: Huang conceded that "China is a big country, with 1.3 billion people, so sure, definitely, there is some violation of the law." He could not refer to any law or provision banning the use of prisoner organs (https://dafoh.org/chinas-participation-vatican-transplant-summit-draws-worldwide-concern-and-sharp-criticism/).

We note that in his evidence to the Senate Inquiry (Hansard 8 June 2018), Professor Coates (Honorary Secretary and President-elect, Transplantation Society of Australia and New Zealand; Director of Transplantation, Royal Adelaide Hospital; and Councillor, Declaration of Istanbul Custodian Group) discussed the lack of data collection on Australian residents who travel overseas for a transplant. Prof Coates reported preliminary results from a survey of transplant professionals that he is running which investigates this question in an anonymous manner. He found that many patients discuss this option with their transplant doctor, and that over 50% of the respondents to the survey (n = 175) had been involved with a case, which is a much higher figure (by a factor of 3-4) than reported in the official ANZDATA registry. He estimated that 20-30 Australians travel overseas each year for a transplant, that the majority of those travelling for transplants are born overseas rather than in Australia, the most common country of birth of those individuals is China, and China is the most common destination for Australian transplant tourists. We highlight this finding because Prof Coates makes the point that there is no comprehensive data on overseas transplants in Australia or many other countries, so assertions about the collapse of transplants for foreigners in China are not based on strong evidence. To date, this report has not been published.[301]

Compassion Not Commerce, 2.56

Dr Martin and Professor O'Connell both stated that China had significantly reduced its intake of transplant tourists, though not necessarily completely

---

[301] The Tribunal notes that the majority of this response is opinion – with which the Tribunal nether agrees nor disagrees – based on facts that it accepts, such as the non-provision of data by Chapman. It notes that the recurring failure to have access to material, from many sources but for which there should be no security concerns justifying secrecy, in the setting of a decade or more of public allegations, is hard to understand and inevitably inclines the Tribunal towards making judgments against the unsupported propositions advanced by, or in effect on behalf of, the PRC.

eliminated the practice. Professor O'Connell described it as having been restricted to a "trickle." Dr Martin described having received only "occasional reports."

ETAC response
See previous response.

Compassion Not Commerce, 2.57
(Dr) Fraser observed that, in the early 2000s, China was a preeminent destination for transplant tourism, noting that "the norm was, if there was a Malaysian patient who required a transplant, they would be officially and formally referred by their doctor to China." (Dr) Fraser indicated that "foreigners can no longer enter China for transplantation." (Dr) Fraser stated that several patients he had interviewed had been prevented from entering China. (Dr) Fraser indicated that it is predominantly Egypt which is now meeting the demand previously filled by China. This is apparently despite the fact that since 2010 it has been a criminal offence in Egypt to buy or sell an organ.

ETAC response
As noted previously, it is not possible to offer a detailed critique of (Dr) Fraser's claims as none of his research is in the public domain. Given his secrecy about his research methods, his results, his sources of funding for research and travel, and the lack of peer scrutiny of any of his claims, we do not accept them at face value.[302]

Compassion Not Commerce, 2.61
In June 2016, the House of Representatives of the United States Congress passed by unanimous consent House Resolution 343. The resolution condemned the practice of "state-sanctioned forced organ harvesting in China" and called on China to "end the practice of organ harvesting from prisoners of conscience." The resolution also called upon the United States Department of State to report annually to Congress on implementation of a

---

[302] The Tribunal could repeat some of its earlier observations but must note in particular that (Dr) Fraser, with others, declined to appear at the Tribunal for no known reason. It would have been clear to (Dr) Fraser that he would have been tested in evidence in ways to which he has not been subjected to date as to the various assertions he has made, always without supporting documentary or other primary evidence.

visa ban to be imposed on persons identified as directly involved with the coercive transplantation of human organs or bodily tissue.

ETAC response
This resolution was passed unanimously by the House, following close examination of The Update by US State Department China specialists. This indicates that these specialists found The Update collation of evidence to be credible.[303]

Compassion Not Commerce, 2.62
Mr Graham Fletcher, First Assistant Secretary, North Asia Division, of the Department of Foreign Affairs and Trade informed the Sub-Committee of the Australian government's position on the allegations that organs are forcibly taken from prisoners of conscience killed in China: ...we are aware of the statistics which allege that there are a very large number of transplants occurring in China, but we do not have any basis for accepting that those statistics are accurate ... we have conducted our own investigations both in China and elsewhere to seek to establish whether the claims made about organ harvesting from prisoners of conscience have any basis, and our conclusion is we have not found evidence that supports them ... we have no evidence that prisoners of conscience are being killed in China.

ETAC response
In the 28 March 2017 hearing, Mr Fletcher is asked for details about DFAT's investigations and the evidence that he might have to disprove claims of 60-100,000 transplants taking place per year. Mr Fletcher replied: "Information we have from Chinese media would say between 10,000 and 20,000. I cannot remember the exact number, but it is in the low thousands." He was then asked by Senator Ludlam: "And that is on the basis of central statistics or record keeping?" to which he replied: "No, that is just two Chinese media reports, one from a government newspaper and one from an economic magazine." (p.2). Mr Fletcher then dismisses figures derived from hospital websites by asserting "There are lots of numbers in China which are not reliable" before conceding that "I am not saying that one [Chinese media] is necessarily more accurate than the other [estimates based on hospital websites]. Information in China is very hard to verify" (p.2).

---

[303] See paragraphs 378 and 379 above

Mr Fletcher later states that the lack of named victims is further evidence that forced organ harvesting does not occur. His reasoning is however faulty, because it is not possible for those whose relatives have disappeared in Chinese detention centre to know whether they were killed for organ harvesting. There are lists of those who are known to have died in detention (for example, on Minghui) but without testimony from those perpetrating the crimes, the cause of those deaths is unknowable.[304]

Compassion Not Commerce, 2.63

Mr Fletcher indicated that the Department of Foreign Affairs and Trade has met with advocacy groups in relation to the allegations. Mr Fletcher added that the Australian government has expressed opposition to the use of the organs of executed prisoners with the Chinese government through the Australia-China human rights dialogue process. The Department has also specially raised allegations relating to the trafficking of organs of prisoners of conscience.

ETAC response

These allegations are raised in the Australia-China human rights dialogues, but, according to Mr Fletcher, are dismissed as "complete nonsense" by the Chinese participants (Senate Inquiry transcript, 8 June 2018, p 53). This dismissal is consistent with the longstanding denial of organ harvesting from prisoners of conscience by the Chinese government.

Compassion Not Commerce, 2.64

Mr Fletcher did not provide further detail on the nature of DFAT's [Department of Foreign Affairs and Trade] own investigations. Mr John Deller, Secretary of the Falun Dafa Association of Australia, drew an analogy to the United Nations Commission of Inquiry on Human Rights in the Democratic People's Republic of Korea. Mr Deller observed of the Hon Michael Kirby AC CMG, who led the Commission of Inquiry: He couldn't get into North Korea; he

---

[304] The Tribunal has viewed the video contributions of Mr Fletcher of the Australian Department of Foreign Affairs to the Sub-Committee and found his doubts about the credibility of the allegations and his assertion that no respectable human rights organisation had given the allegations credence, unreliable and an obvious overstatement. They were also impossible to integrate with his assertion that the Department had no capacity to conduct an independent inquiry. The Tribunal found Fletcher's assertion generally on behalf of his Department of there being insufficient evidence to support the allegations neither convincing nor persuasive.

couldn't get any of that information that we were talking about. He interviewed people who had been abused and tortured, and they gave testimony, and from that he formed a very clear picture and conclusion, which is widely accepted around the world.

ETAC response
See previous response[305]

Compassion Not Commerce, 2.68
(China's Response) On 2 October 2018, shortly before the completion of this report, the Sub-Committee received from the Embassy of the People's Republic of China a submission from the Chinese Organ Transplant Development Foundation. This submission provided a substantive statement of the Chinese government's official position in relation to human organ transplantation and organ donation. The submission states that the Chinese government has "a consistent and clear attitude towards human organ transplantation" and follows "internationally-acknowledged ethical principles of organ transplantation". The Foundation's submission contends that since the introduction in 2007 of the Regulation on Human Organ Transplantation (RHOT), China has developed a reformed human organ donation and transplantation system that "reflects China's identity, culture and governance of society, including donation system, procurement and allocation system, clinical transplant service, post- transplantation registry system and transplant service regulation system."

Compassion Not Commerce, 2.69
(China's Response) The Chinese Organ Transplant Development Foundation's submission identifies the adoption of the RHOT as the beginning of the "legalisation and standardisation" of organ donation and

---

[305] The Tribunal has been guided in its approach to its work by the UN Commission of Inquiry (COI) chaired by the Hon Michael Kirby who, for example, insisted on public hearings of evidence in a way that may not have been intuitively acceptable to the UN, as well as in his approach to evidence assessment generally, as set out in the statement by John Deller – for similarity of approach (see paragraph 425 – Compassion Not Commerce 2.64). In many ways the obdurate refusal by those invited to assist the Tribunal by giving evidence where sources would be exposed runs counter to the underlying principles of all Kirby's guidance to be found in his COI Report.

transplantation practice in China to ensure that the rights of both donors and recipients are protected. The submission also highlights the adoption in 2011 of "the Eighth Amendment to the Criminal Law of the People's Republic of China" which distinguishes organ donation with informed consent from organ trafficking and states that "whoever organises others to sell human organs shall be convicted and punished."

ETAC response

The Chinese Organ Transplant Development Foundation's submission refers to a regulation and a law that no doubt exists. However, a directly contrary law from 1984 allows organ sourcing from prisoners without consent. This 1984 instrument remains the law despite the new 2011 law. As well, since the Communist Party of China controls and directs the police, the investigators, the prosecutors, and the judges, the 2011 law is not applied against the Party or its institutions. It applies, occasionally, against black market marginal outliers who become too obvious, whose prosecutions can then be publicised as evidence that China is "cracking down" on organ trafficking.[306]

Compassion Not Commerce, 2.70

(China's Response) Further, the submission notes the work China has done in conjunction with international organisations around the world: such as WHO, The Transplantation Society (TTS) and the International Society for Donation and Procurement and international experts (including famous Australian organ transplant expert, former TTS president Philip O'Connell) have come to China to participate in and witness the establishment of [China's] human organ donation system.

ETAC response

This is an example of how Chinese officials use their interactions with WHO and TTS to prop up claims of reform. The unjustified TTS and WHO whitewashing of the situation in China impedes progress towards actual reform and real consistency with international standards. The stance of TTS is in fact contradictory, as on the one hand officials such as Prof Delmonico state that TTS is unable to perform inspections and that such inspections are

---

[306]   The Tribunal has been able to check the accuracy of the statement about the 1984 instrument but has not been able to confirm the ETAC comment on the 2011 law being used against the party – see *Robertson et al*, Appendix 2A, Witness 44

not its responsibility, while at the same time, TTS supports Chinese claims of reforms (despite acknowledging that they are unable to verify any evidence of the claimed reforms). This position is incoherent.

Setting aside the sources of organs, China is in obvious breach of other international ethical standards, which again are largely ignored by TTS and WHO. For example, China has no laws, guidelines or compulsory confirmatory tests to determine death although this breaches the Declaration of Istanbul's (DoI) Principle 5 'Each country or jurisdiction should develop and implement legislation and regulations to govern the recovery of organs from deceased and living donors and the practice of transplantation, consistent with international standards.'

Compassion Not Commerce, 2.71
(China's Response) The Foundation's submission strongly emphasises voluntary, informed consent as a key principle underlying China's reformed organ donation and transplantation system, noting that Chinese citizens have the right to donate, or indeed to not donate, their organs: Any organization or individual shall not make others donate their organs by coercion, deception or temptation. Organ donors should have full capacity for civil conduct and written consent is required for organ donation. Donors who already gave consent have the right to withdraw. If a citizen has refused to donate their organs, any organisation or individual shall not donate or procure their organs. If a citizen has not refused to donate, their organ can be donated after their death with the joint written consent of their spouse, children over the age of 18 and parents.

ETAC response
Many of China's "altruistic organ donations" come from hospitals that employ social workers to convince relatives to allow organ procurement from their ICU [intensive care unit] -bound dying relatives by offering significant monetary incentives to cover inflated hospitals expenses.[307] This

---

[307]   The Tribunal is less impressed by ETAC's response on this issue about 'altruistic organ donations' than by the stark fact that the PRC's submission, presented late in the day – October 2018 – to the Australian Sub-Committee was in writing, without oral evidence in support and provided no documentary or other proof of its assertions despite years of international controversy and the Sub-Committee itself having taken evidence concerning forced organ harvesting since March 2017. In regard to the ETAC comment about financial incentives, see Appendix 2A, Witness 47, Torsten Trey.

practice clearly violates Principle 5 of the WHO Guiding Principles in transplantation that demand 'no financial incentives for organs', and likely also violates Principles 6-8. (https://www.who.int/transplantation/Guiding_PrinciplesTransplantation_WHA63.22en.pdf)

For further information on payments to families, see DAFOH (https://dafoh.org/public-organ-donation-system-china-largely-depends-monetary-incentives-families-deceased-relatives/).

Compassion Not Commerce, 2.72

The (Chinese Organ Transplant Development Foundation) submission does not, however, address the allegations of organ harvesting from prisoners of conscience.

ETAC response

This is consistent with all commentary from Chinese officials and representatives in that they deal with evidence and claims by ignoring or denying without offering any countervailing evidence.[308]

Compassion Not Commerce, 2.79

(Sub-Committee conclusions) The Sub-Committee is not in a position to conclusively establish the veracity of the allegations either in relation to past activity or current practice, but, on the balance of evidence, is inclined to conclude that organ trafficking has occurred in China and may continue to occur, albeit on a lesser scale. If the full extent of the allegations made were to be verified, it would represent a systemic campaign of human rights abuse against vulnerable ethnic and spiritual minority groups. These groups have substantial diasporas in the Australian community. The Sub-Committee considers that the Australian government has a responsibility to apply the full extent of its available capability to investigate these allegations as far as possible.

---

[308]   The Tribunal regards ETAC's response as understating the significance of the Sub-Committee's simple comment at 2.72. For the PRC to decide, in its own interests in October 2018, to make representations to the Sub-Committee that had been considering forced organ harvesting from the start of its investigations in March 2017 (as the questioning then of Graham Fletcher reveals), and yet to say not one word about the subject is impossible to understand. It is not something that can add to evidence adverse to the PRC but neither can it encourage the Tribunal to credit the other assertions made by the PRC in its written submission

ETAC response

We agree with the sentiment of this statement by the Sub-Committee but disagree that organ trafficking, including forced organ harvesting from prisoners of conscience, is decreasing. Regarding the Sub-Committee's view that they are 'not in a position to conclusively establish the veracity of allegations', we note that the mandate of the Inquiry was to address multiple issues to do with organ trafficking and organ tourism – a far broader set of questions than those raised by organ harvesting in China alone. We therefore assume the Inquiry would have had limited time and resources to devote to assessing the situation in China, which may explain their lack of a definitive view on recent and current practice. The lack of detailed and meticulous scrutiny of the available evidence about organ harvesting in China has however been a recurring issue internationally and is one of the reasons why ETAC initiated the China Tribunal.[309]

Compassion Not Commerce, 2.80

*(Sub-Committee conclusions) The progress of ethical reforms to the organ matching and transplantation system in China is a matter of dispute. **While reform may be occurring, the Sub-Committee believes the available evidence is insufficient to conclude that China has in fact ceased the use of organs sourced from executed prisoners.** It is not clear whether China remains a major destination for transplant tourism. The Sub-Committee is however concerned that any person travelling to China to receive an organ transplant today may be participating in unethical practice.*

ETAC response

We agree that it would be very premature to say that China has ceased using organs from prisoners, including prisoners of conscience. Regarding the status of China as a destination for Australian organ tourists, we await the results of Prof Coates research ... We have contacted him for an update on his

---

[309]   The Tribunal has no comment to make on ETAC's response and has been guided to its own conclusions by consideration of evidence closely focused on forced organ harvesting. It is impossible for the Tribunal to know what the Sub-Committee members would say to the logical step-by-step approach taken by the Tribunal to reach its Judgment. It was clear from video footage of the Sub-Committee hearings that answers by Mr Fletcher setting out the government 'line' – ultimately adopted in very reduced form by the expression of agnosticism of the Sub-Committee – were not necessarily accepted as convincing or even sincerely held by those parliamentarians questioning Mr Fletcher. Mr Fletcher has since been appointed Australian ambassador to China.

results but have not yet had a response. If we receive one in the near future, we will forward this to the Tribunal. Evidence indicates that transplant tourism to China is still occurring from South East Asian countries and Saudi Arabia.

Compassion Not Commerce, 2.81
*(**Sub-Committee conclusions**) There is sufficient evidence that China used the organs of executed prisoners in the past without their free consent. There are contending views about whether this practice is still occurring – although other evidence points to an ongoing, possibly worsening, regime of repression and human rights violations in China. Given this, the onus is on the Chinese authorities to demonstrate to the world that they are not overseeing or permitting the practice of harvesting organs from executed prisoners without their knowledge and free consent. In the absence of such a demonstration by the Chinese authorities, the world is entitled to question assertions of claims to the contrary.*

ETAC response
We agree with the sentiment of this statement by the Sub-Committee; we note however the omission of mention of prisoners of conscience. We strongly support the view that "the onus is on the Chinese authorities to demonstrate to the world that they are not overseeing or permitting the practice of harvesting organs from executed prisoners without their knowledge and free consent" but would add: **or the killing of prisoners of conscience for their organs**. *In the absence of such a demonstration by the Chinese authorities, the world has a* **responsibility to not only question assertions of claims to the contrary but to urgently take action**.

426. An 'Additional Comment by Dr David Matas' is part of ETAC's response to the Tribunal's request for assistance. It is largely opinion or argument that cannot assist the Tribunal in its forensic function, and so is not set out here. It can be found in the response itself, at https://chinatribunal.com. Its second and third paragraphs contain useful summaries.[310]

427. In its overall assessment of the Australian report and ETAC's response two things are clear to the Tribunal. First, however this fact may have been 'covered-up' or disguised in the interests of the comity of nations, the PRC

---

[310] ETAC's response can be found at https://chinatribunal.com Appendix 4, item 28

denied to the Australian Sub-Committee material that would normally, in any truly rigorous forensic setting, be demanded as essential to deal with allegations as important as those under consideration. None of the essential background material showing consent of patients – or even showing that donors and recipients could be identified at all – was provided; nor was any verifiable material dealing with numbers of operations etc.

428. Doctors speaking in support of the PRC were effectively complicit in the denial by their failure to highlight the fact that essential material was missing. In making presentations to the Sub-Committee they should not have been allowed to get away with failing to produce supporting material, which must have been available if the propositions advanced were accurate.[311]

    The Tribunal detected in the reactions of those Australian parliamentarians questioning witnesses, and in the (only just) agnostic position adopted as a conclusion, the possibility that they experienced frustration of the kind the Tribunal has, in the face of the obdurate failure by the various named doctors to assist in the production of essential raw material.

429. Second, even in the measured responses of ETAC, it is possible to discern from time to time the enthusiasm of those committed to a cause the Tribunal has been alert to guard its own judgments against this.

430. However, looking behind assertions to the Sub-Committee from all sides, and focusing on evidence of value to the Tribunal, it is clear that there is nothing of substance in the Australian report, Compassion Not Commerce, to deter the Tribunal from making the findings that follow; and that there are substantial grounds – in the form of non-disclosure of evidence – to encourage the Tribunal to reject statements favourable to the PRC that are unsupported.

431. Viewing the Compassion Not Commerce report and the ETAC responses overall, the Tribunal finds the responses by ETAC serve to eliminate opinions

---

[311]   It should be noted that the Tribunal's view is not that the **doctors** who gave evidence in favour of the PRC are necessarily to be judged as poorly motivated. It is simply that the report – after analysis and with the ETAC responses available – provides no evidence on which this Tribunal can properly act. The **Tribunal records its disappointment that the doctors named** did not respond to request by the Tribunal to cooperate and to give evidence so that their evidence could be tested.

expressed in the report on: statistics, telephone calls, blood testing (being for communicable diseases), number of transplant operations performed, the value of accompanied visits by doctors to the PRC and the voluntary donation scheme said to be effective and in practice. The absence of supporting evidence from the doctors said to speak favourably of the PRC is a recurring shortcoming of the report as are the various misunderstandings of analysis in the Update. It is clear from the Report itself and from the ETAC responses that there has not been anything approaching a proper detailed analysis from raw data of the kind performed in the Update and by this Tribunal.

432. Thus, although recognising that assessments by countries like the UK or Australia, which express lack of conviction that forced organ harvesting has occurred, could be favourable to the PRC in this inquiry, the Tribunal finds nothing in their assessments that actually favours the PRC. It therefore makes no certain conclusion of any kind – one way or another – from the reports of government committees and similar.

433. The Tribunal recognises that intelligence from spying on the PRC – something done by the UK, the US and Australia for certain – might have revealed that the allegations made against the PRC were correct or that they were completely false. If the latter, then it is at least possible that the Tribunal would have been alerted to the existence of such information. This has not happened so the Tribunal is left to act on the basis of there being no relevant intelligence material favourable to the PRC.

The Response of the PRC Generally

434. There has been little response by the PRC to the allegations made. At paragraph 63 above the Tribunal dealt with the failure of the PRC to react over many years to many reports of forced organ harvesting. The limited extent to which the PRC has advanced counter-arguments has been considered in the immediately preceding paragraphs and found to provide little or no help to the Tribunal. With evidence now reviewed, it is necessary to return to the topic of the PRC's general response, applying the common sense and experience of the world citizen.

435. Although many citizens have not heard of forced organ harvesting in China, a great deal of information has been made public, going back to at least 2001 when a detailed account by Dr Wang Guoqi was given to the US

Subcommittee on Trade of the House Committee on Ways and Means[312]. Although no representative from China is shown to have been present at the meetings of the Subcommittee it is inevitable that the Embassy of the PRC in Washington would have reported back to Beijing about the hearing and what Dr Wang said. The same can be said with equal certainty of all the other meetings referred to in paragraph 20 including the November 2018 Australia Foreign Affairs Committee inquiry (Compassion Not Commerce).

436. Similarly, media reports – infrequent though they may have been – around the world expressing concern about the allegations of organ harvesting that were becoming public, would have been reported back to Beijing by PRC embassies; that is part of their job. And it is clear that the PRC was actively engaged with countering Falun Gong internationally throughout that period, as the document leaked from the Estonian Embassy of the PRC in 2008 shows (paragraph 7 footnote 15 above).

PRC Response to Research Paper by Lavee, Robertson and Hinde

437. At a symposium on Development of Organ Donation and Transplantation in China held in Kunming, the capital of Southwest China's Yunnan Province, attended by Huang Jiefu, head of the China National Organ Donation and Transplantation Committee and reported in Global Times of 7 December, 2019, the head of COTRS (China Organ Transplant Response System), Wang Haibo, referred to a recent academic report. He said that the report, Analysis of Official Deceased Organ Donation Data Casts Doubt on Credibility of China's Organ Transplant Reform, by Jacob Lavee, Matthew P Robertson and Raymond L Hinde, January 26, 2019, published on BMC Medical Ethics (mentioned at paragraph 395 and footnote 280 above)[313]. was a 'serious accusation and China felt the need of answering [such accusation]'. He said China would 'lodge a formal rebuttal to the journal on why such [a] paper was published'.

438. The Lavee et al paper claimed that China's data for increase in organ transplants closely matched figures generated by a binomial/quadratic equation, demonstrating that the data were artificially generated. Wang

---

[312]   Paragraph 20 above

[313]   https://bmcmedethics.biomedcentral.com/articles/10.1186/s12910-019-0406-6

showed slides to prove that data shown on the WHO website, data from the US, Brazil and Iran, all fit the binomial equation that gives upward swing and that data from many other countries fit into their own closely matche[d] equations. 'Every country's data can fit into an equation, because the equation is generated from the data,' said Wang.

439. Jose Núñez, WHO officer in charge of global organ transplantation, told the Global Times that they had received the report produced by Lavee, and it was sent to them repeatedly, twice a week. 'But we didn't respond,' said Núñez, noting that 'China had already provided efficient data with Global Observatory on Donation and Transplantation'.

440. Bjorn Nashan, former president of the German Transplantation Society and now working at First Affiliated Hospital, University of Science and Technology of China in East China's Anhui Province, referred to Lavee's paper as 'scientific misconduct', saying that if the authors have questions about Chinese data, 'they should first of all ask China to provide such data, but they did not'.

441. Although their paper was based on publicly available material, in line with academic standards and in light of Nashan's observation, the researchers, as asked by the journal, emailed every Chinese surgeon and official mentioned by name in the paper and sought their responses. They did this multiple times. No one replied.

442. The Tribunal recognised that China had already provided the (misleading) data and that there was no data fabrication, falsification or plagiarism, which is how scientific misconduct is usually defined.

443. The Tribunal also noted that the 'formal rebuttal' promised has not been published.

444. In these circumstances, the PRC response to the paper is effectively a bare denial, unsupported by additional data or argumentation that could be dealt with by Lavee, Robertson and Hinde or reviewed by the Tribunal itself.

445. Of course it is true that before the PRC acknowledged the use of organs from executed prisoners for transplantation, it was lying both to the world at large and to the medical profession. But the flows of information that were

undoubtedly being reported to Beijing continued and only at the Australian hearing did the PRC put in any 'defence', and then of no substance.

446. Must the Tribunal simply disregard the failure of the PRC to do more? Should the PRC be accorded some form of 'right to silence' matching that of the individual defendant charged with a regular crime in, say, the US?[314] The Tribunal is disinclined to draw any inferences from anything the PRC does *not* do, for example, not responding to the Tribunal's request for engagement.[315] But may the gravity of the allegations, and the extended period over which they have been made, require a different, common sense reaction? Perhaps considering a hypothetical situation may help. Suppose it were said of either the UK or the US that in a prison in Leeds or Philadelphia (cities chosen at random) Muslims were being tortured to death for being Muslims, and suppose the allegation was entirely untrue, although being made by a respectable organisation that had attracted attention in government committees in various countries. Would issuing a simple denial be all that the UK or US would do, on grounds that their word should be enough and it would be to honour an impertinence by doing more? Or would they do a great deal more – including seeking redress from whoever made the totally false, but believable, allegation and throwing open the gates of the prison and offering sight of all records to an appropriate neutral team of observers?

447. The Tribunal cannot go so far as to draw any inferences adverse to the PRC from its failure to rebut an allegation that it protests is totally untrue. It sets out in its conclusion what may, nevertheless, flow from this failure.

---

[314] The right to silence has been effectively abrogated in the UK because inferences can sometimes be drawn from silence in the face of questioning or if declining to give evidence at trial.

[315] Paraph 62 above

The Tribunal's Overall Conclusions on the Facts and on the Law

Primary Conclusions of Forced Organ Harvesting

448. Making overall conclusions is a difficult exercise; difficult because much of what happens in the PRC is obscured by disinclination of the state to be open with those investigating the issue for nearly two decades and because of the size and complexity of the country.

449. Difficulties of this kind can easily translate to doubt and uncertainty, especially if uncertainty is an easier or safer resolution because – as David Kilgour said of governments expressing uncertainty – finding a truthful resolution adverse to the PRC could be 'inconvenient'. Difficulties can also translate to doubt and uncertainty simply because there are so many factual issues where evidence is missing; and equally because questions naturally arising, for example, about how professional people, especially medical practitioners of all kinds, could do the things alleged, can only be answered by the equivalent of guesswork, not by evidence.

450. But difficulty is not impossibility, nor can it justify those commissioned to make a decision becoming fearful of doing so if a conclusion is properly possible by consideration of all available evidence.

451. The most obvious 'difficulties' facing this Tribunal are:

- How can any witnesses giving evidence adverse to the PRC be accepted as truthful and accurate when not tested by questions or challenges put to them by the PRC?

- In a country of the size of China, how can any inference be drawn or conclusion reached about central control of actions by individuals, or individual local institutions (hospitals usually), that are thousands of kilometres away?

- More generally how can the possibility be excluded of alleged crimes being merely the work of 'rogue' institutions or individuals?

- Where it is necessary to establish a mental state for proof of a crime, how can it be proved that the relevant mental state existed in the central government of the PRC, or in the CCP, to trigger an act performed thousands of kilometres away?

- How can the mental state of the PRC or CCP be proved without access to the individuals at the very top of those organisations for the purpose of investigating the individual states of minds or the collective mental state? More generally, how can the Tribunal make judgments about a state known (in common with other authoritarian states) for its use of the 'big lie'?

The PRC has occasionally made truthful statements about organ transplant, most notably in 2006 when it was eventually compelled to acknowledge use of organs from executed prisoners for transplant operations. Its other statements have been accusatory of Falun Gong practitioners, asserting that everything said adverse to the PRC on this issue is propaganda and lies. And it now states that all organs come from volunteer donors or a properly controlled *post-mortem* donor scheme. Should the Tribunal be concerned when such a big state makes such uncompromising statements? As this Judgment is being written, citizens on both sides of the Atlantic have direct experience of senior politicians lying and 'getting away with it', on one view, despite the lies being recognised for what they are.[316] There is not quite the gulf in behaviour between authoritarian states and those that boast of their open and honest democracies; citizens of all countries can cope with firmly expressed untruths from their leaders, and can work out what the truth is – though it may not bring the leaders down.

452. The Tribunal has considered all these difficulties against the simple – and obvious – point that the Tribunal should not be concerned about what it does

---

[316] The administration of President Trump in the US and both sides of the debate in the UK about the UK's leaving the European Union are all assumed to have told lies on a generous scale without leaders being toppled.

not have (and might have had in a conventional investigation). What the Tribunal must do – just as mathematicians, quantum physicists, engineers etc do when confronted by an impasse to a known line of inquiry – is to look elsewhere, examine what is available and follow the deductive trail, testing its conclusions with the same rigour as it would have tested an investigation that had more materials available to it.

453.   With this in mind, and with the need to avoid contamination by what the PRC has obscured or by knowledge of the PRC's known breaches of human rights laws generally, the Tribunal approached its final decision-making process by making conclusions category by category, and where possible strictly limited to the particular category. As noted earlier, it approached each category, where possible, on the basis that the country concerned was not the PRC, but some other or imaginary country with a good human rights record.

454.   The first three categories of evidence considered were: the description of what happens in transplant surgery; telephone calls to hospitals; and the scale of transplant activity in China (including short waiting items).

455.   In shortened form the conclusions for each category were:
        Telephone calls were made to hospitals and individual medical staff including senior surgeons. The hospitals telephoned were offering organs for sale. Those organs were from people who were alive at the time of the calls and were available to the callers at short notice.
        Very large numbers of transplant operations have been carried out in the PRC. The Tribunal assesses as credible numbers of operations between 60,000 and 90,000 per annum in the years 2000-2014. This, when compared to the number of eligible registered donors, which, by 2017, had risen to 5,146, leaves an incomprehensible gap. To achieve the numbers of transplants performed – before and since 2017, the year of most recent estimate, – there must have existed another source or other sources of tissue-typed organs; this in turn shows that there must have existed a group of donors unidentified in PRC material

456.   The conclusions, reached above, lead the Tribunal, without giving any consideration to Falun Gong practitioners, and assuming the evidence relates to a country with nothing to its discredit, to the certain conclusion that:

Hospitals in the PRC have had access to a population of donors whose organs could be extracted according to demand for them.

457. Turning to the conclusion reached on the basis of direct and indirect evidence about forced organ harvesting, and of medical testing:

Forced organ harvesting has happened in multiple places in the PRC and on multiple occasions for a period of at least 20 years and continues to this day.

Medical testing of groups, including Falun Gong and Uyghurs, was related in some way to the group concerned because other prisoners were not tested. The methods of testing are highly suggestive of methods used to assess organ function. The use of ultrasound examinations further suggests testing was focused on the condition of internal organs. No explanation has been given by the PRC for this testing; blood or otherwise.

458. Combining these conclusions with the previous finding leads inexorably to the conclusion that:

There has been a population of donors accessible to hospitals in the PRC whose organs could be extracted according to demand and this has coincided both with the long-term practice in the PRC of forced organ harvesting and with many Falun Gong practitioners, along with Uyghurs, being compelled to have medical tests, focused on their organs.

459. Now considering the conclusions about the torture of Falun Gong practitioners and Uyghurs and the evidence of public statements by the PRC about Falun Gong practitioners:

Acts of torture have been inflicted by the PRC authorities on persons detained for their practice of, support for and defence of Falun Gong and for no other reason. Such acts of torture have taken place at many different sites in the PRC over a long period of time. Acts of torture, generally, reveal an overall consistent attitude and approach of the Chinese state towards practitioners of Falun Gong, which is systematic in nature and designed to punish, ostracise, humiliate, dehumanise, demean and demonise practitioners of Falun Gong into renouncing and abandoning their practice of it. The PRC and its leaders actively incited such persecution for the sole purpose of eliminating the practice of, and belief in, Falun Gong.

Acts of torture have been inflicted on Uyghurs and generally reveal an overall consistent attitude and approach of the PRC towards Uyghurs, which is systematic in nature and designed to punish, ostracise, humiliate, dehumanise and demean Uyghurs. It is clear that Uyghurs have been routinely forced to undergo regular medical testing.

460. Combining conclusions makes it clear that:

There has been a population of donors accessible to hospitals in the PRC whose organs could be extracted according to demand for them, and this has coincided with the long-term practice in the PRC of forced organ harvesting and of many Falun Gong, along with Uyghurs, being compelled to have medical tests, focused on their organs; the PRC would have no difficulty in committing Falun Gong practitioners to any fate and could readily use them as the population of donors accessible to hospitals in the PRC whose organs could be extracted according to demand for them by means of forced organ harvesting.

461. This process of step-by-step reasoning leads inexorably from: the clear evidence of a supply chain of organs over many years but from an unaccountable source; the fact that Falun Gong practitioners once incarcerated *could* be a useable source; and there being no other source identified, to the Tribunal being satisfied that:

In the long-term practice in the PRC of forced organ harvesting it was indeed Falun Gong practitioners who were used as a source – probably the principal source – of organs for forced organ harvesting

462. The remaining categories of particular evidence – evidence about Huang Jiefu and evidence from PRC and CCP officials – do nothing to displace this conclusion; rather the reverse. And the conclusion fits with the conclusions reached at the start of the evidence review by consideration of the general background.

463. **Since 1999 the PRC and the CCP regarded practitioners of Falun Gong as unworthy of any of those universal rights that attach to human beings by reason of their humanity; this regard by the PRC and the CCP and all that followed from it was simply to maintain the PRC's and CCP's power and authority over the Chinese people. Coincident with the developing persecution of practitioners of Falun Gong over time has been an enormous, unexplained provision of transplant infrastructure, in the absence of a voluntary organ donor system.**

464. Further,

Falun Gong practitioners and Uyghurs have been routinely tortured.

The brevity of this sentence is not to mitigate the enormity of what is contained within.

465. **There is insufficient evidence to make a conclusion of forced organ harvesting from the Uyghurs**. But the vulnerability of the Uyghurs to the will of the PRC to establish and maintain complete control over them by incarceration is obvious.[317] The vulnerability of the Uyghurs to being used as a bank of organs is also obvious.[318]

---

[317] Attending to the different arguments about what may happen to the Uyghurs in the future led the Tribunal to broader thinking. Organ transplantation has to date been human to human, with the exception a few famous failed experiments (eg Baby Fae, baboon to human heart transplant). It is in the context of the present need for human-to-human transplants and the inadequate supply of such organs that creates the substrate for forced organ donation, the subject of the China tribunal. The Tribunal has found that forced organ donation has happened in the People's Republic of China, indicating a conspicuous disregard of medical ethics. But perhaps human-to-human transplants will have had their day in the not too distant future. Major advances have been made in xeno-transplantation (animals to human) notably with the development of genetically engineered pigs. The stage is set for the first human experiments of such therapy. Such experiments throw up many and obvious ethical challenges, and the need for transparent and complete reporting of outcomes, short and long-term is self-evident.

A country which is prepared to accept such appalling practices must be subject to international research scrutiny, and any published findings subject to additional doubt. Research is built on a foundation of reproducibility and good ethical practice. Both must be rigorously maintained.

[318] Throughout the time the Tribunal was working on the evidence presented to it, increasing amounts of information about the approach and conduct of the PRC towards the Uyghurs has come to public attention. Mostly it has related to their incarceration, 'brainwashing' and torture. Some more recent reports have referred specifically to forced organ harvesting. One recent example comes from 'extranewsfeed': Muslims Are Being "Slaughtered on Demand" For Their Organs in China CJ Werleman (https://extranewsfeed.com/@cjwerleman) Extranewsfeed (https://extranewsfeed.com/muslims-are-being-slaughtered-on-demand-for-their-organs-in-china-b502133c725) Jan 21, 2020. Werleman refers to Enver Tohti (see paragraph 165 *ante*) and gives an account by an eye witness of the harvesting of Uyghur organs in 2006. https://extranewsfeed.com/muslims-are-being-slaughtered-on-demand-for-their-organs-in-china-b502133c725.

Werleman also quotes Professor Erkin Sidick: "The CCP transported and dispersed more than 1 million Uyghurs to various Han provinces first, then divided them into different groups. One group is for organ harvesting, another for biological experimentation, and others for other purposes, such as distributed killing. The CCP has run out of money to maintain their vast concentration camps, and is resorting to these kinds of means. I constantly get info from high level government officials through several middle men, but it has been impossible for me to make my info official because doing so will put some people in danger, including those government officials,"

466. In reaching its conclusion the Tribunal has not had to apply its knowledge of the multiple breaches of human rights law generally for which the PRC is culpable, although it acknowledges that there is nothing inconsistent between the Tribunal's conclusion and the PRC's human rights record; in reality, the reverse.

Has Forced Organ Harvesting Ended?

467. The most recent evidence of availability of organs on demand is to be found in the telephone calls of 2018[319] and the Korean film of 2017[320] They are not in themselves sufficient to prove continuity of forced organ harvesting on the same scale although they do nothing to disprove it. More important is that the system has been in operation for years despite international evidence-based concerns and criticism, and research asserting that the practice is proved. There is, thus, no particular reason for it to stop and many people's livelihoods in the PRC depend on it. Further, it is clear from the evidence of torture by those who were imprisoned but not 'harvested', that the authorities had objectives for the overall treatment of members of Falun Gong other than the purely commercial purpose of harvesting and selling organs. Further still, it would appear probable that access to a supply of organs has been one of the reasons the PRC has been able to become so formidable in the skills required for transplant surgery and thus to rise – subject to the shadow of these allegations – in the estimation of transplant surgeons elsewhere in the world, several of whom continue to support the PRC in public (as at the Australian Committee hearings for the Compassion Not Commerce report –above). There is no evidence of the practice having been stopped and the Tribunal is satisfied that it is continuing.

Professor Siddick confirmed the accuracy of this account to the Executive Director of ETAC as follows: 'The original source of this info is a high-level government official in China's central government, and I got the info through a middle [man]. But I cannot disclose the middle man. It will cost a lot of Uy ghurs' lives if the middle-man was found out by the CCP.'

The Conclusions the Tribunal reached about Uyghurs have not been changed by material such as this, but there can be little doubt that such material, and the very considerable number of reports about incarceration of and torturing of Uyhgurs, makes even more pressing the need for their suffering past and present to be addressed with the utmost urgency.

[319]   Appendix 2B, item 4. https://chinatribunal.com/wp-content/uploads/2019/06/ WOIPFG-Investigation-Report_NewEvidence_2018.pdf

[320]   Appendix 2B, item 54 https://vimeo.com/280284321

Geographical Spread of the Practice

468. The map Appendix 1B[321] identifies the hospitals spoken of by those tortured and medically tested and hospitals which, when called on the telephone by investigators, responded in ways that revealed organs were available on demand.

---

[321]   Appendix 1B

Conclusions on Criminality

469. As a preface, it might be thought bizarre in the extreme if forced organ harvesting by a state, or state-approved bodies, was established by strong evidence, at a court with jurisdiction covering individual criminal or state responsibility, and the court should then say that for technical reasons no case could be pursued. On hearing this the citizen would realise that the world order offered her or him no protection through legal processes and that impunity was fully in place in the state concerned. The clear reality is that any court seized of such evidence would know that it *had* to find jurisdiction to act in accordance with its statute and rules because to do otherwise would have it condemned to oblivion or to be replaced. This certainty is one that confronts 'uninvolved' states around the world whenever they are faced with strong evidence of the criminality of other states. They would prefer never to have to refer such evidence to legal authorities (manifesting denial of the 'inconvenient truth' spoken of by David Kilgour). Following the Tribunal's Primary Conclusion on Forced Organ Harvesting a priority may be to 'force' facts on to a court with jurisdiction because once facts as grave as those alleged and accepted here *do* reach a proper court, a proper court *will* find a way to act. The issue will simply then be which crime or crimes to charge.

470. The Tribunal comes to the following conclusions based on its factual conclusions spelt out above *and* on the basis of the legal Opinions and Advice received.

Genocide

471. The Tribunal has no doubt whatsoever that physical acts have been carried out that are indicative of the crime of genocide. Reviewing the definition of genocide found in the Genocide Convention, and repeated in the Rome Statute of the ICC, the Tribunal is certain that there has been killing of members of a group,[322] there has been caused serious bodily or mental harm

---

[322]   Genocide Convention 1948, Article II(a).

to members of a group,[323] and there has been the deliberate inflicting on the group of conditions of life calculated to bring about the group's physical destruction in whole or in part.[324]

472. The Tribunal also finds that in relation to the legal understanding of the term 'group', Falun Gong practitioners and the Uyghurs do constitute, respectively, a group. Further they belong to one or more of the groups that are specifically identified in the Genocide Convention as deserving of protection, namely a national, ethnical, racial or religious group.[325]

473. In order to find criminality, there must be a conjunction of both physical acts and mental intent. The question to be asked by the Tribunal is whether the crime of genocide has been committed by way of forced organ harvesting of prisoners of conscience. To arrive at the conclusion that the crime of genocide (as legally defined) has indeed been committed, such forced organ harvesting must have been carried out with the specific intent to destroy, in whole or in part, these groups. The Tribunal has not been able to find such requisite specific intent.

474. The Tribunal notes the intention of eliminating Falun Gong practitioners as enunciated by General Secretary Jiang Zemin to the Political Bureau of the Central Committee of the CCP on 7 June 1999, the 20th anniversary of which has recently passed. Separately, the Tribunal notes the development of the market for organ transplant surgery, with its huge money-making potential. How and when these two lines of events met and/or merged is not clear from the information and evidence available to the Tribunal. This, in turn, meant the Tribunal was unable to conclude with certainty about, or be sure of, the specific intent behind the forced organ harvesting of prisoners of conscience.

475. What concerned the Tribunal was the fact that some practitioners of Falun Gong, and some Uyghurs, while having suffered arrest and detention, were released notwithstanding that they had made, at least with respect to Falun Gong practitioners, no promise nor given any undertaking to cease the practice of Falun Gong. In fact, their repeated arrest and detention, in some cases, is evidence that this was so. Why was this allowed to happen?

---

[323]   Genocide Convention 1948, Article II(b).
[324]   Genocide Convention 1948, Article II(c).
[325]   Genocide Convention 1948, chapeau of Article II.

If the physical and biological extermination of Falun Gong practitioners, or Uyghurs, was the ultimate goal of the CCP, their release should not have occurred. If, however, the goal was primarily organ harvesting for profit, then different considerations would apply. As cautioned by Datuk Sivananthan, the intention to forcefully harvest the organs for the sake of profit is not the same as an intention to forcefully harvest the organs in order to bring about the physical or biological destruction in part or in whole of a protected group.

476. Given that there was no participation of representatives of the PRC or CCP in these hearings to address this issue and given that no explanation has been offered to otherwise account for the release of persons detained, **the Tribunal is constrained from concluding that the crime of genocide had occurred.**

477. An alternative argument considered by the Tribunal was that the determination of the crime of genocide was not affected by the fact that some practitioners of Falun Gong and some Uyghurs were released and/or allowed to leave the PRC, given that the definition of genocide only required that acts of genocide were carried out with the intent to destroy a group 'in part', and not 'in whole'.

478. The Tribunal noted that it was possible to characterise what had occurred as the implementation of a policy to develop the market for organ transplants where Falun Gong practitioners and Uyghurs served unfortunately as a ready and rich resource to meet demand, such that the infliction of forced organ harvesting on these groups was not primarily motivated by the intention to exterminate these groups in whole or in part. Whether or not, despite that, those responsible for forced organ harvesting of members of these groups had the requisite mental state or intent to constitute the crime of genocide is not clear. Whether a knowledge-based approach to criminal intent to commit genocide could be attributed to them is also unclear and, as advised by Datuk Sivananthan, fraught with legal uncertainty.

Crimes against Humanity

479. Adopting the definition of crimes against humanity as set out in the Rome Statute of the ICC[326], the Tribunal is certain so as to be sure beyond reasonable

---

[326]   Rome Statute of the International Criminal Court 1999, Article 7

doubt that attacks have indeed been directed against Falun Gong practitioners and Uyghurs in the PRC, with actual knowledge of the attack by state actors of the government of the PRC. Indeed, these attacks are state-sponsored or -sanctioned, and pursuant to or in furtherance of a state policy to commit such attacks. The Tribunal concurs with the advice offered by Edward Fitzgerald QC that forced organ harvesting is sufficient to constitute an attack. The Tribunal is further satisfied that such attacks are indeed widespread or systematic.

480. The Tribunal is also satisfied beyond reasonable doubt that one or more of the following acts have been committed on Falun Gong practitioners and Uyghurs in the PRC: murder;[327] extermination;[328] imprisonment or other severe deprivation of physical liberty in violation of fundamental rules of international law;[329] torture;[330] rape or any other form of sexual violence of comparable gravity;[331] persecution on racial, national, ethnic, cultural or religious grounds that are universally recognised as impermissible under international law;[332] and enforced disappearance.[333]

481. **Taken together, such attacks and such acts constitute crimes against humanity, which the Tribunal is certain beyond reasonable doubt or 'so as to be sure'[334] has occurred.**

Torture

482. Based on the findings of the Tribunal above in relation to torture in the context of crimes against humanity, **the Tribunal is of the view that it is beyond reasonable doubt that acts of torture have occurred.** In the context of the Convention against Torture, the Tribunal is certain of two things. First, that these were acts:

---

[327] Rome Statute of the International Criminal Court 1999, Article 7(1)(a)
[328] Rome Statute of the International Criminal Court 1999, Article 7(1)(b) and Article 7(2)(b)
[329] Rome Statute of the International Criminal Court 1999, Article 7(1)(e)
[330] Rome Statute of the International Criminal Court 1999, Article 7(1)(f) and Article 7(2)(e)
[331] Rome Statute of the International Criminal Court 1999, Article 7(1)(g)
[332] Rome Statute of the International Criminal Court 1999, Article 7(1)(h) and Article 7(2)(g)
[333] Rome Statute of the International Criminal Court 1999, Article 7(1)(i) and Article 7(2)(j)
[334] In some jurisdictions the 'modern' form of 'beyond reasonable doubt'

by which severe pain or suffering, whether physical or mental, [was] intentionally inflicted on a person ... punishing him [or her] for an act he [or she] ... has committed or is suspected of having committed ... or for any reason based on discrimination of any kind, when such pain or suffering is inflicted by or at the instigation of or with the consent or acquiescence of a public official or other person acting in an official capacity.'[335]

483. Secondly, the exception in respect of *'pain or suffering arising only from, inherent in or incidental to lawful sanction'*[336] does not arise. It is clear that the type of treatment experienced and described by witnesses who appeared before the Tribunal was in no way justified by this exception.

484. In relation to two other groups, Tibetan Buddhists and House Christians in the PRC, the Tribunal is unable to come to any finding as there was insufficient evidence presented to it to satisfy the elements of the possible crimes under consideration.

---

[335] Convention against Torture and Other Cruel, Inhuman or Degrading Treatment or Punishment 1984, Article 1

[336] Convention against Torture and Other Cruel, Inhuman or Degrading Treatment or Punishment 1984, Article 1

Actions to be Taken

485. As has already been mentioned, the Tribunal is acutely aware, both having had regard to the legal Opinions and Advice and from its own collective knowledge, of the jurisdictional hurdles that lie in the way of prosecuting crimes under the international law of genocide, crimes against humanity and torture.

486. In relation to the crime of genocide, and notwithstanding the conclusion arrived at by the Tribunal, it is still open for the UN General Assembly to request from the ICJ an advisory opinion on the issue of forced organ harvesting in the PRC and whether it constitutes genocide. There would be no need for the PRC to consent to such a request. Resolutions calling for the same may be moved by one or more member states for consideration and, if sufficiently supported, adopted by the General Assembly.

487. Action at an international level could also be founded on the basis of the Responsibility to Protect ('R2P' as commonly known). This is a political commitment endorsed by all member states of the United Nations, including the PRC, in 2005 to prevent genocide, war crimes, ethnic cleansing and crimes against humanity (universally endorsed at the 2005 World Summit and re-affirmed in 2006 by the UN).[337] Respect for norms and principles of international law mandate national governments, regional and international communities to initiate action to intervene in such situations. However, intervention requires approval by the UN Security Council, of which the PRC is a permanent member and can therefore exercise a veto.[338]

---

[337] see https://www.un.org/en/genocideprevention/about-responsibility-to-protect.shtml

[338] The unlimited power of the 'P5' members of the Security Council to exercise the veto has been the subject of discussion – see, for example, https://www.globalr2p.org/calling-for-a-unsc-code-of-conduct/ The work of this Tribunal may stimulate further thought of the need for reform

488. It would also be open for the UN Human Rights Council to consider this matter, again based on a resolution proposed by one or more of its 47 member states. Subject to a majority vote in favour by the Council, the Council could create a mandate for a Special Rapporteur to investigate these allegations of forced organ harvesting of prisoners of conscience in the PRC, and to report back to the Council on whether the crimes of genocide, crimes against humanity, and torture have indeed been committed. Despite the time this would inevitably take, this course of action could be given some priority without reducing the importance of all other possible actions.

489. The UN Working Group on Arbitrary Detention might also have a role if necessary – co-operation could be established for an interview with a known arbitrarily detained person.

490. But the risk in identifying too many possible international interventions is that none will receive proper focus, and all may fail.

491. Apart from action at an international level initiated by governments (or possibly others), domestic action in such matters is possible – by asserting universal jurisdiction powers, established in some national courts by national legislation or by international law, to permit individual plaintiffs to file legal actions against particular individuals or even against a sovereign state for acts or conduct that may constitute genocide, crimes against humanity or torture. [339] The Tribunal is aware of an action commenced in, and accepted by, the national courts in Spain in 2013, by a group of Tibetan exiles seeking to bring, among others, former Chinese leader Jiang Zemin to justice for acts of genocide in Tibet. As a result, the Spanish court issued an international arrest warrant for Jiang. The Tribunal is, however, not aware of any recent developments in this case. More recently efforts have been put in train by

---

[339] In the UK, Lord David Alton and Fiona Bruce MP introduced Bills in Parliament that, if voted into law, would allow the citizen some ability to stimulate government action when genocide is suspected. Their Bills – to *provide for the High Court of England and Wales to make a preliminary finding on cases of alleged genocide; and for the subsequent referral of such findings to the International Criminal Court or a special tribunal'* – might restrict the ability of the UK government not to respond to events that called for the possibility of genocide being investigated. The Bills are awaiting government time to make further progress. See, for example, https://www.fionabruce.org.uk/news/fiona-and-lord-alton-liverpool-host-parliamentary-event-question-genocide-determination. Note https://chinatribunal.com/wp-content/uploads/2019/06/Lord-Alton_China-Tribunal-Submission.pdf

lawyers in Melbourne, Australia, to have Aung San Suu Kyi prosecuted for crimes against humanity in respect of the suffering of the Rohingya Muslims; present progress also unknown. The recent success of Gambia against Myanmar at the ICJ for alleged breaches of the Genocide Convention offers no new route to action for either Falun Gong practitioners or the Uyghurs; the PRC's 'Reservation' in respect the jurisdiction of the ICJ for alleged Genocide Convention breaches is not something that, on present authority, could be overcome.

492. The Tribunal has emphasised that its principal role is to identify whether it is satisfied beyond reasonable doubt that crimes have been committed rather than to identify with certainty which individuals may have committed such crimes.[340] Having noted possible courses of action that governments could take, the Tribunal leaves to citizens, activists and motivated politicians the task of pressing governments to do what may be thought their duty to do in the face of revealed wickedness of the kind shown in *any* finding that forced organ harvesting has happened or is continuing to happen in the PRC.

493. The Tribunal notes, with disappointment, that both UK and Australian governments have expressed no desire properly to test the allegations by themselves or through the United Nations. It might be expected that allegations such as these – as grave, on a death for death basis, as any that were proved against the worst political mass murderers of the 20th century – might be thought worthy of the most urgent and potentially beneficial action that the world order would allow. But not to be expected of the UK or Australia, it seems. As noted, the US took a different line.

494. So far as governments are concerned, the Tribunal reverts to what it has said about the PRC's failure to engage with the allegations being made for such a long period of time. Other governments' failures to investigate the allegations sufficiently to find them proved has enabled them to justify doing little or nothing, and certainly never initiating one of the processes that could bring these allegations to formal judicial determination. Over this time the PRC may have deserved better of itself than to let an existing practice continue

---

[340] And the test of 'beyond reasonable doubt' is different from lesser levels of belief or opinion such as that 'there is a case to answer' or similar. For governments to intervene, judgment at these lesser levels are what many would think more than sufficient to require them to act by instituting investigations at international level.

and grow. Countries testing grave allegations and *not* letting the PRC escape oversight could have helped the PRC to understand that the practice in which it was engaged *had* to stop if it was to find a place in the world that was something more than that of an enormously powerful commercial partner, and competitor, of other states. Tragically unchecked action allowed many people to die horribly and unnecessarily in the service of objectives that successors to the present PRC leaders may come to recognise were never essential to the wellbeing or growth in stature, of their state.

495. Finally, assuming governments do not act as it might be thought they should, criminality of the order revealed may allow individuals from around the world to act jointly in pressurising governments so that it becomes impossible for those governments or other international bodies ***not*** to act.

496. Nor should the citizen *as shopper* be overlooked. Boycotting goods started before the American Revolution, by Americans in respect of English products, and has been an intermittent force ever since, against countries such as Israel, the US and South Africa. The effect of boycotting is always uncertain and may be limited. More significant for these events is the fact that for much of its customer base the PRC is a very long way away, and it may be that an individual citizen's willingness to take a stand about what their 'neighbour' is doing is in inverse proportion to how far away that neighbour is.

Recommendations and Final Observation

497. As explained above (paragraphs 36, 124 and 126) the Tribunal sees no need to make general recommendations because there are plenty of individuals, bodies, and governments, that should act given the conclusion that the tribunal has reached.

498. It has given the Tribunal no pleasure to reach this conclusion, to which it was driven by evidence and the application of reason and logic. The conclusion shows that very many people have died indescribably hideous deaths for no reason, that more may suffer in similar ways, and that all of us live on a planet where extreme wickedness may be found in the power of those who are, for the time being, running a country with one of the oldest civilisations known to modern man, which we should be able to respect and from which we should be able to learn.

499. However, this much can be said, and may be a statement long overdue from responsible governments around the world:

    China is a wonderful, diverse, and cultured land, where, today, the state – the PRC and the CCP – may be involved in many more areas of life than is the case in other countries. Any person or organisation that interacts in any substantial way with the PRC – the People's Republic of China – including:

    - doctors and medical institutions;
    - industry, and businesses, most specifically airlines, travel companies, financial services businesses, law firms, and pharmaceutical and insurance companies, together with individual tourists;
    - educational establishments; arts establishments

    should recognise that, to the extent revealed in this document, they are interacting with a criminal state.

Members of the Tribunal
Sir Geoffrey Nice QC (Chair)
Prof Martin Elliott
Andrew Khoo
Regina Paulose
Shadi Sadr
Nicholas Vetch
Prof Arthur Waldron

Date
1 March 2020

Counsel to the Tribunal
Hamid Sabi
Tabitha Nice

Junior Counsel to the Tribunal
Markus Findlay

Assistants to Counsel to the Tribunal
Eliah Alexander
Adetokunbo (Toks) Hussein
Tatiana Lindberg
Eleanor Stephenson

Appendices

Appendix 1A.
Witnesses of Fact: Witness
Statements and Oral Testimony

What follows are copies of the witness statements provided to ETAC. Some of these statements were provided with Chinese characters as well as the English translation. The Chinese characters have been removed. Immediately after each statement is a summary of the additional points made during their oral testimony. For an accurate view of the evidence, each hearing and witness testimony is available on the China Tribunal website.

(All submissions are in original language, not necessarily UK English.)

Witness 1: Dai Ying

Female, age 60. Occupation in China: owner of a private supermarket; current occupation: unemployed.

When you were detained in China was it ever through a court process? If yes, what was the judgement about?
There were legal procedures, but the procedures were not correct. No lawyers were allowed. Sentenced for 3 years in prison. According to the §300 criminal law. Thereafter, sent to Laojiao (education through labor) for 2 years, without any legal procedure.

Detention In China: I was sentenced to 3 years in Laogai (reform through labor), followed by 2 years in Reeducation through labor camp. March 2000, Futian District Detention Center, Shenzhen city. Feb 2003, Sanshui Women's Forced Labor Camp

(Translator's Brief: The following was written when Dai was 48 years old, about 12 years ago.)

My name is Dai Ying and I am 48 years old. During the past seven years of the Chinese regime's persecution of Falun Gong, I was illegally sentenced to three years of forced labor. After that, I was taken to another forced labor camp for two more years. During the past five years, I have suffered cruel torture by the Chinese Communist Party (CCP). Due to the persecution I suffered, I have lost the sight in my left eye, my upper and lower teeth loosened, and my body is deformed. I wish to expose the cruel torture I suffered at the hands of the CCP regime to the international community, so the world will hear the truth about the CCP's persecution of Falun Gong.

Imprisoned
On July 21st 1999, fellow practitioners and I went to the Shenzhen City appeals office to appeal to the government. Instead of finding help, the police arrested us. My husband was secretly detained, but 10 days later, he successfully escaped. On September 29, police officers from Shenzhen City arrested my husband and me. They ransacked our home and detained us at Futian District Detention Center. With our family's help, I was bailed out 15 days later, but my husband was still in detention.

Because my husband, Li Jianhui, remained firm in his belief in "Truthfulness, Compassion, forbearance", Shenzhen government officials reported him to Guangdong Province officials and the 610 Office of the Central CCP. The prosecutor from the Shenzhen City Procuratorate told my husband, "You were not guilty, but we had to sentence you. This was dictated by higher authorities." Before the trial began, I hired a lawyer named Qu from the Shenzhen City New Century Lawyers Office to represent my husband.

My husband's brother hired a lawyer by the name of Ms. Xu. Both of them were supposed to defend my husband. After they read everything in his file, they didn't think that he was guilty. Attorney Qu took this file to Beijing and, during a law seminar, discussed the constitution and other laws in regard to my husband's case. Those experts agreed that my husband had not committed any crime, so Attorneys Qu and Ms. Xu decided to defend my husband and prove his innocence. However, before the trial, Shenzhen City Court learned that lawyers would defend my husband and plead not guilty. Shenzhen municipal government officials used staff at the police bureau to stop Ms. Xu. They did not allow her to defend my husband. In addition, they had the Shenzhen City Juridical Bureau force Ms. Xu to void her contract with me and barred her from representing my husband in court. They did not allow the two lawyers or any members of our family to be in the courtroom. Instead, they appointed a lawyer who pleaded guilty. Futian District Court "illegally sentenced" my husband to a four-year term at the end of February 2000. The trial was illegal under China's Constitution and the procedure was not based on any legal grounds.

Therefore, I wanted to go to the State's Council at Beijing's appeals office. I wanted to speak up for Falun Dafa and its practitioners. (Appealing to the government is also a right granted to every citizen under the Constitution.) On March 5th 2000, I went to Beijing to appeal. Police officers there detained me and took me back to Shenzhen City, where I was detained in Futian District Detention Center.

Torture

In China, under the CCP's rule, there are no human rights to speak of, which is why when the leaders of the CCP are overseas, they openly say in public that they do not speak of human rights, they speak of the right to live – the rights the Chinese government give its citizens are just the right of animals to live, and if you don't obey, even this right will be stripped from you. The courts can disregard the constitution and the law and pronounce you guilty without a shred of evidence. Just because I wanted to help my husband ask the government for justice, I was deemed guilty and detained, awaiting my sentence to be passed.

In order to resist and protest the persecution, I went on a hunger strike. Three days later, police officers from the detention center began to force-feed me. Forced-feeding has become a means for guards to torture Falun Gong practitioners.

They carried me outside. Four or five guards held me down. They put a very rigid tube into my nose until I bled. When the tube did not reach my stomach, they forced my teeth open with a screwdriver. Then they put a bamboo barrel with a very sharp end into my mouth with a lot of force. My mouth hurt immediately. After that, they force-fed me with food or condensed salt-water. I felt like choking. Food and blood came from my mouth and nose and went all over my clothes. After they finished the forced-feeding, I felt as if I had died. I was force-fed every two to three days. One time during the force-feeding, I held my teeth closed very tightly. Doctor Zhou from the detention center used a large screwdriver to force my mouth open. I lost two front teeth and my upper and lower front teeth became loose.

Practitioner Wang Xiaowen also lost two front teeth. I witnessed practitioner Ms. Xue Aimei being forced-fed with chilli oil and chilli powder. After she returned to her cell, her nose and face were all bloody and she was covered with chilli oil and food. Because we hadn't committed any crimes and were being detained illegally, all of us refused to wear the detention center uniforms. Guards Li Xiaozheng, Zhang, Meng and others, about a dozen in total, stripped over 20 female practitioners. The guards pushed naked female practitioner out of her cell to show her to male prisoners, just to humiliate her.

We also had to do hard manual labor daily. We made leather shoes. Our fingers developed blisters and became deformed. These products were exported to the US, Europe, and other countries. We were forced to work from 7:30 a.m. to midnight, and sometimes until 1:00 a.m. We weren't given any breaks during the week or on weekends. A cell was just a little over 30 square meters. There was a washroom, but there were over 30 people in the one cell. We had to sleep on our sides and often with our head next to another's feet. For food we were given mouldy rice. The treatment in the detention center was inhuman.

I was sentenced to a three-year term. On March 8, 2001, I was transferred to Shaoguan Prison (currently Guangdong Province Women's Hospital) for further persecution. Because I refused to give up Falun Dafa, Political Instructor Luo, Dai, Team Leader Zheng Zhue, Team Leader Cai Guangping, and Assistants Lin and Yang took turns talking to me daily. They used hard and soft tactics, threatened and cursed me, and attempted to brainwash me. They often forced me to watch TV programs defaming Dafa and Teacher. When I refused to give up Falun Dafa, they tortured me. They forced me to stand facing the wall, without moving or sitting down. They also deprived me of sleep. Besides talking to me, the only thing they could think of was to make me stand for a long time. Three days passed and I couldn't keep from falling down, but they woke me up and forced me to stand again. Then I fell again, stood up, fell again. Not until I couldn't stand up anymore did, they allow me to sleep. Then they told me to stand again. This went on and on relentlessly. Occasionally, they allowed me to sleep for no more than two hours.

During the few hours that they allowed me to sleep, they had two inmates with contagious diseases sleep beside me on the ground. One had TB and the other had a skin disease. Her body was rotting. The guards wanted me to contract their diseases.

One time in our meeting, I was taken to the platform. Guard Lo said in front of hundreds of people, "She practices Falun Gong. No one is allowed to talk to her nor give her any personal items." I was also deprived of buying any day-to-day items for use in the bathroom. I had to use water as I was not allowed any paper. Generally, I was watched by three to four people when I was eating, using the bathroom, and taking a shower. They monitored me closely. They always found fault with me and swore at and humiliated me. They recorded what I said and then reported it to the guards.

I didn't give up my belief. Therefore, the guards often shocked me with electric batons. They also threatened me, "If you are not 'transformed', you will be taken to the Great Northwest". The Great Northwest is located in the Northwest of China. Not many people live there but there are concentration camps, where many of the detained have disappeared. After just one month of this inhuman torture I developed high blood pressure (before, my blood pressure was normal). It exceeded 220. I felt muddle-headed. Even so, they still forced me to do 14 hours of hard labor daily. When I didn't reach the quota, they didn't allow me to take a break. I made saddles and light chains to hang on Christmas trees. I was totally exhausted. Seeing that I didn't give up practicing Falun Gong, guard Lo said, "I have been treating you too nicely". She threatened to lock me up with a mental patient in solitary confinement and have that mental patient spray urine on me. She asked me to think about it for 15 minutes. After I told her that I didn't care, she gave up.

I Became Blind in One Eye
A few days later, at about 10:00 p.m., guard Li and three criminal inmates carried me to the basement. The inmates pressed me down and tied me so that I couldn't

move. Guard Li was holding an electric baton and began to shock me. He shocked me at my acupuncture points and my sensitive parts. He shocked my Sun and Renzhong acupuncture points, and central nervous system in the cervical vertebra. He shocked me many times. I cried miserably. My heart felt as if it were torn and I was in terrible pain. I couldn't stand up. That time, they shocked me for between 30 and 40 minutes. The next morning, I could no longer see clearly. This was the result of being shocked for a long time. I demanded that team leader Zheng and guard Yang take me to Li City Hospital, which was outside the prison. The diagnosis was that the blood vessels and vision nerves at the bottom of my eyes were injured. I went blind in my left eye, and my vision was 0. The doctor said that it couldn't be healed, and I would lose my vision in that eye completely. In addition, it also would impact my right eye. My right eye was 0.1, and my left eye became 0.

The persecution by the CCP has caused great harm to me and my family. My family was separated and ruined. My husband and I were detained, and my 14-year-old daughter had nobody to take care of her. My mother passed away during this persecution. I was not told about her death.

Liu Cheng, a prisoner who participated in my persecution, said, "You are not treated the most inhumanly. Song Ping was tortured worse than you. What you suffered was only one tenth of what she suffered. When she was shocked, they poured water over her. Once she was wet all over her body, they shocked her with a few electric batons at the same time. She was shocked until she bounced off the wall then bounced back to the ground. Then she was shocked again. She was wounded all over. She could no longer eat. Then she was taken to the hospital."

After being shocked, I became blind. However, Guangdong Women's Hospital still forced me to do hard labour. When my family came to visit, I had to be escorted by two guards. The meeting room is isolated from the outside with walls and windows. We can only communicate through the telephone. Behind me, there was a guard holding another phone to monitor my discussion. He recorded it at the same time.

We were not allowed to inform family members about the persecution we suffered. If we ever said even half a sentence about what was going on inside the jail, our phone would be cut off, and we would lose the chance of being visited ever again. Therefore, if a person was detained in the prison, he was forbidden to hear any outside news, nor could those outside find out what was going on inside. Only two months before my term was due to expire did they agree to have someone bail me out for medical reasons and let my family take me home.

At 10:00 p.m. on February 27th 2003, two months after I returned home, police officer Wang Xiang from the 610 Office in Shenzhen City and over 20 police officers broke into my home. They took my husband and me to Futian District Detention Center, where I met practitioner Ms. Wang Suqin, who was 67 years old. She told me that when police officers from the 610 Office in Shenzhen City interrogated her, they locked her in a small room.

Although it was a very cold winter, they ran fans non-stop for two days and nights and deprived her of food and sleep. She told me that her son, Li Xiaoqiu, was also detained at Futian District Detention Center. Her daughter suffered from inhuman torture from the police officers in the 610 Office of Shenzhen City. Her daughter asked someone to pass a note to her, which said that she would never commit suicide. Even if [the authorities claimed that she had], she would have been tortured to death.

Sanshui Women's Forced Labor Camp

Because I wasn't "transformed", when I had been home for only two months, I was again taken to a forced labor camp for two years. I was detained in the No.3 Team in the No.1 Ward of Sanshui Guangdong Province Women's Forced Labor Camp.

At Sanshui Forced Labor Camp, I was detained in a small cell. The windows and doors were covered so that people could not see what was going on inside. I was tortured by the head of the forced labor camp, Xie, Tang; Divisional Manager Ge; Chen; Team Leader Sun; Tang, Zhang; and guard Liu Ai. They didn't allow me to write letters to my family nor allow my family members to come and visit me. They tried to brainwash me, took turns talking to me, forced me to write my "understandings" daily, deprived me of sleep and forbid me from going to the bathroom. This kind of mental torture and brainwashing was the most painful. I had noticed that some practitioners became very sick after being forced to undergo brainwashing. Some could no longer walk. Over 30 practitioners suffered from high blood pressure. I also saw that a female practitioner was persecuted to the point of mental collapse. The guard didn't notify her family. Some were skin and bones from the torture. Some were transferred to other places where they were cruelly tortured. Every time practitioners were transferred; guards brought other people into their cells and closed the doors. The practitioners who were dying were wrapped in blankets and carried by guards and prisoners secretly downstairs. No one knows what happened to them.

Every day we were forced to do hard labor sorting garbage. The garbage came from Hong Kong. It stank. We had to take all plastic and metal from the garbage. This is the type of work no one else wants to do, but we were forced to do it. Everyone was assigned a quota. If we couldn't meet the quota, our term would be extended.

In April 2004, about 160 practitioners were locked up in one room. Many police officers and doctors from Foshan City People's Hospital gave us injections and performed medical exams. I asked team leader Sun, "How come you are only examining Falun Gong practitioners and not the other prisoners as well?" She said, "Even though they want injections, they will not receive them. This is the special care the government gives you guys." A few police officers brought in a practitioner who had fainted after being injected. After seeing this, all of us resisted and did not cooperate. I was not given an injection, but some practitioners were given injections. Seeing all of us resist it, they stopped giving injections.

A few days later, police officers took a few practitioners to the forced labor camp clinic. Doctors from Foshan City People's Hospital performed exams, took blood for testing, did electrocardiograms, x-rays, and so on. The equipment to carry out these procedures was brought in by staff from Foshan City People's Hospital, and some of it was installed in luxury buses. When the doctors were giving me an electrocardiogram, they appeared to have found a problem. One asked in detail whether I had a heart problem. I said, "I was persecuted for three years, and I suffered cruel punishment. My heart sometimes stopped beating." During this medical check-up, the doctors pressed and tested my kidneys. One asked me, "Do they hurt?" They took a lot of blood. When I asked the doctor why they took so much blood, the doctor said that it was needed to test for a number of things. In the end, every Falun Gong practitioner had been given a medical check-up and had his or her blood tested. Even those who had developed a mental disorder were not exempt.

Other, non-Falun Gong practitioner prisoners didn't have to go through this. At that time, I already knew that the medical check-ups were not for our health. After the exams, I discovered that some practitioners had disappeared; I didn't know where they went. The warden said, "If you don't give up Falun Gong, we transfer you to other places." I never heard from the practitioners who were transferred. I understood the reason for these medical tests after I heard about the CCP harvesting organs from living Falun Gong practitioners. Then I understood the depth of their deceit.

Because of the long-term persecution at Sanshui Women's Forced Labor Camp, I was at the brink of a mental breakdown. My blood pressure was as high as 250. I often felt dizzy. Staff at the forced labor camp realized that my life was in danger and were afraid to take any responsibility. On September 30, 2004, they told my family to pick me up and bail me out for medical reasons.

Leaving the CCP

On the evening of September 7, 2005, police officers from the 610 Office in Shenzhen City started another round of persecution. We were warned before the police officers arrived, so we quickly left home. They arrived at our house soon after we had left. Because they couldn't find us, they searched for us citywide. They tried to track us down with electronic equipment. They set up video cameras on the road and at the exits to and from Shenzhen City in an effort to track us down.

After we left home, we wandered around for nearly two months. We made every effort to get to Thailand. Once we were in Thailand, we went to the UN Refugee Board. We told them the truth about the persecution of Falun Gong in China and our experiences. With their help we escaped the CCP persecution and now live in Norway.

We hereby acknowledge and appreciate the support and help from the UN and the Norwegian government. We also want to appeal to all kind and just people and governments in the world to join together and stop this brutal persecution!

Was there a reason given for why you were tortured?

On March 8, 2001, I was transferred to Shaoguan Prison (currently known as Guangdong Province Women's Prison). Because I refused to give up my belief, Instructor Luo, Director Dai, Chief Zheng Zhu'e, Chief Cai Guangping, Clerk Lin and Clerk Yang lectured me in turn every day. They coupled threats with promises. They threatened me, verbally abused me, and brainwashed me. They often forced me to watch programs that slandered Falun Gong and its founder. They also forced me to face the wall. I was not allowed to move, sit down or sleep. On the third day, I couldn't stand it anymore and my legs gave out beneath me. They woke me up and forced me to stand again. I fell down again, and they forced me to stand once more. This process repeated until I could not stand up again. They allowed me a short nap, but soon made me face the wall once more. They didn't allow me more than two or three hours of sleep for many days.

Even during those two or three hours, they ordered two prisoners with infectious diseases to supervise me as my "personal cangues". One had pulmonary tuberculosis (TB) and the other one had a skin disease.

During a large-scale meeting, the guards took me onto the stage. Instructor Luo told everyone that I practiced Falun Gong, and no one was allowed to talk to or share anything with me.

Every day, three or four personal cangues watched me. They followed me everywhere I went, including when having meals, using the toilet, or taking a bath. They deliberately created trouble and abused and insulted me. They reported my every word and action, throughout all 24 hours of the day, to their chief.

As I refused to be "transformed", the guards frequently shocked me with electric batons. They often threatened me, "If you don't transform, we will send you to the Northwest." Northwest referred to the concentration camps in the remote and secluded regions of north-western China, the area in or around Qinghai Province. Many people who had been sent there had vanished.

Summary of Oral Testimony: 8th December 2018

My lawyer didn't have enough time to read through the file. I hardly had enough opportunity to meet the lawyer.

From the start they already decided I had done the crime. I wasn't allowed to go inside courtroom. I heard that they said my husband had committed the crime.

What they did to my husband was very unlawful. I tried to appeal and find a relevant department. No one would listen to me. I had to go to the Beijing council to appeal. As Falun Gong Practitioner we are not even allowed to come close to those offices. We wanted to meet some foreign journalists. I was arrested in Beijing and then sent to Shenzhen and was sent to a professional bureau in Beijing.

Every day when I had to go to the toilet four criminals followed me and poured cold water on me in the winter. I had to use water to clean myself. I was not allowed toilet tissue. In every way they try to destroy your dignity.

I requested to have an eye test as they damaged my eye. After several requests they took me to an eye clinic. Two police officers came with me, one of their surnames was Deng.

I was in three different places of detention. In one there was about 30 people and I was the only Falun Gong Practitioner. In labour camp there were about 20 people and I was the only Falun Gong Practitioner. They deliberately separated us. It was the same in the reform/education process. I was the only Falun Gong Practitioner.

I didn't see any children.

In the labour camp some did repent of Falun Gong because the torture was unbearable. You go though many terrible experiences. It's not that they wanted too but they were forced to.

Many people don't even know what they're doing after torture. Everyone who repented did so because they were forced to do so.

The guards also have a quota to reach showing their supervisors that they had reformed Falun Gong Practitioners.

I did ask why they are doing this to us and not other criminals.

Falun Gong is derived from Buddhism. There are five different practices and its principles are: truthfulness, forbearance and compassion. When you practice these values you become elevated. When I was young, I was very sick and couldn't even eat fruit. Falun Gong improved my health and the doctors were amazed.

Falun Gong was legal at the time and I was practising and all the people practising had good health. Even the doctor was surprised and convinced that practising Falun Gong is good for health.

My workplace in Shenzhen was very good. When I was working there, I had a health problem and after Falun Gong my health improved. My boss was impressed.

Witness 2: Feng Hollis

Female, age 56. Languages: Mandarin (fluent), English (intermediate). Occupation in China: antique trader; current occupation: unemployed.

Detention in China
1st March 2005 – 11th April 2005 – Beijing Haidian District Detention Centre 11th April 2005 – 25th April 2005 – Beijing Forced Labor Dispatch Center 25th April 2005 – 1st September 2006 – Beijing Women's Forced Labor Camp

What was the reason given by Chinese authorities? Do you have official documentation?
Reason is because I practice Falun Gong. I have scanned copy of official document. Did you witness anything related to forced organ harvesting?

All Falun Gong practitioners in the women's labor camp had regular body checks every 3-4 months. Including: blood pressure check, blood tests, chest X-ray, weight check, kidney ultrasonic wave check.

If you were tortured in detention, please provide details.
Forced to sit on a stool for over 20 hours a day with feet closed, rest hands on knee, back straight, eyes must open and not allowed to move without permission from drug addict inmates.
Limited food each meal. Equal to one slice of bread.
Limited water to drink, even in summer under 40 degree. Was given only 500 ml a day.
Forced to watch videos slandering Falun Gong. Limited sleep. 2-4 hours a day.
Not allowed to wash hair, clothes and take shower. Was only allowed to do so after I went on hunger strike.
Forced to do hard labor.

When you were detained in China, was it ever through a court process? If yes, what was the judgment about?
I was held in a detention centre, and later given two years forced labour in Beijing Women's Forced Labour Camp without any legal procedure.

Was there a reason given for why you were tortured?
When I was held in my local detention centre, police officer Liu Dafeng was in

charge of my case, and he took me to his office every evening after 10pm. Upon entering the office, he began swearing at me using very dirty and obscene language. When he had finished interrogating me, he told me to sign their paperwork to renounce Falun Gong. I refused every time.

Because I refused to sign his paper, one time he grabbed my coat and pushed me against the wall, and at the same time he kicked my legs. I told him that Falun Gong practitioners all tried to be good people living in accordance with the principles of "Truthfulness, Compassion, Tolerance". I had not done anything wrong nor committed any crimes, so I refused to sign.

Before I was given two years forced labour and was still being held in the detention centre, the local domestic Security Division brought in four former practitioners and a few police officers to talk to me, in an attempt to force me to give up practising Falun Gong.

They talked to me from 9am to 9pm daily for three days. Finally, Yang Jian, head of the Haidian Domestic Security Division, came in person. He told me that other practitioners were not treated like this and that he did not want to sentence me. At the time I did not understand what he really meant. I thought it was because I had friends abroad.

After I was taken to the Beijing Women's Forced Labour Camp, he repeatedly came to the camp to talk to me and clearly spelled out their intentions. He asked me to be a special agent and promised me that if I agreed to work for them, they would release me immediately. I refused.

I was taken to the No. 5 Division after arriving Beijing Women's Forced Labour Camp. Two female guards were responsible for brainwashing me in an attempt to get me to renounce my belief. They took turns from 6am until 11pm. I refused to cooperate with them.

Later the head of the division Chen Xiuhua came to talk to me in person in order to force me to give up my belief. She deprived me of sleep, and I was only allowed to sleep for two or three hours per day. In the evening I felt very cold while being forced to sit on a small plastic stool. I requested to put on more clothes, but Chen did not allow it. When Chen left the room one time, I hurried to put on one more layer of clothes. As I was buttoning up my clothes Chen came in. She said, "You tried to cause a scene. Now you lie on the floor." They always tried to humiliate practitioners.

Chen forced me to watch many video programs that framed and slandered Falun Dafa. Everyone else would have a break at noon, including the camp guards. However, I was forced to get up at 4:30am. and go to bed after midnight. At noon I was forced to sit on a child's plastic chair and watch slanderous video programs over and over again.

Later, Chen talked to me almost daily from early in the morning until 2:00 am. the next day. When she took breaks, I was forced to continue watching the slanderous videos.

In June 2005, I was taken to the so-called Intensive Assault Unit. This unit was established specifically to deal with practitioners who refused to renounce their belief.

Usually, practitioners who had not given up their belief within six months would be taken to this unit, but I was sent there two weeks after arriving in the labour camp. Later, I learned that the real reason was because my local domestic security division wanted the forced labour camp to force me to renounce Falun Dafa as soon as possible. They intended to send me overseas as their spy.

In the "Intensive Assault Unit" I was initially tortured by being forced to sit on a plastic stool for at least 18 hours a day. The surface was very rough and after one or two weeks the sores began to rot on my buttocks.

There were very strict rules when sitting on the stool. I had to have both legs and knees close together, with both hands-on top of the knees and the back had to be straight. I was not allowed to close my eyes or move. When I wanted to move, I had to report to the drug addict, the inmate monitoring me, Xue Mei, and ask for permission. If I was thirsty, I had to say, "Report to monitor. I want to have some water." If the drug addict said, "Go ahead", then I could pick up a cup and drink water. When I finished, I had to say, "Report to monitor. I want to put the cup down". If the drug addict said, "Move!" then I could put the cup down. No matter what action, I had to report and ask for permission first. If I moved without permission, they would start shouting and swearing at me.

I was also not given enough food to eat. For each of the three meals a day I was only given a half-piece of steamed sour bun (probably equal to one slice of bread) with no other food. After one week, I became very skinny. I asked guard Li Ziping to increase the amount of food, but Li told me that since I refused to renounce

Falun Gong I was considered as "purposely resisting the Chinese Communist Party (CCP)". Therefore, I would purposely not be given enough food to eat.

I was also deprived of drinking water and restricted use of the toilet. I was taken to the "Intensive Assault Unit" in June 2005. The temperature in Beijing reached 40 degrees Celsius. I was only given about 500ml of water per day. When I was thirsty, I could only moisten my lips with this limited amount of water.

When I needed to use the toilet, I was forced to wait between 30 minutes to 3 hours before being allowed to go. This led my bladder to be in pain. Later, I didn't have a feeling whether I had urinated or not. Every time I needed to use the restroom, two inmates, usually drug addicts, would follow me to the toilet.

I was not allowed to wash my hair, take a shower or wash my clothes for two weeks till I began to hunger strike. Practitioners who had not given up their belief would only be allowed to wash their clothes, take showers or wash their hair once every several months, sometimes up to six months.

There was only one window open and the door was closed in my room. I sweated all the time. After two weeks my clothes became very smelly. I requested to wash them, but my request was rejected. In addition, drug addict Xue Mei swore at me because I made the request.

Because of being short of food and drink, I fainted a few times. The guard then gave me some pills, but they didn't tell me what the pills were. After taking them, I felt my head was so heavy, I then stopped taking them. I had already read many reports that guards put drugs into practitioner's meals to destroy their central nervous system in order to get them to renounce their belief.

In the "Intensive Assault Unit" I was locked in an isolation cell. Three drug addicts monitored me; each being assigned an eight-hour shift. They recorded every detail of my daily activities, such as at what time I drank water, how much I drank, and when I used the toilet, and whether I was passing water or stool. If it was passing water then how much did I pass and what was the colour of the urine, yellow or clear. If I was passing stool, they recorded whether it was dry or liquid. What was my facial expression? Whether I was happy or not happy? What did I say? When I was in bed, did I lie flat or on my side and when I turned over? The purpose of this detailed record was used as a reference for finding a psychological breakthrough.

I also had my body checked every three to four months, including blood tests, chest x-rays, ultrasonic kidneys check, blood pressure test, weight check, electrocardiogram etc. I did not really understand why they did this at the time, and only learned after I came to England, that this might have to do with the harvesting our practitioners' organs.

When you say you were held in a detention centre, and later given two years forced labour in Beijing Women's Forced Labour Camp without any legal procedure. "Who has "given" the two years?
I was held in Haidian District Detention Centre for about 40 days, when a woman with plain clothes came to see me. She stood outside my cell and started calling my name.

I then went to the cell door to acknowledge that I was the person she was calling. I was standing in the cell, while she was standing outside the cell. We could see each other through the bars and wire mesh.

She started reading the verdict that was issued by the Beijing Labour Re-education Committee, saying that I was given two years force labour. She then told me that if I think I am innocent, I can appeal when I arrive at the labour camp.

I was taken to the Beijing Dispatch Centre before being taken to the women's forced labour camp, and I was going to appeal. But when I asked for a pen and paper, the guard Wang (surname) told me that I was not allowed to have them. She said that if I want to appeal, even I wrote the appeal letter, she wouldn't pass on the letter for me.

When I arrived in the Beijing Women's Forced labour Camp, I still wanted to appeal, but I experienced the same response.

In the verdict, it said that I had 400 copies of Falun Gong materials at my home. See attached Chinese version of the verdict – translated into English.

I also have a list of confiscated items that were taken from my home and logged by the Haidian District Police Department. If you need it, I can also email it to you.

Summary of Oral Testimony: 8th December 2018
I had to work until midnight or 1am because I didn't give up Falun Gong. Before I had my own antique shop. I often came to UK on business.

When I was arrested there were international reports and the authorities knew about it.

I never received the results of the medical examination, whether they were normal or whether there was something wrong with us.

All Falun Gong Practitioners were physically examined. We had to get in the brace position. No one knew which hospitals we were taken to. I twice had problems with my feet. I didn't see other inmates who were physically checked. The other inmates would be sleeping whilst we were physically examined.

When I was in labour camp, I had not heard about organ harvesting. There were a lot of senior Falun Gong Practitioners who never renounced their faith and collapsed.

I never saw any children in the prison.

I did not witness any sexual violence against Falun Gong Practitioners in prison. Even if these things did happen, I was isolated from these things. Even drug addicts told me that the police wouldn't allow me to go close to the door.

All Falun Gong Practitioners were examined, including senior members.

We had to stand in a queue and were not allowed to look to either side. I was not aware of who was being examined.

On 24th November my case received attention of UN and inspectors came to see me at the labour camp. I met with Naomi after I was released who told me about the training group.

UN human rights organisations wanted to know how Falun Gong Practitioners were treated in the labour camp. Certain people were dragged away in 4 vans.

Some people shouted saying Falun Gong is good but police shoved cloths in their mouths. I don't know if anyone disappeared.

I also want to add that when I was arrested during my detention we were jailed and put in individual cells and weren't allowed to communicate with other Falun Gong Practitioners. Former Falun Gong Practitioners came to talk to me all day to encourage me to renounce my faith. I was the only Falun Gong Practitioner who received such talks. The leader said they didn't want to sentence me but they didn't tell me why.

The reason I was released was due to international pressure at the time and I was one of the Falun Gong Practitioner who was forced to give up my faith. For this reason, I was released. I am still in contact with Falun Gong Practitioner in China. My fellow Falun Gong Practitioner after their release they were sentenced to a third time to re-education through labour scheme. They were taken to a legal school, like a brain washing training camp. Some of them were in prison. The situation has not changed at all.

Clarification Post Hearing

The witness describes fainting and a nurse being dispatched to check what was wrong. Statement says a guard provided medication. Oral evidence says it was the nurse. Which was it? (If indeed there is a difference)?
When I was taken to the labor camp, we were forced to go to a clinic to have our body checked. I was checked by a person who I believed to be a nurse, as she was wearing a white robe.

After I fainted in my cell, the same woman in a white robe came to see me. That is why I call her "nurse". After the nurse had checked me, she left. When the guard returned to my cell, it was the guard who provided me with the medicine.

Witness 3: Abduweli Ayup

Male, Uyghur.

I am Abduweli Ayup. I was born in Kashgar city in 1973. I am currently residing in Turkey. I was arrested in August 19th, 2013 by the local Chinese State security police, because I promoted linguistic rights of Uyghur people through my online writings and opening a mother language kindergarten in Kashgar. I was arrested when I was planning to open Uyghur mother language kindergarten in Urumchi and Khoten. I was freed on 20th November 2014. On my release I found employment in an English Training Center in Kashgar. But my students became less and less because of my "criminal" background and police pressure. My friends and relatives also felt terrified about contacting me. In Kashgar the police always stopped me to check my ID, because I have experienced terrible torture during my time of detention and imprisonment, I was always terrified whenever I saw a police uniform.

Every time on checking my ID, the police would identify me by my "criminal record" and treat me badly. After being freed from the jail, I was arrested two times because of my "criminal record". First time was in December 2014, they placed me in a cell for approximately four hours. I was ordered to clean the stools away in the toilet in order to humiliate me. The second time was on the 7th July 2015. A police SWAT (special police in Chinese) team knocked me down, slapped and kicked me for about half an hour before taking me to custody having me thrown into a cell for about six hours. Since the last arrest I could not sleep at night, as I always felt nervous about being arrested again.

On the 25th August 2015, I was forced to leave Kashgar, as the police gave me a warning about renting an apartment in the city. This is how I lost the chance to live in my home city, and that is why I decided to leave the country.

When I was arrested, my arms were twisted behind my back and I was handcuffed, at the same time a hood placed over my head before I was thrown into a police van. First, I was taken to a police station where I was forced to sit on what was called 'a Tiger Chair'.

My ankles, wrists and my neck were secured to the chair by chains before my interrogation commenced. During the questioning they hit the palms of my hands while threatening me to admit that I have committed the crimes that they accused me of. Regardless of the beatings and threats I refused to admit anything. I was then taken to a detention centre at around 9:00 pm by three of the men who arrested me. First, I was taken to a hall, where they stripped me naked, there were approximately 20 convicted criminals working there whose crimes were murder, serious robbery, etc. Once I had been stripped naked, they encircled me and attacked me. Then I was thrown into a cubical type cell in which you could not stand up but only move in crouch position. There was an open toilet which give off a putrid smell that was unbearable.

The next day I was transported to Urumqi, arriving at around 9:00 pm, the same procedure of interrogation took place, secured to a tiger chair, beatings of the hands and shoulders and threatening verbal interrogation. After this ordeal, I was taken to a hospital. As I had a hood placed over my head, I don't know which hospital it was. I know they carried out a full body check, X-ray, taking saliva, urine, and blood samples, applying a cold gel before examining different body organs. After which I was then taken to Tengritagh detention centre, I was beaten up on arrival before being placed in a cell. The cell was small and constructed of glass, the detention term for this was called 3D watch, where I was beaten once more.

There were about 20 Uyghur inmates, of whom including myself the three of us were political prisoners. In the Tengritagh detention centre 60% were Uyghurs, 40% were Chinese.

The questions I were asked during my interrogation were: "Why did you return from the USA? Which organisation send you here? What relationship do you have with Uyghur organisations and other international organisations?" The main question that was repeatedly asked was "who sent you from the USA here?"

While in the Tengritagh detention centre, I never shared a cell with anyone who had been sentenced to death, but after I was transferred to Liu Da Wan Prison on the 10th September, in around November, I shared a cell with a Uyghur man called Abdurahman from Ghulja who was sentenced to death. Later I was moved to a different cell. I learned from others that he was executed in December and buried by the authorities in Gulsay Graveyard, his body wasn't returned to his family. I heard that about one month later his family wanted to plant some flowers around his grave, they were told that they didn't have permission to disturb the soil around his grave for one year. I suspect that his organs must have been removed.

Their family were only allowed to see his face before his burial, when they asked to wash his body, they were not given permission. I believe the authorities prevented them from seeing his body as they had a lot to hide. I am also aware that two other Uyghurs were executed, according to others who knew of their execution, the procedure after death was exactly the same. After the execution, the families were only allowed to see their faces, they were not allowed to wash their bodies before burial. That was the common practice at that time.

Summary of Oral Testimony: 9th December 2018

According to Chinese constitution if we are open or set up kindergarten according to law that is legal that is why we thought to make use of the legal protection to protect our mother tongue. That is why I did it. I completed master's degree in linguistics, I believe 3-6 years old is the most important period to learn mother tongue.

Because I know under Chinese constitution language is protected by law and I have written articles to show that you can use the law to protect and promote our language especially ages 3 to 6.

At the same time, I have organised conferences in Urumqi, Kashkar and Khotan mainly about promotion of mother tongue. At the time I not only promoted Uighur but encouraged others to the conference too.

The very first thing that I feel I can never forgive and forget is that I was raped.

When I was taken to Urumqi before transfer to get centre I was taken for health check. As I was black hooded, because they placed that over my head, I don't know which hospital I was taken to. The procedure was first blood, urine samples then saliva. I believe then I went through an X-ray because I remember I felt something on my chest. At the time I didn't know what was happening, I had cold gel on my body, something on top doing the check. After this checkup I was taken to the detention centre.

In Liu Da Wan prison, in September 2013, cell number 1#1 which I shared with Abdurahman from Ghulja.

I shared a cell in September then was moved to a different cell, after release I made enquiries about him, so not certain he was executed in December. After arriving in Turkey, I wrote an article about him for Radio Free Asia. After the article was published friends wrote to me and told me about what happened to him. According to a friend of his who came to Turkey the family was called by the police after the execution and told they could only see his face not his body. According to Uighur Islamic tradition we wash the body before the ritual burial, the parents cried for that right to be given to them so they could wash his body before the burial, the police refused, they said it is not allowed, you have no permission to see the body. A month later, according to Uighur tradition, we plant something, a tree or flower in the grave. When the family went to the graveyard there are people watching who approached them and said they couldn't disturb the soil for at least one year. The family wanted to find out the reason why planting something was not allowed and they were told from people who know this procedure, that most of the prisoners before execution, their organs are completely removed which is why the government, the Chinese authorities would see the body and they will know what happened.

It was published in the Independent newspaper in the UK.

As mentioned in my statement, I was taken to a hole, stripped naked and they ordered 20 convicted criminals and they did it, so it was not one person there were many. I did not mention rape in my statement because you [Rahima, the interpreter] are a woman and I couldn't tell you when I did the statement.

The three prisoners that were executed; one was Abdurahman. I know the name the other one as Kaisar. The third one I only vaguely remember, and hope is not a mistake, Iliar.

Their crime was separatism. I know Kaisar was accused of terrorism. I don't remember clearly about the third, whether his crime was separatism or counter revolutionary, but I don't know.

Witness 4: George Karimi

Male, not a Falun Gong practitioner or Uyghur.
Statement dated October 15, 2018.

On 9ᵗʰ October 2003 I was taken into detention in Beijing, China. In the beginning I was not told why. I was told there was a problem with my friend, and they needed to ask me some questions. After 33 or 37 days, I received notice that I was being charged with resisting arrest. I was being held in the Beijing detention center. My friend, Milap, who was detained the same day as I was tortured extensively. I was taken to an interrogation room in the detention center frequently where I was chained for long hours to a chair, and many times I could hear Milap screaming in a room near mine. He was forced to sign a statement, written by the police, blaming me for counterfeiting American currency. Seven months after my arrest I was still in detention and I was informed that I was being detained for counterfeiting American currency.

Milap was released a few months afterwards. When he returned to India, Indian authorities made a video. Milap had contracted AIDS in the Chinese detention center, and he was very weak and thinking that he might pass away. He did not want this false statement against me on his conscience, so he arranged for Indian authorities to make a video where he gave an affidavit saying that he had been tortured by the Chinese police and had been forced to say that [I] had done counterfeiting. His statement was that there had not been any counterfeiting and the charges were false. I was still in detention in 2006 when I was given a life sentence for counterfeiting American currency.

The court documents specifically mention that I supposedly did this using my small office black and white printer that the police had confiscated. I served 4 years in the Beijing #2 prison, when I was the first foreign prisoner to be transferred out of the country. I was transferred to Sweden, my home country, where I served until 2015, when I was finally released. I vigorously defended myself against all the charges, mainly so the Swedish government representative could know that I was innocent. In China's judicial system one must accept all the charges. If the person wants to meet his family or apply for transfer, then one must accept the charges without defense.

In the old detention center, all those that had to be executed were on the first floor. They generally take those to be executed at 5am. This is the time; we knew from the police officers that they take them at 5am. Some inmates after 11 or 12 at night they were starting to scream. We knew that they did the executions in the morning because we could hear them screaming. I have seen one of the prisoners, where they were dragging him on the floor. He was screaming and the way he was screaming, and his face is something I cannot forget. The most devastating thing to me was that he was being dragged by another prisoner. He was in full chain, handcuffs and feet. They say it is 7 kilos. One of the prisoners was dragging him, with his back on the floor. My Taiwanese translator told me he would be executed the next day. The execution building was another building from the detention center.

Apparently, it is the building where Mao's wife hanged herself. Another Chinese prisoner pointed out the building to me once. We could see it from the shower.

For a brief time, I shared a cell with a high Communist Party official who was later executed. While we were discussing, he said, sometimes they send the CCP members to witness an execution. The reason is to make them understand that if they become traitors in the future, that can happen to them. It creates fear in them. I asked him, where he has witnessed such executions? He told me the same thing as the other Chinese prisoner below the courthouse.

In prison the prisoners talked about organ harvesting. It was very common, but the prison officials did not talk about it. Government officials who were in the prison talked about it. Discussion about organ harvesting was mainly in the detention centers.

Around 1st July 2004 I was transferred to a new detention center, also in Beijing. My prison officer had 2 stars. I don't remember his name. He was in charge of my cell and another 2 or 3 cells. He didn't speak English, so another prisoner from Taiwan would accompany me and he would translate for us. Between April 2005 and May or June 2006, after the guards had arranged the killing of a Sierra Leone prisoner by having the prisoners in his cell beat him. I didn't know what happened to him after that, but I learned later that he had died of internal bleeding. In that period of time, I would meet the prison officer about 1 or 2 times per week to chat even though they were not supposed to speak with prisoners. Each time the Taiwanese prisoner would accompany me to translate. In that time, we discussed forced organ harvesting maybe 5 or 6 times. He said, "In any case, they are criminals, and they will not be needing their organs after execution, so they don't need it, so it doesn't matter". One time he said, "You know they are cremating the bodies of the prisoners who have been executed. So what the families get are just the ashes. So what is the matter if we remove the organs or not. Anyway, the prisoners are going to be executed. They don't have any use of their organs, so it is better to harvest the organs and use for others."

Another time he told me, "Recently a group of 24 or 25 Falun Gong members had to be executed. Only one of them was not executed because he or she was sick". So I asked why he or she was not executed. He proudly explained that, "If the person is sick, so the organs are of no use."

As long as a person is not convicted, he is innocent. But on the Chinese detention and court documents, they write Criminal (submission's name). How can you call someone a criminal when the guy has not been convicted? The prison officers the way they punished us; it was personal. They were enjoying it. For Falun Gong practitioners it was 2 to 3 times worse.

Summary of Oral Testimony: 8th December 2018

I had a private lawyer. Lawyers in China can't defend anybody.

I knew I had a life sentence. It was as if they were distributing chocolates or something.

I couldn't defend myself. My embassy was powerless. We had emails from American embassy, and they couldn't do anything. It doesn't matter how much an embassy is behind that person. Minimum sentence in detention was 15-20 years.

In 2006 organ trafficking issue came up in detention centres. I was talking to the guard to his office for a cigarette, as he wanted to know about Europe. He said executions were taking place in the detention centre not in the court.

They believe in reincarnation. They say no one can be reborn if their organs are missing. We were given cards to purchase food and other things. Three hundred a month. If they were going to be executed, they would remove 20 from their account. This was an indication they were going to be executed as they knew they had to pay for the bullet.

Us foreigners complained about being housed with those who would be executed. Execution is done by being shot in the head.

A lot of negotiation was done on my part, not only from Sweden but from other countries to get me released. My friend Matthew was executed in 2006. Matthew was a CCP member before he was thrown in prison. They explained everything to me, how party members are sent for execution. He said organ harvesting was not spoken about. It was known as monster prison. If someone is already a Falun Gong member it is already a crime.

I told others not to sit like Falun Gong Practitioner's do as they would transfer you to another person. After Falun Gong, it was UG, Tibetans, and then Christians. Falun Gong Practitioner's and foreigners were the only people who protested in the detention centre.

Three or four Muslims were in our cell. Prisons would use prisoners to punish other prisoners. Prisoners forced Muslim prisoners to eat pork. Christians were called underground churches. Mostly it was Falun Gong Practitioners who were persecuted.

There were no children.

They hid everything from foreigners, as we were the only ones who could pass messages out. I don't want to remember what I heard from hospital. It was horrible. A French citizen was with some Falun Gong in the hospital. I can say it was a nightmare against Falun Gong members. He told me they would gut them on the stomach; stitch them up badly so when they coughed blood would jump out.

In China everything is a business. It's a bonus system. This is very important. The way they controlled their inmates – everything was a bonus. If an inmate was behaving well, he would get a 5-point bonus. Everything is a points system.

They are experts at propaganda – better than Hollywood for deceiving the international community.

Medical staff was not allowed in executions.

I heard about organ harvesting from my Matthew who was executed. Mostly it was the prison guards who were taking about this. It wasn't a secret what they were doing. Execution was in the same building. Sometimes they use the trustworthy inmates to bring the prisoners for execution. Cleaners or kitchen staff knew more than us.

I have written a book. I have written a bit about what happened in the hospital. I will write my account and send it to the Tribunal.

Witness 5: Liu Huiqiong

Female. Occupation in China: worked at a company in Beijing, in charge of the company website and various documents. Occupation now: kindergarten teacher.

August 23, 2017
My name is Liu Huiqiong, also known by the name of Zeng Hui, and I started to cultivate Falun Dafa from 1999. I am now settled in Europe. I have been detained without charge by Beijing "610" police and illegally detained for two times and have been forced to have blood tests and the so-called physical tests for 8 times. From March 2001 to September 2001, I was illegally detained in the Beijing Municipal Public Security Bureau Detention Center. From September to October 2001, I was detained in Beijing Dispatching Division. From November 2001 to August 2002 I was detained in Beijing Women's Labor Camp. In September 2005 I was again illegally detained. I was detained for altogether 4 years due to the two illegal imprisonments in the labour camps, during which I experienced forced physical tests 8 times. Each of my physical tests has been recorded and the so-called "medical records" have been numbered. However, I myself or ordinary people have no access to these records, and they are classified as "state secrets".

September 18, 2001
At noon, 7 people – I myself, Liu Qinqin, Qin Peng and Wu Xiangwan and Wang Ying from Qinghua University, Dr Gong Kun and Chen Zhixiang from Academy of Mathematics and Systems Science, Chinese Academy of Sciences – were transferred from Beijing Detention Center to Beijing Daxing Dispatch Division in special police van. The van was like a sealed iron box with a surveillance device inside, and we could talk inside. Before entering the Dispatch Division, we were forcibly taken for health checks. I refused to have my body checked. The police threatened me: "If you do not take the health checks, I will kill you." We were forced to take otorhinolaryngology tests, blood pressure measurements, stethoscope of the heart and the lungs, blood drawing and X-ray of the chest.

October 11, 2001
In this month all Falun Gong practitioners were ordered not to eat in the morning for the morning physical tests. "610" Office ordered the Labor Re-education Department to send a special medical test van for the Falun Gong practitioners, who underwent X-rays of the chest and blood drawing. We were numbered in advance, and each blood sample tube was labeled with our numbers, and a large tube of blood was

218

drawn from us after we were confirmed by our real names. Then we were checked for our internal and external organs. This time, the number of items of health checks was extremely many. Our ears and eyes were examined carefully with a magnifier. We were also forced to have our private parts checked in an insulting way.

On October 16, 2001, more than 40 Falun Gong practitioners were handcuffed and escorted by police in two separate vans to Xin'an Labour Camp and Tuanhe Labor Camp. I was detained in Number 7 Division of Xin'an Labour Camp. The Division Chief Wang Zhaofeng and Section Chief Li Shoufen said to me during the initial days of my arrival: Only your files are yet to be completed; we still do not have your information.

December 2001
In Xin'an Labor Camp, about 700 women Falun Gong practitioners were kept in custody in Division 1 to Division 7. That day we Falun Gong practitioners were forcibly sent to the hospital for health checks. The items checked were similar to those of last time. During the time we were physically checked and tested, SWAT were stationed at the hospital to maintain order.

In Beijing Women's Labor Camp and Tuanhe Men's Labor Camp, there were over 200 riot police (SWAT), who wore helmets, boots, and police uniforms. They carried on their waist military belts two to three electric batons of different lengths. They beat Falun Gong practitioners who protested against persecution whenever they wanted in the name of anti-terrorism or maintaining stability.

In mid-December, an elderly female Dafa disciple aged about 60 who was kept in Division 4, shouted loudly at the Monday ceremony of raising the blood flag of the CCP: Falun Dafa is good, Falun Dafa is good! Dozens of policemen and SWAT officers rushed over and struck and kicked the elderly lady, knocked her to the ground, and then dragged her out of the playground, and locked her in the basement of the Intensive Training Division.

In about May 2002
All the SWAT police and the daily patrol police in Beijing Women's Labour Camp were equipped similarly: boots, police uniforms, special belts, two to three electric batons.

Every time forced health tests were carried out, all the SWAT police were present at the scenes forcing us to obey them to go through what they called physical examinations. That day "610" police and the Labour Re-education Bureau brought in their van the most advanced equipment and forced us to take physical tests, items being tested were the same as those of the previous times.

When I was detained in No.7 Division of Beijing Women's Labor Camp, the Division Chief Wang Zhaofeng and Section Chief Li Shoufen said in front of me and other people: Falun Gong practitioners are kept as spare goods.

September 28, 2005

At 9am that day, as soon as I entered my company in Beijing, a group of policemen from Shuangyushu Police Station under the command of the 610 Office rushed in and blocked the office door. They kidnapped me to Shuangyushu Police Station. "610" Office led police from Shuangyushu Police Station and raided my home at Shuangyushu and locked me on the same night at Haidian Public Security Police Branch Bureau Detention Center. I was forced to take all the so-called health checks and photographs were taken of me on the next day after I was detained there.

October 28, 2005

On this day more than 20 Falun Gong practitioners were sent to Dispatch Division, only I and Li Fei from Beijing were female. The police handcuffed me and Li Fei together and ordered us to sit in the Iveco police car.

The police drove us to Daxing Dispatch Division. Policewomen there took me and Li Fei forcibly for physical tests. The person who tested us was a male police doctor. The door was wide open, and the male police doctor yelled at us: pull up your clothes! We want to check if you have any trauma. We were very embarrassed and refused his request.

The male police doctor was annoyed and shouted at us: Report if you have any trauma. Then we were forced to do all the so-called physical tests.

December 5, 2005

Yesterday notice was given that Falun Gong practitioners would be physically tested today, while other inmates didn't need to have any physical check. In the early morning, orders were issued again that Falun Gong practitioners be not allowed to drink or eat and that more than 40 Falun Gong practitioners held here must all undergo physical checks. The atmosphere in the corridor was very tense. All police wore uniforms and carried batons on their waist. They shouted reproachfully at inmates who were assigned to monitor Falun Gong practitioners: Monitor Falun

Gong closely. If there is one Falun Gong practitioner escaping the physical tests, no inmate will have any chance to be released from the labour camp. Each Falun Gong practitioner was grasped at the arm by one to two criminal inmates and was forcibly lined up from the second floor to the first floor to be drawn blood. This physical test only tests blood. Down to the first floor we saw 10ish medical staff in white coats who had been waiting there. They were divided into two groups, each group of four people. Four tables were assembled together to serve as a temporary worktable for each group of doctors, and test tube racks were already placed on the tables. On the tube racks were clear glass-tubes. Each glass tube was labeled with a number which stands for a Falun Gong practitioner who would be drawn blood for tests. Our name was numbered in advance. When we were drawn blood, our real name was to be checked to ensure its conformity with the number and name as listed in the medical staff's notebooks. The medical staff looked tense.

On December 10, 2005, I left the Dispatch Division. 20 other Falun Gong practitioners and I were sold to Hebei Gaoyang Labor Camp as free labourer at the price of RMB1000 per person by the Beijing Labour Re-education Bureau.

You said, "However, I myself or ordinary people have no access to these records and they are classified as "state secrets"." How do you know they are "state secrets" and what does that term mean to you?
In 2002, when I was in the Beijing Women's Labor Camp, we asked the police many times for our medical exam results. The guards said that those are state secrets, even them cannot know it.

In April 2002, at the Beijing Women's Labor Camp, a guard surnamed Li told a guard surnamed Su that Falun Gong are merchandise, and that tomorrow there would be another shipment.

CCP's policy against Falun Gong is to "eradicate them physically, bankrupt them financially, and if they were beaten to death, it counts as suicide."

They do not allow Falun Gong practitioners to communicate to overseas media about the persecution. I wrote an article titled "The death of Qinghuang Kong" and it was published on minghui.org. The article describes how Qinghuang Kong, a Falun gong practitioner in Yunnan province was persecuted to death. In March 2001, a police officer from Beijing Public Security Bureau openly told me, that my article was a leak of 'state secrets' and that I could be sentenced to 7 years in prison for that. They interrogated me for 3 days. I did not speak a word.

You said, "I have been kidnapped" Questions: Does this mean "detained without charge"? Can you explain what happened and how you were 'kidnapped' and who kidnapped you?

The first time: On Feb. 19, 2001, I was with 3 Falun Gong practitioners in my home. At 11:30pm, the police from the Beijing 610 office broke into my home with "all-purpose keys". They called out my name and asked me to open the door. Some police went inside my home, some stayed outside. The police grabbed our arms, searched our bodies, and ransacked my home. They handcuffed us and took us to the van. We were taken to Beijing Haidian District Police station, then were transferred to Beijing Public Security Bureau. They said, you are Falun Gong. Falun Gong is what our country wants to suppress. We can arrest you for no reason.

In April 2001, police Zihui Hu from Beijing Bureau said, 610 Office has a list of several hundred Falun Gong practitioners. It was Jiang Zemin's order to arrest them. The head of Beijing Public Security Bureau is in charge of this. He took out the name list and asked me, do you know so- and-so (name in the list). If I caught this person, I could have at least 50,000 Yuan reward.

You said, "On December 10th, 2005, I left the Dispatch Division. 20 other Falun Gong practitioners and I were sold to Hebei Gaoyang Labor Camp as free labourer at the price of RMB1000 per person by the Beijing Labour Re-education Bureau." Did you see this transaction? How did you know about these details?

Beijing police told us in private: "Beijing Labor Camp Bureau sells Falun Gong practitioners to other cities as free labors. Four months ago, a group of them were sold to Gaoyang Labor Camp." Gaoyang Labor Camp sent two charter buses to pick us up. On the road, every two people were handcuffed together. We were asked to hide our heads behind the seats. We were not allowed to lift our heads. There were a dozen police in each bus. The police had electric batons and handcuffs.

The guards at Gaoyang Labor Camp also said publicly: "we spent 1000 yuan for you to work here." We were forced to plant potatoes and other vegetables. We were forced to make carpets. We were not paid. The labor camp has a few hundred acres of farmland and a carpet factory.

When you were detained in China was it ever through a court process? If yes, what was the judgement about?

There were no legal proceedings. The police took me from my home and my work to the detention center. I was interrogated for days in the detention center. They asked me, who were the Falun Gong practitioners I know, what Falun Gong activities I participated in. I did not answer and did not sign anything. They sent me to a labor camp where many Falun Gong practitioners were held. I was sent to labor camps twice, 1.5 years and 2.5 years.

Was there a reason given for why you were tortured?
On March 5, 2001, a Beijing police surnamed Hu told me, "you know a lot of Falun Gong, you participated in 9 Falun Gong activities. You will be heavily sentenced." Then six police came to me and started to shout at me: the government has a secret order. We don't have to obey the law when dealing with Falun Gong. We can do whatever we want to do. We can beat you to death. You will not be able to save your head.

One police started to unbutton my clothes. He humiliated me and said, "don't think about going back to your cell. I will sleep with you for sure…."

I was locked up on an interrogation chair for 20 hours without moving. They beat me. They said, "[we will] dig out your organs and burn your body."

On April 19, 2001, police surnamed Hu talked to me in his office for 2 hours. He said, "as long as you give up Falun gong, you can go home immediately. If you are willing to become our spy (and persecute other Falun gong), you will be paid several thousand yuan a month. You could even go abroad and enjoy more benefits." I refused. He said, "If you keep practicing Falun Gong, you are on a one-way street to death."

Summary of Oral Testimony: 9th December 2018
There were 700 female Falun Gong Practitioner's in one labour camp alone in Beijing. 5th March 2001, they continually questioned me for 12 nights and I did not speak because it was my human right to remain silent. 5 police chiefs from 7pm till noon next day kept beating me and swearing at me saying I didn't have human rights. He said that now that the CCP is in charge and they represent the community.

The policeman asked me questions whilst pointing at the stool I was sitting on. He said this was the stool of a death row prisoner. Not many who sat on this stool made it out alive. 5 policemen were around me all the time. One was in charge of beating me.

He unbuttoned my shirt and pushed me down and when I resisted, he pulled my hair and slapped me many times. He poked me many places on my face and my body. My face and body were swollen.

Denied water and couldn't stand up.

I kept weeping but they wouldn't stop torturing me. A policeman named was in charge of interrogating me every day. He took out a notebook and said this is a blacklist of hundreds of Falun Gong Practitioner like you and the list was requested by the president of China. The Chief of Beijing Police ordered these things.

He asked me if I knew a certain person named Lee from university. If I said yes, he would get 100,000 RNB. If they catch him, I'll get 30,000.

I was working at this company [photograph provided]. The next day the police came to my workplace and arrested me. And this time I was in prison for 2.5 years. They confiscated my ID card. My house was registered in Hunan province.

The policeman didn't know I was a Falun Gong Practitioner and that's why I got a new passport. After I got my passport, I figured out a way to get out of the country. In May 2001 the police took me to the hospital affiliated with Beijing public security bureau. The prison doctor who took me there called Lu and I asked him why he was taking me there but couldn't answer.

At the PSB hospital I had checks on my internal organs. The female doctor said to me and said my organs were in excellent condition and I was surprised. I said are you going to take them away? She said she had no other option. Your heart is too good.

After I returned, I began my hunger strike, lost a huge amount of weight and had a haemorrhage under my skin. Doctor Lu told me I had a problem but never asked me if I need any treatment. During this time the police also asked me to leave finger and palm prints.

On the A4 sheet I left my fingerprints and palm prints there was the name of a man in another province. I realised this was the name of the person who would receive my organs. They never came again probably as I was very skinny and had lots of problems. The doctors could only see our number rather than our name.

Yes all of them are [Falun Gong Practitioner]. One of them disappeared. One left China.

[The force shown] is specifically against Falun Gong Practitioner. You may remember a lady shouting Falun Gong is good and the police came to sort her out.

When I was questioned for 20 nights, I heard other Falun Gong Practitioner being beaten. We were treated in the same way as death row prisoners and we felt like one.

Clarification Post Hearing

Oral evidence says March 2001 continually questioned for 12 nights. Statement says three days. Which was it?

I lived with Cao Kai and Li Xiaodong of the Chinese Academy of Sciences and Dr. Li Tianyong of the Agricultural University in Room 102 of Tianhui Yuan in Beijing Hui Longguan District. We were ransacked by the Beijing police and forcibly abducted at 23:30 on February 19, 2001.

At 1:00 am on February 20, we were detained at the branch detention center of the Beijing Haidian Public Security Bureau. From February 20th to 27th, the police interrogated me every night.

On the evening of February 28, four of us and dozens of other Falun Gong practitioners were transferred to the Beijing Public Security Bureau Detention Center.

From March 1st to 4th, police Hu Zihui and another police officer interrogated me every night, they would not let me sleep. Before March 5, I remained silent for 12 days without speaking.

The reason for my silence: I have to tell the police which Falun Gong practitioners I know, where they live. the police said that I participated in nine Falun Gong cases, and each case was enough to sentence me to a big sentence. I can't recognize what they said, so keep silent.

Oral evidence says there was a reward of 100,000 RNB for the police officer if "Lee" was found and the witness would get 30,000. The statement says it was 50,000. Which was it?

In late March, Hu Zihui retrained me in a room on the first floor. There was a computer and a lot of office documents on the desk in the room. There was a printer in the corner of the room.

Hu Zihui took out a big book. Its length, width and height are about (22*30*3) CM. Then he said that this is the blacklist requested by President Jiang Zemin. There are hundreds of Falun Gong practitioners, and the director of the Beijing Municipal Public Security Bureau Qiang-wei Responsible for this matter.

They arrested these people for bonuses, for example, Li Huakai's value is at least 50,000 yuan. He is the Ziguang Group of Tsinghua University.

Li Wendong's value is at least 30,000 yuan. Do you know them and know where they are? If you know that you told me, I can get a sum of money.

There are a few pictures whose contents have been translated into English.

Work photo from 2005. Shown during the hearing, I think as evidence that they were working at the company described. Can the Tribunal please have a copy? (you can photograph the photo with your phone and send)

At the hearings a written account of what happened in the hospital was requested/ offered. Could you please send that but please do keep it as brief as possible.
On this day, I was forcibly taken to the Beijing Public Security Bureau Hospital. A woman who is the same age as me, our hands are tied together by the police. We are not allowed to speak. We were taken to the hospital and sent back together. At the hospital, we were examined by doctors in different rooms. She may also be a Falun Gong.

A middle-aged female doctor took me to the top of the hospital building. I saw a middle-aged man in casual clothes standing in the corridor. He may be an official responsible for human organs.

I was taken into a room in the middle of the corridor. The female doctor used the tool to force me to take blood pressure and do cardio-pulmonary auscultation, and carefully do abdominal touch check. At this point, the room door was pushed open, and the middle-aged man in the corridor entered the room. He stood on the bed and looked at me carefully. I was afraid of this person and wanted to sit up and refuse to check. At this time, the female doctor looked up and looked at the man who had just entered, and she politely said to the man: You should not come in now. The female doctor's eyes hinted at him that you would scare her. Then she looks back at me.

The female doctor said with satisfaction: the organs are very good and the heart is very good!

I said: Before the Falun Gong practice, my heart was not good and my health was not good.

She looked at me, overbearing and fiercely said: Your heart and your body is very good.

I am angry and ask: My heart and body are very good, is it not to take my heart and organs?

She said arrogantly: There is no way, the upper (official) decided. I looked at the door in anger, I want to leave here right away.

She said: I will send you back today.

Additional Documents Provided

https://chinatribunal.com/wp-content/uploads/2019/06/Liu-Huiqiong_Decision-Dismissal-certificate-of-Laojiao-ReducationThroughLabourEnglish.pdf

https://chinatribunal.com/wp-content/uploads/2019/08/Liu-Huiqiong_2_Laojiao-ReducationThroughLabour-Decision-Chinese.jpg-1.pdf

https://chinatribunal.com/wp-content/uploads/2019/08/Liu-Huiqiong_Dismissal-certificate-of-Laojiao-ReducationThroughLabour-Chinese.jpg-1.pdf

Witness 6: Jintai (Tony) Liu

Male, age 38. Languages: Mandarin (fluent)' English (beginner level). Occupation now: plasterer/gyprocker; occupation in China: Application Engineer of a Swiss company. Level of Education in China: Master's degree of Chemical Technology.

Detention in China
From the end of November 2006 to 12 January 2007, Beijing Changping Brainwashing Class.

12th January 2007 to February 2007, Beijing Changping Detention Centre.

February 2007 to 14th May 2007, Beijing Tuanhe Labour Re-education Dispatch Centre. 14th May 2007 to 11th January 2009, Beijing Tuanhe Labour Re-education Camp.

What was the reason given by Chinese authorities? Do you have official documentation?
A group of maybe five or six men from state security and 610 Office came to my classroom, and they found Falun Gong material on my computer and the Nine commentaries on the Communist Party by Epoch Times.

No, I don't have official documentation. When those men searching my computer, I asked them "why are you arresting me?" and "where is your search warrant?". Then one police officer took out a piece of paper and chucked it in front of me and said, "this is the paper that authorises your arrest".

When you were detained in China was it ever through a court process? If yes, what was the judgment about?
No, not through a court process. Without court process, I was illegally detained for two years in a forced labor camp.

Experience in Detention
Every year during my detention, the authorities would force us to have blood taken and X-rays but never notified me of any result. I suspicious that these tests may have been somehow connected to organ harvesting. I had heard about organ harvesting from internet before I was arrested. But it's hard to believe for me. April to 14 May 2007, I was locked in a cell (maybe in No. 6 Team of Beijing Tuanhe Labour

Re-education Dispatch Centre, which was an area which held many drug addicted prisoners) with about 8 drug addicts, who were commonly induced to abuse Falun Gong practitioners. Those drug addicts were rostered on shifts to persecute me by the guards' order. The cell has surveillance camera installed, so the guards know everything happened inside. One day a drug addict inmate was beating my back and waist, another inmate came in from outside yelled at him: "don't injure his organs". I felt strange why these guys did not care about my well-being but cared about my organs. What's more, I knew the drug addict inmate came from outside was just said what the guards' let him say, because without guards' order nobody could came to the cell. One drug addict once told other drug addicts in front of me: a Beijing woman's husband (a Falun Gong practitioner) disappeared after being arrested.

One day of October or November 2007, when I was tortured to give up my belief, a guard (name is Li Wei who was a key person to try and torture Falun Gong cultivators) threatened me privately, he came to see me (almost face to face), stared at me and said "nothing is impossible!" Then left.

In order to let me give up my belief to Falun Dafa, the guards let prisoners tortured me a lot of times.

For example, during September or October 2007, I was transferred from the Fourth Brigade of Tuanhe Re-education Labor Camp to a specially-designed room in another brigade (by guards: Gong Wei, Pan Lin, Yang Bo). The walls and ground of that room were covered with soft sponge in order to prevent inmates from committing suicide. They starved me for three days, and then prisoners dragged me around the room. They claimed that I was on a hunger strike and had the prison doctor force- feed me twice daily. The doctor pushed plastic tubes through my nose into my stomach. They often pulled the tubes in and out several times just to torture me. Prisoner Zhang Guobing also urinated into the sticky fluid used to force-feed me. After two weeks, the guards realized again that their torture methods hadn't changed my resolve, so they transferred me back to the Fourth Brigade to continue my persecution.

November 2007, guards Li Wei and Yang Bo in charge of torturing me to give up my belief. They transferred a specific group of seven or eight prisoners from Beijing Tuanhe Labour Re-education Dispatch Centre to the labor camp. The guards trained them intensively, and then along with prisoner Zhang Guobing, ordered them to take turns with the torture. During the day, four prisoners participated. Zhang

Guobing is the leader and included Zhang Wenbin and Liu Jinsuo. They shoved my feces into my mouth. Zhang Guobing ordered the other three to strip my clothes, and then forced a toilet brush handle into my anus. They pushed the handle so hard that I couldn't defecate. They also handled my genitals and forced my back against an extremely hot heating unit. The other shift of three or four prisoners included one named Du Fu, and another nicknamed "Little Shandong". They stripped me and handled my genitals. "Little Shandong" pulled my pubic hair, and they opened the window to freeze me with the winter's cold air. They also pinched my nipples hard with their nails. A prisoner whose last name is Ma, he led Yuan Li and another prisoner torture me at night. They woke me at night by pouring cold water on me, or by piercing my skin with needles. They then dragged me to the ground, stripped me and poured cold water over me. Yuan Li often used a sharp point on his badge to puncture my nails. I have been tortured like above for two days and two nights.

I have also suffered lots of other tortures in the Fourth Brigade of Tuanhe Re-education Labor Camp. The prisoners forced to me sit still on a small plastic stool for an extended duration. They also forced me to stand motionless for long periods, until my legs and feet were badly swollen. Additionally, there were times that they denied me restroom use, forcing me to urinate and defecate in my pants. I was forced to wear those pants, even during meals. Another time, guard Zhao Weiguang ordered the prisoners subject me to sleep deprivation, allowing only 2-3 hours of sleep a day. They then shortened it to one hour per day, and eventually to no sleep at all. One prisoner tied threads to my eyebrows, then pulled them off. He eventually pulled all the hair off my eyebrows. He then used the same method to pull off my eyelashes and facial hair. Prisoner Zhang Guobing spat on my face and body, and once even forced my mouth open to spit into it. Guards and prisoners tortured and humiliated me physically and mentally.

The "Three Statements" that I have been forced to write as follows: the "Guarantee Statement", the "Dissociation Statement", and the "Repentance Statement".

The Guarantee Statement let me abide by the rules and regulations of the labor camp, do not practice the Falun Gong exercises or spread the FG to others.

The Dissociation Statement asked me to declare my dissociation from the "Falun Gong" association. (Actually, Falun Gong does not have any "association". No one supervises me or forces me to do something.)

The Repentance Statement let me plead guilty to breaking the nation's laws and constitution, feel sorry to my parents, the country and the party.

Let me write three statements is extremely evil. Because Falun gong teaches me Truthfulness, Compassion, Forbearance; asks me to be selfless and considerate of others under all circumstances; gives me a healthy body by practice the Falun Gong's five exercises, etc. Why should I sign those false, mean, shameless "Three Statements"?!

So from being kidnapped to Beijing Changping brainwashing class at the end of November 2006, to being detained to Beijing Tuanhe labor camp in November 2007, I have always refused to write this so-called "Three Statements" no matter how the police and prison guards (or prisoners who follow the guards' order) deceive, threaten, torture me.

However, in November 2007, I finally could not bear the tortures from the labor camp and wrote the "Three Statements" in violation of my heart. Then I was afraid to use my conscience to think about the so-called three statements, because if I use the conscience of a normal person to look at the statements, they are all fakes, they can't be written, I would can't pretended to be transformed. And the guards would let the prisoners torture me again. Under those tortures, I was completely beaten. I feel that I have betrayed my belief, sold my soul and conscience in order not to be persecuted, and live like a walking dead. I feel dead is better. But our Master taught us that we can't kill others or commit suicide. So I wish I could go abroad to expose the persecution of the evil party, that is also an excuse to persuade myself to live.

Were documents provided when you were taken into detention?
Kidnapped from my university to brainwashing class:

Only when I asked them for document at the university, they wrote a piece of paper on site and throw it there; and then they kidnapped me, so I don't know where's that paper later.

From Brainwashing Class to Beijing Changping Detention Centre:

Because I didn't give up my belief, they sent me to the Detention Centre, but gave me nothing and no explanation.

From Beijing Changping Detention Centre to Beijing Tuanhe Labour Re-education Dis- patch Centre, Beijing Tuanhe Labour Re-education Camp:

On January 12th 2007, they transferred me to the Changping Detention Center. I refused to cooperate with them as well and didn't sign any statements, because I firmly believed that there was nothing wrong with practicing Falun Gong. After being held in the Chang-ping Detention Center for over 30 days without legal procedures, officials suddenly announced that I was to be taken to a forced labor camp for two years (from January 12th 2007 to January 11th 2009) without any documents to me. Due to this decision, they immediately transferred me to Beijing Tuanhe Labour Re-education Dispatch Centre, and Beijing Tuanhe Labour Re-education Camp.

Was there a reason given for why you were tortured?
My belief to Falun Dafa is the reason to be arrested and tortured.

At the brainwashing class, they said if I gave up my belief, and wrote the so-called three statements, that would send me back to my university to continue my studies. Because I refused, they transferred me to the Beijing Changping Detention Centre.

At the Detention Centre, they let me tell them where's my Falun Gong books and materials come from? Who I connected with? I refused to tell anything and have been illegally declared two years' labour camp.

At Beijing Tuanhe Labour Re-education Dispatch Centre, they tried to let me wrote the three statements, and said if I won't write the three statements, I must write a guarantee statement to abide by the rules and regulations of the labor camp at least; and then it's the Tuanhe Labour Re-education Camp's duty to let me write the three statements. When I can't bear the tortures there and wrote the guarantee statement to comply with the regulations of labor camps, the Dispatch Centre's guards stopped torturing me.

At Beijing Tuanhe Labour Re-education Camp, almost every time when the guards or inmates torturing me, they would ask "Will you still practice Falun Gong?" or "Will you write the three Statements?" After I bowed down temporarily under the brutal torture, my life became slightly easier. Although I was still forced to watch brainwashing videos, they stopped torturing me in a single cell, let me live in a cell with other forced transformed Falun Gong practitioners and several inmates who monitor Falun Gong practitioners not to talk with each other. And sometimes let me do the labor camp's slave work (better than watching brainwashing videos).

Summary of Oral Testimony: 9th December 2018
During my detention the prison guards used certain words to insult me and Falun Gong, in particular in the brainwashing centre e.g. "your master is a liar who is only

there to collect money", "your master has gone to America and you are suffering because of him", "why does your master let you suffer here? Why doesn't he come and save you?" They had even prepared a video to insult Falun Gong and our teacher. I tried my best not to listen and not remember any of it, to put it out of my mind. I still practise Falun Gong.

After I signed three statements and until January 2009, I was with other people who have been transformed. They were there watching us. I do not really know if anyone disappeared.

There were no underage children there. I was probably the youngest at the time, so they told me. There was the elderly person of 60 or 70. He had bleeding in the brain, so they let him out, I think.

I consider Falun Gong to be just a belief. At the time, other than Falun Gong there was nothing to stop me losing my morale. As for religion, maybe western people think differently. I just want to follow the principles of truthfulness, compassion and forbearance.

When they were beating me, their purpose was to make me write three statements. Before I went in there were reports of organ harvesting. I was very surprised as I thought they might consider my organs as useful. I did not want to believe that. I rather wanted to believe they cared for me a bit.

Witness 7: Hong Chen

Female, age 54. Occupation in China: workshop manager at a textile factory; occupation now: cleaner at the Australian Parliament House.

When you were detained in China was it ever through a court process?
No Court processes for my detention and labour camp imprisonment

What was the reason given by Chinese authorities? Do you have official documentation?
After Jiang Zemin started cracking down on Falun Gong, in order to clarify the truth, I went to Beijing to appeal. On 25th October 1999, I was arrested and detained in Beijing Chaoyang District Detention Centre for 5 days. After that I was transferred to Tianjin Lutai (near my home) Detention Centre and was detained there for 3 days, then I was sent to Tianjin Women's Detention Centre, where I was detained for 10 days, then was sent back to local Lutai Detention Centre and detained for another two days. No documents were given to me for the 20 days detention. On 15th November 1999, I was taken to Lutai Textile Factory of Ninghe County, Tianjin, where I used to work before I lost my job in 1996. I was detained there for 40 days and was released after my husband was called in to sign the Guarantee and paid ￥1000 penalty.

One day in Feb 2000, I went to a photocopy shop to copy some new Jingwen for fellow practitioners. I don't know how this was found out, several days later, on 15th February 2000, I was taken by authorities? at home and taken to Lutai Textile Factory again. This time I went on a hunger strike to protest against the illegal detention. I was released after 32 days.

Between 25 Oct 1999 and 25 Apr 2000, my home was raided 5 times, for only once I was given some paper for the raid.

On 24 April 2000, I was sentenced to one-year re-education through labour, and was imprisoned in Tianjin Banqiao Women's Labour Camp from 24 April 2000 to 23 April 2001 (Certificate available). In the labour camp I was forced to do hard labour work without pay, 14–17 hours every day, sitting on a ma-zha (a folding stool bonded by canvas belts, see illustration below) which caused me anal fissure, prolapse of the anus and hemafecia. I was also blood-tested 3 times in the labour camp, and no explanation or results were given to me.

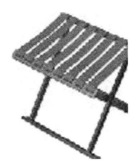

Did you directly witness incidents of forced organ harvesting or were you threatened with forced organ harvesting?

In October 2000 in the labour camp, the Head of Brigade 2, surnamed Ma, said that there was instruction from up above: Those who do not give up practicing Falun Gong will be sent to the north east remote area to die.

In October 2000, a Falun Gong practitioner, surnamed Zou, was brought in the labour camp. I found that her eyes were staring blankly, like in a trance. She happened to sit next to me when we were doing hard labour work. I saw her two palms were all black and purple, so I asked her what was wrong. She suddenly burst out crying, I was shocked. She told me that it was too horrible. She and some other Falun Gong practitioners who refused to say their names, were detained in an unknown place. Each one was given a number. She was forced to sit in an electric chair and her two palms were blackened by the torture of electric needle. Because it was so painful that she cried out loudly. A policeman from the same hometown recognized her dialect and told her secretly: It is a very dangerous place here; you'd better tell your name so that you can survive. Under the help of this policeman, she was sent from that unknown place to my labour camp.

Now living in Australia, I can safely practice Falun Gong. I have been trying my best to help those who are still persecuted in China. In 2016 I learnt that Falun Gong practitioners Yixi Gao and his wife, living in Muling, Mudanjiang City, Heilongjiang Province, were taken from home by police at midnight on 19 April 2016. He died on 29 April. It was reported that he stayed in the Public Security Hospital, Mudanjiang City, for 43 hours and went through dozens of checks and examinations before he died. His body was dissected.

Further notes

On 15 Feb 2000, I was cooking breakfast at home, 4 policemen came to our home. They said they wanted me to go with them to the police station for some investigation, I asked investigation about what, they wouldn't answer, just dragged me into the van. At the policemen station, they asked me whether I had printed Falun Gong materials, I said No. Several hours later, they couldn't get any info from me, so they drove the van to the textile factory I worked and handed me to the Factory Director, saying that he needed to watch me and if I disappear, then he would be the one to take responsibility. So the Factory Director assigned 6 staff members to watch me in three shifts, two at a time, sleeping in the same room with me.

Summary of Oral Testimony: 9ᵗʰ December 2018

I was blood tested two times during my time in the detention centre. I was very tired, overtired during the time in the labour camp due to the labour we were given to do daily. They used our tiredness as an excuse to do medical tests on us. Nobody prescribed any medicine after the blood tests nor reduced our labour.

When I was released, I went to Australia.

I was detained in 1999 because I would not give up my belief in Falun Gong. I can give you a copy of the decision. I also have a copy of the search warrant. [The witness holds up document 1 and 2 to the camera]. I was not threatened with organ harvesting.

Almost every day I call all the government departments to ask them to release detained Falun Gong practitioners. I call hospitals and people who participate in organ harvesting. I do not have any recordings of these phone calls.

Additional Documents Provided

https://chinatribunal.com/wp-content/uploads/2019/06/HongChen_Decision-on-Re-education-through-Labour-English.pdf

https://chinatribunal.com/wp-content/uploads/2019/08/HongChen_Decision-on-Re-education-through-Labour-Chinese.jpg.pdf

https://chinatribunal.com/submissions/hongchen_instructions-on-the-handling-of-chen-hongs-mistakes-chinese-jpg-2/

https://chinatribunal.com/wp-content/uploads/2019/08/HongChen_Instructions-on-the-Handling-of-CHEN-Hong%E2%80%99s-Mistakes-English.jpg.pdf

https://chinatribunal.com/submissions/hongchen_instructionsonremovingchenhongspartymembershipenglish-jpg-2/

https://chinatribunal.com/wp-content/uploads/2019/08/HongChen_List-of-Withheld-Articles-English.jpg.pdf

https://chinatribunal.com/submissions/hongchen_list-of-withheldarticleschinese-jpg-2/

Witness 8: Zhang Yanhua

Female, age 48. Occupation in China: factory worker; current occupation: unemployed.

Detention in China

3rd November 2001, Harbing Female Prison, Heilongjiang Province, 7 years

2005, Jiang'an Police Station, Qiqihar City, Heilongjiang Province, 2 days and 2 nights 21st March 2017, Zhonghua Street Police Station, Qiqihar City, Heilongjiang Province,3 days. Three days later, transferred to Qiqihar City Detention Centre and held there until 4th July 2017.

What was the reason given by Chinese authorities?

For printing materials of Falun Gong truth and putting up posters of Falun Gong truth. Official Documents available: verdict and arrest notice

When you were detained in China was it ever through a court process? If yes, what was the judgement about?

There was some legal proceeding.

When I was arrested in 2001, I was sentenced to 7 years in prison.

On March 21, 2017 when I was arrested there was a "permit to arrest." Then my case was sent to the procuratorate. Because I went on hunger strike and was tortured, my life was in danger. I was released on medical parole on July 4, 2017

Did you witness anyone in the detention centres talking about forced organ harvesting?

Yes. Can't recall detailed time. When in prison, I heard an inmate saying: her hometown is Sujiatun, Shen Yang, it is cheap to do kidney transplant? in her hometown. She also said live organ harvesting exists.

Did you witness anything related to forced organ harvesting?

When in prison, I was forced to have my blood tested. On March 21, 2017, when I was arrested and held at the Detention Centre, I was forced to my blood and my heart tested.

If you were tortured while in detention, please detail briefly below.

Reason: Adherence to belief

At Heilongjiang Female Prison: police directed inmates to torture many times. Tortures include being hung up by handcuffs, freezing, handcuffing to the back for long periods of time, sitting on a small stool for a long time, confining clothes, deprived of sleep, toothpick pricking, not allowed to go to the toilet

At Zhonghua Street Police Station and Detention Centre, Qiqihar City: tortures included: being poured cold water, handcuffing to the back, sitting on a iron chair, being beaten up.

Were you given any reasons for the blood tests and the results?
When I first entered the detention center, the blood test was done with no reason nor results. After I went on hunger strike for 60 days, they took a tube of blood. Then 5 or 6 days later, they took another tube of blood. When the blood test was done for the third time, they took me that they wanted to know what was deficient in my body. But they never showed me the results.

The first time I was in the detention center, they took me directly to the clinic inside the detention center and did blood draw and examined my heart. The second time after 60 days of hunger strike, they took the blood right outside the cell. The third time, it was done just outside the cell. The cell mates saw it, and said, "It's only been a few days in between the blood draw. Even if one eats regularly, one can't reproduce blood this fast. You should start eating. Otherwise, your blood can't be reproduced." At this time, the person who drew my blood said that the purpose was to see what was deficient in my body. But I feel that it was an excuse. Because I was on hunger strike for 60 days already. I only had some fluid through IV. My body was very weak. Two consecutive blood draws did not make sense.

The heart exam was done in the detention center clinic. Three times blood draw, 1 tube each time. The same doctor who works in the detention center did it. I don't know the name. I did not see other people being blood tested. The first time was in the clinic. The 2nd and 3rd times were just outside of the cell. They did not ask me any questions.

Was there a reason for why you were tortured?

In Prison
Since 1999 when the persecution started, the prison is a place to torture and humiliate practitioners.

The purpose of torture is to force practitioners to give up the belief. The torture methods include hanging for a long time on the wrists, freeze, stand still for over 12 hours, sleep deprivation for 7 nights while tied up. I was once locked up in a room from 5am to midnight. The window on the door was covered with paper. A dozen inmates (non-practitioners) and 2 to 3 guards would surround me and defame Falun Gong, humiliate me and torture me. They said, "If you give up Falun Gong, and say it is not good, say you have been deceived, we will not treat you like this. We will let you sleep and rest."

In Police Station
The type of tortures in the police station include being tied up on the iron bench for 2 days and 1 night, the four limbs being tied and stretched for a long time, sleep deprivation.

The purpose was to have me sign a statement. The police said, "The statement is to say that you are guilty for distributing flyers and hanging up posters. You must sign quickly. If not, I will torture you."

In Detention Center
In order to force me to do labor, they stripped off my clothes and poured cold water on me. They asked other inmates to beat me. I said to the police, "the inmates beat me." The police said, "you don't work, you don't obey the rules, that's why they beat you." I said, "you are breaking the law." the police said, "yes."

The tortures include freeze, being handcuffed in the back and feet were also cuffed, sleep deprivation for 7 to 8 days, force feed while I was on hunger strike, the food that was force fed to me contained large amount of salt.

Summary of Oral Testimony: 9th December 2018
On the second day of my detention, I was asked to undergo manual labour, which I refused on the basis that I was being unlawfully persecuted. In the detention centres, physical labour is profitable.

Three or four inmates beat me up for my refusal; they slapped me and beat my head. After they beat me up, the supervising Police Officer entered the room, despite my protestation to him about my ill treatment, he simply told the inmates to "keep beating her". I confronted him that he was violating the law, but he didn't care and left the room.

The next day, whilst I was in the interrogation room with the officer, I asked him: "How could you allow them to treat me like this". He instead warned me to fall in line. The Police Officer indicated that he was off duty for the next two days and he said, with a sinister smile, "I hope you would have fallen in line when I get back".

I knew what was going to happen to me because the I had seen how over the years, the Chinese Communist Party directed people to beat up others illegally. I was certain about my fate. Later on, two to three inmates pulled me from a 1m height and dragged me to toilet which had a transparent glass (so that all could see). I was stripped naked, and the prisoners poured barrels of cold water on me. I was so cold and suffocating – the water went directly to my ears (I hadn't eaten or drank water for five days). I cried out "Master help me" because I couldn't bear it. The weather must have been minus twenty degrees. I resisted the tests based on what I had heard from the inmate as well as what I heard from the outside. The inmate was not a Falun Gong Practitioner but was a criminal.

There was a copy [of the arrest and search warrants] taken from my phone – I didn't bring the original copy. I am able to supply them to the tribunal.

Other inmates threatened me with force organ harvesting. Furthermore, the police also threatened me with electrocution. These threats were made in prison.

After 1999, the persecution of the Falun Gong was very dirty. I had read about it before and was scared. In 2011, when I was kidnapped, I was detained for five days. One policeman uttered very crude language to me. The police said they'd keep me to cook for them. I felt it was too dangerous staying with them. It was very scary.

I was released November 3rd 2008 and served the entire sentence. The police didn't care about my welfare; case in point, when I was on hunger strike and suffocating from freezing cold water. I had to be injected with glucose during my time on hunger strike. In fact, bribery amongst the police was commonplace and my family bribed the police so that I may be granted medical leave.

Additional Documents Provided

https://chinatribunal.com/wp-content/uploads/2019/06/Zhang-Yanhua_Court-Documents-ENGLISH-Wang-Wenlong-Zhang-Yanhua-Wang-Yuxian.pdf

https://chinatribunal.com/wp-content/uploads/2019/08/Zhang-Yanhua_Chinese1.jpg.pdf

https://chinatribunal.com/wp-content/uploads/2019/08/Zhang-Yanhua_Chinese2.jpg.pdf

https://chinatribunal.com/wp-content/uploads/2019/08/Zhang-Yanhua_Chinese3.jpg.pdf

https://chinatribunal.com/wp-content/uploads/2019/08/Zhang-Yanhua_Chinese4.jpg.pdf

https://chinatribunal.com/submissions/zhang-yanhua_chinese5-jpg-2/

Witness 9: Jiang Li

Female, age 44. Occupation in China: baker with Shanghai Airlines; current occupation: newspaper distribution.

My name is Jiang Li, daughter of Jiang Xiqing, a Falun Gong practitioner who has been persecuted to death. The following is my testimony to be submitted to the Independent Tribunal.

On January 28, 2009, my father Jiang Xiqing was persecuted to death by Chongqing government and legal departments. We, Jiang Xiqing's family members, attempted many a time to negotiate with them, but in vain. We had to hire lawyers from Beijing to take legal actions. However, on May 13, the two lawyers from Beijing whom we had hired – Li Chunfu and Zhang Kai – and Jiang Xiqing's family members were handcuffed, then hung up and beaten up cruelly by Chongqing police. This is the case of lawyers being beaten up that shocked the whole world.

As per descriptions from the autopsy report of my father (literally translated), "Number (four), skin of the body (the chest, both elbows and armpits, "deng") scatter, existing, black, purple, regions. The left fourth, fifth, and sixth ribs fractured. Small amount of intercostal bleeding between the left fifth and sixth ribs, and between the sixth and seventh ribs". "Skin of the body" refers to the skin of Jiang Xiqing's corpse. "The chest" does not mean the left of the chest, nor the right of the chest, nor the upper part of the chest, nor the lower part of the chest. It means the whole of the chest. "Scatter" means in different directions and all over. "Existing" means to be really there. "Black" refers to the colour of the skin. "Purple" refers to the colour of the skin. "Regions" means areas or parts of the body. To put all the phrases together, it can be paraphrased as "Patches of black and purple coloured wounds scattered all over the chest of Jiang Xiqing's body."

http://www.aboluowang.com/2009/0520/130074.html
https://www.peacehall.com/news/gb/china/2009/05/200905142226.shtml
http://www.ntdtv.com/xtr/gb/2009/05/15/a295138.html

The character in the bracket "deng" does not mean "equal to". It means "similar to". This is to say that other parts of Jiang Xiqing's body, besides his chest, similarly had patches of wounds scattered all over.

The spots of blood and the patches of black and purple wounds scattered all over Jiang Xiqing's body (1) were not born with, (2) neither were they scars of natural growth, (3) least of all were they possibly caused by operational negligence during the process of emergency treatment, and (4) they were indeed the results of violence and beating.

Therefore, the strongest ribs – left number 4, 5 and 6 ribs – being fractured and small amount of intercostal bleeding between the left fifth and sixth ribs were caused by violent beating. All of my father's internal organs have been extracted and were made into specimens.

Here is a recount of what happened:

My father was abducted by police the third day after the Wenchuan Earthquake in 2008 when he was at home watching TV.

The police didn't present any ID or warrant. He was sent from Youxi Police Station to Jiangjin Detention Centre, then sentenced to Xishanping Labour Camp for a year without having any legal documents. During his detention, my sister Jiang Hong once went to the National Security Bureau and inquired about my father's situation. Mu Chaoheng, a policeman from the National Security Bureau, said that he had the power and that he could persecute whomever he wanted to for as long as he desired. He continued to threaten: "last time (in 2000), when Jiang Xiqing and Luo Zehui were sent to the brainwashing class, your father was not sentenced to detention in the labour camp nor was he jailed at my discretion, because I was considering your father's old age and his difficulty to look for a job, plus expenses and fees that your family had to pay. But this time, I will sentence Jiang Xiqing to one year in the labour camp."

On August 4, 2008, Jiang Hong and several others went to visit my father at the labour camp, but was told that my father was receiving "training" and punishment. Later, Jiang's family members asked for many times to visit Jiang Xiqing, but they were all illegally rejected.

On January 27, 2009, which was the second day of the Chinese New Year, at 3.40pm, I myself, Jiang Hong, Jiang Hongbin, and my niece Jiang Guiyu went to Xishanping Labour Camp to visit Jiang Xiqing, and we met him at the gate of Second Section, Division Seven. Jiang's health was normal.

On January 28, 2009, the third day of the Chinese New Year, at about 3.40pm, Chongqing Xishanping Labour Camp called to notify us that Jiang Xiqing died of acute myocardial infraction at 2.40pm that afternoon.

After several hours of negotiation, at 10.30pm on that day, I myself, Jiang Hong, Jiang Hongbin, Jiang Ping, Zhang Daming, Chen JIxiang and Li Jia went to the mortuary. When Jiang Xiqing was pulled out from the freezer, his body was found to have many bruises on it, but it was still warm on his philtrum and his chest.

All members of our family felt father's body and it was warmer than the hand; my father's upper teeth were tightly biting his lower lip (the expression on his face was full of pain.) This is what our family saw in the mortuary.

We asked for emergency rescue and were declined brutally. Jiang's family members shouted loudly for help and called 110, but they were dragged away from the spot by the many law-enforcement officers by force. Jiang Xiqing, still with obvious signs of life at that time, was pushed back into the freezer in the mortuary. Many of the law enforcement officers smelled of alcohol at that time.

Normally, after a person dies, when he/she is stored in a freezer, it takes no more than 2 to 3 hours for the body to cool down. But when Jiang Xiqing's families found that Jiang Xiqing's body was still warm, it was still almost 10 hours after the Labour Camp announced his death.

On February 8, 2009, Jiang Xiqing's body was forcibly cremated, under the command and supervision of Zhou Bolin and Tan Xi, directors of Prison and Detention Centre Supervision Division of No 1 Branch of Chongqing Municipal People's Procuratorate, before there was an official autopsy and without the approval of Jiang's family. Other people who were involved in eliminating evidence by cremating Jiang's body were: Zheng Guanglun, Deputy Chief of Xishanping Labour Camp; Liu Hua, Section Chief of Management Section of Xishanping Labour Camp; Mao Shaoyong, Deputy Section Chief of Management Section of Xishanping Labour Camp; Tian Xiaohai, Division Chief of No 7 Division of Xishanping Labour Camp; Wang Jing, Section Chief of No 2 Section of No 7 Division of Xishanping Labour Camp; Hu Guihua and Zeng Zhiqi, police officers of No 2 Section of No 7 Division of Xishanping Labour Camp.

All J iang Xiqing' s Organs Have Been Extracted and "Made into Specimens" (Recording available – link to download the audio will be provided)

On the afternoon of January 29, 2009, family members of Jiang Xiqing and the defendants met for negotiations in Room 422 of Yuxun Hotel, Beibei District, Chongqing.

During the negotiation, the plaintiffs and Jiang's families questioned on the many spots of bruises on the right of Jiang's chest. The labour camp authorities and other government and legal departments explained that they were caused by "Gua sha," or scraping. But when Jiang died, it was already winter, and there was no reason for scraping.

On March 27, 2009, Zhou Bolin, director of Prison and Detention Centre Supervision Division of No 1 Branch of Chongqing Municipal People's Procuratorate, delivered to Jiang's families at Yuxun Hotel, Beibei District, Chongqing, an autopsy report – Chong Fa (2009) A Zi No. 2729 – issued by Chongqing Forensic Institute on March 23, 2009. This issuing date was around 40 days away from the autopsy. This report did not have any medical explanation, and imprudently came to a conclusion that Jiang Xiqing died of "coronary atherosclerotic acute heart attack, which caused acute myocardial ischemia, resulting in acute respiratory failure.

When being strongly questioned and protested by the family members of Jiang, the law enforcement officers present explained that the wounds were caused by "chest compressions".

Cardiopulmonary resuscitation (CPR) is an emergency procedure with chest compressions on the middle of the chest, and except for young children, very unlikely causing rib fractures. Even in case of rib fractures, they happen in symmetry, and would not be as described in the autopsy report "The left fourth, fifth, and sixth ribs fractured.

Small amount of intercostal bleeding between the left fifth and sixth ribs, and between the sixth and seventh ribs", which precisely corresponds to the wounds caused by beating.

On March 27, 2009, Jiang's family went to Room 422 of Yuxun Hotel, Chongqing, for the autopsy report of Jiang Xiqing. In the recording, the director of Prison and Detention Centre Supervision Division of No 1 Branch of Chongqing Municipal People's Procuratorate clearly stated that Jiang Xiqing's organs were all extracted and made into specimens.

You said "On the afternoon of January 29, 2009, family members of Jiang Xiqing and the defendants met for negotiations in Room 422 of Yuxun Hotel, Beibei District." Who are the defendants?

'Defendants' refers to the labor camp officials, Procuratorate. "Heaps of people in the room. Others were in plainclothes, public security, etc. But those who were identified were labor camp officials and Procuratorate. It's not a court process. It was after they grabbed us and tried to make us sign the documents to cremate the body; the purpose of the meeting was they wanted to force us to sign to agree to cremate. This was the first meeting. It was a private meeting".

Summary of Oral Testimony: 9th December 2018

Inside the mortuary, we were briefed on the internal policies. In particular, we were proscribed from seeing the whole of my father's body and could only view his face. Mobile phones or other recording devices were restricted and a body search was required as a condition for entry.

We didn't get the chance to evaluate his body [and see if there were stitches or injuries]. There were approximately 20 Police Officers there, of which ten rushed in to pull us out of the room. In particular, one policewoman said, *"In any case we have the death certificate that confirms your father is dead"*. My sister attempted to administer mouth-to-mouth resuscitation on our father. However, they said any efforts would be useless and we were forcefully removed from the room. The whole process lasted about five minutes.

We didn't sign the [autopsy] report. No I do not know when the autopsy was carried out. The autopsy report was issued to my sister and uncle after a month of them chasing for it. The report was error-ridden: the first version had a doctor's signature and listed my father's age as 66, whilst the second version did not have a doctor's signature and listed his age as 45.

We visited my father around 3pm [on January 28th 2009] and when we talked to him, his health was very good. Indeed, his health was always good. I had asked him if he had been subject to torture or physical abuse. He indicated that he had been forced to stand and wasn't allowed to shower; he was locked up in a very small cell from morning till afternoon. I don't think at the time of my visit he was subject to any physical abuse that might have caused earlier bruises.

On 14 May 2008 my father was arrested but we were not told why. Up to 20 Police Officers stormed in. My mother was arrested first and then my father. In addition, their home was raided by the police afterwards and they found Falun Gong material. I do not know why they took my father's organs [as Zhou Bolin said, that they had been made into "specimens"]. He was in good health when we saw him. Why didn't they allow us to check his body? Even if his organs were transplanted, we would not be told that – they would say it was for specimens.

I am a practitioner of Falun Gong. I also think Falun Gong is a belief.

Additional Documents Provided

https://chinatribunal.com/wp-content/uploads/2019/06/JiangLi_AudioTransciption_English.pdf

Witness 10: Huang Guohua (David)

Male, Aged 46. Profession in China: sales; current profession: owner of a flooring company. Languages: Mandarin, intermediate English.

Detention in China

Place of incarceration: No 1 Re-education through labour camp, Guangzhou City, Guangdong Province

Date of incarceration: Oct 31, 2000 to Jan 30, 2001, Nov 20, 2002 to Dec 16, 2003

What was the reason given by Chinese authorities?

They said I had 'disturbed social order'. I have the sentencing document to labour camp and the release document.

Did you witness anything related to forced organ harvesting?

I was blood tested three times to check my liver function within 24 hours by the clinic inside the labour camp. It was summer 2001.

One day in the summer of 2001, I had a slight cough, the guard named Chen Fumin, who was in charge of Falun Gong, took me to the clinic inside the labor camp for a "check-up." When we got there, Chen told me that I would be blood tested for liver function. I asked, "I only have some slight coughs, it makes sense to check my lungs, but why liver?" Chen answered blatantly, "This is an order! Don't ask why!!" They took 50cc of my blood. I was sent back. One hour later, Chen came to me again and said that the first tube of blood was broken, and that I had to be blood drawn again.

The next morning before breakfast, Chen took me for the third time to have my blood drawn. He said it was all for my own good. Two weeks passed and I did not get any results of the blood tests. When a physician visited the camp, I asked her about my blood test results. She said that my blood was very thin and was like that of a 70 or 80 year-old man. From then on, they never checked on my health again.

I also strongly suspect my wife, Luo Zhixiang was organ harvested. (see end of submission).

Were you tortured while in detention?

Yes, the purpose of torturing us was to make us give up our belief in Falun Gong. They continually demanded that I give up my spiritual belief. When I refused they would intensive the beating and torture. I will give 4 examples of what happened during these torture sessions.

Example 1

One day in December 2002, (I forgot which day) in Haizhu District Detention Center, the "610" policeman wanted me to give up my belief in Falun Gong. I rejected their unreasonable request as one cannot simply just give up their spiritual beliefs. The "610" policeman was very angry. They moved me to another room and locked me on the "death bed" or "dead person's bed". I was locked there for more than 12 hours. After that, the policeman locked my four limbs with a heavy chain that was nailed to the floor for more than 7 days. I wasn't allowed to go to the bathroom and had to release myself right where I was cuffed.

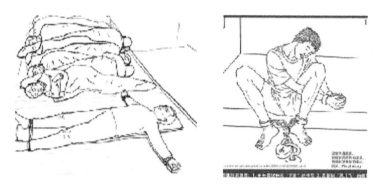

Example 2

In 31 December 2002(I remember the day was the last day of 2002) "610" policeman transferred me into Guanzhou Forced Labor Camp, the Second brigade. That policeman Bi Dejun asked me to write a letter of guarantee to give up Falun Gong, of course I rejected him. At this time, three people who were known to be particularly vicious, appeared. Their names are Wang Feng, Cui Yucai, and Jiang Yong. They were all black-handed drug dealers who used drugs.

They deported me to a remote room. At the first, they're punched and kicked me, hit my abdomen with their knees, and hit my back with their elbows. Then they twisted my arm and pressed my head on the concrete floor. A person jumped up and used his weight to smash my head with his foot. It felt like my head will be crushed at any time. They had already taken off my shoes earlier. The other torturer jumped and stomped on my fingers and toes. It felt like my fingers and toes were crushed. The last torturer fiercely hit my back with his fists. I don't know how long they beat me, they only stopping once they've become exhausted and sat on the ground.

Example 3

After that, I was held alone for more than 6 months in a room with no sunlight. Eight people were on duty for 24 hours, guarding me. They also recorded down all my words and deeds–and even my behaviour after sleeping was recorded to try and decipher my thoughts. Every day they forced me to watch a lot of videos that slandered Falun Gong to mentally break me. This kind of mental and spiritual torture was crueler than any physical torture I had suffered.

Example 4

Six months later, the policeman released me out from that small dark room. However, the policeman forced me to kneel down to them and say "Thank you for saving my life" every morning until I was released out of labour camp. If I did not smile and say "Thank you for saving me life" to the policeman, they would force me to watch more videotapes that slandered Falun Gong.

I strongly suspect my wife, Luo Zhixiang was organ harvested.[341]

At 1:00 p.m. on November 20, 2002, my wife Luo Zhixiang and I were sleeping in our rented room at #201, Building No. 5, the fifth branch of the Shangchong cun Zhongyue Road in the Haizhu District of Guangzhou City. Suddenly four or five Shangchongcun security guards broke into our room and searched our personal belongings. When they found our Falun Gong books, they immediately called the Nanzhou Street Police Station in the Haizhu District. About half an hour later, Li Zhizhong, the head of the police station (badge number: 024430, phone: 86-20-84204836), and another policeman bound my hands behind my back with an electrical cord.

They only discovered a few Falun Gong books, but probably to obtain a bigger bonus (anyone that arrests a Falun Gong practitioner is awarded a 5,000 yuan[342] bonus, while anyone locating a Falun Gong materials site receives a greater reward), they tried to make it look like more. They added a few dozen of my movie and music CD's and claimed they were Falun Gong truth-clarification CD's. When I exposed their scheme, the policeman who was videotaping turned red in the face and refused to look at me.

---

[341]   Family names have been removed

[342]   5000 yuan is about 600 US dollars

At 3:00 p.m. on November 20, 2002, my wife and I were taken to the police department and interrogated. We refused to cooperate with their illegal conduct. In the end, they got no information. That evening we were thrown into two separate cells. At that time my wife Luo Zhixiang was three months pregnant.

Two nights later, just after midnight on November 22, 2002, we were transferred to the Haizhu District Detention Center. To protest our illegal arrest, we went on a hunger strike starting on 20 Nov, the day we were illegally arrested. The police started force-feeding us on November 24. We were force fed in an emergency treatment room of the Number 177 China Navy Hospital on Chigang Street in the Haizhu District of Guangzhou City. A nurse named Tang Ying participated in force- feeding us. They forced a tube about one meter long from our nose down into our stomachs. It was extremely painful when they shoved the tube in, and the tube was bloody when they pulled out.

We were force-fed once every day or two until November 28. Because my wife Luo Zhixiang was pregnant, she was taken away from the Haizhu District Detention Center by Xinhua Street "610" officials from the Tianhe District in Guangzhou City on an "awaiting interrogation" warrant. She was put into the Huangpu Brainwashing Class, known as the most brutal in Guangzhou City. Luo Zhixiang was very weak, having begun her hunger strike on November 20 and maintaining it until she was killed on December 4.

After they released me from the Labour camp, I visited my sister-in-law's home. Then she told me what happened to Luo Zhixiang starting from November 28 up until the date my wife passed away, December 4.

On November 29 my wife was moved to the Tianhe District Chinese Medicine Hospital for injections.

She was in a double room on the third floor. The outside room had two beds, one for Luo Zhixinag and one for the person who monitored her, and a video camera mounted above the bed. The inside room housed two security guards with a monitoring device. The bathroom was in the hall.

On November 30, the Xinghua Street "610 Office"[343] notified my wife's elder sister, to come see her. They said that my wife was terminally ill. Her sister wanted to take

343   "610 Office" is an agency specifically created to persecute Falun Gong, with absolute power over each level of administration in the Party and all other political and judiciary systems

her home, but Cheng Di, a "610" official, denied her request. They did not want to release her because she refused to write a pledge to give up Falun Gong, but they did not want to take responsibility for her death either. If she died, they could claim that her sister was with her.

Although my wife was closely monitored, she secretly told her sister that she intended to escape. Around 6:00 p.m., my wife pulled out her intravenous needle and walked out when the monitoring staff was in the inside room. When she got to the elevator entrance, however, she was intercepted. She did not have the energy to run away since she had not eaten in so long. After this the "610 Office" intensified their surveillance.

Around 9:00 pm, her sister drank some water from the carafe in her room and quickly fell asleep. My sister in law said that she is a very light sleeper and awakens at the slightest noise. That night, however, she slept heavily until awakened by the sound of running footsteps around 1:00 am. She did not see her sister and thought that maybe she had escaped, so she prepared to go home.

Suddenly a security guard rushed into the bathroom then ran downstairs. My wife's sister felt something terrible must have happened. She hurried into the bathroom and saw the window open. She looked out of the window and saw her sister Luo Zhixiang lying unconscious directly below. Since so many people had already gathered on the scene, she realized that it must have been some time since her sister fell. At this time my sister in law notified my parents.

She then rushed downstairs, crying. She saw a person taking pictures of my wife, Luo Zhixiang. She begged them to help her sister, but no one listened to her pleading, nor did anyone look worried. After the pictures were taken, doctors carried my wife in to take X-rays and do an ultrasound. After they had examined her the doctor came out and told my sister in law about the condition of my wife. The doctor said that she had no fractured bones, and the baby in her uterus was normal. There was a small amount of blood on the ground where she fell. A subdural hematoma (a blood clot on the surface of the skull) was discovered under the rear left part of her skull where she had hit the ground.

My sister in law asked to see my wife, the doctor told her she was already being transported to the emergency ward. When my sister-in-law went to the emergency ward, she saw my wife being wheeled into an emergency room.

About twenty people, including "610" officials, a security guard, doctors, and nurses entered the emergency room, but her sister was not allowed in. A few minutes later, my sister in law heard my wife's terrible cry from the emergency room. Her sister saw through a crack in the door that someone was removing Luo Zhixiang pants. Then someone in the emergency room saw her looking through the crack and drove her away. She said her mind was racing because she didn't know what they were doing in the emergency room and why she had made that loud cry.

Someone reported the incident to the local police, who soon arrived. Cheng Di, the head of the Xinghua Street "610 Office" was angry and shouted, "Who called the police?". The police took a report from my sister in law, which took about 40 minutes.

They told her that Luo Zhixiang had been transferred to Guangzhou Overseas Chinese Hospital at Jinan University, and offered her a ride there.

When my sister in law arrived at the hospital at 3:00 am on December 1, the doctors at Guangzhou Overseas Chinese Hospital told her that their examination revealed two injuries at the rear of my wife's brain, one on the left and another on the right. The left injury was caused by the fall from the third floor, but the result was only clotted blood in the brain covering, which should heal after relieving the pressure. The injury on the right side, however, was very deep. Even if it did heal, she would probably be a vegetable.

My sister in law was confused, in Tianhe China Medicine Hospital, they did not say anything about two injuries to Luo Zhixiang head. She was advised to ask the people who had transported Luo Zhixiang. Xinhua Street "610" officials Cheng Di and Gui Jia explained that her fall from the third floor was interrupted by the air conditioner on the second floor. Her head hit the ground and bounced up, injuring the right rear brain. My sister in law could not believe that a rebound injury could be more severe than that from a three-story fall.

The police told my sister in law that my wife had attempted suicide. It is well known that Falun Gong prohibits killing life, including your own. Besides, she was pregnant. Luo Zhixiang had even called her mother-in-law in Shandong Province to tell her about her pregnancy.

With one female and two male guards in the room and her sister, how was it possible for this extremely ill person, who had been on a hunger strike for 11 days to jump from the window of the bathroom on third floor for no reason. In addition, the two sisters had been under surveillance by the "610 Office" 24 hours a day including visits to the bathroom.

It was not until December 4 after my wife was confirmed dead, that her sister's surveillance was discontinued.

Around 8am, December 4, Guangzhou Overseas Chinese Hospital's doctor said to my sister in law that my wife was brain dead and they had switched off the machines.

Before this had happened, her sister saw that Luo Zhixiang's breathing was being supported, but it appeared that her heartbeat was working as normal.

After a few hours, about 12pm, the hospital staff came to remove Luo Zhixiang away. From then on, no relatives were allowed to see my wife again. On the 4th Dec, my brother in law went to Guangzhou City to meet my wife's sister.

My parents came to Guangzhou Overseas Chinese Hospital on December 5 and asked to see my wife's body. The hospital said that "610" prohibits all family members from seeing Luo Zhixiang's body.

On December 5, my parents and our daughter Huang Ying went to Guangzhou City. "610" officials anxiously demanded that Luo Zhixiang's sister sign a cremation authorization which she refused to sign.

On the same day December 5, the "610" officials ordered my parents to sign the authorization. My parents firmly refused when they were told that their daughter-in-law died as the result of suicide. The "610" officials stayed in a hotel in Tianhe District for about seven days, forcing my parents and daughter out of the hotel. One of the officials from the Tianhe District political commission had paid the hotel bill. My parents and our daughter went to the Xinhua Jie "610 Office" to ask why, but they were driven away by a dozen people at the orders of Cheng Di, director of the "610 Office." (They were homeless in Guangzhou City for almost four months.).

A few days later, my parents went back to the Tianhe District, Xinghua street "610 Office" for the second time as they wanted to find out why "610 Offices" had illegally arrested my wife. As well as how my wife fell down a three-story building, why they persecuted and killed my wife and why the "610 Office" forbid them from seeing her body. My parents wanted to know why no one was taking responsibility for the death of Luo Zhixiang.

The officials ignored all these questions and the director ordered them to sign a document stating that my wife had committed suicide. They refused, the Tianhe District, "610" director Liu (phone: 86-20-38622610) then said, "It doesn't matter if you don't sign. The result will be the same. She will be cremated either way."

During this time Luo Zhixiang's brother and elder sister also appealed to the "610 Office" of the Political and Judicial Commission of Guangdong Province and Guangzhou City, the Police Department, and the People's Representative Committee of Guangzhou City on behalf of Luo Zhixiang, claiming she had been tortured to death by the Tianhe District and Guanghua Street "610 Offices". The Tianhe District "610" office colluded with higher governmental authorities to put pressure on Luo Zhixiang's brother in order to cover up the facts. The Political and Judicial Committee of Guangdong Province pressured Huizhou City, then Boluo County, then the Police Department of Boluo County. Finally, an envoy from the Police Department of Boluo County delivered a secret message to Luo Zhixiang's brother in Guangzhou. Once he read the message, they took it back. Afterwards, they said to Luo Zhixiang's older brother, "Consider your future before you appeal for your sister".

My wife's older brother knew well that Jiang Zemin's regime could do terrible things, and he dared not appeal. He was very angry but felt he could do nothing about his sister's murder, so the appeal was delayed.

The "610 Office" originally did not want me to know of my wife's death. When the situation became so obvious that they could no longer hide it, they told me the news. At that time, I was in the forced labour camp and under their control. They ordered me to sign the cremation document. They threatened that if I did not sign, my term in the forced labor camp would be indefinitely extended, and my wife's body would be cremated without the signature. In addition, they threatened to punish my wife's older brother.

On April 2, 2003, the Tianhe District "610" officials came to the Guanzhou Forced Labor Camp and announced the news of my wife's death. This announcement had been delayed for four months. They took me to the Yinhe Yuan funeral home in Tianhe District of Guangzhou City to see my wife's body. Her body was so shrivelled, emaciated and distorted that I hardly recognized her. Within two minutes,

I was pulled out of the room by Zhou Jianhong, the captain of the second brigade, and policeman Li Weicheng. The Tianhe District "610" officials had prepared a cremation document and directed me to sign it. I saw there was already a signature, they claimed it was my wife's sister's signature, but it was obviously a forgery, her name was not spelt correctly.

When I exposed this mistake, they became enraged and ordered me to sign. I appealed to them, "How can I sign this without discussing it with my wife's older brother and elder sister. If your wife was dead, would you cremate her body without talking it over with her parents and family?" They had no reply and stopped trying to make me sign. They agreed that I must see my wife's older brother and elder sister.

About 10 a.m. the next day, a guard from the second brigade asked me to come to the reception room of the forced labor camp. My wife's older brother and elder sister had arrived, but my parents and my daughter were not allowed to come because they are also Falun Gong practitioners. At the same time, about twenty people came in from the Tianhe District and Xinhua Street "610" offices. I questioned how my wife died. They insisted that she had committed suicide. I said, "That is impossible for the following reasons: 1. Falun Gong prohibits killing, 2. She was pregnant, 3. Why didn't she commit suicide when she was caught outside of the hospital? The only logical conclusion is that you killed her." They dared not say any more. I then asked why they didn't allow my wife's sister to bring her back home while she was alive.

The "610" officials gave the excuse that she was not following the China Family Plan[344]. I protested that that was a matter for the Family Planning Committee and had nothing to do with the "610 Office". Again, they could not argue.

Meanwhile, my wife's sister informed me that her brother had been severely pressured by the "610 Office" officials and the Political and Judicial Committee. I understood his tough situation: he dared not say that he would not sign, nor that he would sign, because his sister was murdered by the "610" officials, and they could easily ruin his life as well. He did not know what to do and so remained silent. In the end, in order to relieve the huge strain on my wife's brother, I unwillingly signed the document.

---

[344] The "China Family Plan" is a policy of the Chinese government to control the population that requests each couple have only one child.

The above is my detailed account revealing how my wife Luo Zhixiang brutally murdered by the Tianhe District "610" officials. More information remains to be discovered. I believe that one day this will all be disclosed and the criminal acts of these murderers will be exposed.

Summary of Oral Testimony: 9th December 2018

At the time, Guangzhou Overseas Chinese Hospital at Jinan University was included in the list of the hospitals that carried out organ harvesting. Jinan University had enough time to carry out all the necessary examinations. I was very suspicious.

There was a contract out to catch my wife. A 610 Officer confided in me that the authorities were invested in finding my wife. Spies were hired to track her movements. One of my friends was propositioned to spy on my wife but he responded, "Your money is too dirty – I won't take it". The police also flew to Guangzhou (the cost was 1000 Yuan) in order to approach my parents. I believe the police had no intention of keeping her alive.

I was told by a police officer in prison – [the police bonus system] ranges up to 5000 Yuan and can be higher for those that are hard to find such as my wife. The amount of Falun Gong paraphernalia seized by the police, in particular DVDs, was also a determining factor for bonuses.

My wife was considered to be out of control. In the Communist regime, one could be killed just for having a cold. Post revolution, there was a point-based system for dealing with enemies. It could be two or even three points allocated to 610 Office. If you caught someone, you'd get a bonus. The pressure on the 610 Office made my wife valuable.

Falun Gong are forbidden from committing suicide and it is tantamount to murder according to our Master. During her detention, she called my mother to say that she was determined to give birth to the baby.

Clarification Post Hearing

The oral evidence said that the doctors instructed that there was no need for an x-ray and this contradicts the statement.
I did not get an X-Ray, but my wife Luo Zhixiang did at both hospitals they transported her to. The doctors told my wife's elder sister that my wife would be getting x-rays but they did not give her nor me any of the x-ray results.

Witness 11: Yu Xinhui

Male, restaurant worker.

My email is [removed]. During my detention in the Guangdong Sihui detention centre, around the end of 2001, I was subject to physical check-ups and blood-tests. The prison personnel said these were for the purpose of seeing whether we had AIDS or any contagious diseases.

The amount of blood they took out was enough to fill a tube; the holder for the tubes probably had seven to eight in a rack. Each person's blood went into eight or so. The prison ward doctors were in white uniforms. Military police stood there watching, they don't get involved, they just watched. They were there throughout the entire check-up process, they weren't there usually.

I was also subjected to chest X-rays. I had chest x-rays three times, the exact same procedure. Only once, they just looked at me a little, other times, they took the whole X-ray.

The first time, they used the machine and looked a little. I don't know if they took the X-ray or not, but I feel that they were just doing a preliminary check-up. The other times after that however, they did the full check-up, taking the X-ray and processing it. Once, they had a urine test. The three times were in late 2003, summer of 2004, and February or March of 2005.

They didn't look at my mouth or ask me to open my mouth; they looked at my eyes. They took a rubber tube and stuck it down my mouth. It was a black tube. It went all the way down to my stomach, as thick as a finger. I think they were doing examinations. I don't know why. I did not have physical wounds at the time. They don't care about illnesses. They didn't ask me anything about my health.

In late 2004 one of the prisoners who was assigned to surround me and make me renounce my beliefs once said: "If you don't do what we say then we'll torture you to death and sell your organs." That was a criminal saying that. They tried to threaten us with that one time. I felt that he knew that the government does organ harvesting, so he was threatening me with that.

Everyone in the prison knows about this. Usually in the prison, regardless of whether the person is deceased, if he is sent to the prison hospital, he faces the reality of having his organs removed at any moment.

Everyone in prison knows that there exists a list of names. People [are] taken away, and no one will return. Every year it's like this. They always take away a group of people.

Not too many. Sometimes several dozen, sometimes under twenty, from every place they call a "prison ward". The harshest time was in the middle of 2006. I remember it was at midnight. Suddenly we heard the noise of a vehicle starting outside. We were very curious, because the whole prison was very quiet. So, I stuck my head out of the window to look, as did some other prisoners. We saw parked outside were three or four large buses, with iron bars blocking the windows. There were also a few armed police's military vehicles, as well as the prison guards' cars and some ambulances like the ones from the hospital, but they were not official. Then in several columns the armed police and the prison guards entered into the prison ward I was in.

Then, starting from the first floor, noises kept arising. When it finally reached our floor, the third floor, I heard that the guards and the police were scolding the prisoners, "Don't look. Turn your face. Lie on the bed." "When your name is called, come out immediately. You are not allowed to bring anything." Then only names were called, one after another.

Sometimes only one name would be called for a prison cell. When they reached my cell, they called away three prisoners.

I saw that everyone's eyes were filled with fear. One night, a lot of prisoners were forcibly taken away and they were put into the same jail as me. A few buses parked here. The armed police were guarded outside with their cars parked here too. And then the prison guards and the armed police entered the empty courtyard of the building I lived in, afterwards they entered into the building and made the prisoners come out group by group. Then they led them onto the buses outside of the walls. Then they quickly took them away.

I once asked a prison doctor, because this particular doctor was very sympathetic to us Falun Gong practitioners. He was especially sympathetic towards me, because we were from the same hometown. Once he told me secretly, saying, "Don't go against the Communist Party. Don't resist them. Whatever they tell you to do, just do it. Don't go against them forcefully. If you do, then when the time comes, you won't even know how you will have died. When it happens, where your heart, liver, spleen, and lungs will be taken, you won't even know either."

At that time the doctor also told me, "Falun Gong practitioners, they all practice qigong.

They often exercise their bodies, so their bodies are very good. So think about it, those organs are of course very good also. So do you think we rather pick you practitioners or those other prisoners? Those prisoners all abuse drugs or alcohol. Otherwise they still have many unhealthy habits. It might happen that, when you take their organs, they are damaged beyond repair. You practitioners' organs are the best."

See full submission with images: https://chinatribunal.com/wp-content/uploads/2019/11/Yu-Xinhui.pdf

Summary of Oral Testimony: 9th December 2018

I was detained on June 7, 2001 because I was a Falun Gong Practitioner. I did not have any legal representation. In our section, I was detained alone and so were other Falun Gong practitioners. We were not allowed to see each other.

I did not get the results of the blood test.

A non-Falun Gong prisoner was assigned by the Police authorities to torture me. In total, there were six inmates appointed to torture Falun Gong Practitioners.

He told me if you fail to transform yourself we will sell your organs. That was an inmate.

He [the doctor] was sympathetic to Falun Gong Practitioners especially me because he is from my hometown, and discretely told me to co-operate with the Communist Party. If you don't co-operate you won't know where your heart of liver goes. I believe the doctor witnessed this directly.

It was almost daily that we would be tortured in order to get us to renounce the Falun Gong. The degree of severity as well as the length of time varied. For example, one would be forced to sit on the 'Tiger Bench' for a day or be sleep and food-deprived, as well as deprived of toilet facilities. In addition, torture instruments were deployed, as well as the use of cruel language. They wouldn't let you live well and they wouldn't let you die; their ultimate purpose was for us to renounce Falun Gong.

No one ever saw the list [of names] in prison. Out of the three inmates that were taken away, one was a Falun Gong Practitioner. The Falun Gong Practitioner was middle-aged (around 40 years old) whilst the other two inmates were young. These prisoners were not on death row.

Witness 12: Huang Wanqing

News editor living in the United States.

My brother, Xiong HUANG, was born on 6th February 1978. He was a college graduate and resident of Wan'an County, Jiangxi Province.

Xiong started practicing a spiritual practice called Falun Gong in 1996. After it became very popular in China, JIANG Zemin the then head of the Chinese Communist Party launched a brutal persecution against Falun Gong practitioners in 1999. Xiong was in Beijing at that time, he went to petition the authorities about this unjust persecution and was apprehended by police there several times.

On February 11, 2000, Huang Xiong visited a fellow practitioner, Mr. LIANG Chaohui in Beijing. They were both arrested and beaten by the Beijing police. Huang Xiong was then escorted back to Jiangxi Province, where he was received two years of forced labor in the Ji'an County Labor Camp. During his detention, he was tortured (After his release, his sister saw injuries on Xiong's foot. Xiong didn't talk much about what he experienced in the Labor Camp. He did say routine beating was the established norm, and the most painful was psychological abuse and the degrading treatment he received) and forced to attend brainwashing sessions.

In the summer of (i.e. mid) 2001, Huang Xiong was released early on condition. Whilst out on condition, he was forced to attend brainwashing sessions at the local police station, and his personal freedom was restricted. To avoid further persecution, he left home and became homeless as he travelled city to city wondering the streets for almost two years.

Upon learning that Huang Xiong had left home, Xiong's sister and brother in his hometown were detained overnight and questioned about Huang Xiong's whereabouts.

His brother-in-law was suspended from his work, and the local police forced him to go to many different places in order to find and capture Huang Xiong. On one occasion, the local government and police station sent 13 teams of officers out to search for Huang Xiong. The communist authorities in Jiangxi Province and the local Ji'an government frequently came to his home to harass and threaten his family members.

They ransacked his home trying to locate where he was. The search and monitor was not only carried out inside China. The Chinese public security office also targeted me, Huang Xiong's older brother; I am a Falun Gong practitioner previously based in Georgia in the U.S., currently in New York City. They investigated three generations of my family and their activities. They also interviewed my university classmates in order to learn everything they could about my situation before and after my arrival in the U.S.

When Xiong left home, He dared not to contact his family members in China, and used different alias, like YUAN Kuan. So, he travelled from city to city around in China. He went to Sichuan, Guangzhou, Shanghai and finally Yunnan, to distribute DVDs about Falun Gong's truth to people. To avoid being arrested, he could not stay long in each place. The police issued a nationwide warrant for his arrest because he continued to talk with members of the public about the true situation regarding the persecution of Falun Gong practitioners by the Chinese Communist Party and Public Security Bureau (police).

In the winter (end) of 2002, Huang Xiong started to send some of his personal items to me in the US. He told me that he was planning to have interstitial videos on TV to clarify the truth about Falun Gong, in order to break the Communist Party monopoly on media.

In April 2003, Huang Xiong returned to Shanghai to collect equipment for broadcasting the interstitial videos into the Communist state television from an overseas practitioner.

He got the equipment and was planning to return to Yunnan. On April 19, 2003, Huang Xiong called me from a public phone booth in Shanghai. Huang Xiong told me that he suspects that he is been monitored and trailed by the Shanghai police and that he was going to Yunnan the next day, and he would call me again to report his whereabouts.

We had established this method of communication – he calls me from a public phone – for several years, and I was often contacted by him every three or so months. The last time he called me was on 19th April 2003 from Shanghai. Xiong's case was investigated by Epoch Times which interviewed local Party officials.

In one interview, Mr. Hu, head of the National Security Department First Division, from the public security sub-bureau of Yangpu District in Shanghai, indicated that he knew Yuan Kuan's situation very well. The reporter asked: "Why did you not inform his family members when you arrested him?" Mr. Hu said: "I know, but I cannot talk about it... We did it like this because we have our reasons." (This reporter is in New Zealand and she is agreeable to be contacted) (see the interview transcript below.) Further, a lawyer friend of mine has confirmed through his friend in Shanghai Public Security that Xiong has indeed abducted in 2003, but he wasn't able to find out the whereabouts and the fate of my brother.

Several months after Huang Xiong's disappearance, I made Xiong's disappearance public and started calling for public attention and help in this case. All of his family members have been searching for Huang Xiong through the Internet, newspapers and on TV. We've posted articles and messages everywhere looking for Huang Xiong. We've repeatedly called the Public Security Office, and all of the police stations in Shanghai, Jiangxi Province and Sichuan Province. However, none of these authorities took responsibility for Huang Xiong's disappearance.

On August 9, 2004, the U.S. Congressman John Linder wrote to me indicating that he had sent a letter to the U.S. Consulate in Beijing about Huang Xiong's disappearance. The U.S. Consulate in Beijing also sent an official letter to the Chinese Ministry of Foreign Affairs to request information regarding Huang Xiong's case.

View letters:
https://chinatribunal.com/wp-content/uploads/2020/02/WanqingHuang_John Finder-20040809.pdf

https://chinatribunal.com/wp-content/uploads/2020/02/WanqingHuang_Letter_ Embassy.pdf

Also, in August and September 2004, Senator Well Miller made inquiries with the Embassy of United States in Beijing, the American Embassy has contacted Chinese ministry of foreign affairs to request information regarding Huang Xiong's case at least twice, but there is no result.

In August 2004, we hired a lawyer, Mr. GUO Guoting, for assistance in this case. Guo Guoting later said about his attempts to find Huang Xiong, "For my investigation, I went to visit several (government) units and that took half a year. The relevant departments I went for investigation all treated me very politely, but they were all passing the buck. Finally, I found the director of the National

Security Department of the Yangpu District Police Station in Shanghai. They all found various excuses to refuse to see me as his lawyer. They didn't allow me to get involved.

Then, I was calling them several times per week, and they were stalling for 4-5 months and were refusing to see me. Since we knew from a news source that this director knew the whereabouts of Huang Xiong, I later went to the Tilanqiao Prison to find out his whereabouts. This is because if you disappear in Shanghai, you would be in one of two situations. You would be either doing forced labor or be sentenced to prison terms. If you are sentenced, your info can definitely be found in Tilanqiao Prison. Your basic information can all be found there. A computer search turned out three Huang Xiongs, but none of them was him.

Before my investigation was over, I was forced to suspend my business for one year and was defrauded of my lawyer's qualification certificate. So, the case remained unsettled."

On April 4, 2005, The Falun Gong Human Rights Working Group submitted a report to the UN Working Group on Arbitrary Detention.

In November 2005, before the U.S. President Bush's visit to China, I sent a letter to the President, asking for his help to find Huang Xiong when he met with Chinese President Hu Jintao and to demand the Chinese communist authorities to stop persecuting Falun Gong.

The World Organization to Investigate the Persecution of Falun Gong (WOIPFG) has also sent a circular about its investigation into Huang Xiong's case.

In August 2016, I submitted a criminal complaint to prosecute Jiang Zemin, the ringleader that ordered the persecution of Falun Gong, to China's Supreme People's Procuratorate and the Supreme Court.

Interview Transcript
Next is a summary of the interview with the National Security Department's First Division head Hu, from the public security sub-bureau of Yangpu district (Tongji University is in this district), Shanghai from the reporter of Epoch Times.

> Reporter: (dialed 86-21-65431000 extension 31090) May I ask who is speaking?
> Hu: My surname is Hu. Do you have anything to say?

Reporter: You are the Department Head Hu? Hu: Yes.

Reporter: I have two matters. First, before I called you, I called the phone # (31091) of the office work branch. A young lady answered the phone. When she found out I am a reporter from Epoch Times, she became abusive immediately. I hope your subordinate, the government worker of national security, knows the minimum manners for work and how to treat guests politely.

Hu: I will inquire about this matter.

Reporter: The second, I'd like to ask you for help. Hu: About what?

Reporter: Why did you arrest Yuan Kuan? (In order to avoid being arrested, Mr. Huang used the alias.) for over one year, you did not inform his family members. According to which law did you do this? Do you know Yuan Kuan?

Hu: I certainly do. How do you know of this matter? How did his family members contact your newspaper?

Reporter: Actually I have not contacted Mr. Yuan Kuan's family members, because probably they do not know anything. Do you know there is a World Organization to Investigate the Persecution of Falun Gong in the United States? They have reports every week. I learned it from them. Department Head Hu, why did you arrest him? Why have you not informed his family members for such a long time?

Hu: I cannot tell you. I know Yuan Kuan's situation very well, but I cannot tell you anything.

Reporter: Why?

Hu: I cannot talk to you on the telephone.

Reporter: I won't take a very long time. You are personnel of law enforcement. You should know the law more clearly than me. Doesn't it violate the legal regulations if you arrest a person but do not inform his/her family members?

Hu: We have our own reasons.

Reporter: But "the reasons" cannot violate the law.

Hu: You should not discuss the matter of legal affairs with me. In this aspect, I know more clearly than you.

Reporter: That is right. Why don't you inform his family members, then?

Hu: I know, but I cannot say. We have procedures laying out how we can accept interviews. You may apply for an interview from the news section of Shanghai Public Security Bureau. If they agree, I will receive your interview.

See full submission: https://chinatribunal.com/wp-content/uploads/2019/11/Huang-Wanqing.pdf

Summary of Oral Testimony: 9th December 2019

Mr Hu must have agreed to the interview because he might have assumed that the reporter was from the local Chinese media and he admitted knowledge of my brother's case (alias Yuan Kuan).

When another call was made to Mr Hu, he denied such knowledge.

There is a lot of evidence [of Jiang Zemin ordering the persecution of Falun Gong]. Firstly, Jiang Zemin claimed Falun Gong is a cult and his edict to crackdown the Falun Gong was obeyed. Secondly, there is evidence of the police beating the Falun Gong and they'd say Jiang Zemin gave the order. Actually, there are lots of report on how Jiang Zemin initially ordered persecution of the Falun Gong such as his letter written to the Chinese Communist Party to wage war with the Falun Gong. Jiang Zemin is wholly responsible for the persecution of the Falun Gong.

When my brother was detained in the Labour Camp, he was beaten and other Falun Gong Practitioners received the worst treatment. The orders were from the 610 office (610 is a secret Government agent to crack down the Falun Gong) and paid by Jiang Zemin; they are Jiang Zemin's allies.

I think the persecution continues but the information is hidden from the public.

Falun Gong is too popular with over 100 million followers in China. It outnumbers membership of the Chinese Communist Party which they consider as a threat. Falun Gong follows truth, compassion and forbearance. It's not just Falun Gong, even underground Christians are persecuted. Just last week there were reports of church bombings. The Chinese Communist Party wants to control everything, and religious beliefs are forbidden.

They [the government] said they wanted to eradicate Falun Gong in three months.

Falun Gong is not a religion. We don't call it a religion. In Western society, it'd be called religion. We don't have church and collect tithes. You can practise it anywhere. Nobody will control you. It is very loose and there is no order like in a traditional religion. Falun Gong have beliefs and exercises and unique; different from other groups. It's not a political group.

Falun Gong is a traditional practice of meditation – it's new. I think in future it will be viewed as religion. Presently, Falun Gong is viewed as qigong.

I have friends of other faiths, but I know very little of their faith. I think Falun Gong is different from other religions. We believe in truth, compassion and forbearance. The Chinese Communist Party does not believe in deities or higher powers as other religions do.

It's complicated [escaping or being released]. My brother used an alias and bought a fake ID which can be bought in China. If you have money, you can escape but my brother didn't want to leave the country. If he wanted to leave, he could have gone abroad, possibly Thailand.

For some people with no money, they have to stay in the country. Most people cannot escape and are persecuted.

Witness 13: Enver Tohti

Dear Your Honour, ladies and gentlemen:

My name is Enver Tohti, a former surgeon who has extracted organs from an executed prisoner. I was born in the town called: Komul, which is in the eastern part of East Turkistan, where Chinese referred as Xinjiang.

The organ pillaging can be traced back to 1990. Location: the new city district of Urumchi, Xinjiang, China. The Railway Central Hospital, I was then a young surgeon seating in the outpatient department for my turn. Located to the north of the city and far from the city centre, where come in contact with indigenous people, since I was one of the very few doctors who speaks native language that indigenous people came to me for medical examination.

One day, a man brought his teenage boy and asked me to examine the boy if there is any organ has gone missing, I asked him why? He said that he has seen teenagers from his village have gone missing for few months, then found that they had their organ been stolen. He lost his son three months ago, while he was shopping with his son in the local Sunday market. Someone took back his son last week, since he is so worried if his son too, had organ been taken away. I simply did not find any scar which indicates there has been any insertion, so I told him everything was fine. However, during that six months period I have seen three boys with huge scar on their body, all of them in the shape of U, the unique shape for kidney surgery.

Then, summer 1995, it must be a Wednesday, I was the only one had no scheduled a surgery, so I was supposed to be free on that day. My two chief surgeons called me into their office one day before, asking me if I would like to do something wild, I was than a young surgeon with passion, I was actually so excited to hear what they said, 'you go to the theatre and ask for the largest mobile operation kit, bring your two assistants and two nurses, inform anaesthesiology department for two anaesthesiologists as back up, then report to me at 0930 tomorrow morning at our hospital gate together with our ambulance,' which is, in fact just a van with a bed in it.

Next day morning, we have assembled at the gate, two chief surgeons appeared in a car and told us to follow. The convoy then on its way to the direction of the west. We had a branch hospital in the Western Mountain district, I guessed we were going there. Halfway through our journey, we saw the car turned left and our driver said: this is the way to the western mountain execution ground.

I felt chilly even in the hot summer. There was a hill, and our two chief surgeons were there, they said: you wait here, come around when you hear gun shot. I was scared, wondering why we were here? We have been trained to follow the order without asking why!

There were gun shots, not machine gun shots but many rifles shoot at same time I urged my team jumped into the van driving towards the entrance to the field. There were many bodies, 10? 20? Do not know how many, looking through the windscreen and the driver side window, I was seating next to him, 5 or 6 corpses were visible to me to the left, on the slop of the hill. Shaved heads with prison uniform, the foreheads were blown up, a police officer shouted at us: to the right, far right, the last one is yours. Confused, why is ours? Not time for that, moved to the location, our surgeons hold me and told me: hurry up, extract the liver and two kidneys.

I turned into a robot trained to carry out its duty. Those police officers and my assistants put the body on the bed inside van already. The victim was a man in his 30s, unshaved with long hair and civilian clothes. The bullet gone through his right chest.

The nurses have prepared the body, two chief surgeons standing on my left observing my movement, I asked to apply anaesthesia, they said no need "We will apply if it is needed". It meant they will observe if the man is not moving and then they will do something. The man seems already dead anyway, so I started my insertion, the cut designed as upside-down "T" shape, to expose internal organs as wide and possible. My scalpel finds its way cutting his skin, blood could be seen, it implies that his heart was still pumping blood, he was alive! My chief surgeon whispered to me: hurry up! His word was the command and also, I felt it was a kind of assurance that I did this by his order.

Whole operation took around 30-40 minutes, chief surgeons were happily put those organs into weird looking box, and said "ok, now you take your team back to hospital, remember there was nothing happened today". I knew, this is another command too.

No one talked about it ever since.

Until I saw Ethan Gutmann in Westminster, I finally revealed this dark secret to the world.

Looking back, I could see a vast wasteland, East Turkistan, or Xinjiang, one sixth of China's map. Has been designated as the experimental field, in another word, a gigantic open-top human laboratory.

The Chinese Communist Party was determined to build nuclear arsenal. For this purpose, they chose Xinjiang and turn it into a gigantic experimental ground that this world has ever seen.

Since 16th October 1964 to 29th July 1996 48 nuclear devices been tested, of which two failed to detonate. 46 nuclear explosions have been achieved, 23 in air and 23 underground. This has resulted that the largest provincial tumor hospital located in the sparsely populated area.

A former Colonel Ken Alibek, of the Russian Red Army laboratory in Kazakhstan reported in his book that Chinese may have tested bioweapon in Xinjiang in 1980. I certainly remember that, that was the first year of my medical university, that many students were late for registration because of the barricade from plague and typhoid fever in southern part of Xinjiang.

It is not acceptable that normal buy-one-get-one-free shopping pattern can be seen in organ transplantation. Predate for your heart transplantation means that they make someone dead for you. Giving away organs to promote business means they have unlimited supply of organs. This can only be achieved if those organs are carried in the living bodies waiting to be taken on demand.

A news broke out June 2016, that the CCP is giving Uyghur people in Xinjiang free national health check-up. With no further explanation. I suspect that the CCP is building their national database for organ trade. It is also widely reported that the CCP is carrying DNA test in the region under a glorified title of improving the quality of life of Uyghurs, and that is, I believe, a lie.

According to the Chinese media that the number of samples have been collected has exceeded 17 million.

Recent development in Xinjiang give further evidence for the claim that how the CCP is covering their organ stealing operation, they have established hundreds if not thousands so called re-education camps across the country, millions of people are sent to those camps, and large portion of them simply disappear inside the camp, and so far, there is no report of releasing people. Those who got out of the camps only because they are ill or unable to look after themselves inside the camp.

(This photo is the direct indication of that Xinjiang is producing human organs, and in massive scale. This photo was taken in an airport. From its content that we can work out that it is from Xinjiang, because of the combination of languages only can be seen in Xinjiang, and it says: special passenger, human organs transportation pass-way).

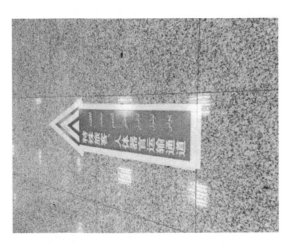

I have given many talk and testimonies around the world. Apart from my own experience, Mr. Guo wengui, (is a Chinese billionaire businessman who later became a political activist) revealed that how the CCP is taking organs from Xinjiang: http://ca.ntdtv.com/xtr/gb/2017/09/29/a1344393.html

October 2017, Taipei, after I gave a talk on organ harvesting, a Taiwanese man approached me said: my brother went to Tianjing for kidney transplant, since he was aware of Falun Gong situation, he asked his surgeon that he does not want Falun gong organs. His surgeon assured him that: "now, all organs are coming from Xinjiang!"

Summary of Oral Testimony: 10th December 2018
I found this surgery is much easier than the normal surgery because normally surgery had to be careful, you had to be very careful not damage anything else, but in this case the only thing you don't want damaged is the liver and the rest is not your concern.

[Witness shows page 2 of paper 2]. Here we have two cases of heart and lungs combined transplanting experience. It is from experience of Yen hospital from a cardiologist surgery. When was it printed – Yun Yen medicine in 2008, 29th Volume, 5th Version. This is a chilling demonstration – it describes the operation procedure. The donor brought into theatre, it is described as a standard operation and general anaesthetic applied, as well as a tranquiliser. This indicates that the donor is alive, otherwise they don't need anaesthetic. But if this a kidney transplantation I have no rejection I can sell one of my kidneys take my kidneys and go home. This is combined heart and lung transplantation. They clearly indicate donor was alive, don't say what happened to donors. They forgot to hide the evidence – they are killing the evidence inside medical theatre.

[Witness pointing to second image] In this image we see a buy-one-get-one-free. Buy-one-get-one-free should not be seen in transplantation industry. This is from Huguna province, where the people's hospital is trying to promote their business by giving away 20 organs for free. How can China afford to give organs away for free? This is a clear indication that they have unlimited supply of organs. To achieve this, you must keep the organs inside human beings and keep them locked up in a cage waiting for their organs to be taken on demand.

In the Chinese medical system prior to the reform in 2002, the whole China has one employer, the state and everybody else apart from farmer and peasant are working for the state. State is the only employer and beside this, the railway system in whole China is sub-militarized system. We as doctors have two sets of uniform. One white for hospital and another is greenish/blueish which we were using as stop on the rail- way system. The system is operated by military system, you don't ask questions you only take order. So, in the hospital, you had to be first house officer, then physician, then junior consultant, then consultant. At that time, I was physician and I had two chief surgeons as my heads. This is in the North of Urumqi, it was called the Railway Hospital, but now 5th Branch of x. This happened in 1995. The senior surgeons came with me to the execution site, so they were maintaining the ordering until the last min. hey also came because I had never done this, so they stood next to me on the left, they said, "cut this, go through there, the whole operation was under the guidance, or leadership, they were telling me."

No [idea of the ethnic origin of the person operated on] and since people in Urumqi have many different colours and shape it was in impossible to tell if he was Mongolian, Uyghur or Chinese. That is why I come to this country. I go to many places to pray: Mosque, church, to pray for him, as one of them will hear for him. [In relation to tissue type and matching] as I stated, this is sub-militarized system, when they had been told to not say anything, they will not say anything. They will follow the order. We never spoke of it. There is little indication that the driver of the van has been to the execution ground because he knew the way. At that time, I had no idea about this organ harvesting, I thought they were conducting an experiment and since I was a physician and considered and lower-ranking surgeon I was not qualified to know that much, so what happened before hand and what happened after they took organs, I had no idea.

[In relation to knowledge of transplantations taking place at railway hospital] Not at that time, but as early as 1990 people were stealing organs.

I made this conclusion [about organs being taken from the Uyghur population] like this – If they can find an organ in as short as 4 hours' time, it means they have plenty of stock in the back of the building. Organs are not like meat you can buy from supermarket and eat later, the longest you can keep it out is probably only 10hrs, so how can you achieve this? The only indication is that you have plenty of human beings and where do these human beings come from? The secretary of the world Uyghur congress said in his speech in 2007 that since 1995 until 2007 more than 100,000 Uyghur people have gone missing and they still do not know where they are. I suspect, they have gone missing and they have gone to this organ pool. Since we started our Campaign with Gutmann and Matas on the Falun Gong issue then people were well aware of this in with the world. So, then the Chinese needed a new source, so in June 2016, they launched a campaign in the name of improving the minorities health they started taking blood samples from the Uyghur population. They said this was for a national health check-up, but you only do that if there is unknown disease, or unknown endemic, but there is not this issue with them, so for no-reason you don't do health check-up since it is a very expensive thing to do. They only did it to the Uyghur ethnic group, despite there being many Chinese and other minorities living in the area. I think this is to build up the online database, so they can find match tissue from the screen.

In 2007 this campaign became DNA collection, they said this under the need for anti- terrorism, again, DNA can be collected with a swab, but they were still taking blood sample, so I think they are doing tissue match under the disguise of DNA sample collection. Recently they have locked up many Uyghur people and this gives them source of organs. When you are behind the bars you are nobody, outside you cannot ask question.

The Chinese regime is such a regime they have their hand on you even if you are living in the west. Think like this, every person from mainland china has an invisible gun pointing at their head, but the gun is not visible to the west. They know what will happen, so they have no choice but to keep silent and try to avoid any trouble.

In 1990, I was intern in the outpatient hospital, local people come to me for medical examination. One day a man came with his teenage son. He asked him to examine his son to see if the organ has gone missing. There is a rumour in the air that organs are being stolen. I didn't see any scar on his sons' body, so I said everything seems fine. But during that period, at the outpatient department I saw more than 100 children. Three of them had such U-shaped scars on their body, such a scar can only be used to remove a kidney, since the kidney is so deep. That was in 1990. So, I believe that this massive organ pillaging started as early as 1990.

[The teenagers mentioned] They were rather younger, probably under 15.

I was the only one picked by chance [to do the operation] and since I kept quiet was never asked to do it again.

I receive indirect threats from China. [Witness chose not to discuss detail].

Witness 14: Liu Yumei

Female, age 61. Occupation in China: public servant; occupation now: housewife.

Were you ever placed in detention in China?

Yes

> Places: Fushun House of Detention, Fushun Detention Centre, Fushun Labour Camp, Fushun Women Re-education School.
> Time: July 20, 1999 to July 21, 1999; July 23, 1999 to September 22, 2000; March 3, 2001 to February 9-21, 2002; April 1-25, 2005 Places and time:
> Guangzhou Shahe Detention Centre from November 23, 1999;
> Beijing Xuanwu District Detention Centre 33 days from December 31, 2000 to February 3, 2001;
> Liaoning Tieling Detention Centre 62 days from October 8, 2002 to December 9, 2002

When you were detained in China was it ever through a court process? If yes, what was the judgment about?

There were no legal proceedings. They came to my house at night to ransack my house and to kidnap me. I was tortured until I almost died. There were only 2 documents. One was detention paper (because there was Falun Gong materials at home). One was 3 years in labor camp (because they found materials on suing Jiang Zemin, then CCP head who started the persecution.) They verbally told me that I disturbed social orders.

What was the reason given by Chinese authorities? Do you have official documentation?

Reasons: I cultivate Falun Gong. I keep materials of Falun Gong. I have sued Jiang Zemin in China.

Did you witness anything related to forced organ harvesting that you would like to tell the Tribunal about?

I was threatened to be organ harvested.

In January 2001, I went to Beijing State Office of Letters and Visits to ask for petitioning. I was kidnapped by police in Beijing and was sent to Xuanwu District

Detention Centre and was detained there. Police there said to me, "if you do not tell us your name and address, all your organs will be harvested, and your family will not be able to find your body." Other people present included 4 other policemen and 3 men who were detained.

Were you tortured in detention?
I have been tortured by over 30 ways of torturing, including being electric shocked on my face and mouth by electric batons, fist hitting and feet kicking, dragging of my hair, beating my face with wood slab, being handcuffed and fettered, being chained on the neck and the iron ring on my neck was fixed to the ground by a lock, my arms handcuffed to the back, both hands and both feet chained together by handcuffs and chains, my body and limbs being forced stretched to all directions and pressed down to the ground in this posture, not allowed to sleep, being forced to sit on a board for long hours, being forced to stand for long hours, being pinched on my armpits, my teeth being pried by iron pliers, being forced fed with a tube inserted through my nose, being poured cigarette ashes into my mouth, being spat, being poured dirty wash from clothes washing, being medicated with unknown drugs that are harmful to cranial nerves.

If a person continues to practice Falun Gong then they will stay in jail and may become insane from the treatment or be killed.

Summary of Oral Evidence: 10th December 2018

[Detained] 9 times. About 10 detention centres but concretely out of the 9 times, yes over 10. No [legal representation], in China this is not allowed.

It was when I went to petition in Beijing on the 31st Dec 2000. I went to say Falun Gong was good and I was taken away by the police and they beat me. They took me away in a van and they took me to a detention centre in Beijing city, they asked for my name and address. I did not give them this. I was then given a form and they asked me to fill it in, I filled it in. I gave true information but hesitating about the name because if I gave them my real name, I would have bad consequence, so I didn't give them my name. Initially I gave them my pet name in my family and when they check it didn't exist because the official name didn't exist. They took photos of me, and asked me to write a written confession, I refused the photos to be taken of me. I thought it was a method of threat, so I did not say. That is what the police told me. Afterwards I was locked in a cell with prisoners, the door was iron, the inmates there they asked me what my name was and for what reason I got in. I said I didn't give the policemen my name, they said oh you are in trouble then as now they will bother you.

They performed medical checks on me. I didn't know about the others; they drew my blood. At the time, there were 10 people in the queue. They asked me to put my hands behind my head and crouch down. I said I am not a prisoner I can't do this. The policeman came to me and kicked me into the crouching position and I was unable to get up. I went to the place for physical checks. The doctor was a prison doctor belonging to the detention centre. She took my blood. I saw through the window there were many people analysing something. I did not know what they were looking for.

From the cell I could not see anything from the outside. They say you are in trouble because usually when the prisoners were sent there for one of two days they would disappear.

[Detention] 1999 for the 4th time. July 20th, 1999 was the first time, afterwards the police came July 23rd, then in 1999 November 23rd in Guangzhou after persecution, because there was the conference on experience sharing and then I was kidnapped because I didn't tell them my address, so they did some recording.

No [never heard about organ harvesting of Falun Gong before 1999].

At the time it was all prisoners other than Falun Gong practitioners – so many people were practicing Falun Gong. The prisons would release other prisoners to accommodate the Falun Gong practitioners.

[Re: suing Jiang Zemin] Yes, in September 2002, there was a rights activist and two other Falun Gong practitioners that tried because there was no way to sue him because he was the leader of the country, but we were persecuted so cruelly. My sister was persecuted to death in April 2004, and after so many times of kidnapping me, because I resisted and protested, that is why someone came to me to sue Jiang Zemin. Wherever I went the door was closed on me, then in the end these three people took a video of me, at the time my parents were in their 70s they had white hair, my bones were broken, that is why they took a video of me to send to the international court.

At the time over 100 people put down their real names, and they were telling the truth about the prisoners and the detention centres. Then the Chinese police took the video away, and then we were mass detained in prison. At the time Jiang Zemin was in power and said that we need to eradicate all these people till the very last one and with the use of any torturing methods. During that time there were many who were persecuted to death, many prisoners went insane because of persecution and torture.

[Re: refusing to confirm identity] It is not just in January 2002, once you go to Beijing, and tell them your real name and address you will be punished including your family members, the people in your work place associated with you will be negatively impacted, as well as residents and local council. I didn't want all these people to get into trouble because of me.

I received medical checks, I was on hunger strike, they tested my blood pressure and came to the realisation I was on the verge of death.

Locally people were aware of my name, but in Beijing and Tie-ling – they were not aware of my name or age.

Yes, most of them did [pursue anonymity], as you would be taken away to be re-educated. The consequences on other people were hard. Other people would not have a chance to raise your case in future. They would rather go through such misfortunes alone because then other people also go through such things.

Yes [an anonymous group of prisoners could be used by the authorities]. Personally, I was checked in the clinic in hospital both times.

[Torture, discretion of witness to describe]. I received cruel treatment, they used electric batons because they asked me to tell other practitioners names, they said tell me other names, if I don't, they put the baton into my mouth. In Beijing they used wooden slate. It is very wide and 7-8 centimetres long and slapped it on my face. They tied me on a bed and treat me cruelly. My neck was fitted with an iron ring with a lock, this kind of lock was chained to the floor. There was a little iron ring between the lock. I was chained by neck to the floor. They fixed me onto this bed by the floor for 10 hours. Also, they handcuffed both hands and pulled my arms, so I was on the bed and I was all stretched out, my leg was also fixed by iron to the floor. I couldn't move at all for 58 days. They force fed me because I was on hunger strike. I am not a criminal, I am a good person, I am not guilty, so I did a hunger strike. They force fed me through a tube in my nose into my stomach. They used one container, they put urine and washed water of rice and they spit into that container.

It was all of these liquids and also the ashes of their cigarettes. They forced fed me all these liquids 2 or 3 times a day. They left the tube in my body. In the end they pulled out this tube. It was white, but above the stomach the tube became yellow colour and then black colour. They fixed me there and force fed me for 58 days. My eyes, my ears, my throat – I lost my hearing ability, my eyes, because when they were force feeding me, I resisted but they pulled my hair and forced me to the floor. They asked a male prisoner to ride on my body. They are hooligans!

After I was kidnapped, they touched me, they touched my body. Yes, including the policemen. Not only criminals. Also, the policemen because I received such a severe persecution. Had I not received such a persecution I would not have realised that these police communist are such a bad person. I am already such an old person.

I want to thank you because there are no human rights in China, I can only use this tribunal to say thank you so much, I want to speak on behalf of those who cannot speak up for themselves. I appreciate on behalf of all of these people. I want to say about live organ harvesting, my two other sisters in Masanjia were illegally sentenced while I was detained. The practitioners detained with them told me when they were there, because my sister didn't let us know the situation because they didn't want the family to worry so I didn't tell my family about these things. They told me that they went through so much ill treatment which effected their health. They told me the health check was systematic and very thorough.

Witness 15: Li Lin Lin

Female. Occupation in China: web programmer; occupation now: housewife.

Dear Sir Geoffrey Nice,

I am from Shandong, China. I am currently a resident in Flushing, New York.

In the beginning of 2005, while I was working in Shanghai, China, I was illegally sentenced to 3 years 6 months' imprisonment by China's public security apparatus for distributing Falun Gong truth-clarification materials to the public. On 15 September 2005, I was sent to Shanghai's Songjiang Women's Prison.

While I was imprisoned there, around end-October 2005 (I have forgotten the exact date), *[Name of person removed for privacy]* (another Falun Gong practitioner who refused to recant her beliefs) and I were brought to a mobile medical vehicle outfitted with advanced equipment to have our organs and blood checked. This medical vehicle was parked at the door of the building where we were imprisoned.

I remember clearly that this examination was only done on Falun Gong practitioners who recently entered the prison and have not given up their faith. The vehicle was well-equipped, and the examination was done mainly on our chest, internal organs and blood. At that time, I even wondered why did they only perform this examination on both of us healthy Falun Gong practitioners who haven't renounced our faith? And not check the other prisoners who had severe illnesses? If this check-up was only done for new prisoners, this can't be the case either, because there were many others who were sent to the prison together with us.

Later, while I was detained there, I learnt that there was an infirmary within Shanghai Women's prison where minor sicknesses would usually be treated, and their medicines dispensed. Those who had more severe illnesses would be sent to Shanghai's Tilanqiao prison for treatment, where they had basic medical facilities and could perform examinations on your blood and organs for example.

If prisoners wished to see the doctor, they had to submit a written request to their respective officer-in-charge, and after it was approved, it would be reported to the infirmary, and after the infirmary had arranged a suitable time slot, only then could they see the doctor. To seek medical attention at Tilanqiao was even more complicated, and I will not go into the details here. That was why I felt that the unusual medical examination of our bodies we went through was even more out of the norm than usual.

Over the years, this incident remained a mystery buried in my heart. It was only until 2008 when I finished my prison sentence and returned home, after I knew of the live organ harvesting of Falun Gong practitioners, only then did I realize what that unusual body examination probably meant. Although what I experienced while I was at Shanghai's Women Prison is not first-hand evidence of live organ harvesting, but it can serve as indirect evidence.

I affirm with my life that every sentence that I said is the truth. Thank you.

Falun Gong practitioner: Li Lin Lin 10/25/2018

You said your "internal organs" were examined. Can you please describe how this was done? and was any medical equipment used?
I was taken to a well-equipped medical van for the medical exams. Chest exam, abdominal exam and blood draw. I don't know the name of the equipment, but I knew clearly that my internal organs were examined. Because the examiner asked me to have my chest near the equipment. The medical van drove directly into the Women's Prison and stopped in front of the building where female inmates were held.

When you were detained in China was it ever through a court process?
There was legal proceeding. But the law they utilized to charge me was illegal. The so-called crime was disrupting the implementation of law using cult. They sentenced me 3.5 years. I distributed Falun Gong materials. The crime does not fit me. I did not sign.

Was there a reason given for why you were tortured?
I was sent to solitary confinement. It was a very small room about 2 square meters by the stairs. Other inmates did not know what happened inside.

I was monitored 24 hours by 4 inmates, who wrote down everything I did and I said. They did not allow me to speak to anyone else other than them. They did not allow me to shower. I didn't write anything against Falun Gong as they ordered, they did not allow me to sleep.

I didn't give up Falun Gong. They threatened to increase my term, and to send to to Xinjiang province, where they said there were concentration camps [holding Falun Gong practitioners]. I was forced to watch videos defaming Falun Gong.

I was forced to read articles defaming Falun Gong. I was forced to write a report about my thoughts daily. If I wrote my true thoughts (to continue practicing) they threatened to increase my term.

I was forced to sit on a stool for a long time with my hands on my legs and not allow to move. This resulted in losing balance when I walk. I was under tremendous mental pressure, which caused my period to stop for 3 to 4 months. They forced me to take contraceptive medicine.

The guards made other inmates suffer because I refused to give up practicing Falun Gong. Other inmates often scolded me and my family.

This kind of mental torture was worse than physical torture. The guards used other inmates to persecute me, promising them to decrease their terms. Because of this, the other inmates persecuted Falun Gong practitioners without any reservations.

Summary of Oral Testimony: 10th December 2018

[Process of being sentenced] the public security bureau arrested me in August 2005 was the first trial, but they don't allow the lawyer to plead not guilty. September 15th 2008 I was sent to Shanghai's Songjiang Women's Prison Female Prison to be detained until 7th July 2008. All together is 3.6. They sentenced me to because I undermine information in the law, but I didn't undermine the law, I simply told the truth about Falun Gong. I didn't sign the paper they asked me to sign because I committed no crime.

At that time, it was approximately October 2005 I had two pieces of clothes. They said they wanted to do a health check because they care about our health. We did not renounce our belief, so they took us for health check. I asked myself why it was just for us two? They said it was because they care about us, because we were very healthy. The criminals were not in good health, but they were not being taken to a health check. The van drove to the prison directly and was parked downstairs. The criminal's health check is not like this. Normally, the inmate the reports to the officers in charge, they have to say first I am not feeling well. We didn't make any request and we were taken to the van. The van was filled with very advanced equipment, they checked our organs, they took our blood. I felt very strange at that time.

I was detained in a small room, 2 square meters. 4 inmates monitored me at all times. I was not allowed to use the toilet instead it was humiliating because I had to use a small container. If I didn't follow their commands, they would not let me sleep. I had to write a report on my thoughts, I had to watch abuse of Falun Gong daily, they made me read anti-Falun Gong books. They didn't allow families to see me, or to buy us anything. I was kept on a small stool, so I got blisters on my butt after so long sitting there. So, there was much physical torture but his was not as bad as the mental torture. Every day it was very stressful and under such extreme pressure I missed my period for several months, they forced me to take pills. If I don't follow their commands strictly, they would slander my master, slander me. I felt all this pain in my body, but it was the mental abuse that was too much. I feel that I couldn't bear anymore at that time. Had I not had the belief I don't think I could have endured it. I can recall this situation, but I am too nervous to recall more.

[Re the infirmary for minor illness, and where Falun Gong were sent to]. I was sent to a Tilanqiao prison before. I forgot, I was sent there twice, but I forget because it was long time ago and I forget the specifics. I can only remember it was twice.

No [never told about organ harvesting in prison], although no one told me, the inmates would sometime mysteriously talk about something. I was told I would be sent to North-Western part of China and they seemed to be implying something but at the time I didn't understand what they meant. I was very scared and nervous during the time that I was there.

Juan wi was with me at that time. I checked Ming net, I know that other practitioners went through a similar situation, they did not allow me to talk to other Falun Gong practitioners. I could only talk to those who had transformed. I never saw any other group receiving special medical attention. The medical examinations were special for the Falun Gong.

I did not do a hunger strike, but there were several times it was too hard to live longer but my master told me that we cannot commit suicide, so I hang on.

Witness 16: Han Yu

Female, age 33.

Were you ever placed in detention in China?
Yes. I was kidnapped on 20th July 2015 by police and detained for 37 days in Beijing Haidian District Detention Centre.

What was the reason given by Chinese authorities? Do you have official documentation?
Not stating any reason. On July 20th just passed 6am when we just finished Sending Righteous Thoughts ceremony and my roommate was leaving for work, police broke into the bedroom where my roommate and I stayed. Later I reckon, the police kidnapped our landlord outside the house who finished night shift and came back. Then police used landlord's key to open our house before kicking into our bedroom, kidnapping my roommate Cui Li and I, and confiscating electronic items, books and printers.

There weren't any official documents. I don't think I broke any law, nor do I ever would accept what they did to us. I never pled any guilty by signing any documents, including the bail pending trial paper when releasing me. Since I didn't sign anything, no documents were sent to me later either.

Did you witness anything related to forced organ harvesting that you would like to tell the Tribunal about? If yes, please write below.
Based on the information we've got I believe that my father Han Junqing was one of the live organ-harvesting victims. My father and my stepmother were illegally arrested and their home was raided on 28th February 2004 (my father was already illegally arrested like this and stayed in a labor camp before this, and during which he was badly tortured.). My stepmother was released one month after but my father was kept in Fangshan District Detention Centre.

On 4th May 2004 I was notified that my father passed away in Fangshan District Detention Centre. [We were told] Due to unknown death cause, an autopsy was done by default. But my stepmother said she didn't sign to approve [the autopsy], neither did I see any approval documents or signed any legal documents of that sort. But the authority did it anyway without our consent and the body was put in Liangxiang District Xiaozhuang village morgue. Not until 1st June 2004, were we allowed to view my father's body. On the day, Fangshan police station sent out close to a hundred police to watch us – no cameras, no reporters allowed – only two family members [each time] could go in for a body viewing session, under police's watch as well.

When it was my turn, I saw obvious injuries on his face, even after the makeup, the severe bruise below his left eye stood out. Besides that, there was a trace of stiches starting from the throat down to where his clothes covered. So I tried to unbutton the clothes. When I just unbuttoned 2 buttons, police saw what I was doing and quickly dragged me out. Later another family member went in, continued to unbutton all the buttons and found the stitches went all the way to the stomach.

After the viewing, my father's body was hauled to crematorium. Everything was done under the surveillance of police until the cremation was done and the ash was buried.

Do you know where the body was kept from May 4 to June 1?
The corpse was stored at Xiaozhuang Forensic Test Center in Beijing Fangshan District.

There is no way to find out exactly which organ was harvested. Because the cut was very long and my father was very healthy because of his practice of Falun Gong.

After my father died, my stepmother received the notice that said my father died because his heart was fatty and over-sized. This conclusion was said to be the result of autopsy. But at the time, my stepmother was at the detention center, she was not asked if an autopsy could be done. She was only given the death notice. She was not given the autopsy result. After my father died, they did not contact us in time to view the corpse. In addition, the corpse had severe bruising marks from being beaten. On the day of viewing the corpse, Fangshan district police station sent several dozen police to be onsite and to monitor us. We were not allowed to bring reporters. We were not allowed to bring cameras. We were not even allowed to cry when he was buried.

Summary of Oral Testimony: 10ᵗʰ December 2018
I want to make a correction to my statement on the day I saw my father's corpse. I want to change the date June 18ᵗʰ after I was arrested, they took everything from my house – all the books and laptops – two printers, hard drives, everything was confiscated. They pulled us out of bed we were still wearing our pyjamas and taken

straight to the police station. We sat on the chair, there was no windows. I arrived at around 7am, I left in the evening having not eaten or drank all day. Then I was sent straight to the detention centre. I went through a physical examination; I was put into one single cell. I stayed in that cell for 37 days and I had two physical exams during that time. My family got a lawyer for me.

Last time he [my father] was arrested in February 2004. In May 2004 I received a phone call from my stepmother, she told me he passed away. I was shocked at this time. Because he was arrested 28th of Feb to the detention centre we hadn't the chance to see him. They told me they were going to have an autopsy. 18th of June families were allowed to see the corpse, every member is allowed to see the body alternately so at that time me and two others from my family went to see the corpse first. I was with my younger brother. At that time, I saw his corpse he looks much thinner than he was when he first entered into the prison. In his face there were traces of being beaten. He had bruises underneath his left eye, it was apparent he had been beaten because the left of his face was seriously bruised. Starting from his throat there was scars and stitches. I unbuttoned his clothes up to where I could. I could see till his chest. There were switches and scars from having been open up till his chest. When my other family members went in, they continued to unbutton his clothes because when I unbutton his shirt, they stopped me. My uncle continued to unbutton the clothes all the way down till his abdominal. It was very clear because they used the black threads from throat to abdomen.

When I first arrived, we had physical examination but nothing afterwards. When I first went into the detention centre before I entered there were several physical examinations.

I don't know why I was released but I think it was because there was incomplete evidence and because I didn't sign any papers. The situation in China is such, they have to submit files within 30 days if not then they will not accept the case, if not have to be released within 37 days if the evidence is insufficient.

Last time I saw my Father was in 2007 during the Chinese New Year. His health condition was very good [before being arrested], he was very healthy. He was over 40 years old.

They didn't notify me directly [of his death], they notified my stepmother and she just told me my father passed away and there was the autopsy that was all. I found out about my father's death when my stepmother received the notification then she called me. My father passed away on the 4th of May, it was two days after he passed away my stepmother called me.

They didn't allow us to see [our father's body for signs of organ harvesting] but we by ourselves unbuttoned the clothes and when I unbutton the clothes the policemen came forth directly to stop me doing so. It was a mess in that situation, so we pushed our way through and open the clothes they didn't actually allow us. After that there were many policemen coming and dragged us away.

[Whether family asked what the scars were for] Because my father was in the detention centre and they said to find out the reason of death they had to go through the autopsy and that is all they said.

Witness 17: Yin Liping

Female, age 51.

I speak Chinese. I was arrested seven times. I was sentenced to re-education through labor three times.

On August 26, 2013, I fled to Thailand. I arrived in the United States in December 2015.

Detention in China

When I was persecuted in China, what I can recall is that I had been caught and arrested for 7 times and I was sentenced to forced labour re-education for 3 times. The 1st time, I was sentenced to forced labour re-education for one year and a half, but I was detained in total for 20 months. Detention places included 6 forced labour camps in Shenyang, Liaoning Province. One of the labour camps – Zhangshi Labour Camp – has one illegal prison in it, which was a small white building. This illegal prison was especially for keeping female Falun Gong practitioners with male inmates. There was also an underground prison hospital there.

The 2nd time, I was sentenced to 3-year forced labour re-education. I was detained in Masanjia Labour Camp. I was carried home on a medical parole.

The 3rd time, I was sentenced to 3-year forced labour re-education. I was detained in Masanjia Labour Camp. I was released on a medical parole after 3 months of detention.

In total, I was sentenced for 7.5 years of forced labour re-education. I was detained for totally two years and a half.

1. In September,1999, I went to Beijing for petitioning. I was caught by police in Beijing. Beijing police handed me over to the police from my home residence. I was first kept in Longfeng Hotel in Beijing, and two days later I was taken back to Diaobingshan City Detention Centre, Liaoning Province, and I was held there for one month. Diaobingshan City was originally called Tiefa City.

2. In November,1999, I went to Beijing the second time for petitioning. I was caught by plainclothes police in Beijing and kept in Qincheng Detention

Centre for 5 days. The police from Beijing Liaison Office of Liaoning local governments took me from Qincheng Detention Centre back to Diaobingshan City Detention Centre and I was held there for over a month.

3. On January 7,2000, I was secretly taken by armed police of Diaobingshan Police Bureau to Tieling Labour Camp. Only after arrival at the Labour Camp did I know I was sentenced to forced labour re-education for one and a half years.

4. On January 30,2000, I was secretly transferred from Tieling Labour Camp to Liaoyang Labour Camp.

5. In September 2000, I was secretly transferred from Liaoyang Labour Camp to Masanjia Labour Camp.

6. On April 19,2001, I was secretly transferred by Masanjia Labour Camp to the small white building of Zhangshi Labour Camp. I was locked with more than 40 men of unknown identity. When I was raped by these men, there was a man who had recorded the whole raping process with a video camera.

7. On April 23, 2001, I was moved out from the male cell to Shenxin Labour Camp.

8. On May 1,2001, I was transferred from Shenxin Labour Camp to Longshan Labour Camp.

9. On May 10,2001, I was transferred back from Longshan Labour Camp to Shenxin Labour Camp.

10. On May 27, 2001, I was secretly transferred from Shenxin Labour Camp to the underground prison hospital in Shenyang. This hospital used to be an air-raid shelter built underground. It is a horrific underground hospital.

11. On August 10, 2001, police of Shenxin Labour Camp sent me under their escort to my home. I was on the brink of dying at that time. "The inmates helped me. My mother brought my child with her and they both searched for me all the way to Shenyang underground hospital, asking for me. If my mother could not find the underground hospital, and if the inmates had not helped me, I would have died in the underground hospital."

12. At the end of September 2001, I was forced to leave home and wandered about. I went to Beijing to sue these labour camps for their inhuman persecution of me, but I was again arrested in Beijing. They transferred me again to Diaobingshan Police Bureau, which sent me again to Shenxin Labour Camp and robbed me of ¥8300 that I had with me. One week later, I was again on the brink of dying under their inhuman tortures, and was sent back home in this dying state.

13. After 10pm on October 8, 2002, I was arrested by over 10 local police in Tieling. I was sentenced to 3-year forced labour re-education. I was detained in Masanjia Labour Camp for the second time. I underwent 7 months of brutal tortures. Then I was on a medical parole and was sent home in a dying state. This time before being sent into Masanjia Labour Camp, they brought me to Masanjia Hospital and forced me to have blood tests. I refused to have blood tests. Diaobingshan Police Bureau's police and police from Shihuangdi Police Station held my head, grabbed my hair and hit me. Then they pressed my head onto the wall, and tied up my body onto a chair. Female nurses from Masanjia Hospital drew a lot of blood from me.

14. In October 14, 2004, while I was still forced to leave home, I was kidnapped by police from Shihuangdi Police Station which was under the jurisdiction of Diaobingshan Police Bureau while I was putting up posters of Falun Gong truth. Diaobingshan Police Bureau sentenced me to 3 years of forced labour re-education. I was sent to Masanjia Labour Camp the third time.

15. At the end of January 2005, my old mother carried me on her back out of the evil Masanjia Labour Camp. A t that time, I was tortured to the extent that my lower limbs were paralysed and I was out of conscience. I was persecuted so badly that I had mental disorder. My lower limbs had been paralysed for more than half a year. I had been suffering from severe faecal incontinence for over two years.

16. On August 26, 2013, after many years of hiding and recovering from the wounds, I successfully fled to Thailand.

What was the reason given by Chinese authorities? Do you have official documentation?
Because I cultivate Falun Gong.

Official documentation: I haven't been given any official documentation. I personally have heard many death threats.

1) In November,1999, when I was held in Qincheng Detention Centre, Beijing, I heard a middle-aged woman guard yelling at those Falun Gong practitioners who refused to reveal their names and thus had been numbered: "The government has numerous ways to deal with you Falun Gong people refusing to reveal names. If you still don't tell me your names, you will all be sent to Xinjiang, then when you die, you will not have the least idea how you die."

2) In January 2000, I was held in Tieling Labour Camp. Wang Zhibin – police exclusively responsible for persecuting Falun Gong practitioners -pointed to a document and told me: this is an internal document of the government, in which the government had defined Falun Gong as a cult and Jiang Zemin had given out orders to "financially intercept them (Falun Gong practitioners), ruin their reputation and eliminate them physically".

3) In 2001 and 2002, I was detained in Masanjia Labour Camp. I often heard Su Jing – head of the labour camp – say that the state was fighting a war without gunpowder against Falun Gong, and that the expenses the state had applied to this war was equivalent to fighting an international war. Wang Naimin and Zhang Xiurong said, if you didn't want to convert, then you never even dream of being able to walk out of Masania, and your death will be counted as suicide. Zhang Xiurong said that Masanjia Labour Camp had got death quota.

Note: I found that those "converted" Falun Gong practitioners just disappeared. It is not known where they have been sent to, which was similar to my case. As I had been secretly transferred under armed escort, other practitioners of Falun Gong had no idea where I had been sent to. I was lucky because my mother, together with my child, had been looking for me, and there were inmates who revealed information to my mother, and because there were police who helped me secretly. I feel scared now every time I think of the underground hospital in the air-raid shelter.

4) On May 27, 2001, Liu Jing– the head of Shenxin Labour Camp–said to me, and I was kept in a confinement cell, "you don't see how wrong you are – Jiang Zemin has orders, killing you people would only be counted as suicides. If you die, don't put the blame on me. You just go to Jiang Zemin."

After saying this, he asked his assistants Song Xiaoshi and Deng Yang to take me to the underground prison hospital in Shenyang.

Blood Tests and Organ Examinations

In September and November 1999, I was arrested and detained. In January 2000, I was detained for 22 months of forced labour re-education. During these periods, I was not tested blood.

On October 8, 2002, after I was caught by Tieling police, I was transferred to Diaobingshan Detention Centre, and then transferred to Masanjia Labour Camp in Liaoning Province. I was forced to have blood test in Masanjia Hospital for the first time.

Three policemen grabbed me by my hair, as if grabbing a chicken, pressed my head to the wall, and tied my arms and hands to a chair. Two female nurses had drawn many tubes of blood from me against my will.

The following is my testimony for my experience of forced blood tests, urine tests, B-ECG, and electrocardiogram at Masanjia labor camp in Liaoning Province

On October 14, I was arrested by Tieling police and sentenced to three years of re-education through labor at Masanjia. For about seven months until around June 2003, I was held in solitary confinement on the first floor of the Masanjia.

I can't remember the month or the day when Li Shujuan, a policewoman in her 50s who was in charge of transporting Falun Gong practitioners to the hospital, ordered several "Four Defenses" members to drag me onto a white van.

She was accompanied by two other young policewomen, one named Qi Fuying, the other policewoman I do not remember her name, but I remember her appearance. The group escorted me to the hospital in Masanjia. There a middle-to-old aged male doctor took my blood pressure, and then issued the forms for blood tests, urine tests, and electrocardiogram. The nurse also gave me a cup to test my urine. It had my name on it.

They dragged me to the blood test room, and a middle-aged nurse took out a rubber tube that had the length of about one Chinese foot from a young nurse's plate near her. She held it to my arm and looked for blood vessels. My blood vessels were so hard to find that she had to slap my arm. When she found the it, she took out a very large syringe from the plate next to her. I was very scared and had an ominous feeling as I had never seen or experienced a blood test like that. I was so terrified that I struggled and desperately refused to allow the nurse to draw blood for me. So Li Shujuan had those four guards hold my head, arms, and legs. Qi Fuying said, "Cuff her."

Because I was too weak, I had no strength to resist them. I let out a loud cry and said: I did not commit any crime, we did not commit any crime, why treat us like this? I cried and asked him why: why did you arrest us, what crime have I committed? Why did you do that? Why lock us up? Masanjia is persecuting me, Masanjia is persecuting me.

The nurse didn't say anything, and everyone was quietly watching her draw blood for me. They took a large tube of blood. I saw that my blood was dark red and near black. I felt that I have seen a large, thick needle pipe like this somewhere, and then I remembered that I've seen one in the countryside when I was a child. It is what vets used to give an injection to a sick horse. I didn't have the urine test because I was too scared. I said I couldn't pee. The Four Defenses hit me to make me pee, I was determined not to pee. There's nothing they can do about it.

They dragged me to the ultrasound room, where they covered my entire stomach in a lot of white paste. Then a female doctor pressed against my stomach and ribs with a flat round smooth instrument. She kept on pressing, pausing, press, and stroking. She repeatedly paused on the same position and carefully press, and then wiped the compressor on her hand, wiping my stomach every time as she did that and painted more of the white, cool, sticky paste. When the woman doctor pressed on my stomach, she said to the policeman by my side, "She's got nothing in her stomach". That was the only thing she said in front of me.

The CDI took about 15 minutes. Then I was dragged to the place where they did the ECG. I don't know the results of any of these checks. Things like this, the physical examination, has never happened to me when I was arrested in 1999, in the detention center and the six labor camps where I was detained.

The only other time I remembered was in 2001, I don't remember the day or the month, but it was at the Liaoyang Correctional Institution, and 50 female Falun Gong practitioners given a chest X-ray.

The male doctor who performed the x-ray said: this group of Falun Gong's lungs look shining bright. [clean, see through, transparent, bright].

Both times when I was arrested and sent to Masanjia in October 2002 and October 2004, I was forced to take a blood test. At that time I didn't understand it but I was very scared and had ominous feelings.

Torture

I have been tortured in the labour camps for uncountable times. In the periods I was detained, I was forced to received non-stop brainwashing day and night, physical punishment, nail pinching of the back of my hands (hands swollen like steamed buns), pricking my wrists (bleeding and broken) with needles, confining me to small cells and using high decibel noise to torture me, brutal force-feeding in a suffocating manner, electric shock with electric batons, electric needles pricking my head and other body parts, and injecting unidentifiable medicines which caused me temporary memory decline and short-term loss of eyesight.

Guo Yong, a policeman, hit me in my waist and the hard hitting caused my lower limbs paralysed and faecal incontinence. Police intentionally cut my hair to make it a mess and then they said that I went insane by practising Falun Gong. When I was brutally forced fed, patients who were watching were so scared that they convulsed, and a patient with heart disease was scared to receive emergency treatment. I was forced to do overload labour for 9 months, and I was so worn out that I spat blood due to excess workload.

My arms were bleeding from the scratch of metal bars, and my fingerprints were not able to read because my fingers were bleeding and broken due to heavy workload of making fake flowers. As I rejected to wear prison uniforms, a group of policemen and policewomen and male inmates ripped off all my clothes and threw me into a toilet and let male inmates watch me. April 19, 2001 was the worst day of brutal persecution of me.

On that day, Masanjia Labour Camp secretly transferred me to a small white building, where I was put into a room with over 40 men whose identities I do not know. While I was being raped by them, the whole process was recorded by a cameraman. This happened only one month after foreign journalists entered Masanjia Labour Camp for investigation in mid-March 2001.

There were many policemen involved in persecuting me. There are some policemen whose names I don't know, and some whose names I have forgot. I write down here the names of the police who were the leading persecutors: – Sun Lizhong, Yu Dehai, Yang Dongsheng, Zhang Fucai, Liu Futang. They were among the police who executed the many times of arrests of me. – Li Chengqiang. He is a doctor in Diaobingshan Labour Camp. He personally forced fed me and ordered male criminal suspects to force feed me chilli water and unknown liquids.

I was persecuted to almost dying. – Two other doctors who have persecuted me are from Masanjia Labour Camp. One of them carries the surname of Cao. I can't recall his first name. I have forgotten the name of the other doctor. – Li Shujuan. She was especially responsible for escorting me to hospitals. Other police's names I remember: Liu Jing, Deng Yang, Song Xiaoshi, Guo Yong. Guo Yong is the police who hit me in the waist and caused my lower limbs paralysed.

Other police who have persecuted me but whose names I do not know include those police who are responsible for male cells and the underground prison hospital. I don't know the names of the police from Shenyang or Beijing who arrested me. I personally know 10 Falun Gong practitioners who have died in the persecution by the Chinese Communist Party. The death of Zou Guirong still remains a mystery. She was arrested by police from Fushun and she died in a hospital. The cause of her death is still unknown.

During my imprisonment in Masanjia Labour Camp, I often found that Falun Gong practitioners who were persecuted just vanished. No one knows their whereabouts. Masanjia Labour Camp is like a labyrinth. And it is a very common phenomenon.

Summary of Oral Testimony: 10th December 2018

I received no legal representation. I tried to find lawyers but there were no lawyers who dared to defend my case.

In November 1999 – because I was arrested in September when I went to Beijing to petition, I was detained locally for one month. Then they came to arrest me again afterwards, then I was arrested and detained in Beijing Qincheng Detention Centre, Beijing. Late one night I could hear a very loud sound of people being beaten up next door. The supervisor was a policewoman, her voice seemed to be a middle-age woman. She yelled a code and a number, she said "there are plenty of methods to treat you. The country has so many methods to treat you. If you don't report your names, you'll be sent to Xinjiang." These practitioners did not give them their names. I was detained for 5 days in November 1999 and that was what happened during those 5 days.

The worst day 19th April 2004 – this hurt me so much. They called my name and another practitioners name. There were about 10 Falun Gong practitioners' names they called. They transferred us from Masanjia Labour camp to a small white building. They used a big, old, tired van. They put us into the van and sent us to a male detention centre. There was also another Falun Gong practitioner but afterward he died, so one of us for whatever reason was sent to somewhere else but we don't know where that was. We were sent to a small white building; we were distributed into different cells. I was sent to a room. In front of the room there was 9 people guarding the door. There were total 10 rooms. I was sent to the first room. The other person was sent to the next room, in my room there were four men sitting there in the room. When I came to the room, I asked them why don't you leave the room? I told them I want to go to sleep. He said, "I never heard anyone could sleep." They didn't allow me to sleep. He said that there was another Falun Gong practitioner who stayed in that room for 18 days and then he went insane because they didn't let him sleep for 18 days. I told him I wanted to go to the toilet, it was opposite my room. When I saw the toilet there was a temporary partition next to the toilet that can accommodate about one person, when I passed that room, I saw 30 men lying there, some were sitting, or talking at about 10 pm at night. An inmate tried to rush out of the room, I rushed out of the room as well. I didn't see what was going on in the room. In the detention centre no-one was allowed to wear any belts. They pulled down my pants and then stripped me and kept beating me.

Afterwards in the night 10 men came with a camera, one man beating my head and all my memories stayed there. I don't recall anything anymore. I just remember that I was so desperate, I stare up in front of me I saw a man was taking video recording of me and next to me there were three men doing something so humiliating to me. The men were laughing, one man was pulling my feet and told me "don't pretend to be dead." I was sexually harassed by them.

I must tell the world since I am alive, I want to sue you all, I want to tell everyone what kind of inhumane deed you have done. Several times I was persecuted to death, but I need to remain strong and with fortitude, I want to live. Such hooligans are so evil and lawless, they are so brutal so cruel. It was too savage. There was a small white building outside the white building I hope people can go there to investigate. There were other Falun Gong practitioners being sent there. I don't think they will strip down the building. You can check on the 19th of April, I said I would never forget this day, it was 2001 I will sue you and tell the world. I told the police so on that day.

The underground hospital – they said it was a shelter. I was very afraid. When we went down there it was very scary, in front of which there was a desk, but no book.

Under normal circumstances there would be a young man guarding, they were not in uniform, there were many male prisoners being detained there and I could hear people yelling "help, help." One person there went insane. This insane man was a political prisoner of consciousness detained there. When we went down there on the left side there were female prisoners being detained there. There are two rooms there, I was sent to umm I'm not sure if that was room 1 or room 2. I was put into the hallway – next to the room there are several round shape containers and these prisoners are only allowed to use the container for urine twice a day. They were only allowed to use the toilet twice a day, during that time if you want to go to the toilet you can only use that small container. I heard people die there, that's was what I saw and heard about the underground detention centre. It was roughly 2002 but I forget.

On the 10th of May I was secretly transported to a re-education centre. There was one educator, name is Jang X? Because I was transferred to another re-education centre, they didn't want us to die there because my understanding was if we die there it causes extra trouble. I told them about experience of being persecuted, and my experience that the country should not treat Falun Gong like this, when the policemen heard my story, he secretly contacted my mother, she went to the re-education centre. I was able to see my mother at this time.

The police man secretly helped me, at the time my mother told me there was a guy who called me, so I know what happened to you. At that time the only person who could have known was this man, there was another man who helped me, during that time I was coughing with blood. His surname is Yin, and when he saw me spitting blood he said, "drink this soya milk, child please drink this or you will die for no reason." I could tell that he really meant this because he saw the Falun Gong being good people and afterward Yin helped me secretly. However, the re-education centre knew about this policeman helping Falun Gong so then he was sent away. I don't know where he was sent, he was no longer in the same place.

Witness 18: Xuezhen Bao

Female. Occupation in China: engineer when arrested then realtor after; current occupation: retired.

My name is Xuezhen Bao, I was born in Feb.1950 in Shanghai. I am an engineer, university graduated, used to work in a state-owned enterprise sector. I start to practice Falun Gong from 1995 and get great health improvement afterwards. During Chinese communist party's persecution to Falun Gong, I lost my job and was imprisoned from 2001 June 1st for 3.5 years due to not give up my belief.

I was detained in Shanghai women's prison. Below is my experience:
Around the first half year in 2003, all Falun Gong practitioners were requested to go through full body medical check. We saw 4 huge buses at the prison entrance, and full of very advanced imported medical equipment.

In that prison, there were 5 detaining sectors, all Falun Gong practitioners in each sector were forced to line up and get on the bus one by one to go through all checks.

Wardens followed us everywhere to make sure we went through the checks. We have to go through all sorts of checks, from height, weight, eye check, blood test, urine analysis, gynecology check, ultrasound diagnosis, check on internal organs: heart, liver, kidney, etc. The syringes they were using to take blood were much larger than normal blood test ones. When I got to ultrasound diagnosis, the doctor looked very surprised; he called for other doctors and wardens and checked with them. I heard a few sentences: "this one is useless" "it is a mess, full of stones, everywhere, she is useless". Then they asked if I feel any pain at my, I told them it felt alright, then they became quiet.

During the test, the warden in charge of Falun Gong, Lei Shi said, 'see how well the government treat you Falun Gong, this test is only for you people, to check everything. Only you Falun Gong people are treated like this, not even us as police (to get this kind of checks)'.

Such medical test went for several days, there were around 100 Falun Gong practitioners were detained in that prison. The doctors came with the bus, no one knew which hospital them belong to. And we were also not allowed to ask where the doctors came from. If anything came up, the doctors would talk to the warden

300

instead of us. Everything from Falun Gong practitioner was restricted; we were not even allowed to speak to anyone.

At that time, we knew nothing about forced organ harvesting. After that check, quite several Falun Gong practitioners disappeared; most of them only had a number as they refused to give their names. At that time, we thought they were moved to another place, but now when we know about forced organ harvesting, they maybe got killed for their organs.

Another time, I was called out by the warden in the morning, they insist to have my eyes check. I felt quite strange, as there is no reason to do such check, and I felt perfectly fine with my eyes. When I asked why, they told me the check was due to my request, but in fact I did not make any request. I told them I do not need such check as I am feeling fine, and I did not make any check request, they wouldn't say anything anymore.

They managed to bring me out of the prison and wait for their car. But after a long time, the car still did not come. I kept asking what the purpose for such test is, my eyes are fine. But they just wouldn't give my any reason. After another 20 minutes or so they still did not get the car and had no other choice but sent me back to the cell.

The experiences during the detention
Being held in detention center, other Falun Gong practitioners and I received inhuman treatment, and detained together with criminals of theft, robbery, pocket picker, drug addicts and murderers. Some 20 people were squeezed into an eleven-or-twelve-square meter (including toilet) cell and there are no benches or bed inside. Sleeping at night, one can only lie on your side not on your back, and everyone can only sleep on the wet floor very close to the toilet. Things to eat are usually the vegetable to be discarded in the markets, or the rotten vegetables or the vegetable leaves worth no more than several dims or pennies per kilogram. What was used is a dirty iron lunchbox, in which rice mixed with vegetables, no matter whether you want to eat it or not. The police also instructed other criminals to watch us, forbidding us to doing exercises and to say that Falun Gong is good and forbad us to tell the truth of persecution.

Being held for more than one year in the detention center, (because of insufficient evidence), the trial was repeatedly delayed. I was not allowed to see my family or the lawyer. In order to sentence me to prison, the "610 office" conducted the evil and sowed dissension, created lies, induced a confession, forced confessions and defrauded me of the so-called oral statements. This was to swindle the so-called confession. In the trial, under the circumstance of absence of any witnesses and evidence at all, the authority illegally sentenced me to three and a half years in prison just using perjury.

(Appendix 3: Indictment, written judgment, written award)

I was later transferred to the Shanghai Female Prison. In going through the formalities because I did not admit I was a criminal, I suffered physical punishment from the first day onwards and I was locked up in a tiny dark cell, a three-square-meter-small cell room, dining, drinking and excreting inside. Because there are no windows in the cell, it is humid and uncomfortable inside. Such humiliation is beyond any description. Later I was transferred to a slightly larger prison cell, however you have to eat, drink and excrete inside this cell as well. Going to the toilet is at scheduled times. The total amount of water for daily wash and use is only two bowls.

And no toilet is permitted even if you have a period, bathing was not allowed either. Because the weather was hot, there was bad smell.

The police in the jail in turn would slander Falun Gong practitioners about their hygiene. In prison, the Falun Gong practitioners are usually "teamed" with 3 or 4 other criminals (that is close-up watching). Speaking to other Falun Gong practitioners was forbidden. Even eye contact will be reported to the police by other prisoners, and the police will find some excuse to question and admonish you. Sitting in small stool with legs bending in 90 degree angles, crossing and stretching your legs are not permitted. After (sitting for) one day, your body becomes stiff all over. There was not even a little bit of personal freedom, the mental pressure was particular large. In winter, the cells are extremely cold without heating. Iron bars simply cannot stop the wind.

The police in the Shanghai Female Prison persecuted Falun Gong practitioners extremely sinisterly and maliciously. They did not show this openly, but in secret all means were employed including beating, luring and cheating were used. In addition, (police) scold you sarcastically, ridiculing and humiliating you. (Police) instructed other prisoners to play dirty tricks on Falun Gong practitioners, push the table to hit Falun Gong practitioners (and use all the force to push the table to hit your body again, you will be hit until black and blue). In order to persecute Falun Gong practitioners, they picked holes in Falun Gong practitioners deliberately, and punished us by forced standing or by hand copying prison regulations and other means to achieve the goal of persecution.

I was made to stand for long periods of time just because I did not fulfil their requirements to place the thing at the so-called right location. For example, in the cell room all the daily necessities can only be placed in a about 40-square – centimeter -small cupboard. It was not allowed to place them anywhere else. I once placed the hanger below the mattress (I saw others doing the same thing). The other prisoners assigned to me turned over my quilt and mattress and pointed to the hanger and said that I had violated the regulations. They deducted my points and forced me to stand until 11 pm (even when I could not physically stand any longer). My whole body and mind have been harmed tremendously.

In the jail, we must withstand the strong physical labor daily for over ten hours. For example, daily requests to weave two coarse-weave shirts or three vests manually with needles (Appendix 4: photographs of similar clothing samples) or to make 400 to 500 strings of 20-centimeter-long beads accessories or bead jewellery with the needlework and beads (if you are even a little absent-minded you can easily stick the needle into your hand and cause bleeding). Or to make over a dozen pairs of uppers for shoes (the kind shoes with bead piece decoration), or to make more than one hundred plush toys and so on. (Appendix 5: so-called result and fruit). After one day's work, two blood blisters appear on both hands due to friction. On the second day you shoulder cannot not be lift up, but still you must continue to work. In the evening your whole-body aches and feels as if it will fall apart. Sleep was deprived if we were unable to fulfil the production target, but also you will be punished by forcing to stand for long time.

Apart from the physical punishment and the intensive labour, the more brutal manner is the mental or spiritual torture of Falun Gong practitioners. This is more devastating than the physical torture. While in custody, the police in order to transform me, subjected me to over 10 hours of the "endless repetitive wheel war". This consists of uninterrupted forced brainwashing of Falun Gong practitioners in various forms daily. Uninterrupted compelled watching of various videos or other materials slandering Falun gong and Mr. Li Hongzhi.

Everyone was forced to write their thoughts and impressions afterwards. Continuous loudspeakers broadcasting, exerting pressure, forced conversion etc., are unceasing unless you are transformed. I originally recovered from illness due to cultivation but was once again became seriously ill after the persecution. My weight suddenly dropped down to less than 50 kg. Under such high pressure, one practitioner who was imprisoned with me could not stand it and was driven insane. She was already pregnant before her detention. (According to the Chinese law, pregnant female detainees were not allowed to be detained. In reality there is an exception for Falun Gong practitioners).

But the police used the physical examination as an excuse to cheat her and aborted her baby; afterwards she was sentenced to four years in prison. After all of this they still forced her to transform. After being cheated and coerced many times, she became insane. It is only a cover that the police let you go a home after being transformed. They will never let you go even after you are transformed, because they receive a big bonus after arresting a Falun Gong practitioner. Outwardly, they claim that Falun Gong practitioners are sentenced to prison because they refuse to be transformed. Actually, the truth is not like this. Seeing her being driven insane, my heart felt particularly heavy. I repeatedly warned myself, I should not become mad, I should hold on. So I had to bear all kinds of inhumane torture. Life in such an inhumane environment for over one thousand and two hundred days, it is truly like experiencing one minute like a year, one hour like a year.

Summary of Oral Testimony: 10th December 2018

I was sent to X district detention centre. When I was sent there, they checked my whole body, they asked me to take off all my clothes, I did not want to cooperate. It was humiliating. They sent me to an isolation cell till midnight or 2 o'clock, then they allowed me to go back to the prison. It was very small, inside that cell room there were about 20 prisoners, we were all sleeping on their sides, like stacking the bricks.

There was also a toilet, they asked me and interrogated me. They asked me to give up practicing Falun Gong. I have improved so much physically and mentally because of Falun Gong. In the past I had health problem with my heart, after practicing Falun Gong I was healed so I didn't want to give up. My master says: "If there is one moment of grace, it should be paid back with a lifetime." I really appreciate my master. My work was an engineer, but they didn't let me back to my work unit. They couldn't find sufficient evidence of a crime, so they tried to find evidence, but they couldn't find evidence. They didn't have any warrant, there was no legal proceedings, there was no arrest warrant, there was no certificate.

After my sentence I was put in Shanghai women prison. I said I didn't commit any crime, I practice Falun Gong, because of these words, I was put in a small cell. Eating, sleeping, go to toilet, all in the same cell. I was not allowed to greet anyone. I was not allowed to talk to anyone. I was not permitted to go to the toilet.

We could only use a little bucket in each cell. They were very violent to Falun Gong practitioners. They made us work every morning every night. We had to weave the sweaters, this is a very brutal thing, many people could not accomplish these tasks. Whoever cannot finish the job cannot sleep. Even more brutal things. We were deprived of sleep, and they would play video to slander Falun Gong and my master. Sleep was deprived, they force you stay something slanderous. I didn't want to cooperate, so I was detained for 3.5 years.

In 2007 the women's prison notified all the Practitioners that they were going to conduct a health check. There were 4 big busses fitted with very advanced equipment. The windows were covered in the bus. So, every time there was only one practitioner that went onto the bus. One would go into the first bus, then go to the second bus, this a very strange way of doing health check. They do a very comprehensive check, abdominal, internal organs, heart. They tested me and did an Ultrasound. The doctor said, "this person is not going to work, she is a mess." They called another person over, I was laying there and listening, the doctor pressed on my ribs. He said, "how do you feel here"? I said, "I don't feel a thing." They looked at each other, this kind of check went on in the hospital for several days. The police said "Look the only Falun Gong practitioners received this health check". They said they would check my eyes also.

When I was detained there, I didn't know anything about organ harvest. After we did the health check some of the people stayed there but many practitioners from outside of the area they would disappear. Until 2006 organ harvesting was revealed in the news, I recalled my experience of having these two health checks. I was very scared. If at that time my organs and eyes were alright it would have been me. I felt that I was a survivor of the Organ Harvest. I must tell you that organ harvesting indeed exists in China. In addition, in 2015 I called a Chinese hospital to enquire about whether they get organs, I pretended to be someone whose relative need organs and said "how long can you get organs?" They said "very fast as long as you bring your health document, very fast". And they said Zhejiang university and in Shanghai, they have "plenty of stock". So, they didn't say Falun Gong but they said they could do it very quickly, immediately.

Now I recall at that time after the health check there were many people disappearing. I think it is very likely that these people are no longer in this world. Even now there is still something like this happening in China. I hope this tribunal, council, lawyers, who is concerned about organ harvesting in China, I hope you can do something for Falun Gong practitioners. Do justice, please.

This [getting my passport] happened even before 2005. My son was in Denmark for many years, so I didn't see my son. I wanted to go to Denmark to see my son, but they didn't give me my passport. Every time I sent in my application, they refused my application, so I went to other department to ask why I was not given the passport. They said it was because I am Falun Gong.

I looked for public officials and went to the security administration. They all try to kick the responsibility about and did not want to answer my question directly. First, they said entry administration is for the public security bureau so it is them that won't give me my passport. I went them and then they said it was the police station that said no. The police said, "well think about this. Do we have the authority to do this? It was from the higher level that other you are not allowed to do this." They kept kicking the balls between themselves. But I recorded all their names, and all of the conversations, and I posted the story to the Falun Gong Website.

As a citizen of China why was I deprived the right to see my Family abroad? I posted everything on Ming Wey website. Two-weeks later the 610 Office sent someone to come to see me. They said you want to see your son right? Then they gave me conditions and they negotiated with me. They said if you go out you need to do such and such. They asked me why I distribute flyers. I said, "we just want to tell people that Falun Gong does not commit suicide, we don't burn ourselves, so the self-immolation was fake.

The whole thing was staged. In China there is no other way for us to tell the facts. The only way to tell the facts to distribute flyers. This is the only way we can say self-immolation was fake." Police heard about this and they had no response. They said, "okay you can go." So, I said, "I submitted four times and you always reject me. Do you have family daughter, son, parents? It is very normal you want to see parents."

They said, "okay you go ahead." I said, "I didn't want to go anyways." Then they said, "well you go, please go." The next day I went to the police and they gave me a passport. I heard from other people that they wanted me to go because I posted all of these facts. This is causing trouble for the policemen, so they would prefer if I went away. They would prefer I was kept silent and stop spreading all this information. In August 2007 I left and went to Denmark. It took me 2.5 years and four applications before I was allowed to go to Denmark.

Yes, there were many [under the age of 18], university graduates. I was not in labour camp. No sorry, I didn't see anyone age of 18 in Shanghai female prison.

Witness 19: Omir Bekali

Male, Uyghur.

Arrested March 2017 and released January 2018

(Below are 2 parts of the testimony. A short statement followed by an interview transcript.)

I was taken to a medical clinic or a hospital in Pichan, on the 26th March 2017. I heard the conversation between the medical staff and the police: "There are 2, 3 people in front of you for the Urine test, we will let you know when it is your turn to give a sample." They gave me water to drink before taking me to the toilet insisting that I produce for them a urine sample. About half an hour later, they removed my clothes from above my waistline, the first thing they did was to take blood samples from my arm. Then I was placed on a bed for a full body check. They used ultrasound to applying cold gel checked my kidneys, then ECG heart, my lung, I believe they were using ultrasound as a cold gel was placed on different parts of my body. I was moved from side to side and rolled over from off my back to my chest so that I could be tested back and chest. I believe it is possible that they used different equipment when carrying out their tests.

They checked my lungs, as I was told to breath in deeply and out slowly, the tests lasted for about two hours. After their completion, I was taken to a police station where I was given an eye test, my eyelids were held open and I was instructed to look left, right, up and down and at the same time they took photographs of the positions of the irises of my eyes. Then they took my fingerprints, and recording of my voice, this procedure lasted for about one hour. When I was taken to a detention centre it was about 8:00 in the evening.

The second time I had a full body examination was in the Karmay hospital, after I had been interrogated and tortured, I remember clearly that was on the 7th April. That was just before I was thrown into prison in Karmay. The medical examination was exactly the same, as before I had a black hood over my head. I believe the hospital was a large one as we had to travel up and down in a lift to reach different medical departments.

Interview record with Radio Free Asia

"Ömürbek, you are the only free person from among those that were arrested, is that correct?"

"Yes."

"Are you happy to go ahead with our interview?" "Yes, I am happy."

"Could you please briefly introduce yourself?"

"I was born on the 30th April 1976 in Pichan County." "What is your ethnic background?"

"My mother is Uyghur, my father's father is Kazakh, and on my passport, it is written Uyghur. I studied in Uyghur schools." "When did you move to Kazakhstan?"

"12 years ago, I am now a Kazakhstan citizen, a legal immigrant. I became a citizen in 2008. Since then I have been travelling backwards and forwards between the two counties doing business. I have been coming to Urumqi without any hassle, and I have never supported any organisations or groups. Since 2016 I have been working in a tourist company.

As we scheduled a trade exhibition in Astana from the 10th June to the 10th September 2017, in March we went to Urumqi to attend a conference in promoting the event. Having completed the 3 days conference, I went to Pichan to visit my family. The following day at 10 O" clock the police came to the house saying they needed to speak to me. There were 5 policemen in uniform, they said, 'You don't know us, but we know you.'

That was on the 26th March, they took me away without any documentation then imprisoned me without any evidence, I was kept in prison until the 4th November despite me being a Kazakhstan citizen.

Both my parents are aged with my father being 78 and my mother over 60, they live in Pichan."

"What was the reason?"

"They said I was a suspect. They accused me of instigating terrorism, organising terror activities and covering up for the terrorists. After arriving at the police station, they turned the computer on and said there is a warrant for your arrest from the Karmay Public Security Bureau."

"But they didn't have an arrest warrant in their hands, is that correct?"

"Yes, they had no paperwork in their hands. I told them that I had only come to visit my parents and was leaving the next day flying back to Almaty. They said, 'we need to talk to you, it will finish in half an hour'. I was taken to Dariyaz police station, where we talked for nearly two hours, during which they didn't take away my passport or telephone. So I contacted my wife and some close friends telling them that there is a warrant for my arrest from Karmay, and I was held at the police station.

They became very worried when I told them what was happening.

They then changed my phone settings, so it stopped working, they said that the county officials need to see me, so they are taking me to the Pichan County Police Station.

They handcuffed me and placed a black hood over my head. When I asked them why they were doing that to me, they said that is the rule, and they do it to everyone. They were all young men and asked me to cooperate with them. I was taken to a hospital (or a clinic) first, where I was examined, and blood samples were taken, and it was a full body examination with my hood was never removed. When I heard them speaking about my examination, I was terrified that they might open me alive to remove some of my organs to sell them. It was a very traumatic experience!

After the procedure had been completed, I was taken to a prison, where I had to change into a prison uniform before being placed in a cell among 13 other young men. They were all Uyghur men in shackles. I was kept there in shackles for 8 days. On the first day, three men – one Uyghur and two Chinese came from Karmay to question me. They said: 'You assisted people with their visa applications, also you took money from them claiming you could obtain a passport for them. Where did you spend all that money? We will carry out further investigation with you in Karmay.'

On the 3rd April, I was taken to Karmay."

"How were you transported to Karmay from Pichan, was a hood placed over your head and were you in shackles?"

"I was in handcuff and shackles, but no hood.

I was taken to the Jarenbulaq Police Station and placed in a basement cell. The following day the police chief came to question me, I will never forget what he said as he opened his mouth. 'Kazakhstan is equal to my xxx' (I am embarrassed to say the rude word he used)."

"Was he Han Chinese?" "Yes, his surname is Liu."

"I didn't react to what he said, as I knew if I said anything or argued I would get myself into more trouble.

They started to question me about the 43 years of my life. I told them everything, as I had nothing to hide. I was not allowed to sleep for two days as I was continually questioned.

They repeatedly asked, 'are you going to tell us?' What can I tell you? I replied. 'Which organisations are you in contact with? What is your purpose for entering the country, what service have you been providing to the people in Karmay? There are many people who have left from Karmay to Turkey, Syria, and Europe, you have been assisting them. Also, you are giving money to organisations.'

I denied everything they accused me of, after which I spent over an hour reading their statements of my replies before signing it.

They said, 'You are lucky that you are a foreign national, otherwise you would have experienced our wrath.'

Then on the 17th April, I was taken to Karmay City Prison."

"During that period, didn't anyone visit you from the Kazakhstan Embassy?"

"In June, during the month of Ramadan, I was told that officials from the Kazakhstan Embassy were coming to visit me, they asked me if I wanted to see them.

I said, 'yes, of course, I must see them.' After the Ramadan was finished, and when the Eid celebration had been completed, on the 16th 17th July they came, a diplomat from the Beijing Embassy and along with another diplomat from Urumqi. We spoke for one and half hours. They explained my rights and the responsibilities of prison to me before leaving.

In explaining my rights, they stated that first of all they have no rights whatsoever to torture me; secondly, they have no rights to force me to do heavy labour work.

In explaining the prison's responsibilities, they said if I am ill they must provide medical treatment, and also ensure I receive three meals a day."

"Is that because you are a Kazakhstan National, therefore, you have those rights?" "The worst experience I encountered in prison was that from the time I arrived in that prison (in Karmay), my ankles were shackled together and then one ankle was chained to the bed. I was to spend every day and night until the 13th June eating, sleeping and carrying out my ablutions on the bed with the occasional wash by the young guards. And I remember that day vividly because they now used a metre of chain attached to my upper arm and ankle to bring me into a crouching position.

It was so agonisingly uncomfortable and I had to live in that position until the 4th November when I left prison. Later I was to find out that my mother and sister had campaigned for my release asking help from the Kazakhstan Embassy, also my friends and members of the public submitted letters of complaint and demanding my release. In the end diplomats from the Consulate approached the Chinese authorities saying that I should be released into their authority whether or they are going to put me on trial.

On the day when the diplomats visited me in July, that was the only time I was free of my shackles for about an hour and a half. When I stood up, I was not able to balance as I walked, I staggered like a drunken man. I know I was innocent; I have not broken any rules or laws I was confident that I was not guilty of any crime. However, when I was locked up in prison, I lost all hope of surviving. On 4th November, I was asked to sign the document, which stated the conditions of my bail. I thought I must leave this hellhole even if it is just to make contact with the outside world, and I signed the paper. People normally count hours or days, in prison, we count the minutes and seconds.

I was then taken to a re-education camp where I remained for 20 days."

"Having spent many months in terrible conditions in prison, how long did you spend in a re-education camp?"

"I was transferred from prison to re-education camp in Karmay on the evening of the 4th November 2017. And I regained my freedom on the 24th November. I spent 20 days there. The place was just like a prison, there are guards at the gate, once passing through the gate, I was taken for a medical examination. My blood pressure read 185 over 115, the lowest point being 115. I have never suffered from any illness or high blood pressure before."

"After arriving at the camp, were you allowed to contact your family?"

"I arrived late at night and was told that they would arrange for me to call my family the following day, but I waited many days before the arrangement was made."

"How many people were sharing one room?" "There were 23 in my room."

"How big was the room?"

"The room we shared was not crowded. There were cameras installed in the room, so we were under observation all the time. People who were kept there were from the age of 16 to 20, middle age as well as old people, and they were from all different backgrounds. There were government employees, teachers, I also saw a whole family – father mother and child. People who had completed their prison sentence were transferred there for re-education. The government employees were accused of being two-faced, which was the most convenient accusation to use.

There were even people brought in because they used Urumqi time. As I was leaving, I heard comments from the cadres that it was now the time to bring in people who work within the legal system. There were doctors, teachers, and lawyers starting to be detained."

"Are they all Uyghur?"

"There were 70 to 80 per cent Uyghur, 30 to 20 per cent Kazakh, and no other ethnic people. According to what I heard, there were over 1000 young men. The camp was comprised of three different areas, designated A, B, and C. I was in area C, along with approximately 300 other men."

"What do you have to do once you have been admitted?"

"The sleeping hours are from 12 am to 6:00 am. In the morning all beds have to be made of military style. If one failed to do it as requested, it will be considered as failing their ideology.

We must attend the flag raising ceremony at 7:30. After that we must wash and then go for breakfast before which we have to sing a red song, such as 'where there is no communist party there is no new China', or 'Socialism is good'. Everyone must sing one of these red songs. Also, before starting to eat, we must say, 'thanks to the party, thanks to the country, thanks to President Xi, I wish him good health; I wish president Xi live long and stay young.' There is another long statement we must read as well, I skipped reading it, so on the third day, I was ordered to stand at the back for refusing to read the statement. After I spoke to them in Russian and Uyghur, they realised I was a foreigner, and they told me to sit down."

"Do you have to repeat those words every day before eating?" "Yes, that is the rules, and you must follow them."

"What lessons do you have to attend?"

"Those who don't know Chinese well, they are taught Chinese. Other lessons include party laws and regulations, the red songs – which praise the party. All lessons are taught in Mandarin, and there is an exam every week.

Also, during lessons, they inform you of cases that have taken place in court and sentences that have been given and what for. This is to create fear, in a way they use of these examples to tell people what a heavy price they will pay if they do not follow the rules. In between lessons, there is 2 hours of military training, marching, standing to attention, and following ordered commands immediately what I have experienced I now suffer from post-traumatic disorder, up till now I cannot sleep properly. It damages one's psychology."

"Have you seen anyone leave the camp when you were there?" "No."

"The cadres told me that it will take one year at least to complete the re-education program."

"So you are a special case as you are a Kazakhstan National, you were treated differently. The re-education Camp started in March, April, didn't it?"

"In Karmay it started in March, at the beginning, people were taken to camps outside Karmay for one or two months. Later they converted government buildings and schools into re-education camps."

"How many camps are there in total in Karmay? And do you have any information regarding them?"

"One in Jarenbulak District, where I was kept, and there are two or three in Karmay I heard. I also heard that they told the government ethnic minority employees that they must complete a re-education program to correct their ideology. The cadres informed their staff that it was directive from the central government, and they have no power not to comply."

"What is the food like in the camp?"

"It was slightly better than the prison. Breakfast is rice soup. Lunch and dinner have some meat. I think they sent me there because they wanted me to improve before returning because I had lost 40 kilos in weight in prison."

"While in the camp, what freedom do you have?"

"When I arrived there, after the lessons we were free to go get water from the washroom. But just before I was leaving, detainees were told they must stay in their rooms after lessons, they installed padlock and chains on the doors. I don't know what happened to cause the sudden change, but I felt there was a sense of emergency."

"How many times were you allowed to shower?" "Once a week."

"Have you noticed anyone ill, not coping with the pressure and showing signs of mental health problems?"

"I saw old men with walking sticks, and other people limping. Regarding mental health, it is hard to know how people felt inside. They brought in people regardless of their disability or old age, claiming that they needed re-education."

"In everyday life, people need essential items such as soap and toothpaste, if families are not allowed to visit, how did people obtain such items?"

"In the camp, you can wear your own underwear, but you must wear their outer clothing. In Karmay, they distributed winter clothing and shoes. Inside the camp, these is a shop only sells underwear and washing products. If you fell ill, you only receive treatment if you could pay for it."

"What if you don't have money?"

"Then you don't get treatment. In the beginning, they refused to provide me with medication, I argued that it was their responsibility to provide me with treatment. As my blood pressure was very high in the end, I was given blood pressure medicine."

"Were there any incidents of deaths, have you seen or heard of?" "No. I don't know of any."

"So, you attended the re-education programme according to their rules and regulations, is that right?"

"It is compulsory; therefore, it is impossible for us to refuse any orders. Regardless of me being a foreigner and all the others, no one has the right to reject any orders. Because there are armed police, some of which carries wooden batons if you show any signs of disobedience they will come immediately and give you a severe beating. Therefore, there is no choice but to obey any given order. When I first arrived, I refused to speak Chinese; they said I was doing that deliberately. So during lessons, I was ordered to stand at the rear of the room. On the 7th day, when I leaned against the bookshelf, one of the officials pushed me shouting words telling me that I must not lean against it. There were other cadres present in the class as well, I shouted back saying don't interfere! After that police came and removed me from the class and locked me in a cell.

In lessons, on my notebook I would only write my full name in Russian, nothing else, which caused outrage. They said I refused to re-educate myself, deliberately refusing to speak and write in Chinese, they demoralised me by swearing at me. So, I shouted back.

The police came, taking me and two other young men, I don't know what they had done possibly they have refused a cadre's order. Also, 5 other men and I don't know the reason why they were removed. In total 8 of us were locked up. Normally after classes you are allowed to get water from the watershed, by locking us up they said we must learn a lesson and admit our wrongdoings. In order to be reunited with their family, and not sent to prison, they are forced to obey all the unfair rules and memorise that they have been taught for their exams because there is no other way out.

They claim that through re-education they can liberate people's mind to embrace the party and love the country, to obey all the party rules and regulations. It was very difficult for me to comprehend the fact that just being an Uyghur or Kazakh, you were forced to undertake such a re-education regime in a prison. Seeing so many innocent people were being treated in such a cruel way, I was deeply saddened; at the same time, it affected me mentally. During my time in prison, being chained and not being able to see the sun, suffering from the prangs of hunger, it is not possible to accept that your dignity is being stomped upon.

All of this will stay with me forever. I was not allowed to make a telephone call until the 19th day, despite being told on my arrival that I would be able to contact my family the following day.

However, they refused to make any arrangement for me to make a call, they made excuses every day. In the end, I requested the contact details of the head of the Karmay city court or the head of the City Judiciary, they said they would supply the details to me, but nothing happened. On the 19th day, the manager in charge said: "If you speak Chinese, he will come to see you immediately." I shouted back: 'Shoot me or take me back to prison, I am not going to learn your teachings.'

Three policemen came, twisted my arm behind my back placing me in handcuffs, and took me to a cell and locked me up. I screamed while kicking the door, the head of security came shouting for me to stop. I shouted back in Uyghur, pretending not to understand Chinese. I tried so hard to free my hands from the handcuffs, as a result, my wrists started bleeding, and they became numb. Eventually, they removed the handcuffs, but they didn't give me food for two days. On the following day, a policeman came asking me if I want food. I said, what crime did I commit to be punished like this? Normally you offer food to someone even before taking them for execution. He then brought me five or six spoonfuls of food, which was given by the detainees whom I shared of my old room. On the third day, I was returned to my old room. My roommates asked me if I had eaten any food, I said, 'no but only the five or six spoonfuls you sent me, but it helped, thank you.' On hearing what I said, they looked surprised saying: 'what are you saying brother, we filled a plate from our meals and sent it to you.' Only then did I realise that the police had thrown away most of it.

I was given a new quilt when I arrived there, and it was very difficult to fold into the required standard, so one of the young men gave me his quilt, which was easier to fold and in that it saved me from further punishment. I was deeply moved by the kindness shown by the people in every way, as they tried to show humanity to one another.

At about 3:00 O'clock in the afternoon, I heard my name being called, I was then told to collect my belongings and be ready to go. I said to my roommates: 'I might be taken to prison or freed, take care of yourselves.'

I was collected by a policeman who told me I would be released. I said don't joke with me, shake my hand if it is true.

Shaking my hand, he said, 'it is true. We are releasing you and you are returning to Kazakhstan.'

I said, 'I have been mistreated unfairly all this time, I am an educated man who can speak four languages. I know your language like my mother tongue as I studied it since being in primary school. I am qualified to be a teacher in your language.'

They were all surprised when I said this, saying, 'Oh you know Chinese.'

I said, 'yes, I have mastered it. I don't need education from uncivilised and uncultured people.' Before passing through the gate, I said to the policemen: 'I will make my complaints to all levels of government, and all the way up to the Beijing central government. I will clear my name of all the accusations that have been made against me. I will make sure they pay me compensation; also I will make sure the head of the department who ordered my arrest loses his job.'

I was sent to my sister's house; they were all in tears upon seeing me. From my point of view, they are hoping that the re-educating these people will make them come out like lambs, but on the contrary, they are planting the seeds of hatred and turning them into enemies. This is not just my view, the majority of the people who are in the camp, from the young to the old, of which 90 per cent of them are educated; they all have a sense of justice.

In my case. I made a decision that I will pursue the cause of justice." "Did anything happen to your family members?"

"I don't know if they will be punished on hearing this, but I knew my brother was taken in one month after I left."

"Where was he?" "He was in Pichan."

Summary of Oral Testimony: 10th December 2018

In 2006 I moved to Kazakhstan and I have obtained a Kazakhstani passport in 2008. There was no explanation as to why I was arrested. I was handcuffed.

I was terrified of live organ harvesting when I went to hospital. After the urine test, they drew a lot of blood from my arm. They also put a cold gel on my body and checked different part of my body.

In mid-July two officials from Beijing embassy visited me.

As well as hearing some from friends in Kazakhstan I have access to YouTube and social media and read some information about organ harvesting.

Every month during my time in prison they drew blood from me. I had a black hood over my head. When I was taken from prison it was late afternoon, when I returned to prison it was around 9pm. Test took about two hours. I believe they recorded everything on a computer.

I don't believe that my torture affected my organs because the beatings were often inflicted on muscles and parts of the body that don't damage internal organs.

From what I saw inside there was a difference in treatment because I was a foreign citizen and the torture, I suffered was different. I've seen people tortured to death in prison. I know their names. I witnessed also young men passing blood urine because of the beatings.

All prisoners must go for a medical test before being placed in detention.

Everyone has experienced the same procedure. I was in 5/6 cells over that period and everyone went through same medical test. 3 or 4 Kazaks were with me in prison.

Every week 3 or 4 people were taken away. I expected it was for release or re-education. I believe they disappeared without trace.

The youngest person in prison with me was 15 years old. There was one or two that age in each cell I was in. Most prisoners were between 15- and 40-years age.

I believe I was released because of diplomatic pressure from Kazakhstan. I believe they would have otherwise taken my organs. I don't believe that those who were taken from the prison were simply released.

Witness 20: Yu Jing

Age 58.

Were you detained in China? If so, what was the reason and do you have official documentation?
I was illegally locked for 3 times in the persecution targeting Falun Gong.

> First Time: February 2000 – I was detained in Langfang Detention Centre, Hebei Province for 33 days.
> Second Time: August 2000 – I was detained in Langfang Detention Centre, Hebei Province for over 20 days.
> Third Time: September 2000 – I was detained in Langfang Detention Centre, Hebei Province for 10 days.

Then I was transferred to Yuecheng Brainwashing Class in Langfang, Hebei Province and was held there for over 20 days. I was tortured to half death by the police of the brainwashing class and then carried to Hebei Langfang China Petrol Natural Gas Plumbing Bureau Central Hospital for emergency treatment. Doctors did magnetic resonance imaging of me and said I had coronary heart disease.

The reason I was detained was that I cultivate Falun Gong.

I have one "Release Certificate" issued in March 2000. I have no further official documentation after that.

The following is what I have experienced and witnessed.

In September 2000, I was tortured very badly in the brainwashing class. After I went back home, my family were very much afraid that I would be taken away by them (the CCP) again. So, my family decided that my brother's sister escort me to Shanghai. I stayed in Shanghai from December 25, 2002 to December 2007. In Shanghai, I established a courier service company which was called "Jixian Courier Company". I went back to Langfang 5 years later.

What I want to state is that I was very shocked upon reading news in April 2006, of Falun Gong practitioners being live organ harvested that was published on Minghui website. I went to Shanghai Zhongshan Hospital to investigate how organ transplants were done in this hospital. I entered the ground floor lobby of Zhongshan Hospital Building, and then went to the reception on the ground floor. I asked the receptionist, I have a friend, his family needs to have an organ transplant. Which department should he visit? A man at the age of 70+, a doctor in a white robe, replied that it was very troublesome because it needs matching and many tests need to be done. I said, those are things to be done by you doctors, what do the patient's family need to do? He replied: money. I told him that money is not a problem. Then he said, bring the patient here. I replied: it depends on what time you can do organ transplant surgery. The patient will come ahead of that time. But if it takes you 3 years, 5 years, 8 years, 10 years before you get an organ, it wouldn't be good for the patient to come so much in advance. He said: if it takes that long, the patient would be dead already. In our hospital, it takes only half a month for an organ transplant. I again asked, if you use an organ from an elderly person of the age of 70 or 80, the organ would not last for too long, and then what could we do? He said, no, the organs are all good organs from young people, just ask the patient to come. I asked if we need to give any money to the person who donates his organ or if we need to thank his or her family. He replied that it was not necessary – we only need to pay the hospital. I asked him how much does it cost to have a kidney? He said, ￥400,000, maybe over ￥400,000. It would be safer if you have ￥500,000. Then he asked where the patient was. I told him the patient was in Hebei. He said, tell the patient to come quickly.

After this investigation I have done personally, I started to collect information of doctors and mailed them truth materials of Falun Gong practitioners being live organ harvested. I took advantage of my business to deliver materials of Falun Gong practitioners being live organ harvested so that more people come to know the evil nature of the Chinese Communist Party.

Summary of Oral Testimony: 6th April 2019
I visited the Zhongshan hospital in April 2006.

Initially I enquired about obtaining an organ transplant in general. When the doctor asked to be more specific about what I wanted I said I needed a kidney.

Minghui website is run by Falun Gong Practitioners.

There is often a backstory with things in China. Things are not transparent at all. I went to the hospital because I used to see television adverts which advocated how successful the hospital was at organ transplants.

During detention I did not hear anything about organ harvesting. However, fingerprints were taken, my teeth and the shape of my face was checked. The details were noted down. No bloods were ever drawn. I thought these were routine checks. Falun Gong practitioners were sent into the room one by one.

In my experience it is highly likely the source of the organs is Falun Gong practitioners. In my home city there are a high number of Falun Gong practitioners and many of them have told me that when they were detained, they were taken for the tests. No one ever explained to them why the tests were necessary. Armed police were sometimes watching over them when the tests were being carried out. This is why I suspect that the tests were related to organ harvesting; if the tests were for beneficial for them, they would have been told the same rather than the doctors/ police refusing to provide any explanation.

I found the doctors' information on a notice board at the hospital. I never received a response from the doctors to whom I had sent the information.

I do not think the authorities are aware of what I was doing. If they did, I would not be alive today.

Most of the detainees in my first two detentions were Falun Gong. In my third detention, most of the detainees were not Falun Gong Practitioners.

There were 36 detainees during my first detention (in the same building) and 33 of them were Falun Gong practitioners. During the last two detentions there were approximately 20 of them. Some of my fellow Falun Gong practitioners' detainees had their blood taken, the shape of their face noted down and their teeth checked.

The release certificate was given to me after my first detention. The authorities should have provided me with other documentation after the other releases but nothing was provided.

During my last two detentions, several Falun Gong Practitioners came in after me and only spent one night in the centre. They then disappeared and no one knew were they went. There were other practitioners who spent a couple of nights and then disappeared. I do not know whether they were released or taken to labour camps, re-education centres or jails.

Witness 21: Yang Jinhua

Female, age 46.

Were you ever placed in detention in China?

Yes

On July 21st 1999, I was detained in a cinema in Tianjin for 1 day.

On July 22nd 1999, I was detained in Laixi Asylum Centre in Qingdao, Shandong Province, and was kept there for 8 days. The Asylum Centre was exclusively for patients with mental illnesses.

On July 29th 1999, I was detained in Psychiatric Department of Laixi No 2 People's Hospital, Qingdao, Shandong Province, and I was kept there for 20 days.

At the end of October 1999, I was detained in Liaison Office of local government in Beijing for 1 night. The Liaison Office is a place where local governments illegally keep petitioners who have come to Beijing for airing their grievances.

From end of October to end of December in 1999, I was held for 2 months in Laixi Asylum Centre in Qingdao, Shandong Province.

In February 2000, I was held in Laixi Detention Centre, Qingdao, Shandong Province, and I was kept there for 7 days.

In May 2000, I was held in Laixi Chengguan Police Station, Qingdao, Shandong Province, and I was held there for 12 hours.

On May 20th 2000, I was detained in Laixi Asylum Centre, Qingdao, Shandong Province, and I was kept there for 4 days.

On June 8th 2000, I was detained in a big basement of Qianmeng Police Station, Beijing, for 7 hours.

On June 10th 2000, from noon, I was detained in Qianmen Police Station for 7 hours. On June 10th 2000, at night, I was held in Beijing Shijingshan Police Station and was held there for 7 days.

On June 18th 2000, I was detained in Laixi Detention Centre, Qingdao, Shandong Province, and was held there for 15 days.

On July 19th 2000, at night, I was detained in Yuyuantan Park Police Station, Beijing, for 1 day and 1 night.

On July 20th 2000, at night, I was detained in a remote detention centre in Shijiazhuang City, Hebei Province, and I was kept there for 10 days.

323

On July 30th 2000, at night, I was detained in Laixi Detention Centre, Qingdao, Shandong Province, and I was held there for 15 days.

From April 12 to May 8th 2002, I was detained in Dashan Detention Centre, Qingdao, Shandong Province, and I was held here for 27 days.

On May 8th 2002, I was kept in Wangcun No 2 Female Labour Camp, Zibo City, Shandong Province, and was kept there for 2 years and 6 months.

On February 2nd 2005, I was detained in Laixi Detention Centre, Qingdao, Shandong Province, and was kept there for 5 days.

On February 7th 2005, I was detained in Wangcun No 2 Female Labour Camp, Zibo City, Shandong Province, and was kept there for 1 year and 9 months.

What was the reason given by Chinese authorities? Do you have official documentation?

The reason given was that I continued with cultivation of Falun Gong and went to Beijing State Bureau of Letters and Visits for petitioning for Falun Gong.

I do not have official documentation.

Did you witness anything related to forced organ harvesting?

On May 8th 2002, on the way to be sent to No 2 Female Labour Camp in Shandong Province, I was taken into a hospital for comprehensive physical tests. Later, when I was also tested physically for several times at the clinic in the labour camp (I can't recall how many times altogether). I remember one morning, at the end of September 2004, I was ordered by the Division Chief Police Officer to go to the courtyard, where parked a big bus. I was ordered to get on the bus. When I got on the bus, I found there were already many other inmates from the labour camp. There were two policemen to monitor us. All windows of the bus were covered, and we could not see the outside. I didn't know how far the bus had driven before it stopped in a certain courtyard. The policemen on the bus ordered us to get off the bus and then separated us. I was taken into a room with a table. A policeman who wasn't wearing police uniform took me to another room and held my hand to force me to leave my fingerprints. After obtaining my fingerprints, he sent me to another room, in which a woman in a white robe measured my blood pressure and used stethoscope to listen to my heart sounds. Then she asked me to sit next to a table nearby. A woman asked me to extend my arms and she drew a large tube of blood from my wrist. After these tests, I was sent back onto the bus and taken back to the labour camp. After coming back, I felt very weird about the physical tests. So, I asked the chief police officer why. He replied it was just a physical test. I did not take it seriously. At that time, I was not aware of live organ harvesting. On

October 12, 2004, I had served the whole length of force labour re-education, but I was not released. At that time, my mother fell down and broke her leg. She was in the hospital, and she needed someone to take care of her. My younger sister, my relatives and friends didn't see me released, so they kept calling the labour camp, demanding release of me. The police bureau also called the labour camp and asked them to let me leave. I was released after in a dozen of days.

If you were tortured while in detention, please detail briefly below.
Yes, I was tortured during the detention periods.

I was tortured by 9 torturing methods. My body still aches, suffering from the unknown pains.

1.   Handcuffing: 3 times, for 37 hours and 30 minutes.

    a)   On July 19, 2000, I was handcuffed for 3 hours to a big tree in the courtyard of Beijing Yuyuantan Police Station by a policeman (I don't know his name).

    b)   On August 1, 2000, Shen Tao and Liu Guanghong – two police from Laixi Police Bureau – handcuffed me and kidnapped me with my hands cuffed all the way from Liaison Office of Laixi City Government in Beijing by train to Laixi Police Bureau and then to Laixi Detention Centre. I was cuffed for 24 hours.

    c)   On the morning of May 8, 2002, Shen Tao, Sui Guoqin and Zhang Luning handcuffed me all the way from Dashan Detention Centre, Qingdao, Shandong Province, to No 2 Female Labour Camp at Wangcun, Zibo City, Shandong Province. I was handcuffed for 10 hours and 30 minutes.

2.   Handcuffing with hands at the back diagonally: On the night of July 20, 1999, a policeman from Shijiazhuang Detention Centre (I don't know his name) handcuffed my hands at the back in a diagonal shape to the chair back, and then hurled the handcuffs onto the ground. He tortured me this way for 30 minutes.

3.   Electric shock by electricity from a hand telephone: On the night of July 20, 1999, a policeman from Shijiazhuang Detention Centre (I don't know his name) handcuffed me, tied my upper body to a chair with cloth, and tied my legs to a bench with cloth. Then he wired all my fingers and toes to a hand telephone.

He shocked me with the electricity generated by rotating the handles of the telephone. He shocked me for 3 times, each time lasting for 10 minutes. I would like to point out that Zhao Jinhua, a Falun Gong practitioner from Zhaoyuan, Yantai City, Shandong Province, was tortured to death by this torture method.

4. Lashed by a whip: on the morning of July 21, 1999, at Shijiazhuang Detention Centre, Hebei Province, an inmate chosen by police to monitor Falun Gong practitioners saw me practising Falun Gong exercises. He then used a special leather whip and flogged me very hard on my upper body for 20 minutes.

5. Hit by a leather boot: In November 1999, in Laixi Asylum Centre, a political supervisor from Laixi Chengguan Police Station (his surname was Wu) knocked me down onto the ground and used his boot to hit me, hitting me all over, for 30 minutes.

6. Force feeding: On the afternoon of June 14, 1999, two policemen from Beijing Shijingshan Detention Centre dragged me to a room, in which 4 policemen immobilized my limbs and head, two women doctors from the prison clinic inserted a tube into my nostril and tortured me for 1 hour and 30 minutes.

7. Stewing the eagle: During the period from May 8, 2002 to November 2006, I suffered from the torture which was called "stew the eagle", that is, I was not allowed to sleep, or to eat, or to go to the toilet. I suffered this torture for 60 days when I was held at No 2 Female Labour Camp at Wangcun, Zibo City, Shandong Province.

8. Sitting on a stool: From May 8, 2002 to November 2006, I was held in both the Second Division and the First Division of No 2 Female Labour Camp at Wangcun, Zibo City, Shandong Province for 1570 days, equaling 23542 hours.

9. High intensity physical labour: going out to work from 5am and getting off work at 10pm.

I did 13 types of handcrafted work: gluing handbags, assembling pens, assembling pencils, knitting sweaters, sewing beads onto clothes, sewing animal dolls, cutting clothes thread ends, making Chinese knots, weaving carpets, sewing quilts, making mooncake paper boxes, winding coils, making decorative flowers with poisonous glues that are exported to foreign countries.

List of the police who have persecuted me.

- Liu Changzeng, Police ID Number: 3734001, Former Chief Police Officer of the Labour Camp,
- Wang Huili, Division Chief
- Zhao Wenhui (female), Police ID Number: 3734049, Division Chief
- Sun Zhenhong, Police ID Number: 3734155, Deputy Division Chief
- Zhao Lili, Police ID Number: 3734134, Deputy Division Chief
- Dong Xinying, Police ID Number: 3734124, police
- Shi Wei, Police ID Number: 3734123, police
- Song Lijuan, Police ID Number: 3734068
- Xia Li, Police ID Number: 3734071
- Liu Guizhen, Police ID Number: 3734062
- Zhou Hongmei, Police ID Number: 3734163
- Other police: Li Ling, Fang Xiuzhen, Wang Yin, Liu Ying, Zhang Yan, Shen Hongxiu, Li Yue, Li Wei, Chen Qianmei, Wang Lijie, Li Hongmei, Cai Jing, Zhang Ran, Zhang Wenbo, Shen Ran

Director of 610 Office in Laixi: Yu Ruizhen
Party Secretary of the Political and Legislative Affairs Committee: Jiang Hongxing
Former Section Chief of Political Security Section: Shao Jun

Medical professionals who have persecuted me: On July 29, 1999, when I was kept at the Psychiatric Department of Laixi No 2 People's Hospital, Qingdao, Shandong Province, I was forced to take for 20 days a large amount of medicines that were harmful to the nervous system of the brain, after each meal.

The attending doctor: Zhang Wenhua. Nurse: Wang Bo

What was the 'reason' given for the torture?
Because I have never given up my belief in Falun Dafa, believing in that Falun Dafa is good and Zhen Shan Ren (Truth Compassion, Tolerance) is good

Summary of Oral Testimony: 6th April 2019

There were other people who were driven on the bus to the location where the tests were performed on me. I did not know who they were. No one explained to them where they were going and why the tests were being done.

The reason they tortured me whilst in custody was because I insisted on practising Falun Gong and because I refused to tell them my name. They wanted to know where I lived and my identity.

After many hours of being handcuffed on one occasion I suffered from numbness to my arm and hands and from back pain. The doctors in the clinic force fed me and did not explain why.

The doctors forced me to take large quantities of medicine and treated me as if I was a patient with a mental illness – they held me at a psychiatric department. I did not want to create trouble and wanted to prove that as a Falun Gong practitioner I upheld the beliefs of Falun Gong and would do as they said.

I never heard of forced organ harvesting whilst I was in detention. I was never threatened with forced organ harvesting.

The tube which they used to take blood was this size [shows size]. I remember it clearly as I had never had so much blood taken from her before. I had blood taken or physical examinations occasionally and irregularly.

I do not know if the other people who were medically tested were Falun Gong practitioners or from other backgrounds.

My family started to look for me when they realised that I had not been home, and they subsequently phoned the police station every day and appealed for my release.

No explanation was given for the medical tests carried out on me.

Witness 22: Yu Ming

Age 47. Languages: Chinese Mandarin

Detention in China

I have been detained for four times in China. Three times were for forced labour re-education, adding up to 8 years in total, and one imprisonment of 4 years. I was illegally kept for altogether 12 years.

> In January 2001 and November 2003, I was detained in Beijing Tuanhe Labour Camp.
> In March 2006, I was locked up in Masanjia Labour Camp in Shenyang.
> In September 2013, I was sentenced to imprisonment in Benxi City Prison in Liaoning province. (2013-2017)

I was arrested just because I am a Falun Gong practitioner. I don't keep the notice for the labor camp. Those are just notice, not formal legal documents. I have formal verdict for the sentence to prison. In the verdict, it listed my previous times in the labor camp.

I have the formal verdict, which I have submitted to the Tribunal.

Blood tests and threatened

In April 2002, in the so-called "Storm Fortification" Building of Beijing Tuanhe Labour Camp, police officer Jiang Haiquan, who is the deputy section chief of Education Section of Tuanhe Labour Camp, threatened to kill me. He had people draw blood from me for blood tests. They drew two tubes of blood from me. Police officers who were present: police officers from Tuanhe Labour Camp Liu Xincheng, Liu Guoxi (he is the division chief, his police ID number is 1153176), Tian Yu. There were some criminals present as well.

In September 2008, in Division Chief's office of Shenyang Masanjia Labour Camp, Liaoning Province, Yu Jiang, who is the Division Chief, threatened to kill me. He also had people draw blood of about 10ml from me. There were many police officers present, including Yu Jiang, Li Meng, Su Jufeng, Liu Jun, Wang Hanyu, and many others.

I and other Falun Gong practitioners were forced to get blood test many times in the labor camp and prison while other non-Falun Gong inmates didn't have the same 'treatment'.

This kind of blood tests were forced, and all carried out in police's offices. My body was tied up, and normally two full tubes of blood were taken. They did not tell me why they drew blood from me. Blood tests results were never given to me. There was a period that they repeatedly drew blood from me, approximately once in a week.

Torture and being forced to give up beliefs
This scenario has happened many times. The following are typical examples:

1. In April 2002, in Number 2 Building of Tuanhe Labour Camp, due to the execution of forced conversion, the police brutally tortured all Falun Gong practitioners who refused to be converted. Police officer Jiang Haiquan, who is the deputy section chief of Education Section of Tuanhe Labour Camp, threatened to kill me during that period. Jiang Haiquan, together with Liu Xincheng, Liu Guoxi (police ID number 1153176) and Tian Yu, assisted by many criminals, ripped off all my clothes and tied me up with ropes. They then used electric batons of over 30,000 voltage to electric shock me many times. They also inserted a tube into my stomach and brutally forced feeding me. They tied me onto a bed and fixed me there for over a month. As I refused to convert, they claimed that I "rejected to be re-educated" and they added 10 months to my forced labour period. They sent me, a man, to Beijing Women's Labour Camp and locked me up there for 10 months until the end of the forced labour period. This adding of the forced labour period was only announced orally, without going through any legal procedure. The basic idea of their oral announcement is as follows: "You must sign to agree to conversion. Otherwise, you will negatively impact our conversion rate and our bonuses. If you don't convert today, you are not going to live till tomorrow." "Then you will not be given a fixed labour re-education period. Otherwise, your re-education period will be prolonged, and you will be punished! Until you agree to give up your belief! We wouldn't allow you to affect our wages, just because of your refusing to convert!"

2. During the Beijing Olympic Games in 2008, all the prisons and forced labour re-education units in China carried out orders to reform all detainees. Falun Gong practitioners and other religious believers were forced to give up their

belief and they were forced to uphold the communist party. I was detained in Shenyang Masanjia Labour Camp, in Liaoning Province, during that period. In mid-September 2008, as I refused to give up my belief, deputy division chief Yu Jiang together with other police officers Li Meng, Su Jufeng, Liu Jun, Wang Hanyu and several others brutally electric shocked me with high-voltage electric batons many times. This caused many massive burns on my body. Later, also because of my refusal to give up my belief, they prolonged the imprisonment period forced on me by one more year. One of the officers said something with the following main ideas: during Beijing Olympic Games, there is a conversion rate throughout Chinese labour camps and prisons. And all the labour camps and prisons are assigned death quotas. Masanjia Labour Camp has been given two quotas, and you are one of the quotas. I was told this not by just one police in the labour camp. Some other kind detainees in the labour camp also told me that they had heard police say this.

3.   In 2013, I was kidnapped because Shenyang was to host the 12th National University Students' Sports Meet. I have obtained a confidential document that has not been made public, yet which can explain and prove this secretive suppression of Falun Gong and other religious believers by the Chinese Communist Party.

I was kidnapped on August 30, 2013. I was locked up in Cell 109 of Shenyang Detention Centre. At about 7pm on (date missing), 2013, Ma Lixin, sub-division chief of Shenyang State Security Sub-division took me out of Cell 109, handcuffed me, and brought me to the Special Interrogation Room on the 1st floor of Shenyang Detention Centre. He first talked with me. That interrogation room was not set up with any monitoring facilities as regulated by the Chinese laws, and the interrogation was carried out illegally during the night-time. I was locked to an iron chair. He firstly asked me to give up my belief and to plead guilty. If I obeyed, he would guarantee that I could go home after one month's detention. Otherwise, I would face a very miserable ending. I refused to give up my belief. Ma Lix in directed his inferior State Security police to interrogate me illegally for two nights. They used toothpicks to prick into my nails. They beat and hit me with their fists. They put books on top of my chest and back and then used hammers to smash on my chest and back. With the books on the top, the smashing caused many internal wounds, but they could not be seen from the surface. I stilled refused to give up my belief. They then re-ported my case to the Procuratorate and the court, and I was sentenced to 4-years' imprisonment.

(The attached document is a confidential internal document, signed personally by the mayor of Shenyang City. It is this document that has caused me and many others to be kidnapped and sentenced to imprisonment.

Did you witness anything related to forced organ harvesting that you would like to tell the Tribunal about?
I have two cases with evidence to provide to the tribunal:

Case one
One of my friends Mr Yixi Gao, a Falun Gong practitioner from Mudanjiang city, Heilongjiang province, was arrested at around 11pm April 19, 2016. Five police, including LV Hongfeng,YU Yang, Li Xuejun broke into his home and took Mr. Gao Yixi and his wife SUN Fengxia without showing any warrant or other legal documents. Police aso took laptop and printer. Mr GAO and his wife were put into the second detention center of Mudanjiang. Mr GAO lost his life in the detention center within 10 days. On April 26, 2016, when Gao's family members went to the detention center, they were told that Mr GAO was already dead. He was only 45 years old.

A family member of Gao Yixi is a friend of mine. And this family member of Gao is still in China. He/She has seen Gao's corpse, which was not yet cremated.

Investigation audio recording No. 1: investigation Comprehensive Section Chief Zhu Jiabin from "610 Office"

Investigation time: June 21, 2016

On April 19, 2016, Gao Yixi, a practitioner of Falun Gong in Mudajiang City, Heilongjiang Province, was kidnapped illegally by deputy team leader Lv Hongfeng and four other police from Yuanming Community Police Office of Xianfeng Police Branch Office, Mudanjiang Police Bureau. He was then detained in No 2 Detention Centre of Mudanjiang. On April 30, the police sent notice to his families that Gao was dead, and his body was kept in Sidao Cremation Factory of Mu-danjiang and was performed an "autopsy".

On June 21, 2016, Zhu Jiabin, Section Chief of the Comprehensive Section of Mudanjiang "610" Office, acknowledged openly to the investigator that they had live harvested Gao Yixi's organs, and he said that the organs had been "sold". We have an audio recording that proves this is true.

When his family saw his body, they saw Mr Gao's eyes opened wide, his fists tight and handcuffed trace on his wrists, his chest swelled high. But his stomach was deflated with no organs inside.

On May 5th 2015, Mr Gao's attorney CHEN Zhiyong went to various police departments and prosecution office and told them the death of GAO Yixi and request them to investigate. But by now Mr GAO Yixi's body is still in the freezer in Mudanjiang funeral parlor.

Torture in detention in China
I have been tortured many times during my detention. I could not remember how many times. These include numerous 300,000 volt electric baton shocks. My hands were hanged on the door with the tips of my feet barely on the ground for more than a month. The brutal forced feeding made me have permanent pain in the esophagus and stomach. The needles with electricity were inserted into the acupuncture point on the head. I was forced to eat unknown medicine. I was tied on a bed with my arms and legs split for nearly a month. I was locked on an iron chair for three months. The awl and the toothpick were inserted into my fingers, and so on. There is a big scar of more than 10 cm long on my head. There are countless other kinds of tortures. Just because I don't give up my faith in Falun Gong.

Among the people who tortured me were Liu Guojun (Captain) of Beijing Tuanhe Labor Camp, police number 1153176, Wei Guoping, police number 1153229, Gong Wei, Guo Jinhe, Jiang Haiquan, Tian Yu, Liu Xincheng, and Ni Zhenxiong.

Those who tortured me in Masanjia Labor Camp of Liaoning Province: Gao Hongchang, director of the Masanjia labor camp, Yu Jiang, Li Meng, Su Jufeng, Wang Yuyu, Liu Jun. These people are all police from the labour camp.

Shenyang Police: Ma Lixin, the captain of the detachment, Zhang Tingyan, the captain of the National Security Team of Shenhe District, Liu Licheng, the deputy head of the National Security Bureau of Shenhe District, Zhao Chen, the police of the National Insurance Team, and the former political commissar of the Shenyang Municipal Detention Center, Shan Baolin, Shenyang Detention center.

Documentation, audio, video, photographs to support the submission
In the labor camps and prison, I secretly recorded a lot of footages of Falun Gong practitioners being persecuted. I also photographed many internal scenes of prison and labor camp. These materials can be provided to the tribunal. This is the first

time in recent years that the international community expose the persecution of human rights.

Since many of my friends have lost their lives and are suspected to have their organs harvested, I have done the investigation in hospitals across China since October 2018. I will provide the court with the investigation video I secretly recorded at major military hospitals and armed police hospital. It is clear that Mainland China is still doing these organ transplants. The shortest waiting time is only one month to get matching organs successfully. And there are pictures of doctors doing this kind of surgery.

Is there anything else you would like to tell the Tribunal about your experience?
1. When I was in prison and labor camps, I have encountered five death penalty prisoners who have been executed. In the end of 2013, when I was in Shenyang detention center, I met a general manager of a funeral parlor who was arrested for corruption. I was detained in the same cell with him when I was kept in Shenyang Detention Camp. When asked by a death penalty prisoner for details of death execution, he told us how a death execution was performed.

His last name is Li. He told me that before the death penalty is executed, the inmate is forced to sign a voluntary donation of body organs. At that time, I and another prisoner who was sentenced to death asked Li what the execution of the death penalty was like.

The funeral parlor manager said that when the death penalty was executed, two injections were given. The first injection is an anaesthetic injection, and the second one is fatal. However, the second injection is generally not used. That means the person had not actually died but was anesthetized. Sometimes the first injection sometimes is not given according to the needs. For death execution, two injections are given successively. The first injection was only an anaesthetic injection, for making people unconscious, not fatal. The second injection is the deadly drug injection.

When the court executes the death penalty, it first informs the Shenyang Army General Hospital and their funeral parlor to the designated place. The people in their funeral parlors waited for the doctors in the hospital to handle the corpses.

That means taking the organs first and then the corpses were collected by the funeral parlors. Sometimes the incomplete bodies of several people were put into one corpse bag and cremation is carried out. Only a pile of ashes is given to the family members, and few family members care about this. Some family members even do not pick up the ashes. In this case, the funeral parlors will dispose of the ashes on their own.

2. During the process of imprisonment, I met several people who executed the death: Xia Junfeng, Gong Zhaopeng, Yang Hanlin, Han Wei, Niu (I can't remember his first name).

The names mentioned above are all criminals who have been executed to death. They were all kept in the same cell with me when I was detained in Shenyang Detention Centre.

Second Artillery Hospital Hepatobiliary Clinic. Doctor Zhang Tao was asked to look for Doctor Yu Delei, from the inpatient section on the 11th floor:

Exhibit A
Time: 23:19.9

Z: Is Doctor Yu here?
P: He's not here
Z: Can we do it here?
P: We can't now; it seems that it's done at the Armed Police hospital. We haven't done it recently.
Z: Do you know how much it costs?
P: 800,000 to 1 million.
Z: Liver?
P: All
Z: Are you referring to the surgery?
P: The Armed Police hospital does it.
Z: You did this previously right?
P: Yes
Z: When did that stop?
P: I forgot which year — but the hospital no longer allowed it.
Z: Was it from the beginning of this year that the second artillery hospital quit?
P: No, maybe from 2017! At other places, the Armed Police hospitals are still active.
Z: So, it stopped in 2017? Did it not continue afterwards?

P: I do not know. It depends if it is allowed; if they allowed it we'd do it. There is the military reform, remember – isn't the army reforming!?

Z: So, it stopped in 2017, that means it's already a year now.

P: About that.

Time: 23: 21: 15

Z: Then it will be little use for me to find Doctor Yu. The clinic asked me to talk to him, but there won't be any operation so there's no use looking for him.

P: Doctor Li Chaoyang is in charge of the matter, but he's not here.

Z: So, isn't it the case that we're not doing it?

P: [He] can contact other hospitals who will do it!

Z: Ah, so he can connect me. What was the name, something Chaoyang?

P: Li.

Z: I went to 309 [military hospital] but they wouldn't allow it. The leader had been arrested, and it was meant to be connected with prisoners.

P: It was to do with military reform. No relation to prisoners.

Two resumes by the name of Li Chaoyang are found. One is listed under the second Artillery and the other is listed under the Second Artillery hospital. It is unknown if these two resumes belong to the same person. Note: The Second Artillery refers to China's strategic missile forces.

Exhibit B
Video: Patient who had kidney transplantation z: investigator p: patient

Z: Are you here for transplantation? Are you done with the surgery?

P: I had a kidney [transplant].

Z: How much was it?

P: The kidney itself cost about RMB 350,000 [US$52,000]

Z: What about for the entire surgery?

P: The surgery was around RMB 100,000; I paid RMB 86,000

Z: And the total cost for everything?

P: Well, have to pay extra to the doctor – for that I gave a RMB 50,000 bonus.

Z: You mean a red envelope?

P: Everyone gives RMB 50,000.

Z: So, you put the red envelope directly in the doctor's hands? Outside of the bill statement?

P: Normally you just give it to Director Wang.

Z: Does he not need to say anything, or does it have to come out and ask for it?

P: There's the matter of whether it's urgent or not.

Z: I'm urgent!

P: If you're in a rush, you better give them some money! If you're not, then just wait; maybe it'll be a year or 18 months then.

P: What's your blood type?

Z: Type A

P: It shouldn't take long for Type A patient. I know someone who has type A blood. He's the one who brought me here. He is Type A. It was only 7 days.

Z: Seven days? That fast?

P: After he paid the gift money, he only waited 7 days. Normally it's two weeks, or at most a month.

Z: So basically, if I don't pay anything, then it might take a while, but how long might it drag out?

P: It depends on your luck. It could be a long time, or several months, sometimes a month or two and so on, and some are even two or three years.

Z: How long have you been waiting?

P: My blood type is O, so it's slower.

Z: Right, right, I heard it's hard to find a match for Type O people.

P: It takes about two months.

Z: So, it cost you about RMB600,000

P: Around RMB 470,000 or RMB 480,000 including the gift money. It depends. Sometimes it costs less than that, but there's not that much difference. It costs an extra RMB 20,000 or RMB 30,000 at most.

Z: What about the situation here – they have abundant kidney sources?

P: They have plenty here. I had my kidney transplantation done on January 28. They did it for 4 people that day.

Z: They did kidney transplantation surgery for 4 patients at the same time?

P: Right

Z: Sounds like they have a lot of kidneys available!

P: They're doing that every day, or at least during the New Year they were doing it every day.

P: Whatever they case, they have a lot of patients.

P: There are more patients on Tuesdays and Thursdays when Director Wang is on duty. Mondays and Wednesday are normal.

Z: How old are you?

P: 31.

17:17:00

Z: Was that kidney you received good? Do you know who it came from? Is that something one can find out?

P: If you give them cash, they'll answer your questions in detail.

Z: How about for your case?

P: I didn't ask.

Z: How could you not ask? What if they gave you an old man's kidney?

P: It seems like mine was small [i.e. from a young person]. My creatinine levels are currently 300; you should be at around 100 when discharged.

Z: So at least they told you it was from a young person.

P: If you pay, they'll make a few guarantees. They'll guarantee it's fast, and you can be sure it's high quality. If you give them the cash, they'll definitely get you a good one. That's the point.

Z: Right! So just to be safe, we're happy to pay up.

17.18.20

Z: I heard transplantation surgery could fail sometimes, and you have to have it done again and again. Sometimes people might have several transplants

P: As far as kidney transplantation goes, it's impossible that you could only have it done once. A kidney can last 20-30 years for many people, and for others about 10 years. From this hospital, one kidney might last 20-30 years.

Z: You asked?

P: Yeah.

Video: Kidney transplantation patient Yang Fei

Z: Mentioned human rights issue

P: In the past, they obtained organs from executed prisoners Patient Yang Fei is visiting the hospital.

Exhibit C

The lawyer may be this person: (link redacted), same name, based in Beijing. There's an email and phone number there. May be possible to confirm identity in some fashion. Not sure if helpful or necessary though.]

17.24.09

Patient Dong Renyou, 64 years old, from Jilin Province. Dong is a lawyer and has his own law firm. He is returning the hospital for a checkup after surgery and prescriptions.

Z: Secret investigator

P: Patient, Mr. Dong Renyou

Z: How long does one have to wait to do liver transplantation here?

P: It depends; it depends on the liver source. Where are you from? Different people have different experiences. I came here in May last year [2018], did the registration, and paid the money; they did it [the liver transplantation] on June 20, 2018.

Z: So, it took about a month?

P: I was in a very serious situation then. At the stage they had plenty of livers available.

Z: Wow, so it depends on when you come?

P: Of course, you've got to have a source for the liver. If you don't have a liver source

Z: Aren't they abundant?

P: This hospital generally has fairly abundant sources compared with other hospitals nationwide. They've done it for many years, and on top of that they have some special means that remain secret to get liver sources – actually they buy them. They'll pay whoever can get the livers.

P: In June [2018] it cost about RMB 400,000 to get on the waiting list. The surgery cost about 300,000 to 350,000.

Z: You mean you have to pay RMB400,000 to get in line? So, there's a waiting list?

P: You pay RMB100,000 first, and when it's your turn you pay the remaining RMB300,000. That makes the total RMB400,000. That's the amount that I paid. When it comes to surgery time, you have to pay extra to the doctor and the anesthetist, so you are looking at about RMB500,000 in total.

Z: You have to pay that much to the anesthetist?

P: This is a must. For such a big surgery, you have to make sure nothing falls through the cracks no matter who you are. You just have to make sure nothing goes wrong. So, it matters where you're from; if you come down from Beijing, it might be easier, otherwise there is no way you could have it done.

Z: [Will] the doctors only tell me the cost for the liver source?

P: RMB400,000

Z: They did not explain the other parts, that there will be more costs come surgery time?

P: The surgery alone costs RMB300,000 to RMB350,000. If you add RMB400,000 extra fees, you can have it done with RMB800,000. This is if there are no special circumstances. Last year I paid over RMB1 million, and I had to be resuscitated at one point. The emergency cost a lot of money before I even had the liver transplantation.

Z: I just asked that young guy if you want to have it done faster, will it work to just give a red envelope [of cash]?

P: Depends on which team is going to perform your surgery. I can introduce you to Director Zhou's team. Director Chen is the chief surgeon. Director Zhou is Chen's assistant. The assistant is responsible for three teams. I had mine done with Director Zhou's team. If you want to do it fast, I can talk to Zhou and you can just pay RMB100,000 so you get ahead.

Z: You pay Zhou directly?

P: No

Z: Who do you give the money to?

P: They have people for taking it. All this is above board, but the red envelope is under the table, to get you ahead of the line.

Z: Who do you give red envelope to?

P: They let you know when it's time to pay; there are doctors who will receive you.

Z: Is RMB100,000 enough?

P: More than enough.

Z: That young fellow just told me RMB50,000 is enough.

P: It depends. I paid RMB100,000. This is in addition to my official payment on the invoice. I wanted a good liver source, so I paid up. For a 3-person team, that's 10,000 to each person. Director Chen doesn't need it. You pay RMB5,000 to anesthetist and the person who is in charge of the blood bank; you want a high-quality liver source.

Z: I first want to know whether they actually have livers available.

P: They certainly do.

Z: How much is it?

P: RMB 400,000 for immediate availability. That woman [referring to another patient] offered RMB500,000, then paid another RMB60,000 or RMB70,000 for surgery, then gave as gift money RMB60,000 to RMB70,000. You can have it done with about RMB560,000 or RMB570,000.

Z: The wait is really a few months?

P: No – they can do it in a month. Go talk to Director Zhou now and he'll be able to do it in a month.

Z: We went to the 309 [PLA] hospital and were told they can't do it anymore because they can't get liver sources from executed prisoners, so it seems the sources are prisoners – it's not like they're getting them from pigs and cows.

P: So, why'd I pay so much? Because I wanted a good one.

Z: So, that's why I want to know whether we can pick our sources? I want a young one! Do you know whose liver you got?

340

P: I know; I don't know the donor's name, but I know their circumstances, like age, height, all that.

Z: So, you even know the height!

P: It's internal information

Z: So, it looks like paying the money is well worth it!

P: Money does the job. Don't be stingy when it comes to the liver source. With a good liver source, you can live another 10 years.

Z: Really?

P: This is no joke. When it comes to this, everyone is equal regardless of your title.

Z: So, you need to have a lot of money.

P: I know how things work here. I know the former heads of the Ministry of Health, like Chen Minliang, Cui Yueli, very well. Also, I've helped them out on some things, so as for the Ministry... also, I have a friend whose wife works in the Ministry, so I know how it all works. I know all about what goes on behind the scenes.

Z: They say they can get livers from young people, from qigong practitioners. They say the best source is qigong practitioners – and didn't Jiang Zemin ban Falun Gong? [Patient smiles.]

P: What if the liver were to be in good condition, for example from someone who had an accident and who they failed to resuscitate after a day or two, and was under the age of 30?

Z: Are there really that many [such cases]?

P: So, what if the person practiced qigong – the type that cultivates the body, not the martial arts type?

Z: Are these the Falun Gong ones they're talking about?

P: No, those are just rumours – [these donors] do breathing exercises, purely using qi to improve their bodies.

Z: Are there really [so many] young people practicing this [qigong]?

P: Just too many. Don't worry about the one with the so-called Master people believe. Normally for the breathing exercises, all the cells in their liver have opened up – they don't even have the form of cells. The chemical indicators are the same, but the quality is different; the numbers are the same, but the livers of those who practice qigong are opened. The qi is in the blood, all through the fat, and throughout the heart.

Z: I'm going to slip them cash, I want to stipulate a condition: I want a good one, a Falun Gong one.

P: You don't need to mention it – you're a local. Talk to Director Zhu, he's in charge of finding matches; he's also the deputy director. Director Chen is the leading director, and he won't want a cent. He's absolutely upright, he doesn't want anything. Say that you spoke to a previous patient so-and-so [i.e. Dong Renyou, the speaker] and he referred you, but that you want quality supplies. Don't mention the other stuff. Then, give him 50,000 yuan, give Li Zhiqiang 20,000, and give 10,000 to the anesthetist and blood transfusion people.

Z: Where are you from? What do you do for living?

P: Jilin, but I've been in Beijing over 30 years. I'm a lawyer. They don't hide things from me; I know everything. Director Zhu has the final say when it comes to matching the liver, like whose liver you'll get. Director Zou will confirm that the match is feasible. So go and talk to Director Zhu directly.

Z: I've heard that there's meant to be a difference – like, some of them practice qigong, so the body is healthy and young.

P: So, hopefully you'll be able to get a match that does qigong and breathing exercises. [But] don't mention practicing qigong. It's dangerous.

Z: As long as they do Falun Gong, it'll be fine!

P: If they do Falun Gong, that'd work too – the whole thing is just a breathing exercise qigong practice. I want the donor to be under 30 years old, and their [body] size has to be about right, as well as the blood type. If you get all those matched up, you won't have any trouble with rejection.

Z: How old are you?

P: I'm 64. I had no choice but to get the transplant. I was once in the hospital for two years, and I've had cancer for six years. It came back three times, and I had four surgeries to remove the cancer.

Z: If [transplants] are regulated in the future, what will happen?

P: That's only happening in Shanghai, Guangdong, and Beijing. The 301 [military] hospital is still fine.

Z: I heard there's a group doing this

P: It's become an industrial chain. Here [referring to the Armed Police Hospital] they have more liver sources than patients.

P: If Director Zou is doesn't come out, you'll want to see Li Zhiqiang

Z: It seems that there were many more patients in the past than now.

P: The regulations now aren't like they were before; now it's been distributed down, and you can get treatment lower down [the hierarchy of hospitals]. For example, some people not from Beijing, like from Hebei, they don't have to come up here anymore, [they can get treatment at] a local hospital. In the past they all had to come to Beijing. I think the number of annual patients has gone down.

Summary of Oral Testimony: 6th April 2019

I came to the USA on 27th January 2019.

In August 2013 in Shenyang there was a national sports meeting held for this reason I was put in prison for four years, released in October 2017.

This photo was taken in detention after I received torture and this one as well.

It was not because of the so-called confidential files that I held. The confidential material that I held was actually collected me after these incidents. I was kidnapped or held for no obvious reason at all. I think it was because they needed to maintain stability during what I already mentioned, the sports meeting period. Because President Xi during that time needed to inspect the community district next to where I used to live.

In this picture [picture shown to camera] am the one waving to the camera. This is where I was kidnapped. I refused to wear prisoners' clothes at that time because I was not a criminal.

I have to say sorry for not being able to share the information regarding this letter signed by the mayor [of Shenyang] because it relates to other people's safety but I am willing to share it with you in private if it's necessary.

The director of the 6:10 office who held a meeting in Liaoning to discuss how to crack down on Falun Gong Practitioner and how to deal with them and how to re-educate and convert them. I started to collect information and evidence after I came to the USA especially.

The document I can't share has a title which is how to deal with cults. The director of 6:10 office came to our city to host this meeting on 11th July. Liaoning Province needs to strengthen its measures in cracking down on cults such as Falun Gong. To implement the direction and policy laid out by the director of the 6:10 office. In order to make sure the smooth going of the national sport's meeting we have to do the following: one of the tasks is to crack down on Falun Gong. We were to need the cooperation of the provincial and national security bureau and the judicial system on the conversion of Falun Gong Practitioner. Not long after this meeting held on 23rd July 2013, in August, I was arrested. This was a watershed in the persecution of Falun Gong Practitioner. That's the summary of the document.

The families of the Falun Gong Practitioner Gao Yixi saw his corpse. His eyes wide open and his body deflated – obviously his organs were missing. We made a video of the footage.

Yes, I have a recording of Zhu Jiabin saying he is a butcher and admitting he sold organs of the victim. We (F-G Practitioners) made a phone call to Zhu Jiabin director of the 6:10 office, he didn't know we were recording and admitted openly that he was a butcher.

During my detention in the detention centre and the jails I was threatened by the police that they would kill me by live harvesting my organs. Some of the fellow Falun Gong Practitioners disappeared for no reason. More than 10 Falun Gong Practitioners died in this persecution and also there were reports on the emergence of hospitals and factories dedicated to live organ harvest from Falun Gong Practitioner in Shenyang, Liaoning. And after this I decided to conduct investigations across China including Beijing. As a result, I found some inside stories and I used audio-video or pictures to record everything and make people more aware of what had happened.

We managed to obtain the phone number belonging to Zhu Jiabin and also, we had video evidence to show that Zhu Jiabin worked at the 6:10 office. And also, during the appeals of fellow Falun Gong Practitioners we could prove that these people are related to CCP authorities.

I have the video that testifies that everything happened at the time. I can play this video to everyone if it is necessary and because I knew the family of the victim before this happened. After I was released in 2018, I obtained this video as proof.

The people who received the death penalty referred to at the end of my statement were not Falun Gong Practitioner.

I do have a copy of my own witness statement in my own language. My statement is a bi-lingual statement.

Clarification Post Hearing

Please tell us about the date at the bottom of the footage? When were the videos filmed, and by who?
Some videos are not taken by me. It was filmed in February and March of this

year. However, the photographer forgot to adjust the time at that time, sometimes shooting the day directly. Then Beijing's monitoring equipment will grab them according to the video time. So I asked the later editors to help adjust and cover up. The blue background behind the subtitles is actually the actual shooting time. Some videos are adjusted by the photographer to the future during photography. It may not be important for later editing, so it will not be overwritten with blue subtitles. List is below of the videos and dates of filming.

Did your lawyer get in trouble?

Yes. My lawyer is China's "709 kidnapping lawyers", the first kidnapped lawyer Wang Yu and Wang Quanzhang lawyer. They defended our Falun Gong practitioners and were sentenced by the Chinese government in the name of disturbing the court order. At present, Wang Quanzhang is still being held in the Tianjin Detention Center. I have provided the document that is the judgment of the court with the name of the defense lawyer. (see attached)

See screenshots: "This was broadcast by CCTV. When I was tried in court, defense lawyers Wang Yu and Wang Quanzhang were kidnapped by the court, video screenshots (screen shot file names 'Yu Ming Defence Lawyer 1' 'Yu Ming Defence Lawyer 2')

New – See video: 'This is a video of when I was taken from the detention center to the court. The person who raised his hand is me.' (File name: YuMing_enteringCourtfromDetentionCentre)

In your testimony to the China Tribunal you say "We made a phone call to Zhu Jiabin, director of the 610 office." What do you mean by "we"?

A lady investigator who is also a Falun Gong practitioner gave the call to Zhu Jiabin.

What are the dates of the videos?

File name: YuMing_PLA309_Nov2018_recipient_Clip1 and Clip 2 excerpts are in the dropbox folder- this video was not shown in April)

这个是在 2018 年 11 月中旬拍摄，其中有使用 Iphone8 手机拍摄，是其他人配合我拍摄。This was filmed in mid-November 2018, which was shot with an Iphone8 phone, and was shot by others with me. This has the transplant recipient talking about how quick it is to get a transplant and the payments and number of transplants that happened when he was in the hospital.

File name:

Video excerpts:

'YuMing_BillboradAdvertising Transplants_2018)

'YuMIng_2018_recipients'

'YuMing_2018_SpeakingWithSurgeon.mp4' (Will provide more info on this person in private)

这个是2018年11月底，我在解放军二炮医院里面的医生宿舍拍摄。

These three are at the end of November 2018, I was filming in the doctor's dormitory inside the Second Artillery Hospital of the People's Liberation Army.

File name: 4-本溪监狱-胡國艦-Masanjia-Hu-Guojian_died.mp4 (Tribunal viewed in April)

Hu Guojian, who was shooting in March, April, and May of 2017, was my own use of miniature video equipment to smuggle into Benxi Prison.

File name: FG_beaten_labourCamp马三家被迫害的學員 Masanjia-short-slave-labor-persecution. (Tribunal viewed in April)

This is in 2008, during the Beijing Olympic Games, at the Ma Sanjia Labor Camp, I used micro video equipment to record.

File name: 本溪監獄路遠峰-Benxi-Prison-walls-compound-Lu-Yuanfeng-letter.mp4 – (Tribunal viewed in April)

This is the letter of complaint/accusation I asked LU Yuanfeng to write in November 2016, after he was beaten by policemen in Benxi Prison. The letter stated who had beaten him.

File name: 黑勞工-Masanjia-forced-labor-diodes – (Tribunal viewed in April)

This video was taken during the Beijing Olympic Games in 2008. I was filmed at the Masanjia Labor Camp.

Additional Documents Provided

https://chinatribunal.com/submissions/yu-ming_release-certificate-scan%e9%87%
8a%e6%94%be%e8%af%81%e6%89%ab%e6%8f%8f-jpg/

https://chinatribunal.com/wp-content/uploads/2019/06/Yu-Ming_Release-Certificate_
ENGLISH-%E7%BF%BB%E8%AF%91%E6%96%87%E4%BB%B603-%E9%
87%8A%E6%94%BE%E8%AF%81.pdf

https://chinatribunal.com/wp-content/uploads/2019/06/Yu-Ming_Shenhe-District-Law-Judgment_ENGLISH_%E7%BF%BB%E8%AF%91%E6%96%87%E4%BB%B601-%E6%B2%88%E6%B2%B3%E5%8C%BA%E6%B3%95%E5%88%A4%E5%86%B3.pdf

https://chinatribunal.com/wp-content/uploads/2019/06/Yu-Ming_Shenhe-District-Law-Judgment_%E6%B2%88%E6%B2%B3%E5%8C%BA%E6%B3%95%E5%88%A4%E5%86%B3%E4%B9%A6.pdf.pdf

https://chinatribunal.com/wp-content/uploads/2019/06/Yu-MIng_Shenyang-City-Chinese-Law-Judgment_ENGLISH_%E7%BF%BB%E8%AF%91%E6%96%87%E4%BB%B602-%E6%B2%88%E9%98%B3%E5%B8%82%E4%B8%AD%E6%B3%95%E5%88%A4%E5%86%B3-%E8%AF%91%E6%96%87.pdf

https://chinatribunal.com/wp-content/uploads/2019/06/Yu-Ming_Shenyang-City-Chinese-Law-Judgment_%E6%B2%88%E9%98%B3%E5%B8%82%E4%B8%AD%E6%B3%95%E5%88%A4%E5%86%B3%E4%B9%A6.pdf.pdf

https://chinatribunal.com/wp-content/uploads/2019/06/YuMing_Defence LawyerTakenFromCourt1.png.pdf

https://chinatribunal.com/wp-content/uploads/2019/06/YuMing_Defence LawyerTakenFromCourt2.png.pdf

Witness 23: Wang Chunying

Age 64

Were you ever placed in detention in China? If yes, where, when and for how long? (please include the name of the detention facility if you know it).

Yes, I have been detained twice at Masanjia (Liaoning, China) correctional facility for 5 years 3 months. The first time was from 1 January 2002 to January 2005 (3 years); the second time was from August 2008 to November 2011 (2 years 3 months).

Did you witness anyone in the detention centres talking about forced organ harvesting?
Xin Shu Hua, a fellow Falun Gong practitioner who came from the same area as I (near a river), who was detained together with me, told me that she had gone through many rounds of torture from 2002 to 2004 but refused to renounce her faith in "truthfulness, compassion and forbearance", until finally the political commissar of Masanjia, Wang Nai Min, said, "You cultivate compassion, right? Why don't you donate your heart then?" Xin Shu Hua said, "I have to live in order to cultivate." Wang Nai Min then said, "This is not up to you, I will send you to Su Jia Tun". The wicked policeman then called Su Jia Tun hospital. The person at the hospital said a vehicle would be dispatched to fetch her at 9 pm that night. In the end, the vehicle didn't appear. The next day, Wang Nai Min called the hospital again, and the hospital said the vehicle would arrive in the afternoon. But the vehicle didn't turn up that day either. The third day, he called again and waited but the vehicle still didn't turn up. In the end, the matter was set aside.

Did you witness anything related to forced organ harvesting that you would like to tell the Tribunal about?
In the afternoon on 12 May 2008, around 200 Falun Gong practitioners from the first and second divisions of Masanjia, were all called to have their blood tested. At that time, I refused, because on 8 March 2006, the overseas media had exposed the systematic forced live organ harvesting of Falun Gong practitioners, thus I knew that they needed to conduct blood tests as part of the organ harvesting process. But at the end, I was forced on the bed by 9 policemen and had 5 ml of blood drawn from me. From my 30 years of experience as a nurse doing medical examinations, I know that when conducting biochemical tests, only 2 ml of blood are required to

conduct tests for liver and kidney functions, yet they drew 5 ml from me, which means that they must have other tests to be carried out.

If you were tortured while in detention, please detail briefly below.
I was tortured twice. Once was the "diagonal hanging", I was positioned between two iron beds, my arms were handcuffed to the beds – one was handcuffed to the upper bed while the other was handcuffed to the lower bed, and I was stretched tight. I could neither stand nor squat for 16 hours. The second time was the "large stretch" when I was stretched for 23 hours – my body was stretched from the head of the bed almost to the end of the bed, my mouth was sealed with tape, my ankles and knees were bound by cloth belts, and both hands were handcuffed separately to the end of the bed (this was reported on Minghui). Those who tortured me: camp head Yang Jian, division leader Wang Xiao Feng, Zhang Chun Guang, officer Zhai Yan Hui, and captain Chen Qiu Mei. Reason was because of the signature on the admission-of- guilt form.

Summary of Oral Testimony: 6th April 2019
I was in prison with other Falun Gong Practitioners.

On 12th May 2008 I was working and all of a sudden, the policeman called us and there was a big bus we were then being sent onto the bus and sent to the labour camp.

We were being called to the correctional facility at Masanjia, Liaoning. There were three to four policemen wearing white clothes and there were men and women policemen there.

So, the policemen asked us to stand alongside the wall telling us that they were going to take some tests. Then I asked them what kind of blood test you are going to do. They said they were doing it for a disease. I said what kind of disease. And he said why are you asking questions and talking nonsense? When I asked you to get the blood test you will do so as I said.

I've been a nurse for 30 years usually if there is a test, 2 ML is very sufficient. However, they took almost three times that amount, nearly the complete syringe, so that's in my common sense, that's very over the normal amount that's needed.

Yes, I know about organ harvesting. On 8th March 2006, overseas media exposed live organ harvesting happening in China, so I was aware of that. So I was suspecting that the blood tests that they conducted on us was about organ harvesting.

I did not give up my practice of Falun Gong so they tortured me, they used a way called 'diagonal hanging' and the 'large stretch' to torture me.

Yes, that's right, nine policemen forced me onto a bed so they could take the blood. At that time, I asked them why did you take our blood test so they asked people to get the blood tested first, I was put at the end of the line to get blood test. I was arrested five times. I was imprisoned twice.

My friend in detention said she was threatened with a heart donation. She told me in person, and she told me that if there are opportunities coming up, she is very willing to be the witness to expose this matter.

So, I was detained in 2001. I knew about the organ harvesting in 2000. I was pressed [unclear, can a translator check this?] by nine policemen in my second detention.

No other incidents where forced organ harvesting was threatened in my first period of detention.

The second time it was a more serious matter because I already knew about the matters about organ harvesting. So, I resisted very strongly about the blood test. I was holding onto the door handle so there were several policemen trying to put me on to the bed for the blood test. That was in May 2008. I was referring to what I said before. There were nine policemen.

My second period of detention was actually from August 2007 until November 2009. Over 2 years' time. So, I was detained from August 2007 until November 2009. Two years and three months altogether. The date I was forced to take blood test was on 12th May 2008 in the afternoon. The 12th May 2008 incident was during the second period of detention.

Some inmates were being sent away I had no way of knowing if they were sent away back home or not.

I did not experience torture of a sexual nature.

Yes, I was a nurse in China. When I was a nurse for those 30 years there were very few organ transplant hospitals. I learnt about it in 2006 and was detained in 2002.

I was a nurse in Dalian, Liaoning that is a large hospital considered to be a 3rd grade hospital.

I have something important to add. Is that ok? Several months ago I had a chance to meet a person, her father was a victim of organ harvesting. So this person tried to expose his own experience but because this person is under surveillance and being chased by the CCP so I am not at liberty to disclose this person's identity.

I am very willing to put this person in touch with the Tribunal.

Clarification Post Hearing
Dates of detention/arrest are inaccurate in the statement.

The officials made a mistake on the second document regarding my age.

Although the release papers says released on Jan 14, 2005, I was actually released 6 days early on Jan 8th, 2005. Is this the date inaccuracy?

Additional Documents Provided
https://chinatribunal.com/submissions/chunying-wang_certificatesofrelease_2005 2009english/

https://chinatribunal.com/wp-content/uploads/2019/06/Chunying_Certificate-of-Release_2005.jpeg.pdf

https://chinatribunal.com/submissions/chunying_certificate-of-release_2009-jpeg/

Witness 24: Lijuan Tang

Female, age 67

Were you ever placed in detention in China?
Yes

If yes, where, when and for how long? (What was the reason given by Chinese authorities? Do you have official documentation?
I was illegally detained in mainland China in Guangdong Women's Prison for 3 years and a half, from April 4, 2008 to October 25, 2011.

The reason was that I cultivate Falun Gong. I have official documentation.

Did you witness anything related to forced organ harvesting that you would like to tell the Tribunal about?
Not long after I was sent into the prison, I sent to a hospital for physical tests and blood tests. I was forced to take irregular physical tests and blood tests. I can't recall how many times I was tested my blood when I was held in the prison, no less than 5 to 6 times. In addition, when my body was checked, my abdomen was pressed and checked very carefully, and my corneas were also checked. I remember once when the prison authorities hired a doctor from an outside hospital to carry out checks of eyes. I was told to have my eyes checked as well. He did very careful examinations of my eyes. When thinking back, I believe these tests were preparing me as a target for live organ harvesting. If my sister had not called the prison very constantly, telling them that she would not let them get away if I were not to be released alive, I would have been probably dead.

If you were tortured while in detention, please detail briefly below.
Yes

I was detained illegally by the Chinese Communist Party in Guangdong Women's Prison for 3 years and a half, and I had been tortured by all kinds of brutal methods of torturing. The "reason" for their torturing me was that I would not abjure my belief.

Methods of torturing I have experienced include the following:

1)   Not allowed to eat they said food was for criminals only

2)   Not allowed to go to the toilet: I had to urinate sometimes in my pants. Pants became dry due to my body heat. I was not allowed to take any shower or wash. As it is tropical climate in Guangdong, my body stank as a result. Then the police directed inmates to find fault with me.

3)   Not allowed to sleep: once I was not allowed to sleep for almost 20 days. When my eyes closed, they used a nib to prick my body and my legs. The pricking caused red blood dots which festered, and flesh stuck with pants.

4)   Forced to take drugs: they claimed these were antihypertensive agents. I had no idea whether they were true or not; my health just went from bad to worse, and my weight dropped from over 70kgs to less than 50kgs.

5)   Humiliation: there was no dignity at all when I was detained illegally. They slandered Falun Gong and made up lies about Falun Gong. I was forced to admit that I was a criminal. They beat me and scolded me at their will. They even took off all my clothes to search my body. Words of humiliation were seen everywhere.

Summary of Oral Testimony: 6th April 2019

It is normal that when you arrive in prison, they conduct a physical test. When they do further tests, it becomes strange. They carried out at least 5 blood tests on me. No results were ever sent to me. It was the principal doctor in the hospital prison who checked my abdomen. I was aware of forced organ harvesting before I was detained.

On one occasion they force fed me and I developed a severe stomach ache so they sent me to an infirmary in the prison where they conducted a physical examination. After this they sent me to an outside hospital (Wu Jing Hospital) where they did CT and blood test. They took me to the police and military hospital outside of the prison and then called my sister. My sister was in Helen Jong Province at that time and they told her that I had cancer. Her sister said they should therefore release her and send her to a hospital. They refused and said I was not qualified to be released. My sister threatened them and said that she would not let them get away with it if I did not come out alive. My health then improved, and they told me to call my sister and tell her. The Falun Gong practitioners at this time were not usually allowed to make calls to their families. I was then sent back to the prison. I have never since been treated for cancer and my health has always been very normal since then.

They did an eye examination on me once in the prison. The doctor who conducted the tests was an external doctor. I asked him if there was a problem with my eyes and he said something about a cornea infection. Nothing else happened and I was sent back to my cell.

During the eye examination they took me from my cell to a very dark room so I could not see much. There was a device there.

I learned about forced organ harvesting on a website in 2006. After I came out of China, I saw a film which was called Hard to Believe. The experiences of the people in the film reminded me of my experiences in the labour camp in relation to the blood tests and how hard they pressed on my abdomen.

I was not aware of anyone else who had experienced organ harvesting and did not see anyone disappearing from the detention centres.

Witness 25: Gulbahar Jelilova

Female, Uyghur

My name is Gulbahar Jelilova, I was born in Almaty Kazakhstan on the 4th of April 1964. I have been in clothing business for nearly 20 years buying from Chinese manufactures and exporting to Kazakhstan. In May 2017 I received a phone call from my business associate's daughter who told me that my Goods had arrived from Mainland China and I need to go to Urumqi as soon as possible to arrange the shipment to Kazakhstan as the storage charge is very high. I travelled by bus from Almaty to Urumqi, arriving on the evening of the 21st of May and stayed in a Hotel. The next morning three policemen arrested me in my Hotel room. I was taken to the police station where I was interrogated the whole day before I was taken to No.3 prison in Urumqi at around 11:30 pm.

They took my Kazakhstani passport away and replaced it with what appeared like an official Chinese ID card that had my photo. They stated that it proves I am a Uyghur from Xinjiang. They pressured me to memorize my new ID number.

The police accused me of transferring 17,000 yuan (£2000) from China to an organisation referred as Nur, which is based in Turkey. I told the police that I have never heard of such organisation and I have never transferred money from China to Turkey. But the police insisted that I was lying, after many hours of interrogation forcing me to confess to their accusations, I refused to admit to any of them as I have never been involved in such things. I told them: "You can kill me; you can do whatever you want. I'm just a businesswoman." At the end they said: "We will let you think this over." I was forced changing into a yellow prison uniform before being handcuffed and a black hood placed over my head and taken to so called Sankan, the Number 3 prison in Urumqi which was turned into an all-female camp a week prior to my arrival. I was held there for three months then taken to No. 2 detention centre in Urumqi before being transferred to a women's prison until I was released in September 2018.

The conditions of all three detention centres were overcrowded and dirty, there were girls as young as 14 and women as old as 80 in my cell. There were over 30 inmates cramped in a 14 square metre cell, we took turns to sleep every night because there wasn't enough space for everyone to lie down. A dozen or more women stood while others slept in shifts throughout the night. And the food was nothing that a human being should eat, the bread as hard as stone and soup made of water and cornflour. It was hardly enough to survive on. We were given three tiny meals a day: One small steamed bun and watery cornmeal soup for breakfast, one small steamed bun and watery cabbage soup for lunch, and one small steamed bun and watery cabbage soup for dinner. On one occasion we were given uncooked steamed buns, it just stuck in our mouths. We buzzed the prison guard on the intercom and informed them we can't eat the steamed buns. They replied saying, 'this is a detention center not your home. Don't you know where you are? In your home you can pick and choose but here you eat what is given. Perhaps you're too full that is why you're being fussy. Following this complain they punished us by giving us only steamed buns and water for one week, no soup. And then they accused us of speaking Uyghur. For one month they punished us by giving us only water and steamed buns. They also punished people in other cells for a similar reason. They said, 'you are forbidden to speak Uyghur, only speak Chinese.' They would feed us only if we spoke Chinese.

What made the circumstances much more intolerable was that we were not allowed to wash regularly. We could only have a shower once a week in which we all had to finish within 40 minutes. They gave us just one bar of soap. Each time, two people showered together. It was not really possible to wash properly in such short period of time and with such a limited amount of soap. Because of the lack of hygiene filthiness, we developed body sores.

In all detention centres, there are no areas free from the surveillance of closed-circuit cameras. We were not permitted to talk to one another. Most of the time during the day, we had to stare at the blank walls. The only exception being when we had political and Chinese language instruction from a monitor when we were given pens and paper. We were only permitted to write and converse in Chinese.

We were forced to take pills which had the effect of disorientation, loss of concentration, subdued, you couldn't even think about your parents or children. These tablets additionally stopped our menstrual cycle.

A number of women suffered serious complications. They fainted from the lack of food, had seizure, and mental breakdowns. I witnessed younger ladies screaming, and hitting their heads against the wall, smearing faeces on the wall, and refusing commands. Those ladies were taken away and disappeared.

I was released in September 2018, I learned that soon after I disappeared in May 2017, my family back in Kazakhstan began petitioning for my release. Each day they sent letters to the authorities in Kazakhstan and China. In the end Kazakhstan government managed to influence the Chinese authorities to secure my release.

On the day of my release, they called me from the cell placing a hood over my head. I was ordered to stretch out my arms which were shackled. I was taken to the prison hospital where I had physical check. It seemed like the police consulted with the doctor, who said that I couldn't be put on a airplane back to Kazakhstan. I had lost a lot of weight and was very weak. I was kept in the hospital for two days where I was given vitamins and drips. Two days later, the police officer responsible for me came and said. 'You are acquitted.' She removed the shackles.

Xinjiang governor Shohrat Zakir told state-run Xinhua news agency that people detained in the camps "will advance from learning the country's common language to learning legal knowledge and vocational skills."

During the time of my 15 months detention I moved from detention camp to camp, room to room, and never saw anybody spending any time learning something."

Medical examination
On the night of arrival at the No.3 prison, I was stripped naked for a medical examination. They took blood sample and urine sample before placing me in a cell. In less than one week, I along with other prisoners with black hoods over our heads were taken to an unknown place, there was medical equipment in the corridor, we were examined, and blood samples were taken, and we also had ultrasound tests. We were examined once a week stripped naked. I fainted once when I was in the No.3 prison, I was taken to the prison hospital where I saw many other prisoners and we all had medical examinations almost daily. In the No. 2 prison, there is a big medical clinic, we were examined regularly taking blood samples and ultrasound tests. We had injection once every 10 days. On the 27th of August 2018 before I was due to be released, I was taken to a big prison hospital for a check-up.

Summary of Oral Testimony: 6th April 2019
I never had Chinese nationality.

I requested a lawyer from the beginning of my detention because I could not read Uighur or Chinese. They said I could not have a lawyer; and I have to go to court on my own.

I was detained for 1 year, 3 months and 10 days.

They gave me a Chinese ID and forced me to remember the Chinese ID number.

They never explained to anyone what they were doing. They put shackles on our ankles and put black hoods on our heads every time we were taken anywhere. We were taken to the police headquarters. Three armed female police soldiers accompanied us.

At least once a month we were taken to a special hospital. Usually three or four buses arrived and took us away and always in the same manner; black hoods were placed over our heads and handcuffs and chains were used. Whilst I was in No. 2 prison, I was examined in a clinic within that hospital.

We were given medicine once a week. We were called over the loud speaker and forced to line up and handed three tablets each time. We were also given an injection once every 10 days.

I and everyone else had a full check-up once a month and I had an ultrasound scan three times. They also performed an x-ray to check my lungs. This was every month. I questioned them about what they were doing and I was told to "shut-up" and that I was not allowed to question them. [Identifying scars].

I suffered from a skin condition when I was in the camps. Almost everybody did. I still suffer from the itching now.

I did not know what the injections or drugs that I received were. We were not permitted to ask what they were.

90% of the prisoners were Uighurs and 10% were from other Muslim minorities, Kyrgyz or Kazkahs for example. If there were 40 in a cell, 38 would be Uighur and 2 Kazakhstan for example. I was the only foreign national there.

Everyone there was innocent. We were there because we were Uighurs or Muslim. For example, there was a Uighur female doctor who was 47 years old and she was detained because they found a Uighur song on her phone. She was told the song was banned.

There was another 51-year-old lady who was Uighur and she sent a message to her son that they had run out of flour. She was accused of sending him a secret message and that was the reason she was detained.

I heard from the ladies there that there was organ harvesting taking place. Many ladies were taken from the cells (including from my cell) and they did not come back. I was taken away for interrogation which lasted 24 hours but returned to the cell. Many other women never returned after being taken away for questioning.

I do not know why I was released. I found out later that they had sent letter to my home whilst I was in prison accusing me of being a terrorist. [The witness showed the letters during her in testimony].

My children repeatedly wrote to China and relevant places explaining to the authorities that I was a simple businesswoman and that I had never been involved in "any other matters". They replied stating that I was under investigation relating to terrorist charges.

When she was taken for questioning there were usually 3 police present. If there were 2 Uighurs, the other would be Chinese.

I never witnessed sexual violence against women, but I did hear that was taking place during interrogations. I was told that things were happening that were too shameful to be spoken about. During one of my interrogations they threatened me with sexual violence and said that if I did not admit "this or that" then certain things would happen.

After I was taken to prison me, and my fellow prisoners developed lice. Consequently, our hair was forcefully shaven off. There was another occasion in which they injected one lady and they said the injection was to put her to sleep.

Clarification Post Hearing

What was meant at the end (when one of the audience members helped translation) about medication being given to help people "go to sleep" and what was the reference to wrist bands?
When I was at the prison hospital, I met women wearing orange wrist bands waiting their turn to put to sleep.

People who were sentenced to death wear orange wrist band, and they wait for their turns to put to sleep (Lethal death) at the prison hospital.

How many women did you see who had orange wrist bands?
Two

Were the people with the wrist bands she saw Uyghurs?
Young Uyghur ladies. One of them told me that she has been given death sentence and waiting for her turn to be put to sleep.

Had the ones with the wristbands been through a court process of any kind? What was their 'crime'?
I don't know because we were not allowed to speak to one another, but I suspected that they must have been accused of involving in terrorist activities which is a common accusation without any proper legal procedures.

Additional Documents Provided

https://chinatribunal.com/wp-content/uploads/2019/06/JeliovaGulbahar_Document AccusingTerrorism.pdf

Witness 26: Private Witness 1 (name redacted)

To the members of the China Tribunal:

Please find attached a translated account of my experience regarding forced organ harvesting in China in the 1990s. It was first published in the Chinese edition of The Epoch Times newspaper in March 2015; the following version has a number of expansions from the original as submitted, in particular on the identity of the forced donor and more. An English-language version of the article was published in March 2019 by the English edition of The Epoch Times. The links to those articles are:

Chinese: http://www.epochtimes.com/gb/15/3/5/n4379800.htm

English: https://www.theepochtimes.com/former-intern-recalls-horrific-experience-of-witnessing-live-organ-harvesting-in-china_2821357.html

The attached document is based on the English translation by The Epoch Times, with some expansions made.

Thank you for your attention.

Secret Military Assignment

The events I'm about to describe occurred in the 1990s. At that time, I was a student about to graduate from a certain military medical school in China. I was interning at the Department of Urology, Shenyang Army General Hospital. One day, the hospital received a phone call from the Shenyang Military Region in northern China saying there was an order for some medical personnel to immediately board a vehicle and go carry out a military task.

The group of six who were chosen included two female nurses, three male military doctors, and me, an intern. The department head gave an order: From that moment on, we were to cut off all contact with the outside world, including relatives and friends.

We immediately boarded a van, the inside of which was completely covered with a light blue swath of fabric. The hospital also dispatched a military vehicle. The door was not yet closed and inside I could see a soldier holding a gun.

361

The military vehicle led the way. After getting on the expressway, the military vehicle put on its siren and all the cars gave way. We drove at a very high speed.

Eventually, we arrived at our destination, and after we exited the van, we found ourselves in a place surrounded by mountains. Soldiers were standing guard around a building. A military officer who came to receive us said the building was an army prison close to Dalian City in northeastern China.

A Nightmare Begins

That night, we stayed at the local military guesthouse; soldiers stood guard outside our room. In the morning, a nurse and two soldiers went to the prison to collect blood and classify the blood type. After they returned with the blood, we all boarded the van and sped off.

After we stopped, I looked through a crack in the door and could see soldiers surrounding the van, all holding submachine guns. They were facing outward with their backs toward us.

Our van was stopped some distance away from where the actual shooting of the prisoner took place. We heard a gunshot, but I do not know if the bullet actually hit the prisoner. When we saw the prisoner, as I explain below, his neck was bleeding profusely – but whether this is because he was shot in the neck, or cut, I do not know.

We waited in the van; no movement was allowed. Suddenly, there was a knock. I opened the door and saw four soldiers holding a man who had rope tied around his feet and neck, with his hands tied behind his back. The man was unresponsive.

The man was lifted into the van and laid on a black plastic bag that had been placed on the floor earlier. The bag completely covered the floor, and at a glance, I could tell it was specially made.

The rope the man was tied up with was very thin the kind that will cut into the flesh if pressured. He was tied in such a way that if you stepped on the rope that went from his neck to his wrists at the back, he would be unable to move or struggle. If he did, the rope would tighten, and he would be strangled.

One of the doctors told me to step on the rope and also hold the man so that he couldn't move. When I held his leg, I could feel that his body temperature was hot. I also saw that his throat was full of blood. It wasn't obvious where he was wounded, but there was most definitely a wound.

The Horror Unfolds

At this time, all the medical staff quickly put on surgical attire. The head nurse cut the man's clothes open with a scissors and then swabbed him with a disinfectant from his entire abdominal region to his chest a total of three times.

Then one of the doctors took a scalpel and made a long incision from under the sternum all the way to the umbilicus. The man's legs began to twitch. Then the doctor opened his entire abdominal cavity. Blood and intestines gushed out at once. The doctor pushed his intestines aside and quickly removed a kidney; the doctor opposite removed a kidney from his other side. They were very skilled, experienced, and fast.

The doctor told me to cut the veins and arteries. When I cut, blood immediately spurted out. There was blood spurting from all over his hands and body. This blood was flowing, verifying without a doubt that this man was alive.

By this time, both kidneys that had been taken out were put in an organ transport container that the nurse was holding.

Brutal Removal of Eyeballs

Next, the doctor opposite me asked me to remove the man's eyeballs. I sat down and leaned closer. At that moment, his eyelids moved and he looked at me. I held his gaze briefly. There was sheer terror in his eyes, the kind of terror that can't be expressed with words.

My mind went blank and my whole body began to shake. I felt terrified. I was paralyzed. I told the doctor that I couldn't do it.

All of a sudden, the doctor roughly grabbed the man's head with his left hand and, while using two fingers to hold his eyelids open, used the hemostatic forceps he already had in his right hand to gouge the eyeballs out. It was done in one motion.

At that point, I was shaking and sweating profusely from head to toe. I felt I was about to collapse.

I remembered that at the guesthouse the night before, a military officer came to talk to our director. There was one thing he said that stuck in my mind: "Under 18 years old, the body is very healthy." Was he referring to this man?

After the doctor alerted the officer in the passenger seat that we were done, the rear door opened and four soldiers got in the van, wrapped the man in a big plastic bag, and dragged him to a military truck parked nearby.

Right away, our van took off, and we drove very fast back to the hospital, again with the military vehicle leading the way. All the surgical gowns, surgical caps, and rubber gloves we had worn were put together to be destroyed when we got back.

Upon arrival, the organs from the man were immediately sent to the operating room where a group of surgeons was waiting, ready to begin transplanting them into a patient on the operating table. I didn't take note of how many surgeons there were, but there were more nurses than surgeons in the operating room.

I did not see the face of the recipient, because there was a white cloth pinned up blocking it. Only the anesthetist was back there, monitoring things. I only saw the rest of the body, where the recipient had been cut open for the transplantation of the kidney. Though they removed two kidneys from the donor, only one of them was used. They evaluated them both in the operating room to determine which was best. Presumably the other one was disposed of. They transplanted the new kidney without removing the original one.

By this time, I could no longer do anything; my entire body felt utterly weak. The director saw my state and allowed me to rest on the side. I laid down, but I was still able to see them perform the surgery.

Background on the Prisoner

I became aware of the rough identity of the individual who was killed that day. Previously, I was one of the individuals who accompanied a nurse to take blood from a soldier in military detention. This soldier had assaulted his superior officer, who he accused of bullying him; for this he was detained, awaiting further punishment or a court martial.

At the same time, however, another military officer had been given the assignment of finding a suitable kidney for a higher-ranking military cadre. As part of this search, he ordered that blood be removed from this prisoner. Apparently, the search for a matching kidney had been dragging on for some time and given that this soldier was found to be a match [kidney matching requires both blood and tissue type by compatible – Ed.], he was selected to be killed. I was told this story by the officer who had located him and ordered the blood test, as he informed a number of us over lunch once we drew the blood.

To be clear, the victim had not been sentenced to death via court martial. This was an illegal, secret killing conducted by the military. No one questioned the process. Those with power in the military system are able to act as they please, and under communism there are simply different concepts of the value of human life. Those with the power can kill.

A Dreadful Burden

I soon left my job at the hospital and returned home. I was still extremely feeble and also developed a high fever. My mother asked what was going on, but I kept my explanation vague as I dared not divulge the matter to anyone.

But the pain was far from over. On the one hand, the entire experience was too horrible to even think about, let alone talk about. I had seen the brutal murder of a fellow human being first-hand, and my heart was extremely uneasy. I was also worried that I would be chased down and killed by the authorities. The burden of it all made me absolutely miserable.

For a long time, the scene in the van that day played over and over in my mind, how a living being just like us had his organs ripped out while he was still alive, and the frightful pain and fear in his eyes as he looked up at me. My heart couldn't bear it. I felt like I was going crazy, and constantly felt on the verge of collapse.

I was able to avoid being tracked down and questioned about the incident because after I went home, I told my relatives – who had been high-ranking military officers themselves – that I wasn't going to continue the internship because I had a better opportunity to get a job elsewhere, making more money than the military system. I never mentioned a word of this incident to them, because it was a military secret. My family told the superior officer at the base that I had other connections to get a better compensated job, and I presume this officer would have had no idea I had been involved in this procedure either. This was a secret military operation, and anyone who divulged it could have been in danger.

Many years have passed since then, but that horrible memory still cannot be erased. All those years, I didn't want to touch it and purposefully avoided it. Because whenever I mentioned it, I could not hold myself together.

When the media began exposing the forced harvesting of organs from Falun Dafa prisoners of conscience in China, I at once understood everything: All of this is true, and forced organ harvesting already long existed in the Chinese Communist Party's military system. It's only that the persecution campaign against Falun Dafa provided a much larger source of organs.

Summary of Oral Testimony: 6ᵗʰ April 2019

The incident occurred between 1994 and 1995 when I was an intern at the hospital.

In between study and graduation, you have one year of work experience at the hospital.

Yes, I do practise medicine, but I dare not to go to a military hospital to work. It's not a military hospital but it was a division of the national defence.

So, I was an intern at the military hospital so if I qualify this practice as an intern, I would be able to wear military uniform but after the incident I decided not to.

Yes, they were qualified doctors. You don't live in China, so you don't understand life in a totalitarian state.

The main doctors may know about it. No this was not the first time. Organ harvesting is a systematic process. Eyeballs were extracted from another location, but I was sent here to remove a kidney. The surgeons are very familiar with the whole process. They were very aloof and didn't have much expression; we were only exchanging a few words. I stood outside the cell whilst the nurse took bloods from the person.

No. I never learnt about organ transplantation in the medical system. The victim was just a soldier.

No, I was not aware of other non-military incidents. I tried my best not to be involved with such incidents and leave as soon as possible.

Organ transplants were popular in hospitals in China. You can go to local hospitals to enquire about it.

I wasn't aware of forced organ harvesting. Afterwards I was transferred to the children's department.

Witness 27: Mihrigul Tursun

Female, Uyghur

My name is Mihrigul Tursun and I was born in 1989 in Cherchen County in the Southern region of East Turkistan (officially called the Xinjiang Uyghur Autonomous Region). I am of Uyghur ethnicity. When I was 12 years old, I was taken to Guangzhou for middle school, under the Chinese government's programme to move Uyghur children to inner China at a young age. The aim of such programme is part of the Chinese assimilation policy to immerse Uyghur children in Han Chinese institutions, far from their native language and cultural environment so they embrace the Chinese way of life. However, my experience in this state programme actually made me more conscious of my ethnic identity. The constant discrimination and humiliation I experienced as a young Uyghur at a Chinese school in a Chinese city made me realise that I was different from the majority Han population.

I went on to study Economics at Guangzhou University and then worked for a private company that does business with Arab countries. In December 2011 I enrolled in the British University in Egypt to study English, where I met my husband. In March 2015, I gave birth to healthy triplets, two boys and a girl, who are Egyptian citizens. I had difficulty taking care of my three babies and on 13 May 2015, I left for China with my three two-month-old triplets to seek help from my parents.

As soon as I came to the border control counter at the airport in Urumqi, I was taken to a room for questioning and my babies were taken away from me. The authorities repeatedly asked me whom I met and talked to in Egypt. Then, they handcuffed me, placed a black hood over my head, and took me to a detention centre where I was held for three months. One day in July I was told that I had been "paroled" because my children were sick. They told me I could stay with them until their health improved, but they warned me that I was still under investigation. They held onto my passport, identification cards, and mobile phone.

I went directly to the hospital to see my children. My oldest son was in an emergency care facility and I could only see him through a glass window from far away. I was not allowed to go near him. The next day, the doctors told me that my son had died due to health complication and they gave me his dead body.

I noticed that all my three babies had been operated on their neck area, when I was in prison. I was told they were fed through a tube which went through their neck since they could not eat. I did not understand why, because I was breastfeeding without any issues before we left Egypt. My other two children had developed health complications and I spent the next few months seeking medical treatment for them, including an eye surgery for my daughter.

I was unable to return to Egypt because all of my documents had been confiscated by the authorities and I had been blacklisted. My ID card was barcoded, which beeped wherever I used it in a hospital, pharmacy, and even on a bus, so the police would check my card and had to approve every step I took.

In April 2017, I was living at home in Cherchen County when the police took me to a detention centre for the second time to interrogate me about what I did in Egypt. The security department officials tortured me by interrogating me for about four days and nights without sleep. They shaved my head and physically examined me. They locked me up for around three months before releasing me to a mental hospital because I kept having seizures and losing consciousness. My father was later able to take me home and look after me and I gradually recovered.

In January 2018, I was detained for the third time for no reason. The authorities handcuffed and placed ankle shackles on me. Also, a black hood was placed over my head before I was taken direct to a hospital. I was stripped naked and put under a big computerised machine. One female and two male officials examined my body while I was still naked and then dressed me in a blue prison uniform. It had the number 54 on it. A Chinese official reminded me that this outfit is usually worn by serious criminals who face capital punishment or life-time sentence in prison, and that "54" in Chinese also meant "I am dead."

I was very scared thinking this could be it, and I would die in this camp. I was interrogated for about three days and nights. During these interrogations, they asked the same questions: "Who do you know overseas? Who are you close to? Which organisation do you work for?" I think, because I lived overseas and speak a few foreign languages, they tried to label me as a spy. My hands bled from their beatings. They also gave me drugs twice, and checked my mouth with their fingers to make sure I swallowed them. I felt less conscious and lethargic, and lost appetite after taking these drugs.

Then they took me to a cell, which was built underground with no windows. There was an iron gate and the door opened through a computerised lock system. There was a small hole in the ceiling for ventilation and we were never taken outside for fresh air. There was a toilet bowl in the corner out in the open without toilet papers. There were cameras on all four sides so the officials could see every corner of the room, including the toilet area. There was one light that was always on.

There were around 60 people kept in a 40 square metre cell so at nights, 10 to 15 women would stand up while the rest of us would sleep on our side so we could fit, and then we would rotate every 2 hours. There were people who had not taken a shower for over a year.

The first night was very difficult. As I was crammed with other women on the floor with chains on my wrists and ankles also connected with a longer chain, I was thinking what I did wrong. Why am I here without any charges or explanations? What was my crime and why I deserve such inhumane treatment? Why I can't use the bathroom in private and have toilet paper? Why can't I have water to take a shower or simply wash my face? Why don't I get enough bread to eat or water to drink?

We were woken up around 5am each morning with loud alarms. We had to fold the six blankets we shared in the same way. If the blankets were not folded neatly and looked symmetrical, the whole cell would be punished. They would take away the blankets so we would have to sleep on the cement floor.

Before we ate breakfast, which was water with very little rice, we had to sing songs hailing the Communist Chinese Party and repeat these lines in Chinese: "Long live Xi Jinping" and "Leniency for those who repent and punishment for those who resist."

We had 7 days to memorise the rules of the concentration camp and 14 days to memorise all the lines in a book that hails the Communist ideology. Those women whose voice were weak or cannot sing the songs in Chinese or remember the specific rules of the camp were denied food or beaten up. In theory, there were supposed to be three meals but sometimes there was no food all day and when there was food, it was mostly a steam bun. I must note that the steam bun we were eating got smaller and smaller as the number of people in the camp kept increasing. We were never given any fruits or vegetables.

They forced us to take some unknown pills and drink some kind of white liquid. The pill caused us to lose consciousness and reduced our cognition level. The white liquid stopped women's periods, though it caused extreme bleeding in some women and even caused death.

As if my daily life in the cell was not horrific enough, I was taken to a special room with an electric chair, known as the tiger chair. It was the interrogation room that had one light and one chair. There were belts and whips hanging on the wall. I was placed in a high chair that clicked to lock my arms and legs in place and tightened when they press a button. The authorities put a helmet-like thing on my head. Each time I was electrocuted, my whole body would shake violently, and I could feel the pain in my veins.

I thought I would rather die than go through this torture and begged them to kill me. They would insult me with humiliating words and pressure me to admit my guilt. In fact, I had not been involved in any political activity when I was abroad. Then they would attack me psychologically and say "Your mum died the other day and your dad will serve lifetime in prison. Your son was in hospital and he also died. Your daughter's eyes will remain crossed permanently, and she will be thrown into the streets because you cannot take care of them. Your family is torn apart."

This was very hard for a daughter and a mum to take. I felt a huge sense of guilt and worthlessness. I cried and begged them to kill me. I don't remember the rest. White foams came out of my mouth and I began losing my conscious. The last words I remember them saying was, "Being an Uyghur is a crime" and I fainted. When I first entered the cell, which was cell number 210, there were 40 other women, aged between 17 and 62. The cell was getting more and more crowded every day. When I left the cell after about three months, there were 68 women.

I knew most of the women in my cell. They were my neighbours, young daughters of my former teachers, and doctors, including a doctor, who had been educated in the UK and treated me in the past. They were mostly well-educated professionals such as teachers and doctors.

The most horrific days for me were when I witnessed the suffering and death of my cellmates. The nights were the busiest time in the camps; a lot of activities such as transferring people between cells or removing the dead bodies would happen at night. In the silence of the night, we would hear men from other cells groaning in agony. We could hear the beatings, the men screaming, and people being dragged in the hallways because the chains in their wrists and ankles would make terrible noise when they touched the floor. The thought that these men could be our fathers or brothers was unbearable.

Unfortunately, I witnessed nine deaths in my cell of 68 people in those three months alone. If my small cell, cell number 210, in a small county, experienced 9 deaths in 3 months, I cannot imagine how many deaths there must be all over my country.

One victim was a 62-year old woman named Gulnisa. Her hands would tremble, she had red rashes all over her body, and she could not eat anything. She was really sick but the doctors in the camp determined that she was fine. The doctors at the camp were supposed to say the patients were fine because if they said the inmates were sick, they would be perceived as sympathetic or supportive of the patients. One night, Gulnisa was humiliated for not having memorised her lines in Chinese and she was crying when she went to sleep. She did not snore that night and her body was very cold when we tried to wake her up. She had died in her sleep.

There was another 23-year old woman named Patemhan. Her mum had died, and her husband, father, and brother were all taken to the camps. Her crime was attending a wedding in 2014 that was held according to Islamic traditions, where people did not dance, sing, or drink alcohol. She said all of the 400 people who attended that wedding were arrested and taken to the camps. When she was taken to the camp, she had left her two children in the backyard. She had been in the camp for one year and three months and she agonised every day over the whereabouts of her children. She had a bleeding for over a month and was denied any medical treatment. One night while she was standing with other women, she suddenly collapsed and stopped breathing. Several people with masks came, dragged her by her feet, and took her away.

After all the torture and suffering I went through, I never thought I would come out of the cell 210 alive. I still cannot believe it. Two hours before I was told I would be released; they gave me an unknown injection. I thought the shot would slowly kill me and began to count the minutes waiting for my death. I was surprised to be still alive when the authorities gave me a statement to read and sign. I read it and swore to it, and they filmed me doing so. The statement said: "I am a citizen of China and I love China. I will never do anything to harm China. China has raised me. The police never interrogated me or tortured me, or even detained me." The police warned me that I must return to China after taking my kids to Egypt and I must remember that my parents, siblings, and other relatives were at their mercy.

On 5 April 2018, after more than three months, I came out of that cell and was able to finally see my kids. I did not see my parents anywhere and was not allowed to ask about their whereabouts. I left my hometown three days later with my two children and stayed in Beijing for about 20 days because I was denied from boarding the plane three times for allegedly missing documents. On my fourth attempt, I was able to board on the plane and landed in Cairo on 28 April. I was lost and in deep pain. I did not know what to do. My parents and siblings could be in those camps and the Chinese authorities could kill them if I do not return to China, but if I did return, I would go back to die in a camp. The Chinese government could still keep my parents and siblings in the camps or kill them.

I gathered my courage and decided to tell the world about China's hidden concentration camps so those people who tortured me and others would be punished for what they have done.

Thanks to the help of many wonderful people, I was able to come to the United States. I cannot describe with words how I felt when I landed in Virginia on 21 September 2018. I was overwhelmed with the sheer joy of freedom and a deep sense of confusion that day.

I currently live in the United States with my two kids. Even though I am no longer in a concentration camp, I have not been completely free from the traumatic experience and the Chinese government's harassment. My life is still haunted by sudden episodes of fear and anxiety as a reminder of the horrific days I went through in the camps.

My children have physical and psychological health issues. They are scared when someone knocks on the door and afraid of being separated from me. I still have scars on my body from the constant beatings and pain in my wrists and ankles from the chains. I cannot hear in my right ear caused by the heavy beatings I received. I am scared of the dark but also too much light or noise. Police sirens give me anxiety and increase my heartbeat. Sometimes, I get shortness of breath, my whole body goes numb, and my heart hurts. I still have nightmares at night. Even though I was told I am safe here, I am still afraid at night that the Chinese police will knock on my door and take me away and kill me.

I also fear that the Chinese government officials are still monitoring me. Several weeks ago, a group of Chinese men followed me outside and continued to follow after I got into a car.

The Chinese government must have also forced my brother to reach out to me. He left a voicemail on the cell phone I brought from China. My brother said: "How could you do this to your parents, to us? What kind of daughter are you? You should go to the Chinese Embassy right away and denounce all the things you said about the Chinese government in the interviews you gave to the Radio Free Asia and tell them you love China. Tell them you were pressured by the Uyghur organisations in the US to lie about your detention and torture in the camps and take back everything you said. Otherwise China can get you wherever you hide."

I was terrified that the Chinese Government could still threaten me from so far way. As I am trying to start a new life in America, go to school, work, and take care of my son and daughter, I am still scared that the Chinese Government will try to hurt me.

Summary of Oral Testimony: 7ᵗʰ April 2019

I was held at the first detention centre for two and half months. I was released from detention the day that one of my babies died.

I was arrested a second time on 17 April 2017. During this detention, I experienced the electrocution. I also did not eat anything or was not offered any water for these three days.

On 22 April I was taken to the hospital in Chechen Town and a black hood was placed over my head. I could not see which channels or which kind of gates we went through to the examining room. I do know however that I did not go through the normal route where the normal people go to have a health check. Despite having a hood over my head, I knew that they took blood out of my veins twice, but I do not know how much. They also checked my blood pressure and checked my heartbeat. Another machine was used, and I was told to take a deep breath. Then I believe they took me to a basement. I felt I was in a lift, so I am quite sure it was a basement. I was taken into a very dark room and they removed the black hood and the handcuff and the shackles. They stripped me completely naked. They placed equipment above my breast and used another machine and examined my front and back. Then they put a liquid on my forehead and both shoulders and just below my heart, both legs and they then put me into a glass machine and made me circle inside that machine while shouting the number "1,2,3,4 to 10". I could not hear anything while I was in the machine. After I came out, I had no energy. I was exhausted. They then changed me into the prison uniform, and I was taken to another room. I thought that they might have taken my organs when I was in the machine.

The first time I was in the camp was from 13 May 2015 to July 2015. I saw my two babies in the emergency department and one through a glass window.

In March 2017, I was on the blacklist and was monitored at my home by two Chinese police for 24 hours a day and any time the police wanted to ask me a question they took me back to prison. They let me live outside the prison because my children were very sick. In 2017 they took me again to a detention camp. I did not know where my children were or who they were with. I was tortured and forced to take medicine. I fainted and developed a seizure and that was when I was transferred to the mental hospital. The condition in the mental hospital was horrific and there were people there with actual mental health problems and this can have the effect of causing those without mental problems to develop mental problems. My father was terrified that because I was a young woman, they might take my organs. He went to the hospital and requested to take me home and to look after me.

The youngest person in the camp and was 17 and the oldest was 63. There were approximately 13 people that were around 50 years old. The majority of the women were aged 17-30.

Each time when I and others were taken to the camps, prior to being categorised and put into certain cells, they had to go through a detailed health check – a blood test, an ultrasound and the women had to go through a very intimate examination, something is inserted inside.

I know at least flour Uighur people living in Washington who have also been threatened by the Chinese authorities like she was.

There was a lady who was 62 and who had health condition inside the prison. She had swollen feet and hands and rashes all over and she died from that.

I have always suspected organ harvesting. There were young women aged 23-26 and I saw that on occasions when they stopped breathing, they were then dragged by their feet and taken away for example. I also witnessed women between 14-18 years of age being taken away and never returning. I suspect they were the victims of organ harvesting.

I had an orange bracelet.

Clarification Post Hearing

Confirmation of the relevant dates.
13th May arrested at the airport on arrival. Gave birth to her triplets in March 2015.

Witness 28: Jennifer Zeng

Female. Chinese name: Zheng Zeng

Submission to Independent Tribunal into Forced Organ Harvesting of Prisoners of Conscience In China

October 23, 2018

To whom it may concern,

My name is Zheng Zeng, also widely known as Jennifer Zeng. I am the author of "Witnessing History: one women's fight for freedom and Falun Gong (Allen & Unwin, 9781741144000 https://www.allenandunwin.com/browse/books/general-books/biography-autobiography/Witnessing-History-Jennifer-Zeng-translated-by-Sue-Wiles-9781741144000)

And the main character of the award-winning documentary "Free China: The Courage to Believe" (http://freechina.ntdtv.org). I am an Australian citizen currently working in Washington as a journalist for the Epoch Times. (https:// www. theepochtimes.com)

Below is my testimony:

1.   I come from China. I graduated from Beijing University with a Master of Science. I came to Australia in 2001 and was granted refugee status in 2003.

2.   I began to practice Falun Gong in 1997. After the crackdown on Falun Gong began, I was arrested four times and then sentenced without trial to one year's hard labour reform in 2000. The first arrest happened on July 20, 1999, when I was walking on the street near the Appeals Office in Zhongnanhai, in Beijing. The police stopped me and asked if I was a Falun Gong practitioner. When I said "yes", they immediately arrested me and put me onto a bus, which was already full of Falun Gong practitioners. The second arrest happened on December 26, 2000, when I was walking toward the court, where four Falun Gong practitioners would be tried, in an attempt to attend the trial. The police again stopped me and asked if I was a Falun Gong practitioner. When I said "yes", they again immediately arrested me. The third arrest happened in February 2000. This

time the police directly took me away from my workplace. The reason was that they gained information that I had attended a Falun Gong practitioners' gathering in January at a Falun Gong practitioner's home. The fourth arrest happened at about 2:00 am in the morning on April 13, 2000, when I was still fast asleep at home. The police took me away without any explanation. One week later I learnt in the detention center that it was because the Internet police had intercepted an email while it was sending out. The content of the email was a letter I wrote to my parents-in-law to explain why I didn't want to give up Falun Gong even after the crackdown. But that email wasn't sent by me. To this day I still don't know who sent that email but was given one year in forced labour camp and nearly tortured to death because of it.

3. On the morning I was transferred from the Chongwen District Detention House to the Beijing Labour Camp Personnel Dispatch Centre in Da Xing County, I was taken to a place to undergo a general physical check-up before transfer. About 20 other Falun Gong practitioners were sent to the Dispatch Centre on the same day. All of them went through the same process. Each of us was interrogated intensely regarding medical history, including what diseases we had before. I truthfully told the interrogator that I had had hepatitis C before I practiced Falun Gong.

4. About one month after we were transferred from the Dispatch Centre to Beijing Xin'an Female Labour Camp, we were taken by bus to a hospital outside of the labour camp to undergo a more thorough physical check, including X-rays.

5. One to two months later, a police officer one day ordered all inmates in our room to line up in the corridor. She then took us all to the infirmary inside the labour camp, which was about 60-70 meters away from our dormitory. After our blood was drawn into syringes, we were escorted back. There was no explanation and we found this very strange, as in the labour camp we were treated like animals and slaves, and the police never explained orders. In the Dispatch Centre, we were never allowed to raise our heads and look the police in the face. Neither were we allowed to speak to other inmates. We did not know why they would take blood tests or do other health tests at the hospital as if they were concerned about our health.

6. No result of the blood test was ever shown to us; neither did any of us ever question its purpose, as our work load was so heavy that we had long since

lost our ability to think about anything other than how we could achieve our work quota that day and how we would survive to live another day.

7. Inmates of the labour camp were not allowed to exchange contact details, so there was no way to trace each other after we were released. When anyone disappeared from the camp, I would assume that she was released and had gone home. But in reality, that cannot be confirmed, as I had no way to trace others after my release and I now fear they might have been taken to a hospital and had their organs removed without consent and thus killed in the process.

8. When I was held in the detention house, unnamed Falun Gong practitioners would often arrive there, being detained for a few days and then subsequently disappearing. On the day of May 11, 2000 alone, 20-plus unnamed Falun Gong practitioners were sent there. One of them was numbered D3. She was detained in the same cell as me. Twelve or thirteen days later she died as a result of force-feeding. We didn't know her name until and after she died, aware only that she was 45 years old, and that she came from Heilongjiang province. I equally have no knowledge of the fate of all the other unnamed Falun Gong practitioners.

9. There were about 1000 inmates in the camp. Ninety-five per cent were Falun Gong practitioners. Apart from long hours of forced labour, I suffered from inhumane physical torture and mental torture and insults. I was forced to squat motionlessly and continuously under the scorching sun when the temperature of the ground was over fifty degrees Celsius. The longest period lasted more than fifteen hours. I was beaten, dragged along the floor and shocked with two electric batons until I lost consciousness when I insisted on my right to ask for a review of my labour camp sentence. I was forced to stand motionless with my head bowed, looking at my feet for sixteen hours every day, while repeatedly reciting out loud the insulting labour camp regulations. The police and criminal inmates would shock me, curse me or force me to squat at any moment if I failed to do so. As a Falun Gong practitioner, I was under endless pressure to sign a statement to denounce Falun Gong as soon as I arrived. I was watched twenty-four hours a day by criminal inmates, who were given the power to do anything they liked to me in order to make me sign. I was also forced to watch and listen to slandering attacks and lies about Falun Gong almost every day. I then had to write 'thought reports' to the police after each session.

10.   Because of instigation and anti-Falun Gong propaganda, Falun Gong practitioners have been demonized and alienated. This also prevents us from gaining understanding from family members. Hostile attitudes toward Falun Gong practitioners exist everywhere in society in China today due to the constant demonization and lies in the state-controlled media.

11.   I urge for a formal hearing to be conducted, with key representatives/experts who have investigated these allegations to be given due notice to testify on the subject, including the Nobel Peace Prize nominees, Hon David Kilgour, David Matas and Ethan Gutmann, and consider including Dr Zhiyuan Wang, a researcher and spokesperson for the World Organization to Investigate the Persecution of Falun Gong. I myself would also be willing to testify.

Summary of Oral Testimony: 7th April 2019

The first arrest, in 1999, was because I was a Falun Gong Practitioner. I was taken to a sports centre and stayed there for a day.

After the second arrest I was taken to a local police station and then a detention centre for 2 days.

I was never given any legal representation.

I was not subjected to medical testing but physical testing.

In the labour camp we were handcuffed in the bus and told we couldn't escape. We were in a huge hospital. There were ordinary people there seeing doctors.

About 24 of us in the centre were Falun Gong Practitioner – same in the labour camp.

Before they cracked down on Falun Gong Practitioner, 100-200 female Falun Gong Practitioner. We were initially in the male labour camp.

After the crack down on Falun Gong Practitioners, they switched camps. We were taken to a female labour camp, majority of us were Falun Gong Practitioners.

Dates of imprisonment were: July 20th 1999, December 26th 1999, February 2000, April 13th 2000.

Inmates are those who have committed a crime defined by Chinese law.

We did not wear uniforms initially. We then wore uniforms. On day one, everyone asked each other what they were here for.

There was a self-management system in the cell. We were called a class.

They were given the power to report to the police what we were doing. Variety of different scenarios. Some are very vicious and tortured us.

Don't have to buy things in the labour camp. There was a score you were given according to the labour you did and your behaviour. Other inmates would do anything to get a high score in order to be released earlier.

Falun Gong Practitioners weren't allowed family visits and weren't allowed to buy things from the prison.

Yes, I did know about sexual violence in the dispatch centre. A female Falun Gong Practitioner from Peking University, she insisted on practising Falun Gong. She was shocked in her private parts and couldn't walk for several months.

Witness 28A: Private Witness 2 (name redacted)

Re: Testimony of being blood tested in jail as a Falun Gong practitioner in 2016
Male, age 63.
Occupation in China: electrical engineer.

To whom it may concern,

My name is (name redacted). I am a Falun Gong practitioner.

On Jan 29th 2016 I was arrested from my home after I signed my name to an online lawsuit against the former CCP dictator Jiang Zemin who it is alleged was responsible for the illegal persecution of Falun Gong.

I was taken to the police station where I was beaten, slapped in the face, punched and kicked during interrogation. They wanted me to give them names of other Dafa practitioners that I knew in my area but I refused. Dafa is another name for Falun Gong.

The next day on Jan 30th I was taken to the Yiatai number 2 detention center where I stayed for almost one year awaiting my trial.

The first week of my arrival I was interrogated further. The guards would not let me sleep for 4 days. I was beaten and not given food. I was put into a small cell with other inmates. I was the only Falun Gong practitioner in the cell.

The police would come to visit me often. I was put into a room and interrogated. They tried to force me to sign statements to slander my belief in Falun Gong.

One time when I refused the policeman went crazy. He took the pen off the table and stabbed it into my hand over and over. I screamed in pain and the blood was everywhere.

One day, after a few months of suffering this abuse a nurse came to my cell with some guards. She wrapped a rubber band around my arm and took two glass tubes of my blood.

At the time I didn't know what was going on. It happened so fast and I was afraid of being beaten.

On December 2nd I was sentenced to 2 years in Jail. 6 months later on August 10th 2016, I was transferred to a jail in Shangdon province.

In jail I was beaten and abused more often. They would interrogate me and try to force me to sign statements to slander my belief in Falun Dafa. I was slapped, punched, kicked and yelled at, but they never hit me in the organs. (It was my belief looking back that this was intentional so as to not damage my organs.)

On the days when I wasn't being beaten or interrogated, I was forced to sit on a small wooden stool from the time I awoke to bedtime. I could not move or get up. If I moved, I was slapped or punched or kicked. I was only allowed to go to the toilet and to eat for a very short time. My legs, back and neck hurt terribly. Day after day this happened to me. It was unbearable.

One day after a few months of being in the jail guards came to my cell and took me to the jail hospital. I was forced to put my arm through a hole in a window. The nurse then wrapped a rubber band around my arm and put a needle into my vein and took another two glass tubes of my blood.

Only Falun Gong practitioners were subject to blood tests. I am a very healthy man and because I practice Falun Dafa I do not drink alcohol or smoke cigarettes.

After they took my blood the second time, I suddenly realized why they did it and I was very afraid that I would be killed for my organs. I didn't sleep well after that and lived in fear that I would be killed until my release on January 29th 2017.

Before my arrest I had already obtained my travel visa. As soon as I got out of jail, I made plans to leave China. On March 17th 2018 I went to the airport and left for Canada.

When you were detained in China was it ever through a court process? If yes, what was the judgment about?
There was a court proceeding. I was sentenced to two years. The crime was disrupting the implementation of law using a cult. I have the sentencing paper and the release paper.

Please provide examples of how the torture was related to not giving up Falun Gong.
Their only goal was to make me give up. In the police station and detention center, I was beaten. In the detention center, they did not allow me to sleep and gave me very little to eat. In the prison, in the first month, they asked me to sign a statement

to renounce Falun Gong. I did not sign. They would beat me and use the pen to stab my hand. I still have the scar on my hand. They said that it was their responsibility to make me sign. In prison, the prison guard said that if I died, no one will know how, that they just tell my family that I was ill and wasn't saved.

Appendix 1B. Maps: Detention Centres and Hospitals

Detention Cluster Map

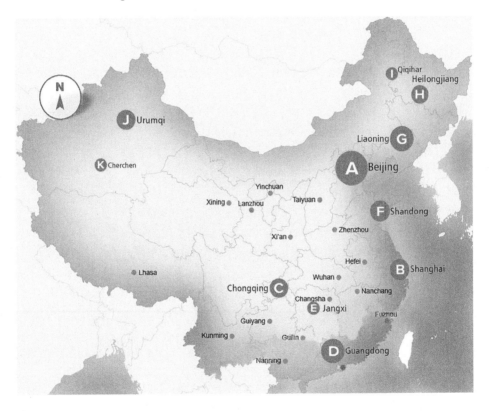

Detention Centre Cluster Map List

A

- Beijing Women's Forced Labour Camp（北京市女子劳教所）– Edward McMillan-Scott
- Beijing Forced Labour Dispatch Centre（北京市劳教调遣处）– Feng Hollis

- Beijing Women's Forced Labour Camp（北京市女子劳教所）, Intensive Assault Unit – Feng Hollis
- Beijing Second Prison （北京市第二监狱）, Chaoyang District, Beijing George Karimi
- Beijing Haidian District detention centre – Han Yu
- Beijing Fangshan District Detention Centre – Han Yu
- Beijing Chaoyang District Detention Centre （北京市朝阳区看守所）– Hong Chen
- Beijing Municipal Public Security Bureau Detention Centre （北京市公安局拘留所）– Liu Huiqiong
- Beijing Dispatching Division （北京市劳教调遣处）– Liu Huiqiong
- Beijing Women's Labour Camp （北京市女子劳教所）, No 7 Division – Liu Huiqiong
- Xin'an Forced Labour Camp, Daxing District, Beijing (大兴新安劳教所) – Liu Huiqiong
- Tuanhe Men's Labour Camp （团河劳教所）, Beijing – Liu Huiqiong
- Beijing Haidian Public Security Police Branch Bureau Detention Centre （海淀区公安局看守所）– Liu Huiqiong
- Daxing District Labour Camp Dispatch Division （大兴劳教调遣处）, Beijing – Liu Huiqiong
- Beijing Xuanwu District Detention – Liu Yumei
- Beijing Changping Detention Centre （北京市昌平区看守所）– Tony Liu
- Changping Brainwashing centre, Beijing （北京市昌平区洗脑班）– Tony Liu
- Beijing Tuanhe labour camp （北京市团河劳教所）– Tony Liu
- Beijing Tuanhe Labour Re-education Dispatch Centre （北京市团河劳教调遣处）– Tony Liu
- The Fourth Brigade of Beijing Tuanhe Labour Re-education Camp （北京市团河劳教所四大队）– Tony Liu
- Qianmen Police Station, Beijing （北京市前门派出所）– Yang Jinhua
- District Detention Centre （北京市海淀区看守所）, No 5 Division – Feng Hollis
- Beijing Shijingshan Police Station （北京市石景山派出所）– Yang Jinhua
- Beijing Yuyuantan Police Station (北京市玉渊潭派出所) – Yang Jinhua
- Beijing Qincheng Detention Centre, Changping District – Yin Liping
- Beijing Tuanhe Labour Camp （北京市团河劳教所）– Yu Ming
- Beijing Labour Camp Personnel Dispatch Centre in Da Xing County – Zheng Zeng
- Beijing Xin'an Female Labour Camp – Zheng Zeng

- Gaoyang Forced Labour Camp （河北省高阳劳教所）, Hebei Province – Liu Huiqiong
- Gaoyang Forced Labour Camp （河北省高阳劳教所）, Hebei Province – Liu Huiqiong
- Shijiazhuang First Detention Centre, Hebei Province （河北省石家庄市看守所） – Yang Jinhua
- Langfang Detention Centre, Hebei Province (河北省廊坊看守所) – Yu Jing
- Yuecheng Brainwashing Centre （岳城镇洗脑班）, Langfang, Hebei province – Yu Jing
- Lutai Detention Centre, Tianjin （天津市芦台看守所） – Hong Chen
- Tianjin Women's Detention Centre （天津市女子看守所） – Hong Chen
- Tianjin Banqiao Women's Labour Camp （天津市板桥女子劳教所） – Hong Chen

B

- Songjiang Women's Prison, Shanghai – Li Lin Lin
- Shanghai women's prison – Xuezhen Bao

C

- Chongqing Jiangjin Detention Centre （重庆市江津看守所） – Jiang Li
- Xishanping Forced Labour Camp (西山坪劳教所), Chongqing – Liu Huiqiong
- Liu Da Wan Prison, Sichuan province – Abduweli Ayup

D

- Futian Detention Centre （福田看守所）, Guangdong Province – Dai Ying
- Sanshui Women's Forced Labour Camp （三水女子劳教所）, Guangdong Province – Dai Ying
- Shaoguan Prison (韶关监狱), Guangdong province – Dai Ying
- Futian District Detention Centre, Shenzhen （深圳市福田区看守所), Guangdong province – Dai Ying
- The First Labour Camp, Guangzhou, Guangdong Province （广州市第一劳教所） – Huang Guohua
- Haizhu District Detention Centre （广州市海珠区看守所, Guangzhou, Guangdong province – Huang Guohua

385

- Guangdong Women's Prison （广东女子监狱） – Lijuan Tang
- Shahe Detention Centre, Guangzhou, Guangdong – Liu Yumei
- Guangdong Sihui Detention Centrev（广东省四会市看守所） – Yu Xinhui

E

- Ji'an County Labour Camp, Jiangxi province – Huang Wanqing

F

- Laixi Chengguan Police Station, Qingdao, Shandong Province （山东省青岛市莱西城关公安局） Yang Jinhua
- Dashan Detention Centre, Qingdao, Shandong （青岛市大山看守所） – Yang Jinhua
- Wangcun No 2 Female Labour Camp, Zibo City, Shandong Province （山东省淄博市第二女子劳教所，即王村劳教所） – Yang Jinhua

G

- Fushun Labour Camp, Liaoning province – Liu Yumei
- Tieling City Detention Centre, Liaoning province – Liu Yumei
- Masanjia Labour Camp – Yin Liping
- Zhangshi Labour Camp, Shenyang, Liaoning Province – Yin Liping
- Diaobingshan City Detention Centre, Liaoning Province – Yin Liping
- Tieling City Forced Labour Camp, Liaoning Province – Yin Liping
- Liaoyang Labour Camp – Yin Liping
- Shenyang Shenxin Labour Camp – Yin Liping
- Longshan Forced Labour Camp, Shenyang, Liaoning Province – Yin Liping
- Benxi Prison, Liaoning province – Yu Ming
- Shenyang Detention Centre – Yu Ming

H

- Second Detention Centre, Mudanjiang, Heilongjiang province – Yu Ming
- Heilongjiang Women's Prison （黑龙江省女子监狱）, Harbin – Zhang Yahua

I

- Qiqihar City Detention Centre （齐齐哈尔市看守所）, Heilongjiang province – Zhang Yahua

J

- Sankan No 3 Prison, Urumqi （乌鲁木齐市第三监狱）– Gulbahar Jeliova
- Urumqi City Second Detention Centre （乌鲁木齐市第二看守所）– Gulbahar Jeliova
- Urumqi City First Detention Centre （乌鲁木齐市一看守所）– Mihrigul Tursun
- Karmay City Prison, Xinjiang province – Ömir Bekali

K

- Cherchen (且末; Qiěmò) Detention Centre, Xinjiang – Mihrigul Tursun

Hospital Pointer Map

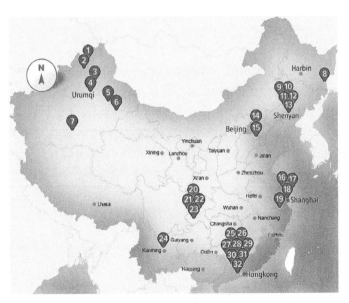

Hospital Pointer Map List

1. Karamay Hospital – Ömir Bekali
2. Karamay City Prison – Ömir Bekali

3. Hospital within No. 2 Prison in Urumqi 乌鲁木齐市第二看守所 – Gulbahar Jeliova
4. The Railway Central Hospital, Urumchi, Xinjiang – Enver Tohti
5. Liu Da Wan Prison hospital – Abduweli Ayup
6. Hospital in Piqan (Pichan) – Ömir Bekali
7. Hospital in Cherchen Town – Mihrigul Tursun
8. Public Security Hospital in Mudanjiang City – Hong Chen
9. Zhangshi Labour Camp Hospital, Shenyang – Yin Liping
10. Masanjia Labour Camp Hospital – Yin Liping
11. Underground prison hospital in Shenyang – Yin Liping
12. Sujiatun Hospital （苏家屯医院） – Dr David Matas
13. Sujiatun Hospital – Liu Huiqiong
14. Hebei Langfang China Petrol Natural Gas Plumbing Bureau Hospital – Yu Jing
15. Central hospital in Tianjin Central – Korean Journalist
16. Shanghai Zhongshan Hospital (上海市中山医院) – Yu Jing
17. Shanghai University Hospital – Xuezhen Bao
18. Zhejiang University Hospital – Xuezhen Bao
19. Zhejiang First Affiliated Hospital （浙江大学第一附属医院） – Matthew Robertson
20. Third Military Medical University （第三军医大学附属西南医院） – Dr David Matas
21. Third Military Medical University case2
22. Chongqing Institute of Forensic Science （重庆法医学院） – Jiang Li
23. Chongqing Institute of Forensic Science – Liu Huiqiong
24. Wuding Hospital （武定医院） – Lijuan Tang
25. Guangzhou Overseas Chinese Hospital (广州市华侨医院） – Liu Huiqiong
26. The First Affiliated Hospital of Sun Yat-Sen University (中山大学第一附属医院) – Dr David Matas
27. The First Affiliated Hospital of Sun Yat-Sen University – Liu Huiqiong – livers ordered
28. No 177 China Navy Hospital （广州市海军医院·解放军177医院） – Huang Guohua
29. No 177 China Navy Hospital – Liu Huiqiong
30. Guangdong Womens Hospital （广东省女子医院） – Dai Ying
31. Foshan City First People's Hospital （广东省女子医院） – Dai Ying
32. Tianhe China Medicine Hospital – Liu Huiqiong

Appendix 2A.
Expert Witnesses:
Witness Statements and
Oral Testimony

(All submissions are in original language, not necessarily UK English.)

Witness 29: Dr David Matas

Evidence statement on organ transplant abuse in China
David Matas

I am a lawyer in Winnipeg, Manitoba, Canada. My clients are primarily refugee claimants seeking protection in Canada. I have been engaged in this work for almost all my professional career.

Because my clients flee human rights violations, I have become familiar with the human rights situation in many countries, including China. I try, as best I can, not only to assist my clients in obtaining protection, but also to combat the human rights violations which caused them to flee. In addition to tribunal and court work for individual clients, I have become involved in research, writing, and advocacy in the broader human rights scene.

A woman with the pseudonym Annie made a public statement in Washington DC in March 2006 that her ex-husband had been harvesting corneas of Falun Gong practitioners in Sujiatun Hospital in Shenyang City in Liaoning province from 2003 to 2005. Other doctors had been harvesting other organs. The Falun Gong practitioners were killed through the organ extraction and their bodies were cremated. The Chinese government denied what Annie said.

A Washington based NGO, the Coalition to Investigate the Persecution against the Falun Gong, asked me and David Kilgour to investigate whether what Annie said was true. It is common for me to be asked to assist in human rights work. This request though was unusual though because of the difficulties it posed.

I knew that Falun Gong was a set of exercises with a spiritual foundation, started in 1992 with the teachings of Li Hong Zhi. I knew that it was initially encouraged by the Communist Party but then repressed in 1999 after it got too popular. That repression though did not mean that they were being persecuted in this particular way, being killed for their organs.

The Coalition who asked us to do the research did not give us any data, money or instructions. Annie's story presented a conundrum. How was it possible to know whether what Annie was saying was true or not? The question was not just, how do we prove what Annie said if it is true? The question was also, how do we disprove what Annie said if it is not true?

What Annie was saying meant that there were no victims to interview because the victims were all killed. There were no bodies to autopsy because the bodies were cremated. There was no crime scene to visit, since the crime scene, an operating theatre, would have been cleaned up immediately afterwards. There were no accessible records, since what records there are belong to Chinese hospitals and prisons, labour camps and detention centres, none of which are publicly available. The sole witnesses available were perpetrators who were unlikely publicly to confess to crimes that they had committed.

The question whether what Annie said was true was difficult enough that it was unlikely to get much of a response either from human rights NGOs or inter-governmental organizations or the media. Human rights NGOs, though they have some research capacity, are for the most part campaign organizations. They look for the easily verifiable, not just because it makes research easier, but also because it makes campaigning easier. Inter-governmental organizations have little internal research capacity and tend to rely on the work of NGOs. As for the media, they cater to readers, listeners and viewers with short attention spans. If a story cannot be told quickly and simply, it normally cannot be told at all.

Addressing a claim of human rights violations with little or no evidence is a situation to which I am quite accustomed. That is my daily work as a refugee lawyer. Refugee claimants come to my office with stories of horror, the clothes on their backs and little else. They of course have this advantage that they are witnesses to what happened to them. Yet, they are often faced with skeptical refugee judges who suspect that they are economic migrants making up stories in order to move from a poor country to a rich country.

Are the stories these clients tell true or not true? Answering that sort of question is not that different from assessing the truth of the story Annie told.

Often when victims or their representatives come to me for general assistance to combat a human rights situation abroad, I can send them off to the media or the local Member of Parliament or a human rights NGO or a UN human rights mechanism. I realized though that, for what Annie said, that would not do. If something was going to be done, David Kilgour and I were going to have to do it ourselves.

But the question was what was that something to be? I began constructing imaginary evidentiary trails, trails that would either prove or disprove all the allegations. In doing so, I followed four principles.

One was never to rely on rumour or hearsay. If someone told me what someone else told him or her, I put the information to one side.

Second, I refused to rely on information from perpetrators. In the course of our work, some perpetrators did come forward to offer testimony, subject to various conditions. I turned all such offers aside, partly because I wanted to have nothing to do with perpetrators and partly because I have in the past found in other contexts perpetrator information to be self-exonerating and unreliable.

Third, I insisted that all information I saw anyone else could see. No one, after our work was done, had to rely on our conclusions. Anyone who wanted to do so could look at the information we considered and come to his or her own conclusions.

Fourth, I determined not to draw conclusions either one way or the other based on one bit of evidence only. Rather I intended to have regard to all the evidence before coming to any conclusion.

The conclusion was that Falun Gong practitioners have been and are being killed for their organs. The basis of this conclusion is set out in books, articles and internet posted research. Some of the evidence on which the conclusion is based is this:

- Investigators made calls to hospitals throughout China, claiming to be relatives of patients needing transplants, asking if the hospitals had organs of Falun Gong practitioners for sale on the basis that, since Falun Gong through their exercises are healthy, the organs would be healthy. We obtained on tape, transcribed and translated admissions throughout China.
- Falun Gong practitioners and non-Falun Gong practitioners alike who were detained and who then got out of detention and out of China told that

    1. Falun Gong practitioners were systematically blood tested and organ examined while in detention. Other detainees were not. The blood testing and organ examination could not have been for the health of the Falun Gong practitioners since they had been tortured; but it would have been necessary for organ transplants.

2. Falun Gong practitioners who came from all over the country to Tiananmen Square in Beijing to appeal or protest were systematically arrested. Those who revealed their identities to their captors would be shipped back to their home localities. Their immediate environment would be implicated in their Falun Gong activities and penalized.

To avoid harm to people in their locality, many detained Falun Gong practitioners declined to identify themselves. The result was a large Falun Gong practitioner population in detention whose identities the authorities did not know. As well, no one who knew them knew where they were. This population is a remarkably undefended group of people, even by Chinese standards. This population provided a ready source for harvested organs.

3. The Party has engaged in a prolonged, persistent, vitriolic national and international campaign of incitement to hatred against Falun Gong. The campaign has prompted their marginalization, depersonalization and dehumanization in the eyes of many Chinese nationals. To their jailors, Falun Gong are not human beings entitled to respect for their human rights and dignity.

Patients we interviewed who went to China for transplants told that:

1. Waiting times for transplants of organs in China are days and weeks. Everywhere else in the world waiting times are months and years. A short waiting time for a deceased donor transplant means that someone is being killed for that transplant.

2. There is a heavy militarization of transplantation in China. Hospitals with a ready supply of available organs are often military hospitals. Even in civilian hospitals, the doctors performing operations are often military personnel. The military have a common culture with prison guards and readier access to prisoners as organ sources than civilian hospitals and civilian personnel do.

In China, the military is a conglomerate business and the sale of organs is a prime source of funds. Military hospital web sites used to boast this fact before we started quoting them. Though they have since taken down the boasts, we archived this information so that independent researchers can still see them.

3. There is an inordinate secrecy surrounding transplantation in China. The names of doctors are not identified. Patients are not allowed to bring their own doctors with them. Before our 2006 report came out, Chinese doctors used to provide letters to patients indicating the treatment given and counselled. The letters ceased after the publication of our report.

- The standards and mechanisms which should be in place to prevent the abuse are not in place, neither in China nor abroad. International organ transplant abuse ideally should be treated like international child sex tourism, an offence everywhere with extraterritorial effect. However, so far that is not the case.

On the one hand, we have organ transplant abuse which is possible without legal consequences. On the other hand, we have huge money to be made from this abuse, as well as desperate patients in need of transplants. This combination is a recipe for victimization of the vulnerable.

- There is no other explanation for the transplant numbers than sourcing from Falun Gong practitioners. Chinese Government official figures for transplants are substantially below the real numbers we can tabulate by adding up reported volumes of individual hospitals. Even if we limit ourselves to official figures, China is the second largest transplant country in the world by volume after the US.

Yet, until 2010 China did not have a deceased donation system and even today that system produces donations which are relatively small. Until 2013, China did not have an organ distribution system. The organ distribution in place today is limited to the relatively small donated organs and does not distribute organs from prisoners. The living donor sources are limited in law to relatives of donors and officially discouraged because live donors suffer health complications from giving up an organ.

The Government of China at first took the position that all organs came from donations, even though at the time they did not have a donation system. They then acknowledged that the overwhelming proportion of organs for transplants in China came from prisoners but asserted that the prisoners who are the sources of organs are all sentenced to death. Falun Gong practitioners have been given short sentences for disrupting social order or sentenced to nothing.

Yet, the number of prisoners sentenced to death and then executed that would be necessary to supply the volume of transplants in China is far greater than even the most exaggerated death penalty statistics and estimates. Moreover, in recent years, death penalty volumes have gone down, but official transplant volumes, except for a short blip in 2007, remained constant or went up. The Government of China has refused to provide death penalty statistics on the basis that they are state secrets.

The UN rapporteur on torture, the UN rapporteur on religious intolerance and the UN Committee on Torture all have asked China to explain the discrepancy between its volume of transplants and its volume of sources. There is no other explanation than prisoners of conscience.

https://chinatribunal.com/wp-content/uploads/2019/06/MagnitskySubmission_OfficialsSurgeons_Final.pdf

Summary of oral testimony: 8th December 2018

I understand it is of benefit to give truthful answers.

Yes, this is my statement. I would not like to make any changes. I did publish my findings in a book. The book is the third version of a report I did with David Kilgour – third version in 2009.

The conclusion [of the report] was that the numbers were large. The problem was we were dealing with everything across China, not just one hospital. We would get anecdotal evidence, whistle-blower evidence, every piece of individual evidence relating to each individual experience. The questions we had was how systemic was this? What was the scale and what were the numbers? And this was a continuing issue.

China initially alleged that the organs were from donations, but they didn't have a donation system. Then after our report came out the official position was said that they came from prisoners sentenced to death and then executed. But the question then became how many persons are being sentenced to death and then executed? But the Chinese government wouldn't then, and doesn't now, release those statistics.

But the notion that it could come from prisoners sentenced to death and then executed was problematic because there was no organ distribution at the time, so all organs had to be sourced locally. The law said execution had to be done seven days after sentence, but people could book transplants in advance and there was no coordination among patients. Plus, there was a high rate of Hepatitis B amongst the prison populations, which made many of their organs unusable. Then of course you need blood type and tissue type compatibility; you couldn't just use any prisoner for any patient. So, this just wasn't an adequate explanation.

Amnesty International were still doing death penalty estimates in China. There was another NGO in Italy at the time called Hands Off Cain that was doing the same. So, we were dealing with it in that way.

Generally, CCP statistics are not reliable. So why should we accept the 10,000 estimate a year statistic that they were generating?

We looked at that statistic. We started going to the websites of individual hospitals (David Kilgour, myself and Ethan Gutmann), and adding up what the individual hospitals were doing. They also had a registration system with minimum capacity, so we could also see what the minimum allowable was.

Instead of getting 10,000 a year, we were getting 60,000 to 100,000 a year with the lower numbers in the earlier years, and as capacity increased going up to 100,000 a year. And of course, the death penalty in this period, number of offences, and number of executions was going down so that reinforced and amplified our conclusions about volume.

I was questioning my own evidence, the evidence that I saw. The Chinese government of course rejected it. But their responses were not very responsive to the evidence. They said I was anti-China, that my reports were based on rumours, that I'm being manipulated by the Falun Gong. That may serve some propagandistic purpose, but I knew I wasn't anti-China. We got investigators to pose as potential recipients. We got admissions of Falun Gong being the source in 10 – 15 % of the case.

The Government made a documentary on Phoenix TV based on our report. They interviewed one of the people we called, Lu Guo Ping. He was presented with a transcript of the video, though not aware of the recording. He denied saying some words and the Government essentially tried to portray us as having distorted the transcript. The fact that Guo Ping acknowledged the call validates our work.

We came to conclusions based on findings. I had to assess the evidence my own way. I have audio recordings of my own evidence. The Chinese government made a documentary about our report and the calls we made. They interviewed the people we called who admitted they said everything we did, but the bit about Falun Gong persecution.

Magnitsky is the namesake of the Act. Legislation adopted by 6 countries, which provides for the listing of perpetrators of human rights violations and the subsequent freezing of their assets. Some in Canada have prepared a Magnitsky brief for perpetrators of Falun Gong repression. Huang Jiefu is involved in organ transplantation.

Organ extraction and insertion are a separate process. Those that insert the organs are guilty of wilful blindness by not asking about the source of organs. Insertion is more complicated than extraction. Dr Enver Tohti in England has been involved in extraction. People in prison have been immobilised. Their blood types have been identified. Huang Jiefu used a process that involved prisoners being immobilised by drugs. Doctors showed up with lists to show who matched their blood types. Once drugged, they would be taken in a white van to a prison where their organs would be extracted, and then they would be cremated.

The system would have to know about the organ but the person inserting it may just assume that the organ is compatible. Organ brokers are just businesspeople. What they see is an inexhaustible supply of organs. They don't need the data to supply the organs. The hospitals would supply the organs. Organs can be ordered online.

There is a map in our book that shows that this is taking place throughout China.

I didn't speak to Annie's husband directly. They're divorced I heard he's in Canada. Whether or not that's true I couldn't say. After our report, China enacted the law requiring consent during transplantation. I am yet to see anybody verify consent. There is a 1984 Law that doesn't require consent. The Law has never been repealed. The notion of consent is not real.

A total figure of enforced transplants at highest would be hard to say. There were about 1,000 hospitals doing organ transplants before the report kicked in. Other hospitals continued doing transplants in an underground kind of way. I couldn't say this is the exact estimate. Numbers started going up during the time of Falun Gong persecution. Liver transplant volumes also went up massively during this time. 100,000 is an identifiable figure. With the unidentifiable it could go beyond that.

State evidence shows transplant surgery was a priority for China. Money must be coming from people requesting organs. Money would go to the broker and the hospital and prison staff. There was a shift from socialism to capitalism, health system was losing money at this time due to shift and needed alternative source of funds – this was primarily from transplants. Hospitals would say their primary source of funds was from transplants. The amount they were charging was very large.

There is a fluctuating ratio [of numbers of organs from different groups]. At the beginning there was no donation system. Chinese did set up a donation system after our report. These seem to be generating tiny numbers. They have set up something, which they call a donation system but as far as I can tell it's a purchase and sale system. They will pay relatives of patients who are accident victims that are brain dead and cardiac alive and ask the relatives to consent to the donation of this accident victim.

The Chinese say now that their transplant volumes are all coming from donations, none from executed prisoners. What they call donations are these purchased organs from relatives. They cost often 39 times annual income. If they're accidented to the point of death their organs will often be unusable. We estimated 2,500 prisoners were sentenced to death and the rest were prisoners of conscience. Once a report came out on total volumes, 60,000 – 100,000 a year, the reaction of the Chinese government was the figures weren't real even though it was coming from their own hospitals and the figures were cross-checked across a variety of data streams.

Even if everything is coming from donations, what they say is coming from donations is maybe 10,000, 30,000 a year. Not 100,000 a year. Organs from prisoners of conscience is maybe 77,000.

About 1000 hospitals were doing transplants in China pre-registration system. 800 of the 1000 applied for licences of which 165 were granted licences to do transplants. Many of the unlicensed hospitals continue to do transplants underground. So, it's difficult to estimate.

China has four different registries for heart, lung, liver and kidney at four different locations. Only the liver registry was publicly accessible at the time of our report. Although, access to the data was eventually blocked after our publication. The identifiable figure would be 100,000 transplants.

After our report China did pass a law requiring consent at point of donation. They have an earlier 1984 law permitting transplant without consent and this law has never been repealed.

Huang Jiefu's reaction to being asked about the 1984 law was: "How do you know about that?"

The notion of consent is cosmetic, it's not real.

The 77,000 estimates mean 77,000 organs not 77,000 people.

[Proximity to source of evidence] David Kilgour talked to the patient who told him what he saw. It was a gruesome story. They kept on trying different kidneys. They went through 8 kidneys before they got a match for this person.

Witness 30: Dr Zhiyuan Wang

View submission: https://chinatribunal.com/wpcontent/uploads/2019/04/WOIPFG_DrWang.zip

Summary of oral testimony: 8th December 2018

WOIPFG's moto is to investigate all organisations and individuals who persecute Falun Gong. We always publish reports on our findings. I can tell everyone about the results of our recent findings on the current situation of Falun Gong practitioners, from the 2nd of this month [December 2018] and the results are shocking.

Evidence no.13 (in detail): a policeman witnessed the entire live organ harvesting. After that he came to us and reported to us the details of what he saw. The victim was a woman – a Falun Gong practitioner in her 30s. Her heart, kidney and liver were taken. He said that apart from the organ harvesting there was extraction of the brains and even more cruel than this, but he did not tell us the details. So, I would like to let everyone know that the persecution of Falun Gong practitioners in China is much worse than what we know now.

There is a transcript of another witness statement, a young military man present during this period. He asks the investigator to distribute the information, 9th April 2002. Young woman already delirious [tortured]. There were two military servicemen there, and no anaesthetics were used on the woman during this operation. The military men's hands were not shaking at all while they did this, and she shouted that Falun Dafa is good. At that moment the military surgeon hesitated, the superior nodded and then he continued. [Reference to the transcript of the telephone conversation].

Evidence no.1 and no.2: (with reference to the suggestion that there is acknowledgement of these actions by some of the senior members of the state, who were aware of it). It is possible they are trying to avoid responsibility because this is too serious. Once exposed it threatens their power so they would evade responsibility. They evade responsibility by CCP always denying it. Secondly, they try to destroy evidence that is included in our reports and those of our organisation. For example, the major responsible people, like the highest chief to execute the live organ harvesting policy was accused of corruption to get rid of him but they do it to destroy evidence and to decrease the anger from the citizens of china towards these people. Thirdly, they asked people themselves to confirm that organs come from voluntary donation, from death row prisoners and show to the world that they are death row prisoners. Fourth, they are using voluntary donation from citizens, after it was exposed in 2006 their pre-text was death row prisoners, but as the international community has paid more and more attention to this, and to the use of death row prisoners which is also not ethical, in 2010 the CCP started to say that the organs came from voluntary donation of citizens. In 2016 their discourse is that all come from voluntary donations, but I don't think that they can cover this completely and I think that in the end it will come back to them. Especially when they have to prove it, like a list of donors, but they have not been able to provide such a list. For example, last month we published a report on the Red Cross, from municipal to county bureau, until now they have not published the report but now there are 23 hospitals in Beijing alone that perform organ harvesting.

In relation to the existence of the brokers, this is another technique that the CCP uses to escape responsibility. I personally telephoned Dr Li in hospital in Beijing and he clearly said that they use certain organs from the brokers and also healthy organs from Falun Gong practitioners. He said yes to this so let me tell everyone that brokers are still an excuse for them to evade responsibility. Now let me tell you something that has been investigated but not reported. On the internet there are reports about brokers, everyone knows that the CCP usually filters everything that is against their benefits but there is still such evidence on the internet.

I am myself a Falun Gong practitioner and have been practicing since February 1998. I have deeply felt its benefits from spirit to body. It improves mental and physical health.

The number of Falun Gong practitioners in prison is numerous and far more than we can imagine. I am not able to tell you the exact number now. The reason why I think the number is great is because it is a state crime, it was the order of Jiang Zemin (the ex-president of China), it was executed by highest levels of the CCP, it was a top-down policy and it was assisted by the army, hospitals, etc. based on evidence in our investigation.

The hospitals all over China over the last 10 years have always been doing organ harvesting, but this is very secretive because the victims die inevitably, they cannot go forward to speak up. That is why I cannot tell you the exact number, but this is the evil that has never occurred in humanity.

The CCP view on Falun Gong, as far as I understand it, they should know that Falun Gong has no political ambition and is not like other religions, it is a faith group who uphold truthfulness, compassion and tolerance – the highest principles of humanity. The reason why Falun Gong is persecuted is because the faith of Falun Gong and its influence on the society scares the CCP because the CCP is atheist. The CCP does not allow its citizens to have faith and it does not allow any faith group to grow powerful. It is a fundamental conflict of interest. The CCP fears the truthfulness, compassion and tolerance.

It [the suppression of Falun Gong] is because Jiang Zemin is the highest leader of the CCP so fundamentally will not allow the faith groups whose beliefs are different from the CCP's to grow. He did not want so many people to believe in deities and uphold the principles of truthfulness, compassion and tolerance as that it could threaten his power.

The second reason was that he was jealous as he thought that so many people would listen to Falun Gong instead of him, which was different to what he wanted to do.

Thirdly, personally I think when Jiang Zemin came into power and politics, he had no foundation like his predecessors, he needed to strategically persecute a group of people to create terror in the society in order to establish his authority. These Falun Gong practitioners did not have political ambition and would not resist. That is why he decided to persecute them but he realised that reality was contrary to what he thought.

In my view, genocide is to kill humans. This genocide mobilised by the state machinery all over China. Every victim after organ harvesting died that is why it is a genocide that lasted more than 10 years. That is why it is the most evil mass murder, genocide. The scale and the importance of the definition lies in the fact that it has lasted more than 10 years. The goal is not a minority, which is scattered in a scattered way. They would want a complete physical annihilation, physical annihilation of all Falun Gong practitioners through renunciation of their faith. The goal is the annihilation of the entire group of people.

by way of addition, from 19th October until 2nd of December this year, I have investigated major hospitals of China, which perform live organ harvesting. Two days ago published the latest report on the CCP's crime of organ harvesting, which included several recording – 11 provinces and cities including Beijing, 16 people were investigated who were the chiefs of big hospitals, some are influential intentionally. Eleven of them directly admitted that they are still using Falun Gong practitioners, the others denied.

Witness 31: Dr Jacob Lavee

Testimonial Submission
Independent Tribunal into Forced Organ Harvesting of Prisoners of Conscience in China
Jacob Lavee, M.D.
Immediate Past President, Israel Transplantation Society Professor of Surgery
Director, Heart Transplantation Unit
Deputy Director, Department of Cardiac Surgery Leviev Heart Center, Sheba Medical Center, Tel Hashomer (phone number redacted) Sackler Faculty of Medicine
Tel Aviv University, Ramat Aviv, Israel

I submit the attached chapter I wrote for the book State Organs as my written testimonial.

In addition, during my appearance before the Tribunal panel in December, I can share my experience, as past member of the ethics committee of the Transplantation Society and past member of the Board of Councilors of the Declaration of Istanbul Custodian Group, in regards to the transformation of attitude of the international transplant community towards China in response to the alleged claims of reform.

Whilst I have submitted a new research paper for publication on the current Chinese organ donation figures, according to academic rules its content cannot be revealed or discussed prior to publication. Therefore, unless it is accepted before my testimony on December 8, I will unfortunately be unable to discuss it at this stage.

Finally, I will be happy to share with the Tribunal any general information regarding technicalities of organ donation and transplantation so as to help familiarise Tribunal panel members with the process.

Please excuse not being able to submit any additional written material at this time due to overburdened clinical activities.

Thank you.

The Impact of the Use of Organs from Executed Prisoners in China on the New Organ Transplantation Law in Israel
Jacob Lavee, MD

In 2005, I was approached one day by a patient of mine with an unusual message. This patient had been continuously hospitalized in my department for more than one year with severe heart failure and had been a top priority candidate on the Israeli waiting list for heart transplantation. He reported to me he was fed up with the endless wait for a suitable heart donor and was told by his medical insurance company to go to China in two weeks' time as he was scheduled to undergo heart transplantation on a specific date. When asked how such an operation could be scheduled ahead of time, the patient responded he did not bother to inquire. The patient, indeed, went to China and underwent the operation on the exact date as promised ahead of time.

This was the first time I had been made aware of the possibility of undergoing heart transplantation in China as no Israeli patient had ever gone there for this operation before. For years, I have heard stories from my kidney transplant colleagues about Israeli patients going to China to get kidney transplants and, never bothering really to inquire, it was my assumption that the source of these kidneys was poor people selling one of their kidneys in order to improve their economic status. The fact that you can also get a heart transplant in China and, moreover, get it on a specific pre-scheduled date was a total surprise to me and got me researching.

It did not take me long to find out the gruesome details of the abhorrent Chinese practice used since the 1980s, whereby the source of most of the transplanted organs are prisoners sentenced to death or prisoners of conscience, whose consent is either non-existent or ethically invalid and whose demise might be timed for the convenience of the waiting recipient who could afford the cost of buying an organ. When I started my research in 2005, this practice was still officially denied by the Chinese authorities. Therefore, the sources of information were mainly the testimony of Dr Wang Guoqi, a former doctor in the Police Tianjin General Brigade Hospital, who fled to the U.S. and spoke in a hearing before the subcommittee on International Operations and Human Rights of the Committee on International Relations, House of Representatives, in June 2001.[1] As I was about to publish my research findings, Dr Huang Jiefu, Vice Minister of Health of the People's Republic of China (PRC), publicly admitted for the first time in December 2005 that apart from a small portion of traffic victims, most of the cadaveric organs in China came from executed prisoners, albeit claiming that the only prisoners who were subject to capital punishment in the PRC are convicted criminals and that prisoners or their family provided informed consent for donation of organs after execution.

The results of my research were first published in October 2006 in the *Journal of the Israeli Medical Association*,[2] and I have added a call for the cessation of the Israeli participation in the process as I have found out that, of all transplant tourists gathering to China from all over the world to get organs, Israeli patients were probably the only ones fully reimbursed by their insurance companies. I have referred to this reimbursement as providing de facto recognition of the Chinese transplant activities as being legal and ethical and have called upon Israeli authorities to immediately ban it all together and denounce any Israeli participation in the atrocious process.

On July 2006, when my paper had already been sent for publication, Matas and Kilgour published their first version of the *Bloody Harvest* report, and I had therefore published an extended version of my original plea in another Israeli medical journal,[3] this time adding the chilling information regarding the use of executed Falun Gong practitioners as a major source of organs in China. Following the publication of these papers, the Israeli lay press picked up my call, and an extensive investigative story of the trade in executed prisoners' organs in China was published in Israel's most widespread newspaper.

An Op-ed on the same topic which I had published in the most popular local news portal *YNet* and a follow-up TV report all contributed to the public awareness of the issue.

Together with my friend and associate to the public campaign, the transplant surgeon Prof. Eytan Mor, we convened in June 2007 a special conference on ethical dilemmas in solving the organ shortage in Israel under the auspices of Israel's National Transplant Center and the Israel Society of Transplantation. Among the invited speakers were Prof. Francis Delmonico, then a special advisor on transplantation to the World Health Organization; Amnon Vidan, director of the Israeli branch of Amnesty International; Dr Yoram Blashar, then chairman of Israel Medical Association; Prof. Gabriel Danovitch, renowned director of the kidney transplant program at UCLA Medical Center, and David Matas who gave the large audience a summary of the *Bloody Harvest* report. A day before the planned conference, we found ourselves in the midst of a diplomatic incident when we were asked by our Ministry of Health to consider cancelling Matas' presentation in response to a request forwarded by the Chinese embassy to our Ministry of Foreign Affairs. We rejected this request and were henceforth kindly asked to at least balance his presentation with a presentation by a representative of the Chinese embassy in Israel in order to avoid diplomatic discomfort. This presentation was indeed delivered in which the source of organs in China was not mentioned at all and the *Bloody Harvest* report was portrayed as just an attempt to slander China. The Chinese speaker was literally booed by the audience.

An interesting and unexpected public support to my call, at that time, came from one of the most respected rabbis in Israel, Rabbi Shalom Elyashiv, who has traditionally headed the minority of orthodox rabbis who ruled against accepting brain death as a legitimate form of death and hence, object to organ donation following brain death. While usually permissive of accepting organ donation from gentile donors who have been proclaimed brain dead, Rabbi Elyashiv surprised many when he openly declared that the use of organs from executed prisoners in China and the selling of those organs to anybody who could afford it was considered by Judaism as a form of God's desecration and should be avoided by all means, even if its avoidance would result in the death of the potential candidate for transplantation.

Following the intensive public discussion, a special meeting of the Health Committee of the Israeli Parliament convened to which representatives of all stakeholders were invited including candidates for organ transplantation, transplant physicians, directors of insurance companies and HMOs, Israeli Falun Gong practitioners and the Ministry of Health. After hearing all sides, the committee unanimously expressed its revulsion of the abhorrent practice in China and issued a call to stop sending Israeli patients for organ transplantation to China.

The committee went further, and together with the Ministry of Health, made sure that the new Organ Transplant Law, which was formulated during the same time, included a unique chapter[4] which bans any reimbursement of organ transplantation performed abroad if it involved illegal organ procurement or organ trade. The new law was passed into legislation by the Parliament in March 2008 and, shortly afterwards, rules were issued ordering all Israeli insurance companies to stop reimbursing any organ transplants performed in countries in which illegal organ procurement or organ trade are known to take place. These rules were immediately implemented by the insurance companies which brought transplant tourism from Israel to China to a complete and abrupt halt. These rules have also helped minimize the total number of transplant tourists from Israel to other venues in the world, cutting this number from 155 in 2006 to only 26 patients in 2011.

The Israeli Organ Transplant Law does not only close the gates for transplant tourism from Israel. In parallel, it includes several unique clauses which pave new ways to increase national organ donation, both from deceased and from living related donors, and thereby promotes national self-sufficiency in organ donation as highlighted by the Declaration of Istanbul.[5] Based on my recommendation to the steering committee of the Israeli National Transplant Center, the law has adopted a unique new policy granting priority in organ allocation to candidates who have been previously registered donors.[6] This unprecedented organ allocation policy was aimed towards abolishing the "free riders" phenomenon of candidates for organ transplantation who, for various reasons, object to organ donation and is based on the ethics principal of reciprocal altruism.

Other aspects of the law provide modest reimbursements for living donors which serve to remove disincentives to living donation.

These include the following non-fungible benefits reimbursements to any live donor who has been authorized by the Ethics Committee, all made by the government: earning loss reimbursement of 40 days, based on the donor's average income during the last 3 months prior to donation (an unemployed donor will be reimbursed according to the minimum salary in the market at the time of donation); a fixed sum transportation refund to cover all commuting to and from the hospital for the donor and his relatives for the entire hospitalization and follow-up period; a 7 day recovery reimbursement within 3 months after donation; five years reimbursement of medical, work capability loss and life insurance, all to be refunded upon submission of appropriate insurance policies and payment receipts, and reimbursement of five psychological consultations and treatments upon submission of appropriate receipts. All these measures have already borne fruits as organ donation, during 2011, has significantly increased by 68% compared to 2010.

Influencing any country to change its unethical and immoral conduct in organ retrieval and transplantation is a daunting task, especially in an enormous and secluded country like China. No single measure can be expected to make this shift and it is only through concerted variety of global efforts aimed at different levels of the atrocious chain which provides organs from executed prisoners and Falun Gong practitioners to wealthy candidates for organ transplantation from all over the world or even to local citizens, before this chain can hopefully be disassembled. The Israeli legal approach has successfully managed to disengage Israeli candidates for organ transplantation from getting their organs in China. If similar measures are enforced by other countries whose patients flock to China to receive their organs, there is a good chance that dwindling this major financial source will ultimately contribute to the dismantling of this widely condemned chain.

References

1. "Organs for Sale: China's growing trade and ultimate violation of prisoners' rights," Hearing before the subcommittee on International Operations and Human Rights of the Committee on International Relations, House of Representatives, June 27, 2001. Viewed at: http://commdocs.house.gov/committees/intlrel/hfa73452.000/hfa73452_0f.htm

2. Lavee J. "Organ transplantation using organs taken from executed prisoners in China – a call for the cessation of Israeli participation in the process," [Hebrew] Harefuah. 2006;145:749-52

3. Lavee J. "Shooting and cutting," [Hebrew]. *Medicine Cardiology*. 2:12-15, 2007. Viewed at: http://www.themedical.co.il/Upload/Magazines/Documents/23/medicine%20heart2.pdf

4. Israel Transplant Law – Organ Transplant Act, 2008. Viewed at: http://www.declarationofistanbul.org/index.php?option=com_content&view=article&id=267:israel-transplant-law-organ-transplant-act-

5. The Declaration of Istanbul. Viewed at: http://www.declarationofistanbul.org/

6. Lavee J, Ashkenazi T, Gurman G, Steinberg D. "A new law for allocation of donor organs in Israel," *Lancet* (2010): 375(9720):1131-3

Summary of oral testimony: 8th December 2018

[The first Israeli patient to undergo heart transplantation in China] was hospitalised in 2005 in our department at the Sheba medical centre, which is the largest medical centre and heart transplantation centre in Israel, for almost a year. The patient was on the top list of heart transplant candidates for heart transplantation. We could not find a heart transplant for him. One day he approached me and told me that his insurance company set up a heart transplant operation in two weeks in China.

I know that no one can schedule a heart transplant operation ahead of time as a donor has to die. Then there are only 24 hours for the operation to be conducted. My patient said he did not know how it was arranged, but that was exactly what had happened. That particular person went to China on that specific date and had a heart transplant at the arranged time.

I heard of the cases when patients had a kidney operation in China, but the heart transplantation caught me by surprise, and I started my research in this issue. I then learned about the well-established transplantation practice in China that went back to 1984. At that time the Chinese passed a secret law that enabled them to harvest organs from executed prisoners and transplant in the other people.

That particular heart transplant patient was followed by approximately 10 more Israeli patients and had their heart transplants on a scheduled date. What puzzled me and pushed me into a public campaign was that we did not have any transplant law in Israel and as a result the Israeli patients were fully reimbursed for these operations which were perceived as lawful in the absence of any restricting law.

Following that case, I started a public campaign and published several papers to at least ban the reimbursement of such operations. As a result of tedious debates and discussions with experts, including me, the Israeli parliament passed the law on 31st of March 2008, which bans the Israeli patients getting reimbursement from transplant operations if it is performed against the local law and if the rules are in breach of the organ trade law as defined by the Israeli law. Since then no Israeli patient went to China anymore.

Out of ten patients, who underwent the heart transplant operations in China, four died. The medical records from China for those who returned came back very brief and with no mentioning of any consent, type of donor or its source. It is just said generally that a certain heart became available. The reports did not contain much detail about the operation itself.

I consider a 40% mortality rate very high. Something definitely went wrong during those operations whether in selection of a donor or during the operation itself.

I do not know much about how the organs were obtained or how the organs were preserved during such transplant operations. The only actual testimony comes from a person who testified in front of the US Senate about a kidney in 2001. He described that an ambulance was set up in the yard of the prison. Immediately after a prisoner was shot, the still half alive body of the prisoner was rushed into the ambulance, which was equipped as a small operating room, and the kidneys were very quickly procured. Even after the removal of kidneys the body was not dead enough and was sent to the crematory half alive. This is not the way to procure the heart. I do not know how exactly the heart was procured for my patients.

I think in addition to a regular blood test the blood tests will normally be taken from the donors for basic viral severe infections such as Hepatitis B and C, HIV viruses, CMV Toxoplasma, which are essential. Also, a donor needs to undergo a variety of viral examinations to be a safe donor. Some of my colleagues told me that their patients, who went to China for kidney transplants, returned with infections of Hepatitis B and C and even HIV. It is not only the high mortality rate that I mentioned earlier, but also the high rate of incidents of viral infections of those kidney patients. My heart patients who returned to Israel did not have any viral infection though.

My Israeli patients did not bring any blood tests results with them from China. We handed all medical information to China, but did not get much from China, only a one-page report consisting of two or three paragraphs and stating just the facts of the operation itself, what drugs were given and during which period.

Before 2008 when the reimbursement of transplant operations was allowed and as far as I know each insurance company in Israel, which sent the patients to China, had a local broker who arranged everything with the hospital in China.

The Israeli patients did not dare to ask about the source of donors and how exactly the arrangements in China were made or about the role of brokers.

During my research I have received a number of threats coming either via telephone calls or emails, including from an Israeli lawyer who threatened a lawsuit if I continued my research. In China I was also proclaimed persona non grata.

From my own research the official number of transplants of roughly 10,000 a year is absolutely wrong. I am not ready to comment on the number of transplants now as it is contained in my new report, which is about to be published soon. Once the report is published, I will submit an additional statement to you.

The national organisation usually takes care of donors through their coordinators. Once the death is pronounced/defined by the physicians, the coordinators approach the family for permission. Even in the countries with opt-out systems, the families will still be asked to agree to organ donation. Only then can an organ be allocated to a person according to the national list.

From my experience, I do not believe that China could quickly switch from a no-donation-system into a voluntary donation country and jump magically into a high volume of transplants within 2-3 years from practically zero.

There is no doubt that there is a financial incentive for judges, prison guards, doctors etc., but the underlying motive has to be something else too. I do not believe that the country executes only for the purpose of money. It is not easy to create such a huge monstrous system, there has to be something beyond it.

I have not seen anything that would indicate that it is not possible that organ harvesting is to do with the destruction of a particular group. I once visited Taiwan and I had an opportunity to speak to a Chinese heart transplant surgeon who worked earlier on the mainland. He confessed that he was part of the team that procured the hearts. I asked him about their motivation, and he told me that they were absolutely blanked by their superiors and they were forced to think that these people were sub-human.

Witness 32: Clive Ansley

View submission: https://chinatribunal.com/wp-content/uploads/2019/04/Clive-Ansley_Submission_Report.pdf

Summary of oral testimony: 8th December 2018

There is no such thing as an independent judiciary in China. Judges at all levels in China are appointed by the People's congress of that particular level and they serve at pleasure of the People's congress. So, they can be removed at any time as well as appointed. The People's congresses are composed of the deputies who are either members of the CCP or they have been approved to stand as candidates by the CCP. In effect the constitutional provision that the courts are responsible to the People's congresses, which appointed them, in fact means that they are responsible to the CCP. They can be removed at any time and I had a personal opportunity to observe that.

Another factor of the lack of independence is illustrated by the court's structure in an appeal process, which is the same at any level. There is an appeal system set out but something that is never mentioned is that there is a political and legal committee, which is a committee of the CCP. A chairman of that committee stands at the top of the structure, and in practice he can overrule any finding by any court at his level. Normally this particular person has no legal training involved; he is a purely political appointment.

[In the absence of any judiciary independence the overview of what will happen to a person from detention to the trial]. A person can be detained by a number of different agencies nowadays in China, but according to the criminal procedural law normally he will be detained by the police or public security bureau. A detention is not the same thing as an arrest, where a person may be detained for a very lengthy period, e.g., months, without being arrested. Various time frames are set out by the procedural code, when a decision to arrest has to be made. Within this time the suspect will be interrogated by the public security bureau and often also by the prosecutors and he will have no access to his counsel at that time. He will also be routinely subjected to torture.

The Article 3.3 of the Code of the criminal procedure specifies that he may have the right to meet with legal counsel after the interrogation is finished, by which time the interrogators will usually have a confession. In practice the suspect is not allowed to meet with the counsel even after the interrogation. The lawyer, whom he may wish to retain, will often be refused an access by the guard of the detention centre.

One thing I remember reading about years ago and since then I have encountered that fairly frequently with lawyers, a lawyer will typically turn up once the interrogation has finished (and the lawyer has now supposedly the right to meet his client) and the guard will tell him that it is not convenient today or that a particular police officer who must be present is not available today. The lawyer would refer the guard to the provision in the Code regarding his right to meet with the client and the guard would typically respond that the lawyer is not refused his right under the Code of criminal procedure but is refused under the internal regulations of that detention centre.

Once the trial is set up, the trial is based on the witness statements against the accused, which are written and signed by the witnesses who are not present at the trial, and these statements will be read by a police officer or a prosecutor. So, the defence has no chance to cross-examine the witnesses.

Article 59 of the Code of criminal procedure specifies that in order that a witness testimony be accepted by the court, a witness must appear personally in the court and must be cross-examined by both sides. If that does not happen the evidence is inadmissible. But in practice this has never happened. We see the witness statements admitted by simply being read out by prosecutors or police officers and there is no opportunity for cross-examination.

There is no presumption of innocence in China and it is a greatly misunderstood issue outside of China. It is not written into the law whereas many believe presumption of innocence is in the procedural code. It is not written into the law as it stands. Second, it is difficult to find a judge in China who is interested in what the Code of criminal procedure says in any case.

There is an interesting history behind this. The Chinese legal system has come under heavy criticisms under the western jurists and legal scholars for many years. One of the things that kept coming up over and over again is that there is no presumption of innocence. In 1997 when the Code of criminal procedure was reviewed, China purportedly answered this criticism and they inserted Article 12 under the code and this article had been heralded ever since as being the enshrinement of the presumption of innocence. In fact, Article 12 simply says that no one shall be guilty of the crime until they have been found guilty by the Chinese court. That says nothing at all about the presumption of innocence.

Most Chinese lawyers, and I must say Chinese lawyers are not the weakness of the system, they are very selected group, where only 9% of law students would pass the bar exams. Chinese lawyers are brilliant, and their standards and values are very high. They are not weak elements of the society. It is the system that defeats them, it is not their inferiority.

Most Chinese lawyers whom I met talk about the presumption of innocence, and almost with pride. This is something that was acknowledged at least in theory by the authorities in 1997.

It is not frequent to see the policy of the governments subject of a criminal case. The whole system is not set up to have an independent investigation by the police to start and then to proceed in the court in order to look at evidence and look at the facts and try to find the truth. The system is from the beginning to the end geared towards compiling evidence against a suspect who has been selected. That is the way it works.

When the persecution of Falun Gong first began in 1999, there was the creation of the 610 office (stands for the 10th of June when the persecution started). The whole process of crushing Falun Gong and removal from the society would be handled by the 610 office. All other organisations such as courts, prosecutors, police, everyone involved in the criminal justice system should defer to the 610 office. The 610 office is not an office consisting of legally trained people or having any legal status in law. So, there is a court system set up on one side and the government claiming the rule of law. Then the government arbitrarily called upon a group of Falun Gong to be crushed. For this the government has created a special office 610 to take care of this problem and the courts do not need to be involved.

In my materials I oversimplified, saying that the normal process is for the police officer to issue a decree and to send somebody to a labour camp. When the 610 office became involved, they did not necessarily start to perform the same functions. In some cases, they used police officers, in some they brought the judges to have some sort of hearing. The judges and the courts took the directions of the 610 office.

It is true to say that a number of Falun Gong practitioners travelled to Beijing or other main cities to appeal to the authorities to change their policy believing that this right was guaranteed under the Constitution. This is a very interesting concept of the right to petition. Long before the CCP took over, long before the modern codes, that right to petition existed in the old dynastic and legal system. It started at the local level. There was a structure, called the Yaman, consisted of the local magistrate's residence and the facility where he held the court. The citizens had a recognised right to come and beat on a drum before the magistrate's structure and present their grievances if they were unfairly treated by local officials, by tax collectors, whoever it was. They could petition at that level. If they did not get a satisfaction there, they were now entitled to go to Beijing and directly petition the Emperor. Today there is no Emperor, but this right has been preserved in Article 41 of the Constitution. This article does not use the word petition, but it addresses the right to come to a bureau and submit grievances against the officials, who they think have wronged them or any kind of injustice that was carried out against them. Over the years leading up to the present because of the gross corruption and the abuses of power in China there has been a rising tide of petitioning. I do not have any actual statistics on it, but I believe there were millions of people every year that have come to Beijing for this purpose. Perhaps because there are so many of them the reaction of the government and the party was essentially to put a lid on it. They do not want to hear from these people or these people coming to Beijing. As a result, they put a lot of pressure on the police forces in the cities and towns throughout China to prevent anybody from their jurisdictions getting on the train and coming to Beijing to petition. Nevertheless, a lot of them are coming through and the local authorities would send the police to Beijing to pick the people up before they could submit their grievances.

In terms of the current position of the Chinese law on ownership of the body and the organs of someone executed in accordance with the Chinese capital punishment law there have been a number of laws dating back to the 1980s on the use of organs from the Chinese criminal prisoners. I am not sure on that subject; I cannot cite any particular governing law right now. But the most important position has always been the official position of the Chinese Communist Party. That position was put forward by Huang Jiefu who is the former Vice Minister of Health in China and he is a person who I think is credited with about 5,000 liver transplants himself. He is a transplant surgeon, but he has been responsible for the entire program of organ transplants in China. So, he stated the legal position on the 1st of January 2015 that there would no longer be any organ sourced from prisoners and that would become illegal. China just very recently has claimed to have a volunteer organ donation system but as far as any of the leading researchers can find there have been very few voluntary donors we have heard of.

In terms of how if at all does the People's Republic of China acknowledge the non-binding validity of the Universal Declaration of Human Rights, I am not aware of any particular statement made.

In terms of genocide definition and persecution of Falun Gong practitioners, genocide doesn't have to be necessarily the attempt to physically wipe out an entire group of people such as in the Holocaust. I think it is enough to look at the statements from Jiang Zemin who started this particular program and other Communist Party statements as well, that the goal is to entirely remove Falun Gong practitioners from Chinese society to essentially achieve a situation where there are zero Falun Gong practitioners.

There are many ways of doing that and there is overwhelming evidence of physical attempts to do that of the numbers of Falun Gong people who have disappeared without a trace and who some of them have been documenting the effects of torture on their body. We have seen a lot of the physical evidence but on top of that the use of retraining or re-education centres to force Falun Gong practitioners to renounce their beliefs and to end the Falun Gong movement. Many of them appeared on television with bowed heads denouncing Falun Gong. There are also prohibitions against employers employing Falun Gong people and seizures of their property. So, in my definition I was looking well beyond just the physical elimination.

In relation to dehumanisation of Falun Gong practitioners, I did contribute the chapter on this issue. It dealt with the last few years when I was in China. There had been the absolute blitz in the mass media for a period of time just totally focusing on Falun Gong. Falun Gong practitioners were demonized. It did remind me of the demonization of the Jews under the Third Reich in Germany because you could not open a newspaper, you could not turn on a TV or listen to a radio without hearing about this non-stop attack on Falun Gong and how the founder of Falun Gong Li Hongzhi was a totally evil person and he had led people to commit all kinds of diabolical deeds. They claimed that studying the works of Li Hongzhi led to people committing murders, rapes, mass murders through poisoning and all kinds of things.

In terms of how effective the process of dehumanisation within the various classes of society was, my opinion is that it was extremely effective.

One of the things that always puzzled me in China was that in my view the overwhelming majority of the population had no respect for the Chinese Communist Party at all. They ridiculed it in private conversation, they attacked it for corruption, they attacked it for lying and yet if you had a discussion about capital punishment for example, in my experience nearly a hundred percent of Chinese people are in favour of capital punishment. When you would talk to them about the possibility of the courts convicting an innocent person they would say *"well, he would not have been in court if he was not guilty"*. These are the very people who told me about the evils of the party and how it controls the media and the courts.

The same applies to Falun Gong practitioners. The people who hate the Communist Party and attack their credibility would be quoting the Communist Party for their opinions of Falun Gong. They were being filled full of these stories like a man in Nanjing who was being executed for having put poison in the food at the noodle restaurant and I think 42 people had died. Everybody knew this story and everybody was attributing it to Falun Gong because the last idea in the news report that announced that this person was going to be executed and taken off for execution was *"Oh and by the way he was a Falun Gong practitioner and had been studying the works of Li Hongzhi"*.

In China there are a number of specialised special courts such as military, railway, maritime and forestry courts. The hearings in the military courts are not public and neither they are in the ordinary courts even though the Code of Criminal Procedure says they must be public. There is an exception made for anything involving state secrets and among the many definitions of state secrets is any information from a criminal investigation. That is why most ordinary criminal courts are not public. When the hearings are made occasionally public it is because the Communist Party will want to hold a show trial. They will want to demonstrate something, and they have the TV cameras there, then they will fill up all the seats and it will look like a public hearing. The only thing is that you must have a ticket to get into those trials. Most often, even the relatives of the defendant will not be able to get a ticket to get in.

Witness 33: Sarah Cook

Dear Sir Geoffrey Nice and members of the tribunal,

My name is Sarah Cook. I am a senior research analyst for East Asia at Freedom House, a non- profit organization dedicated to the promotion of democracy and human rights around the world. I have worked for Freedom House for 11 years and have served as the organization's chief analyst on China for eight. I reside in New York and received a Bachelor's Degree in International Relations from Pomona College and as a Marshall Scholar, completed two masters degrees in politics and international law at the School of Oriental and African Studies in London. I have been involved with human rights causes and research related to China since 2001.

My recent work at Freedom House has included authoring a 140-page special report on religious freedom in China published in February 2017, titled: *The Battle for China's Spirit: Religious Revival, Repression, and Resistance under Xi Jinping.*

Enclosed for your reference is a copy of that report. You may find the following pages of particular relevance to your inquiry and as context on the broader situation of religious persecution in China:

- Executive summary: pgs 1-3.
- Evolving mechanisms of religious control essay, including sections on indoctrination, imprisonment, and economic exploitation: Pgs 15-23.
- Uighur sections of Islam chapter: Pgs 66-85.
- Falun Gong chapter: Pgs 108-129.

Although the question of forced organ harvesting was not a primary focus of the study, my research team and I did review evidence available at the time and conducted a number of our own interviews with several relevant individuals. The following are the specific sections of the report relaying our findings:

Excerpt from Evolving Mechanisms of Religious Control essay (pg 21)
[T]here is evidence suggesting that religious prisoners have been killed extrajudicially to provide organs for China's booming organ transplant industry. Numerous circumstantial facts, expert analyses, and eyewitness accounts point to the victimization of Falun Gong practitioners in particular. Large numbers of transplants continue to be performed with short waiting times, despite a shrinking

420

number of judicial executions and a still miniscule number of voluntary donors. In this context, the large-scale disappearance of young Uighur men, accounts of routine blood-testing of Uighur political prisoners, and reports of mysterious deaths of Tibetans and Uighurs in custody should raise alarm that these populations may also be victims of involuntary organ harvesting. *[Endnote for this paragraph: For example, a Uighur Muslim released from an Urumqi prison in 2011 gave Freedom House a detailed account of monthly blood tests administered to Uighur political and religious prisoners and not to Chinese criminal inmates. He and two Tibetan interviewees cited reports of mysterious deaths of fellow believers in custody. Interview with Uighur refugee now living in Turkey who wished to remain anonymous, October 2016.]*

Excerpt from Falun Gong chapter "Key Findings" (pgs. 108-109)

Economic exploitation: The party-state invests hundreds of millions of dollars annually in the campaign to crush Falun Gong, while simultaneously engaging in exploitative and lucrative forms of abuse against practitioners, including extortion and prison labor. Available evidence suggests that forced extraction of organs from Falun Gong detainees for sale in transplant operations has occurred on a large scale and may be continuing.

Excerpt from Falun Gong chapter "The money trail" section (pgs 120-121)

It is in the context of dehumanizing propaganda, severe abuse in custody, and economic inducements that the ultimate form of financial exploitation has been reported: the killing of Falun Gong detainees and the extraction of their organs to be sold at high prices to Chinese patients and foreign "transplant tourists" as part of a multibillion-dollar industry. The allegations first surfaced in 2006, and several investigations by foreign journalists and legal specialists have found them to be credible;[1] some members of the medical community have voiced their own concerns.[2]

There are indubitably serious problems surrounding the sources of organs for transplants in China.[3] A thorough investigation into these sources is beyond the scope of this study. Nevertheless, Freedom House reviewed available evidence compiled by other investigators (including phone calls made to Chinese doctors), interviewed former Falun Gong prisoners of conscience who provided detailed accounts of blood tests in custody, spoke to a Taiwanese doctor whose patients have traveled to China for transplants, and met with the friend of a military hospital employee who had firsthand knowledge of organ extraction from a Falun Gong detainee as recently as 2011.[4] The above review found credible evidence suggesting that beginning in the early 2000s, Falun Gong detainees were killed for their organs on a large scale.

There are reasons to believe that such abuses continue. The organ transplant industry in China remains enormous and growing, even as the number of judicially executed prisoners has declined over the past decade.[5] After admitting that extracting organs from executed prisoners was problematic, the Chinese government has initiated a voluntary organ-donor system, but its capacity remains small. Moreover, in 2014, a top health official announced that organs from prisoners would be embedded within the same database, even though prisoners are not in a position to provide free consent for "voluntary" donations.[6]

A detailed June 2016 study of publicly available data on the number of transplants being conducted at medical institutions in China found that the scale is many times greater than the 10,000 transplants per year often cited by officials.[7] This would indicate that the discrepancy between known supply and actual transplant volume may be even larger than previously appreciated, increasing the risk to Falun Gong practitioners, other prisoners of conscience, and criminal detainees."

New concerns over escalated persecution in Xinjiang
Since the conclusion of our research for the report in late 2016, a series of developments in Xinjiang have occurred which could indicate a current or future plan to use Uighur or other Muslim minority detainees as sources for China's booming organ transplant industry, although arguably other explanations may also exist. Specifically:

- **Mass extralegal detention**: A network of "political re-education" camps in the region has expanded rapidly. Human rights groups estimate that one million or more ethnic Uighurs, Kazakh, Uzbek, and Hui citizens are reportedly being detained for indoctrination, seemingly indefinitely, although some have been released or prosecuted judicially. Reports of mistreatment, torture, and deaths in custody at the facilities have already emerged.
- **Widespread DNA testing and other medical examinations:** In December 2017 Human Rights Watch reported that Chinese authorities in Xinjiang were significantly expanding access to biological data of residents by "collecting DNA samples, fingerprints, iris scans, and blood types of all residents in the region between the age of 12 and 65."

- **Crematoria expansion:** In June 2018, Radio Free Asia reported that according to local officials, authorities in Xinjiang "are rapidly constructing crematoria staffed by dozens of security personnel." Between March 2017 and February 2018, the regional government issued tenders for contractors to build nine "burial management centers" in mostly Uighur- populated areas. The article attributed the trend to an official effort to discourage traditional Uighur burial ceremonies, but a Han Chinese staff person at one crematorium told the reporters that police typically make cremation arrangements and that some corpses of individuals who had died at the indoctrination camps had been brought to his center.
- **Transfer of Uighur prisoners from Xinjiang to other provinces**: In recent months, reports have begun to emerge of Uighurs who had been sentenced to prison being transferred in large numbers to detention facilities in other provinces. One interpretation of the transfers is that the purpose is to avoid overcrowding of facilities in Xinjiang, but another possible explanation could be to move potential organ "donors" closer to a wider range of hospitals.

Ongoing organ transplant tourism from the Middle East

In October 2017, a Korean television network conducted an undercover on-site investigation of a prominent transplant hospital in Tianjin.[8] Among the findings of their investigation was that a large number of organ recipients had come from the Middle East alongside patients from South Korea and elsewhere. Hospital staff and patients interviewed reported wait times for organs were between days and weeks. Although ethnic proximity is not essential for successful transplantation, my understanding is that it can improve matching and receptivity. From that perspective, organs extracted from Uighur detainees could be a useful supplement to ones taken from Han prisoners to serve patients traveling from the Middle East or Central Asia.

Given the above, I would encourage the tribunal to seek out other witnesses with relevant regional or medical expertise who may be able to shed light on questions such as:

- Has any expansion occurred or been planned to hospitals within Xinjiang, and particularly to any transplant centers there, such as at Xinjiang Medical University? Analysis of procurement records, which have informed investigations of re-education centers, could potentially be applied to hospitals, as well as other government documents, and may help find an answer to this question.

- What biometric or other medical data is being collected from Uighurs on a large scale, especially those in detention, and would such data be useful for identifying organ "donors" to match recipient patients?
- Is additional information available on the scale – now or projected into the future – of organ transplant tourism from the Middle East and Central Asia? Are wait times for such patients unusually rapid, suggesting reverse matching from an available population of "donors"? Would organs from ethnic Muslim minorities indeed be more desirable than from Han Chinese for such recipient patients?

Thank you for your attention to this critical human rights issue and please let me know if you have any further questions.

(Signature redacted)

Sarah Cook
Senior Research Analyst Freedom House

References

1. Kilgour and Matas, "Bloody Harvest;" Ethan Gutmann, The Slaughter: Mass Killings, Organ Harvesting, and China's Secret Solution to its Dissident Problem (New York: Prometheus Books, 2014).
2. See for example A. Sharif, M. Fiatarone Singh, T. Trey, and J. Lavee, "Organ procurement from executed prisoners in China," American Journal of Transplantation 14, no. 10 (2014): 2246–2252, http://onlinelibrary.wiley.com/doi/10.1111/ajt.12871/pdf.
3. A lack of transparency is exacerbated by Chinese officials' vacillating explanations of their sources. For example, after years of denying that executed prisoners were used to supply organs for transplant, officials admitted in November 2006 – shortly after the emergence of the more damning allegations regarding Falun Gong – that the majority came from prisoners. Mark Magnier and Alan Zarembo, "Death Row is Organ Source, China Admits." Los Angeles Times, November 18, 2006, http://blogs.abcnews.com/theblotter/2006/11/china_admits_se.html
4. Interview with Taiwanese urologist who wished to remain anonymous, March 2016; interview with a technologist and Falun Gong practitioner from Beijing who wished to remain anonymous, June 2016. The Beijing interviewee's friend apparently relayed the highly sensitive incident to him as a warning, knowing that he was a Falun Gong practitioner.

5. Duihua Foundation, "China Executed 2,400 People in 2013," October 20, 2014, https://duihua.org/china-executed-2400-people-in-2013-dui-hua-2/.

6. A. Sharif, M. Fiatarone Singh, T. Trey, and J. Lavee, "Organ procurement from executed prisoners in China,"

7. David Kilgour, Ethan Gutmann, David Matas, "Bloody Harvest/The Slaughter: An Update," June 22, 2016, http://endorganpillaging.org/wp-content/uploads/2016/06/Bloody_Harvest-The_Slaughter-June-23-V2.pdf

8. Kim H, Shin D. TV Chosun, Documentary on Transplant Tourism to China. Hospital visit excerpt with English subtitles by the China Organ Harvesting Research Center: https://vimeo.com/250087127/37c9aedd40 Original full documentary in Korean: https://youtu.be/dDsDfgQSgdg

Additional Documents Provided

https://freedomhouse.org/report/china-religious-freedom

Summary of oral testimony: 8th December 2018

Report on religious freedom in China published in February 2017, titled: The Battle for Chinas Spirit: Religious Revival, Repression and Resistance under Xi Jinping looked at the full gambit of religious groups with a detailed chapter on Falun Gong.

In China it is not considered a religion as they only recognise five. Internationally it could be considered organised religion. It slipped through the cracks initially and then was deregistered. When the Falun Gong tried to register again it was not allowed to do so because it was banned by Chinese Communist Party in 1999. The report really looks within each one of the regions' groups. We examined, the revival and nature of the various forms of repression each religious group faces and examples of repression and resistance. What is clear is that everything applies to the Falun Gong. There are a large number of Chinese verdicts where individuals are being sentences to prison from Jan 1, 2013-2016. We were very interested in the 900 something individuals sentences to prison and extra-legal detention. One of the other things that came up in our research, was the issue of economic exploitation of various forms, as well as the political and economic dynamics that lead into it the question of potential organ harvesting. Strictly, organ harvesting was beyond the scope of independent investigation. However, we looked at various investigations that have been conducted and we spoke to many Falun Gong practitioners. We heard the same kinds of accounts over the years by Falun Gong refugees that I have interviewed. They have experienced the same type of blood tests, ultrasounds and other medical examinations. One of things that really came out of our research was how difficult it is to reform an organ transplant system from an unethical system to an ethical one. This is important to understand about the Chinese governments claims about having transitioned in such a short period to an ethical system.

I conducted an interview with fellow from Beijing which including questions of resistance in China. He was interested in how they were dealing with it especially using mobile phones and the internet to reach people in China to counteract the government propaganda as well as whether they had experienced blood testing in China. But as we got to the topic of organ harvesting, he said how someone he knows had been a former student and had worked at military hospital. This friend of his had been sent on an errand to retrieve an organ and was told that it was from Falun Gong practitioner in 2011, there was other information that added credibility of his account. He was very hesitant because he was concerned about the person he knew which is why we left him anonymous in our report. This is as close as one ever gets to a first-hand account of being targeted for organ harvesting abuse long after the evidence came out in 2006. The last thing I will say, is taking the above review and other information I have received related to the scale we came to the conclusion beginning in the early 2000 the Falun Gong have been killed on a large scale for their organs.

We are also interested in Uyghur Prisoners from Xinjiang.
I have done previous research on the 610 office. It is an extra legal – party committee and security force which was started before Falun Gong was officially banned. It was a part of president's efforts to get things going. Operates in extra-legal arena and is focused on getting Falun Gong to transform. One of the things we looked at was the level of on-going activity. Our evidence suggest that the 610 Office is still active. A fair amount of money being spent by the 610 office during this period. However, it has been part of some of the purges and it has been weakened because its own head had been sentenced to prison. You don't see quite the same level of top down push in 2016 as you did in 2013.

[Whether there is a 610 equivalent for other religions] That's a good question! The 610-office mandate has been expanded it now deals with 23 various quasi-Christian and qigong religions. It is not only the Falun Gong. One of the other things you see happening is the expansion of its mandate to other forms of dissent. You see overlap in bureaucracy with the modelling of the 610 office. It is also based in this party committee and you see some of the same staff.

[To consider a definition religion] We look at the Universal declaration of Human Rights, Article 18. Article 18 includes not only formal religions but various forms of spiritual practice and personal beliefs which is why we included more organised religions such as Christianity and Islam but also the Falun Gong. In general repression against the Falun Gong has become clear in other areas of civil society, and in wide array of various forms of human rights and civil liberties abuses. On the other hand, to some extent Falun Gong was an unusual exception. We found Tibetan, Uyghur Muslims and protestant Christians are those who faced an increase in religious persecution. Catholics have a happier situation whilst the Falun Gong with some of its grass roots resistances, which includes targeting local members of the police has helped to repress the persecution a little bit. However, there is still a very large amount of persecution against the Falun Gong.

[Page 19 of report, link above] I think in general we were looking at the practical reality with laws and regulations especially to a special religious group. We also looked at information related to arrests and detention, information about festivals, children education for example is more tightly controlled. We looked at legal codification, as well as practical behaviour by officials, especially looking at the way some groups which were previously not targeted are becoming very heavily targeted. In some cases, regardless of what the laws are because legal provisions are used to sentence people but in practice there are other legal dynamics that may not have been there before.

Uyghur Muslims from Xinjiang are the most likely to be targeted and since we finished this report the conditions have gotten worse. We did try to see if we if Uyghur prisoners of conscious had been blood tested. One person we interviewed had been detained from 1997-2011 and we asked him if they had been blood tests, and it was interesting because he didn't think it was related to organ harvesting. He was concerned with the prevalence of HIV and unsanitary conditions in hospitals and thought that HIV was being spread in this way. However, what he did say was that were monthly blood tests to Uyghur political prisoners and prisoners of conscious but not for Chinese. That combined with conversations with Tibetan prisoners about mysterious deaths in custody and periodic injections given to people is why we flagged that there should be concern over the fact that they may be victims of involuntary organ harvesting

[Independent verification of HIV case] Because it was not the scope of what we were looking at I have not looked into this further. He saw among his fellow Uyghur prisoners.

[Whether the arrests of, and organ procurement from FG has decreased]. How the organs are sourced across different populations is related to some combination that can vary over time. One of the things that can vary over time, just in general is that those communities are more likely targeted for organ harvesting than those that have gone through the formal system. Perhaps possible that the percentage is less than the early 2000 when there was less international scrutiny. The awareness among Falun Gong practitioners and their family members means that families of those who are newly detained may be more vigilant, but that is some level of speculation. Among the prisoners we have found that people can be detained for a very long period of time, for example 12-18 years and there is some level of judicial system. You have Falun Gong who have been there from some time, large levels of new arrests does not mean that there is less of a residual community of Falun Gong detainees that can be used for organ harvesting.

We found that it (FoH) may be continuing but it is more difficult to find conclusive evidence with the amount of resources and time that we had. In everything we looked at there was a good chance that it is continuing and has not stopped which I thought it may do around the Olympics as the Chinese government became more public about reforming its organ transplant system.

If I could say on the Uyghur question most of it is written testimony. We know that 1 million have been extrajudicially detained and transfer of them to transplants hospitals is highly likely. I would just flag that as I think even since we have finished research on this report Uyghur Muslims are being heavily prosecuted.

Witness 34: Matthew Robertson

Dear committee members of the Independent Tribunal into Forced Organ Harvesting from Prisoners of Conscience in China,

My name is Matthew Robertson. I am currently Research Fellow in China Studies with the Victims of Communism Memorial Foundation. In January 2019 I will commence studies at the Australian National University pursuing a Ph.D. in political science on the topic of China's organ transplantation system. I am professionally proficient in written and spoken Mandarin Chinese.

I have been asked to submit testimony to the Tribunal as to my research on the issue, with a focus on the primary evidence I have examined and witnesses spoken to, etc. The following notes address this.

1.   I have studied China's organ transplantation system since around 2013, when I was a journalist covering Chinese politics and domestic security issues;

2.   Since 2016 I have further pursued the topic as a research fellow and scholar;

3.   I have interviewed, interpreted for, or spoken to about half a dozen eyewitnesses, in person and on the telephone, about their experiences in Chinese prisons or detention centers being examined for what appeared to be the health of their organs, or being subjected to what they felt were suspicious blood tests or physical examinations in custody. Such cases included the close probing of abdominal organs by unidentified nursing staff using an ultrasound wand, or a case in which only the Falun Gong captives in a detention center in northeast China were called into a bus, which had pulled into the courtyard with doctors and nurses, and subjected to blood tests and abdominal examinations;

4.   I have read hundreds of Chinese medical papers about organ transplantation, including on topics such as: the advancement of clinical techniques for organ extraction; internal debates about the ethics surrounding brain death; case reports of organ extraction and transplantation surgeries; post-operative studies; cohort studies; the development and consumption of immunosuppressants, etc. I possess a collection of dozens of Chinese textbooks and nursing and clinical handbooks on organ transplantation. I have collated and read reports

by securities firms analyzing Chinese domestic pharmaceutical companies who manufacture immunosuppressant drugs, etc.;

5.   My research is focused on primary Chinese-language sources, and where possible, is data-driven. I am in the process of collating and analyzing a number of databases on China's organ transplantation system, including: roughly 120,000 medical papers on organ transplantation scraped from Chinese academic databases; thousands of biographies of physicians involved in organ transplantation in China scraped from public data; thousands of Chinese patents related to organ transplantation; data from hundreds of Chinese hospital websites offering organ transplantation services, and more;

6.   I am the lead author, with a statistician and transplant surgeon, of a study awaiting peer and legal review, which conducts a forensic statistical analysis of China's voluntary organ transplant data. The paper (when it is finally published) will be the first peer reviewed report to scrutinize and raise questions about the official data on China's voluntary organ transplantation system. It uses data on voluntary donations myself and colleagues collected from the Red Cross offices of every province in China, as well as central data on voluntary donors in China, and submits them to analysis for statistical integrity. I am the second author of a scoping review, also awaiting publication after peer review, which examines the record of Western medical journals in publishing research from China that uses data obtained from unethically sourced organs;

7.   I have read or am acquainted with a large portion of the secondary English-language academic literature on the death penalty in China, the anti-Falun Gong campaign, China's domestic security apparatus, medical ethics in China, the use of physicians in the abuses of human rights (as seen in psychiatric abuses perpetrated against political prisoners, for instance, or China's birth control policies), and practically all literature on China's organ transplantation system including the allegations of organ harvesting;

8.   My Ph.D. and scholarly research is aimed at bringing the tools of mixed-method social science enquiry to bear on the complex question of China's organ transplantation system and the source of organs that have fueled its growth over the last two decades. The quantitative data I am using is in the form of the aforementioned databases, while qualitative data includes the forensic analysis of clinical papers, interviews with eyewitnesses and Chinese

surgeons, the study of Chinese media reports, and so on. In the jargon of social science research design, my Ph.D. will consist of a case study using the tools of process tracing and data science to answer empirical questions about the dimensions and growth of China's organ transplantation system, and to evaluate the arguments about the source of organs China has used.

Some general findings I have observed from my research include:

1. China's organ transplantation industry embarked on a period of rapid development post-2000, including in the opening of new transplant wards, buildings, and research laboratories; many hospitals performed their first liver, heart, and lung transplants; thousands of new surgeons and nurses were trained and began publishing research; the state began subsidizing immunosuppressant research and manufacturing, and placed domestic immunosuppressants on health insurance subsidy lists; many new organ transplantation-related patents were registered and published; many more transplant- related medical papers were published;

2. I have observed from official Chinese organ registry documents and clinical papers that after the year 2000 there were numerous cases of transplants available on demand; coincident with this, I have observed that hospitals regularly reported being able to perform transplants within weeks; I have read transcripts, listened to audio recordings, and witnessed investigators calling Chinese hospitals eliciting such waiting times from doctors and nurses spoken to;

3. I have observed that the official explanation for organ sourcing in China has changed on several occasions. Prior to 2006 the official stance was that organs came from volunteers. In 2006 this shifted to all organs coming from death row prisoners. In 2015 it was claimed that only volunteers were used;

4. I have observed that human rights research organizations and scholars are of the view that the number of death penalty executions declined almost every year from 2000 onwards, a view also found in Chinese-language judicial sources;

5. I have observed that there was a widely observed and richly documented series of reforms to the review of death penalty cases in China, in which the Supreme People's Court recentralized review authority and beginning in

January 1, 2007, subjected each death sentence to a process of review and approval. This led, according to Chinese and foreign academic sources, to a significant decline in death penalty executions;

6.   I have observed that the growth trajectory of the transplantation system did not slow following this shift in death penalty volume and procedure – a change that one would expect to observe if the two were as tightly linked as claimed;

7.   I have observed that the Chinese government has provided no adequate explanation for the source of organs through most of this period (2000-present) given these opposite trajectories in transplant system growth and availability of the primary source of organs claimed to supply it;

8.   Generally, I have read widely in the Chinese transplant literature and am happy to answer questions on all of the above and related lines of enquiry.

Thank you for your attention to this important issue.

Regards,
Matthew Robertson New York City October 21, 2018
https://chinatribunal.com/wp-content/uploads/2019/06/12_SurgeonProfileOne_ZhengShusen.pdf

Summary of oral testimony: 8th December 2018

I am a research fellow of Chinese, beginning a PhD at the Australian National University and writing a thesis on organ transplantation in China. I am fluent in Chinese.

Conclusion of my studies: forthcoming publication on potential violations of dead donor rule. I collect everything that has been published in Chinese medical journals. I have worked with a data engineer to organise a database, I have 120,000 publications in the database so far. I will analyse this for my database.

I hope to be able to answer any questions you would like to know about the subject. It gets technical and complex.

My approach – there are two issues in consideration of numbers: Volume and trajectory

432

Trajectory over time and whether their numbers are explicable with reference to the official Chinese explanation of death row prisoners. Growth over time. I am looking at post 2000 and 2007.

Whether the transplant figures ranges from 60,000 to 100,000, it's still important to see if it's within the margin of reality. What is the growth over time? I consider the period post 2000 to 2007. The official explanation given in 2007 suggests all transplants are sourced from DRPs.

If there was a drop in 2007 then the continued growth in the transplant system. There is a huge question about where those organs are coming from. Death penalties dropped precipitously post 2007. Therefore, there is suspicion over figures. It is important to consider if there was drop in death penalty executions in 2007, then the continued transplant growth raises questions as to the source of organs. Are they prisoners of conscience?

Voluntary citizen donors – not prisoners of any type. There is more transparency here for obvious reasons. I have a forthcoming paper specifically on this issue. I can't talk about it in detail. The official data is not trustworthy. The full analysis is coming soon. There were 119 voluntary deceased donors until 2009, and that number comes from several doctors which makes it reliable for me.

To explain using DRP, consider SDP judicial review process. There are academics who talk about the process to lawyers, judges. Courts in Qidong have been earnest and forthcoming in publishing DR figures. Years of data have been collected in some provinces which accord with slightly less than 10,000 executions annually.

There is an issue of coordination; there was no system of transporting organs across China.

Also, the issue of blood-borne disease in prisons meant that over 50% or prisoners had hepatitis and were thus unsuitable donors.

There was a need to maintain the conspiracy that DRPs were the main organ sources, but this is complex as you'd need to keep them off the grid. Yet prisoners go through court process. This leads to conclusion that there is an alternate source.

Yes, the criminal procedure requires death penalty executions within 7 days. There's wide-spread immediate availability of organs. The proof of this is seen in so called emergency transplants. From 2007, urgent/emergency transplant (as short as 4 hours) stats were no longer reported.

The plausible conclusion is that there are extra-judicial killings. DRPs are publicly shot at execution site and Human Rights advocates are aware of the short time between sentencing and execution and think it doesn't allow justice. This indicates alternative source of organs.

Medical papers don't deal with international community perception of organ harvesting. International community response would be dealt with in local media reports.

International pressure has caused China to show that they are a rule of law country. As a result of international pressure, statements were made to indicate that it was death row prisoners who provided the source of organs in China.

China claims they follow international medical guidelines.

Reports suggest donors are brain dead. Thoughts about transplant ethics in China – there are countless papers on this topic. It was already claimed that China was adhering to international standards because they relied on consent. Definition of brain dead is an international definition. Individual is still alive but there is neurological damage. There is no brain death law in China but the guidelines service as sufficient for transplantation.

There is a significant difference [between sources of organs and number of executed prisoners], but we don't know what it is. We don't know how many transplants and we don't know how many death sentences there have been. Certainly, it exists. I think there would be a significant gap giving generous estimates to death row population and voluntary donation. But we can only infer from other information.

Ethan Gutmann's report said a peasant waited three months for an organ.

[Relationship between mode of execution, impact on numbers or organs] I've looked at medical textbooks and spoken to surgeons. It's hard to figure it out because these are medical texts written in Chinese. What is clear is that transplantation is taking place in a clinical setting. Brain death is being falsely declared. Moment of death appears to be at the point where the heart is removed. This can't take place in an execution context e.g. being shot in the head.

Execution is taking place in a clinical setting. Medically trained personnel are being involved in the execution. We don't even know that the official registries know what is actually going on in reality. No institutionalisation of medical record keeping until 2009 – it was a wild west. Timing is significant and lines up with FG persecution.

There would be a great many agencies involved in this process and you probably still wouldn't be able to find a record of all the victims.

There are anecdotes from prison guards that tell prisoners to make sure their families come to visit them.

Red Cross data is not reliable.

Continuation of evidence on Day 3: 9th December 2018
Two main considerations for suspecting organs sourced from non-death row population:

Number of transplants
Immediate availability of organs

In terms of the availability there is the well-known incident where Huang Jiefu went to Xinjiang for the national celebration of the 50th anniversary of the Liberation of Xinjiang and did a liver transplant where he took out the liver of the patient, removed tumour and re-implanted it. He had ordered two back up livers for back up from two locations. Back up livers were delivered next day. It's a vivid case that shows it is not a coincidence that there were death row prisoners who were available and had their sentence approved recently. You can't rule out that it could have been a coincidence, or two coincidences in fact so it is simply a matter of the judgment you want to apply to it.

When I recounted this to Dr Michael Millis a western doctor who is familiar with the Chinese system. He said indeed there must have been a coincidence. Indeed, it could have been a coincidence. You can't rule that out factually. 30% of transplants in 2005 were urgent.

I haven't done a systematic comparison [of Chinese and Western systems] – it's hard to get data. 14% of liver transplants in UK. Reason comparison is not necessarily meaningful. UK is small geographically. All hospitals are linked where there is organ sharing. In China that is not the case now. There was certainly nothing of that kind in early 2000's.

No organ sharing system, large geography. They've got them on demand in many hospitals. There has been immediate availability of matched organs. I've seen papers where they suggest that paramilitary hospitals in China share resources. They aren't sharing organs because they have them on demand.

[Waiting times] US: many months to years. If your need is more urgent you'll get the first available organ.

China: key difference is which way the matching is going. They have the donors in a big list and they're just waiting for the recipients to appear and then all they need to do is extract the organ. This is the most reasonable and plausible way of explaining what we've observed.

Chinese medical reports refer to having donors available.

[Consistency with suggestions of brokerage] Consistent to the degree that the brokers have a relationship with hospitals, and they can contract their people at the hospitals to know about the availability of organs.

[Whether urgency is recognised on the waiting lists] It appears that those who are more politically connected and/or can pay more. The more urgent the organ transplant. A well-known case was a Chinese actor received two liver transplants. The first within a month of him needed it. The cancer came back. Then he got the next liver transplant within a week or so. Because he was famous his transplantation was widely remarked upon. His doctor was the famous transplant surgeon, Beijing's transplant surgery founder. So doctors get political capital by servicing famous or wealthy people.

309 military hospital has a very advanced transplant department and is specifically for party members.

[Whether children have been involved] Only anecdotally and not in a way that I was satisfied writing about. I have looked through medical papers now that we have a database. When I searched previously this didn't pan out essentially.

[Reform] For sure there is in my opinion there are actual voluntary deceased donations going on. I strongly believe that to be the case. That's from reading medical papers and watching news reports and 60-minute style documentaries from Chinese state-run documentaries. What I have been is convincing, but it comes with a caveat. One, a hospital in Shanghai, a first-tier city, had a citizen donor, a genuine case, they mobilised 60 medical staff. It is a massive production and the circumstances were just right for this case, but it is certainly not for the scale they have claimed.

Dr Jacob Lavee and I have a paper on this exact issue. The report uses only official data and will put to rest this very issue as regards official data. They're still doing many many transplants from all indications. The paper will give very good answers to this.

The study of this issue is itself a very interesting issue. Essentially until 2014/2015 there wasn't much. There is very little peer-reviewed scholarship on China's organ transplant system. That itself is quite a remarkable thing actually. I have gone through literature on healthcare reform, pharmaceutical, corruption in the hospital system [and more] and there is nothing on the organ transplant system, and that is strange in itself. Even Cambridge books in related areas don't mention much on this issue.

First hand research. The stuff I'm doing is based on Gutmann and FG investigators. They're the ones that did the initial research. I'm applying a social science research methodology. With scientific research you have a recipe. I'm just doing that to a sense to what's already been done.

You get interviews, medical papers, clinical handbooks; nursing handbooks etc. and then you put it all together. Then you can get things from each thing.

Transplants according to Chinese medical papers. How many papers are clinical and how many are not clinical. There is often an overlap. You don't know if the same organs were not used.

There could be an overlap of one organ. It's very complicated. Some of these papers will just say by way of background our hospital has done this many. There is no standardised reporting method. It's almost always incomplete. Eventually we'll have a big rectangle of data. Then we'll have some predictive modelling.

It will be possible to use some process and have some rules that are transparent. Then we'll have a series of numbers. But even then, that will be from a process that is not necessarily accurate.

My foundation's report will have some simple way of showing the data and the growth of the system. We went through all the material and made pivot tables each time a hospital did its first of each type of transplant, building its first ward, transplant lab. Very few hospitals reported doing their first heart transplant and then it just spiked. All that takes off during 2000. That's solid and interesting data and it totally doesn't match with the data on the death penalty. So, the Chinese government has a lot of explaining to do. It wasn't until 2006 when they declared that all those organs were from the death row. But that is not what the data from their own hospital websites says about it. Scholars of death penalty hadn't seen it before and wondered about it as well when it was shown to them.

[Transplants is a discussion about insertion of organs as distinct from harvesting, which is a parallel system] Yes, that's a correct interpretation of what I've described. Although there are many medical papers focused on the extraction process.

I can speculate wildly [about the reluctant of transplant surgeons to acknowledge that there might be an issue]. Huang Jiefu got his PhD from the University of Sydney. He is a perceived to be a known quantity among many people at that university and has networked with the community there [the Australian surgeons] who consider him a colleague and perhaps even an ally against corrupt military hospitals. If they don't make good with him, they have no impact with him they have no way of pushing anything in a positive way. I have spoken to them a bunch and this is my general understanding.

As regards the other side and the prisoner of conscience issue in China it's a FGP issue. Which is politically sensitive and a totally no-go issue. If they were trying to go down that path. It's not like a friendly academic discourse that they would be having. Their condition for engaging with him is not to touch this issue and so they've done so. There's a lot to be said about this. This results in the transplant surgeons being put in a very awkward situation. It means they share the podium with respected liver transplant surgeons in China, and in one with the doctor who heads the anti-cult commission, which was set up next to the 610 office to carry out the anti FG propaganda and prepare the transformation materials for the transformation that we have heard about. He is head of that agency. Frank Delmonico and others find themselves doing the high ten [gestures] and they didn't know that he was that guy.

They didn't know these people are so controversial until bothersome people like me inform them. There is some awkwardness about that. But that is what you sign up to when you decide this issue is off limits.

So, what do these guys genuinely think is going on here? I spoke with him [Jeremy Chapman] and Dr Nancy Asher in Hong Kong. I described the emergency transplant thing. I put it to them that it's probably the case that there's a live organ donor pool or an extraordinary coincidence. Dr Asher didn't know what I was driving at and only gave me 10 minutes and watched the time very officiously. Dr Chapman sad "I said prisoners" as in "I don't buy into the idea that they are only death row prisoners". So that and other comments through back channels seems to me that they must know something is not quite right. I have what he said written down but not with me. It's my impression that they know something is not quite right.

[Knowledge of who the recipients are] I have not spent effort trying to find people like this and interview them. It depends on the country. Taiwan has some data because researchers were able to get access to insurance data and to figure out some numbers. There is a doctor in Malaysia who has a lot of data that had outcomes of transplants such as country of origin, but names aren't mentioned. He had some indication on the quality of the organs. In Malaysia, I forget the medical details but there was an indication of the quality of the organ being the same as with living donor because ischaemic damage was minimal. There is no global way of capturing this or of requiring reporting.

[Countries using legislation to prohibit travel to China for transplants] Yes Taiwan, Israel, something in Spain. In Australia it didn't get past the state level.

[Is there an ethics committee in Chinese hospitals] Yes. Different role though. They just rubber-stamp everything that comes in from surgeons. What the surgeon says goes. Dr Rogers and I have a paper coming out that deals with this explicitly.

[Whether any TV programmes identify the start date for the voluntary programme and explain how the transplant skills were built on by earlier practice] No. And no start date was identified. The party line doesn't differ. By 2015 no prisoner organs were used. The only reason I believe them is that it would be far too elaborate to stage. Barring countervailing evidence, I have nothing to suggest I was fooled but perhaps I was, but I don't think so.

If a Chinese doctor could get his whole family out of China and he had data that would be useful he might disclose it but even then we don't have a smoking gun. How would we know what he's saying is true? The scale is so big. In the public realm it would be more of a PR issue. The Chinese government have been successful in this area.

[Chapman and O'Connell have criticised the work of Matas] I am not aware that I am criticised by them.

[Whether personal threats have been received]. Not me. A few agents asked about me at one point.

Witness 35: Ethan Gutmann

Tribunal Statement

My investigation into Chinese organ harvesting of prisoners of conscience was essentially an accident. I had been writing about Chinese Communist Party (CCP) surveillance of Falun Gong practitioners and other dissidents since 2002, around the time I left Beijing to finish Losing the New China (Encounter Books, 2004). By 2005, I was thinking about my next book and my experience on the ground told me that Falun Gong was the biggest issue in China. Yet there was a gap in the existing literature. Research by Falun Gong practitioners was emotionally charged, while published writing by self-proclaimed "objective" outsiders overcompensated with undue formality, bias against spirituality, or avoiding actual witness accounts in favor of formulaic original research. That partially explains why I maintained a degree of scepticism about the first public organ harvesting allegations from both the Epoch Times and the Kilgour- Matas report, Bloody Harvest in 2006. Yet I was firmly convinced that a comprehensive account of the conflict between the Chinese State and Falun Gong was long overdue, and I began a lengthy interview process to fill that gap.

One of my very first interviews was in Toronto with three women who were fresh out of labor camp. Even in that early stage, I recognized that their stories were relatively routine – demonstrations at Tiananmen followed by capture, incarceration, and attempts to force practitioners to reject Falun Gong using torture, brainwashing, threats to the family, and humiliation. One of the women – call her Wang – was the least articulate but had a very appealing salt-of-the-earth quality. At one point Wang mentioned a "funny" physical exam. I asked her to explain. Wang did not consider the matter important and started to go on with her real story. I persisted – had she been hunger striking? No. Taking Medication? No. Was anyone else examined? Yes, other Falun Gong. What were the tests? A urine sample, a large blood test, an EKG, some tapping around the stomach and groin, x-rays, and then the doctor spent a lot of time shining a light into Wang's eyes. Was there a peripheral vision test? No. Focus or reading test? No. No vision test, nothing involving actual sight? No. Test of ears, nose or throat? Genitals, reflexes? No. In fact, there was nothing that could constitute a proper physical examination. The tests were aimed at the health of her liver, kidneys, heart, and corneas – the major retail organs.

At no point did Wang seem to grasp the implications of what she was relating. Instead Wang was irritated at me, the stupid white guy who kept asking about some insignificant medical examination but didn't understand the significance of her spiritual battle. While I didn't believe at the time that Wang had been seriously considered as a candidate for organ harvesting – probably too old, I thought, although I would ultimately learn that I was wrong about that – I still remember feeling a chill as my comfortable cloak of scepticism fell away.

I mention Wang's interview in detail for three reasons: First, because there is nothing quite like the moment when it dawns on you that this thing might actually be true (and the converse of that is that none of the breakthrough interviews that followed – from Falun Gong refugees to Uyghur medical staff to Taiwanese surgeons – surprised me all that much).

Second, because it indicates that my system was too conservative. After The Slaughter (Prometheus, 2014) was published, my subsequent research for Bloody Harvest/The Slaughter: an Update (ETAC, 2016; referred to as 2016 Update) indicated that China had made far greater strides in transplantation than we had understood at the time and by exploiting techniques such as ECMO, Wang's organs were probably viable for transplant. Third, Wang's interview became a rare and valuable benchmark for me: an interview free from bias.

Bias, the psychological effects of severe trauma, or even unconscious attempts to spin testimony to fit into an organ harvesting storyline was clearly a danger to my investigation. Yet it seemed equally absurd – and possibly even bigoted – for reporters, NGOs and government investigators to simply regard all Falun Gong witness testimony (or Uyghur or Tibetan testimony for that matter) as having little value – essentially devaluing the currency to zero simply because there were counterfeit bills in circulation. So when it came to the 50- plus Falun Gong refugees from the "Laogai System" (labor camps, psychiatric centers, long-term detention centers and black jails) that I interviewed in three continents – my strategy was to avoid revealing any tripwires or special areas of interest such as organ harvesting to the witnesses and simply explain that I was writing a "comprehensive history of the conflict between the Chinese State and Falun Gong." Then I had to live up to that representation by employing a kitchen-sink approach: Questions about their early spiritual background, how they got involved in Falun Gong, their first arrest, and the various tortures they suffered – these were all explored at length. These are subjects that most practitioners who had undergone severe trauma have a strong desire to talk about, but it also would acclimatize them to my demand for a level of detail that they were not accustomed to (The guards knocked you down? What color was the floor?) so that any questions about medical examinations or fellow practitioner disappearances would blend in seamlessly with my ongoing interest in their general physical and mental status throughout their narrative.

That was a highly demanding requirement for everyone involved; it meant time above all. Time to allow the witness to vent, to explore spirituality, to act out emotionally, or even to tell me what they thought I ought to know, rather than what they knew first-hand. And after all that, I would still be there, waiting for their story. This explains why most of my interviews went on for about four hours on average, and a handful of my interviews were carried out over two or three days. (I have made the tapes and notes for these interviews available to the Amnesty International Secretariat, the BBC, and many other press organizations that claimed to be sceptical of the organ harvesting issue. None of them accepted that challenge). In the process, I discovered eight unambiguous cases of Falun Gong refugees that had been tested for potential harvesting of their organs. Most of those cases are in chapter 8 of The Slaughter (although one could easily add the woman I have already spoken of, and Wang Yuzhi in chapter 6 to that list). The calculation of organ harvesting deaths based on that survey method of 50 practitioners is in the appendix.

A word about second-hand methodology – as a former business consultant in Beijing, I carry a deep-rooted distrust of Chinese official numbers. I used to advise my corporate clients that even if they are looking at tapioca production figures, mainland numbers are often coded political messages that barely reflect reality. I don't reject official numbers or methods of analysis that use them outright, but I instinctively look for other ways to get at the information, if only to serve as a point of comparison. The 2016 Update, which relies on the transplant volume accounts of individual hospitals – Sun Yat-sen in Guangzhou, Tianjin Central Hospital – rather than Beijing' so-called official numbers – this is one method. Another method is the witness survey method that I used in The Slaughter.

However, these sorts of estimates don't make much sense if there is no clear motivation by the Chinese State to carry out mass murder. And that is why I did not throw away interviews simply because the subject could shed no light on organ harvesting. Fully six of the chapters in The Slaughter have little to do with the "how" of organ harvesting, but are about the "why," the motivations and the context: What was the appeal of Falun Gong? Why did the CCP target it? Coming from a non-violent spiritual movement, how did practitioners think about fighting back? What were the key moments of escalation, how did the struggle change over time? As I said in The Slaughter, organ harvesting, organ tourism, these are "toxic allegations," and I believe in addressing the motivational question in full – money alone isn't quite enough, although the financial imperative is obvious in the Wang Lijun case (chapter 9) and throughout the 2016 Update. What emerges is that the CCPs motivation for organ harvesting clearly changes over time: from simply carrying out an order to eliminate Falun Gong, to a public and increasingly global struggle against a recalcitrant movement that will not convert, to a mass cover-up of two decades of organ harvesting crimes. Understanding those shifts requires a historical understanding of the CCP, yet it also calls out for a coherent narrative of the last two decades. It demands that we question the narrative that the Falun Gong persecution was an isolated event. The discovery that "Eastern Lightning" House Christians were also being tested for their organs emerged organically from the interviews with Fang Siyi and Jing Tian (chapter 8) yet organ harvesting of death-row prisoners began in the 1980s, and that is why I began to suspect that the Uyghurs were the first prisoners of conscience to be harvested and to look closely at the specific CCP reaction to the Ghulja Incident in 1997 (chapter 1) – and later, the specific challenges of the Tibetan resistance (chapter 8).

A word about anonymity: approximately half of the medical and law enforcement personnel that I quote in The Slaughter insisted on keeping their names and locations secret. Given that they have family in Xinjiang or in other areas of China that request must be respected.

Sometimes going on the record can present problems as well; one of the key affirmations that organ harvesting of Falun Gong was taking place in a Mainland Chinese hospital was made by Dr Ko Wen-je, a surgeon at National Taiwan University in 2008 (see first five pages of chapter 9). Yet Doctor Ko, when he became a candidate for mayor in the Autumn of 2014, tried to publicly deny his own account (I had kept all of our correspondence which you can see in the following video: (https://ethan-gutmann.com/ko-wen-je-interview/). In October 2018, faced with the unchanged text of The Slaughter being published in Mandarin, Mayor Ko attempted to pit his credibility against mine in the Taipei courts; the Taiwanese prosecutor publicly declared two days later that Mayor Ko "had no case" (the phrase has much the same meaning in both Mandarin and English). China is powerful, and the international medical community is no stranger to its gravitational pull, but facts and documentation can prevail over time.

My final comment has to do with the relevance of the Tribunal's work. While much of my work is historical analysis, my recent testimonies at Westminster (ETAC website) have related the following facts: Over the last 18 months, literally every

Uyghur man, woman, and child – about 15 million people – have been blood and DNA tested, and that blood testing is compatible with tissue matching. As the press, and even the UN, has widely reported, there are now approximately one million Uyghurs in re-education camps. Finally, the first of nine planned crematoriums was completed in Urumqi in early 2018 and is apparently manned by 50 security guards.

My involvement in this investigation may have essentially been an accident yet having seen a glimpse into what I can only describe as a real-life hell, I cannot un-see it. And given Beijing's determination to continue this medical practice, I will likely continue my work on this ongoing human rights catastrophe, this cold genocide – call it what you will – until the end of my life.

Ethan Gutmann

Summary of oral testimony: 9th December 2018
The Human Rights Watch brought the information about DNA testing of Uyghur group to our attention. This was backed up by Radio Free Asia. They left something out. It was not just a deterrent against terrorism, which is the advantage of DNA testing. They were also doing blood testing.

I also explored in my book about Falun Gong practitioners. The police would come in their own homes and administer cheek swab and also a blood test. I thought it was a potential for tissue matching. I believe there are 12-15 million of Uyghur.

As the pressure on this issue increased in the press and the UN approximately 300,000 of the Uyghurs disappeared and were taken to other provinces, which may be due to a poor local medical infrastructure. These signs, along with 50 security guards (paid $1200 dollars a month) to guard crematorium was concerning.

In relation to genocide I do not like to use the term of genocide too often because it can be distracting, but I have no comment on that in a legal context. I was quoting someone else when I made a reference to genocide. I call it a slow-motion genocide rather than cold genocide. I am hesitant to define genocide.

In relation to the volume of transplants, I do not have the exact number and I am not even sure that China has that number. There was a rumour about the existence of some large database. One of best witnesses is Dr Ko Wen-Je, a Surgeon at the National Taiwan University. I called him to ask about a database of organs. He refuted the existence of a database and said there is an informal eBay-style system as a doctors' network. It does not strike me as something like the holocaust, which is an exact system. We do not have exact figures, but we use ranges and make estimates. We do have estimates of 60,000 to 100,000 transplants a year. I lowered the estimates as China tends to exaggerate figures.

When we put out our 2016 report, everyone wanted us to write an executive summary, but we refused because we wanted journalists, governments etc. to get a feeling of the figures. We wanted people to wade into the numbers. The 60,000 to 100,000 estimate is a very low estimate and has the basis of one transplant per day in the authorised hospitals. You can still go with the government's figures announced 4 weeks ago. Huang Jiefu said that they will be doing 50,000 transplants by 2020. He has embraced our estimate. He has embraced it for very different reasons, I don't believe it is a real number, but he has said it is up about that number.

The update is less about 'how' but 'why'. The reason or answer to that changes dramatically over time. The crackdown on Falun Gong practitioners is not unusual and is a very public move of China. The initial assumption was that the crackdown would take 3 months, but Falun Gong practitioners put up a strong fight, not a physical one, but in the prisons, they refused food and water and protested. Over time, this can and has inspired Falun Gong practitioners to build infrastructure of resistance to make their fight global.

I interviewed about 150 people. I interviewed about 50 – 75 in depth and 75 peripherally. The interviews with 50 refugees from the labour camps were the most intense because they had a lot to offload.

In terms of regional concentration of transplants, it used to be concentrated in military hospitals in a number of locations. If you look at 2006 report entitled *Bloody Harvest* the spread is quite dramatic. You need a large-scale map and it would show a sea of black dots. Every province is trying to competitively do organ transplants.

There are three factors to consider:

1. The rise of Falun Gong detention and severity of persecution, which increases over time and in particular in 2002.
2. The rise of production of anti-rejection drugs
3. The rise of Extracorporeal Membrane Oxygenation (ECMO) (oxygenation of lungs and hearts) which can preserve organs eight hours after extraction and which increases chances of getting organs to wealthy organ tourists.

In terms of how the 610-office considered Falun Gong – a cult, practice or religion, it was all propaganda. They were considered as the Enemies of the State. I interviewed a 610 officer on several occasions. This was not an issue that came up a lot. He thought that Falun Gong practitioners were a bit nutty. He thought a female Falun Gong victim of torture was tiresome. He eventually defected.

Many Falun Gong practitioners were communist party members. Some were in the public security bureau of China.

I intentionally conducted the interviews in a slow and unfocused manner. With trauma they experienced I am certain that people would not reveal certain issues, e.g., medical examination. Sometimes I asked directly if they were medically examined and they would not remember.

I could determine who was examined and who was not. In 50 unambiguous cases it was said something about the medical examination, but I had to ignore it as they were hunger striking. Around 20 out of 50 said that there was no examination at all, whilst eight were tested.

Several factors should be considered in relation to those medically tested. Firstly, people who did not reveal their names and provinces or otherwise vulnerable people were more likely to be medically examined. They showed a lot of resistance. They would not recant even under torture. Secondly, the younger members would be examined.

The Uyghurs were the first group we know of being systematically harvested for their organs. There were dissident cases in 1970s when the major revolution took place. However, the systematic organ harvesting started in 1997. A doctor I know of did the kidney and blood testing of political prisoners. He is a central witness.

There was a policy against the Uyghurs before Falun Gong, but it was on a small scale. They were the spoils of war following the Uyghurs uprising. 40 people were shot. Falun Gong practitioners were more organised. I have seen any evidence of a final solution document or similar. It was a process that happened over time.

As to the intention against Falun Gong practitioners, it was two-fold. Firstly, it was a military and entrepreneurial operation. China tells the military you are way too big and we cannot afford you. Secondly, it was political to clearly eradicate the enemies of China. There was used the word "recant", so I believe it is a religion.

I am not ready to give you the exact figure for organ transplant. It is all in my Update. China is protected by the fact that they don't record it.

My definition of live organ harvesting is from the famous policeman overseeing organ harvesting. All being done by doctors.

I have 50 interviews in form of tape recording and digitally, which I can provide.

In terms of who did organ harvesting, I do not know in the beginning. Then it has become sort of star system of the medical world as if they enjoyed showing off their cars. The doctors would boast of making 15000 extractions. It may not be true. On the other hand, there was a high suicide rate among surgeons who conducted extraction.

In terms to the intention with regards to Falun Gong practitioners, in the beginning it was to destroy a movement and reputation. Over time it becomes something else because of the FG resistance. It then becomes an attempt to destroy them.

My experience with the Chinese, and I worked 3 years as business consultant in China, is that they always exaggerate. I still think the numbers from the doctors are better than the government numbers, which are very arbitrary. It is not like reading a business balance sheet.

Witness 36: David Li & Dr Huige Li

December 3, 2018

To the Independent Tribunal into Forced Organ Harvesting of Prisoners of Conscience in China:

Thank you for the opportunity to submit evidence to the Tribunal. I am David Li, a researcher at the China Organ Harvest Research Center (COHRC), a non-governmental organization based in the United States. COHRC would like to submit our statement of facts, "Medical Genocide: China's State-Driven, On-Demand, Extrajudicial Mass Killings of Falun Gong Practitioners for Organs."

The statement includes a brief summary of organ transplant abuse in China as reflected by our research, including the on-demand nature of transplants performed in China, the scale of the number of transplants performed (independent of official totals provided by the government), and the sources of organs used to supply these transplants. The statement also describes the role of the communist state in developing a high-volume transplant system without voluntary donations. In addition, we provide the wider context of this form of transplant abuse-its role in the Chinese regime's persecution of Falun Gong, including directives by Communist Party leaders to orchestrate the systematic destruction of this religious group. Finally, the statement applies the Convention on the Prevention and Punishment of the Crime of Genocide to weigh whether the actions taken by the Chinese regime constitutes genocide.

Some in line references in the statement are highlighted in yellow; they refer to separate collections of evidence (video clips) and first-hand witness testimonies that we can furnish when our representative(s) testify before the Tribunal and upon formal request. The separate collections of evidence include (publicly available) video interview clips with Chinese hospital staff describing a transplant case in which they were involved. They also contain screenshots of web pages describing recent cases of on-demand transplantation, including short waiting times, cases of large numbers of simultaneous transplants conducted by individual hospitals in a single day, sourcing of organs from living bodies, and other evidence.

Please let me know if we can provide further assistance.

Sincerely,
David Li
(Signature redacted)
Director of Communications
China Organ Harvest Research Center
https://chinatribunal.com/wp-content/uploads/2019/04/COHRC_Independent-Tribunal-_Statement-of-Facts-Application-to-Law_20181128_Submited.pdf

Summary of oral testimony: 9th December 2018

We both represent the Chinese organ harvest research centre. This is an NGO founded in the US. We have been doing this for about 10 years.

On demand transplant is unique in the world. There are reports that show waiting times for organs are short in China. Liver waiting time is only two weeks. In a Shanghai hospital it was only 1 week for a liver. Additionally, one other website promised organ donors were available anytime.

In 2017 a South Korean journalist went to a transplant centre saying they are waiting for a patient and a nurse, secretly recorded, suggested waiting times for organs ranged from days to weeks (the telephone recordings between 2015 – 17 exist to attest to this fact).

In 2018 Mr Hill, a BBC journalist, called a hospital and was told that he could have a liver within weeks of time. The official government numbers of annual 15000 cannot explain this.

When the doctors take the organs from a living body, they cut them all out at once and then separate the organs.

The scale and capacity of China's transplant system is 70,000 transplants a year and may be more than that. It is based on a minimum transplant requirement of any hospital in China. There are official requirements for a hospital and 167 hospital granted authorisation to do transplants. There is a difference between having the capacity to do transplant surgery, and actually doing it.

We calculate every patient for 1 month in a hospital to make it realistic.

Conservative calculation is based on the official numbers published by China e.g., 12,000 transplantations in 2004. They indicate that they obtained the organs from executed prisoners in that year. There are no official numbers of executed prisoners, but according to Amnesty International it ranges from 2,000 to 10,000 executions.

Assuming the official number is 4,000, you can get 12,000 organs (one liver and two kidneys). However, many prisoners are unsuitable due to being disease carriers, drug addicts or alcohol abusers. At any time, there is no system at all for sharing of the organs.

Also, organ harvesting is a local illegal business, which depends on the doctor's relationship with a judge. The utilisation is in fact low and cannot be 30%.

If we take 12,000 transplantations which is a lowest number. It cannot be explained by its official source. Therefore, the majority of organs must come from a different source.

In terms of the policy of destroying Falun Gong practitioners, to our knowledge there has not been a noticeable change in the persecution of Falun Gong practitioners. We have not analysed the issue raised by Ethan Gutmann, namely that persecution towards Falun Gong practitioners has reduced. We know that brain death was not the source of the organ donations. On their website they say that donors do not come from brain death. There is no documentation, which describes ethnic background or religious profiles of the source.

All Falun Gong practitioners are given the choice between renouncing practice or being put through torture in order to renounce. They have to sign multiple statements that they will make public statements renouncing Falun Gong. For Falun Gong practitioner, the public denouncement of their faith would mean spiritual death.

The samples of torture methods (p14 of our written statement) against Falun Gong practitioners, including electronic shocking, sexual violence and exposure to extreme cold, derive from a collection of published works. There is a systematic abuse of Falun Gong practitioners all over China. We have seen this is common practice across all prisons and labour camps. I have no knowledge of Uyghurs or children.

In terms of who extracted the organs, there were two teams: the procurement team and recipient team deliberately separated from each other. The recipient team would not know where the organs come from. The medical staff do the tests on the organ itself, but not aware of what information they get from the donor.

I believe Falun Gong is a religion. There is a debate about it being a religion between what Chinese Government say and what other people say. Chinese government say it is a cult etc. I am not aware of any other definition of religion. Falun Gong is not an organised religion. They do not have churches etc. But for the purpose of spiritual religion that is a belief.

In terms of how the state authority identify Falun Gong practitioners, they used their prior knowledge (the government have created a blacklist) or looked at physical evidence such as if they do exercises publicly or participated in the distribution of pamphlets. Further, there was a more organised campaign by knocking on doors to ask people if they practised Falun Gong. I believe the government want to destroy Falun Gong.

Witness 37: Dr Huige Li

Live Organ Harvesting in China: A submission to the Independent Tribunal into Forced Organ Harvesting of Prisoners of Conscience in China
Huige Li, MD, PhD
Professor of Pharmacology at the University Medical Center of Mainz, Germany

Live organ harvesting is different from living organ donation. Living organ donors donate an organ or part of an organ, e.g. a single kidney or part of a liver. Living organ donors remain alive after donation. In contrast, vital organs are removed during live organ harvesting and the victims are usually killed by the procedure.

Live organ harvesting doesn't necessarily mean that the organs are procured from conscious individuals without anesthesia. It means that the so-called "donors" are alive (either under anesthesia or not) at the start time point of organ procurement.

There are 4 different types of live organ harvesting practice known from China.

1. Organ harvesting from prisoners incompletely executed by shooting

There are well documented cases in which the gunshot was deliberately fired to the right chest instead to the head of the prisoners during execution. The purpose was to maintain blood circulation for organ harvesting in order to improve quality of the harvest organs.[1] The first documented case was in 1978. Zhong Haiyuan, a schoolteacher from the Jiangxi Province, was sentenced to death for her "counterrevolutionary" thoughts. In addition to the investigation of the book author, one of the execution officers revealed much details. The live organ harvesting in this case was planned in advance.

In 1995, the former surgeon Enver Tohti was ordered to harvest organs from an incompletely executed, still-living prisoner in China. He has testified in many occasions including at a European Parliament hearing on 29 January 2013.

In 2015, Jiang Yanyong, a famous high-ranking military doctor in Beijing, told to Hong Kong journalists that corruption, illegal transplantation and organ trade were common in military hospitals. In his interview, Jiang also revealed the practice of the organ harvesting from still-living bodies. His statement implies that this brutal practice was relatively common.

Unfortunately, there is no systematic studies available so far and the incidence of the practice of incomplete executions in China is unknown.

For details see our recent publication.[1]

2. Organ harvesting from prisoners after lethal injection

Since 1997, execution in China has been increasingly performed by lethal injection in parallel to shooting. Unfortunately, organ procurement from prisoners after lethal injection was performed under a condition that the prisoners were still alive.

This is a systemic failure.

First, the criteria of death determination issued by the state neither conform to current medical science nor to any standard of medical ethics. In the Provision on Issues in Execution by Injection issued by the Supreme People's Court in 2001, death was defined as fulfillment of all of the following three criteria: (1) cessation of heartbeat, (2) cessation of respiration, and (3) dilated and fixed pupils (diameter > 0.5 cm).[2] Although these criteria may be reasonable for determination of natural death, they are inappropriate for lethal injection, because lethal injection-induced death differs significantly in its mechanisms from natural death or death caused by disease. Moreover, death by lethal injection is simply determined by a forensic doctor and the Provision doesn't require any objective verification of death, not even the confirmation of heart arrest by the electrocardiogram (ECG), leaving loopholes for abuse.

Second, the loopholes in the law are systematically exploited.[2] In China, death is pronounced within tens of seconds after starting the lethal injection. At this stage, however, neither the common criteria for cardiopulmonary death (irreversible cessation of heartbeat and breathing) nor that of brain death (irreversible cessation of brain functions) are met.[2] For comparison, the North Carolina warden waits for a flat line appearing on the ECG monitor, and waits for another 5 minutes before declaring death. In total, death is pronounced in the United States in the time range of 14 to 18 minutes after starting the lethal injection.[2]

Because the announcement of death within tens of seconds after starting the lethal injection is a common practice in China,[2] it can be assumed that all the organ procurement after lethal injection happened on still-living bodies.

Furthermore, analysis of postmortem blood thiopental level data from the United States indicates that thiopental, as used in lethal injection, may not provide sufficient surgical anesthesia. The dose of thiopental used in China is kept secret. It cannot be excluded that some of the organ explantation surgeries on prisoners subjected to lethal injection are performed under insufficient anesthesia in China. In such cases, the inmate may potentially experience asphyxiation and pain. Yet this can be easily overlooked by the medical professionals performing the explantation surgery because pancuronium prevents muscle responses to pain, resulting in an extremely inhumane situation.[2]

The two types of live organ harvesting discussed above happened to prisoners sentenced to death. Therefore, an execution (either complete or incomplete) must be performed before organs are procured.

The situation for prisoners of conscience is different. Without death sentence, an execution before organ procurement is not necessary. Therefore, organ procurement from prisoners of conscience is almost always live organ harvesting because killing of the prisoners before organ harvesting would otherwise decrease the organ quality.

3. Execution by organ explantation

It is unclear how organs are procured from prisoners of conscience. However, a case published in the "Henan Medical Journal" may provide a picture how such live organ harvestings may look like.

The operation was performed in a hospital of the People's Armed Police Force in 2001 and the paper published in 2003.[1]

In the section 2.1 of this research paper, the "major points of donor heart removal" included: "systemic heparinization (2 mg/kg); delivery of cold cardioplegia to the heart through the aortic root until the heart stopped beating; cut of the superior vena cava at 4 cm above right atrium ...". Besides blood type and heart weight, no other information about the donor was provided in the paper.

The fact that systemic heparinization was performed and heart beating was stopped by cold cardioplegia implies that the blood was circulating, and the heart was functional before the explantation procedure. Because brain death determination is only performed after 2003 in China, this donor couldn't be a brain death patient. Therefore, the only possibility left is that the donor was not a brain death patient and the cardiac arrest was induced by the cold cardioplegia delivered by the medical professionals. Death of the donor was caused finally by heart removal.

4. Organ harvesting under the pretext of brain death

In 2003, the Ministry of Health drafted *Standards for Determining Brain Death (Adult) (Draft for Comments)* and *Technical Specifications for Determining Brain Death (Adult) (Draft for Comments)* and published them in the Chinese Medical Journal and other journals. This was the start of organ donation after brain death, although these proposed technical specifications do not have legal effect.[3] Until today, there is no brain death legislation in China.

China's clinical criteria for determining brain death require the fulfillment of all the following three conditions: (i) deep coma, (ii) absence of brainstem reflexes, and (iii) no spontaneous respiration (depending on mechanical ventilation to maintain breath completely and apnea test to confirm no spontaneous respiration). Thus, a patient undergoing determination for brain death must already be on a ventilator.

However, in a number of Chinese medical papers, the transplant organs were listed as coming from "brain-dead donors," while the organ procurement processes indicated otherwise. Examples are shown in the table below:

Publication	Hospital	Operation	Excerpt in Chinese	English translation	Comments
Sheng J et al. Journal of Southeast China National Defence Medical Science 2005 (01): 17-18	Fuzhou General Hospital of Nanjing Military Command	Heart transplant (n=5) (2002-2004)	5 例供体均为青年男性。**脑死亡后气管插管**辅助呼吸并维持循环稳定，全身肝素化后阻断主动脉…	All 5 donors were young males. **After brain death, intratracheal intubation was performed** to aid respiration. The circulation was maintained and stabilized. After systemic heparinization, the aorta was clamped…	Apnea test was not performed.
Wu L et al. Chinese Journal of Nursing. 2008 (02): 168-169	Fujian Medical University Union Hospital	Combined heart-lung transplant (n=4) (2004-2007)	供体均为**脑死亡者，行气管插管**，经胸骨正中・胸，肝素化，切除心包…	All donors were **brain death** individuals. **Intratracheal intubation was** performed, a midline incision made, heparinization performed, pericardium excised…	No apnea test. Intubation directly followed by organ procurement.

Publication	Hospital	Operation	Excerpt in Chinese	English translation	Comments
Wang F et al. Journal of Kunming Medical University. 2013; 34 (03): 89-92	Yan'an Hospital Affiliated to Kunming Medical University	Heart transplant (n=7) (2003-2013)	7 例供体均为生前同意捐献遗体的男性**脑死亡者**，年龄 22-45 岁。**供体脑死亡后插入气管导管人工通气**，同时迅速·胸，自主动脉根部注入肝素 3mg/kg 后阻断升主动脉，于主动脉根部灌注 4°C St. Thomas 液 500-1000 mL，**使其迅速停搏**。	Seven donors, aged 22-45 years, were all male **brain death individuals** who agreed to donate their bodies during their lifetime. **After donors' brain death, intratracheal intubation was performed** for mechanical ventilation and, at the same time, thoracotomy was done quickly. After injection of 3 mg/kg heparin into the aortic root, the ascending aorta was clamped. 500-1000 mL 4°C St. Thomas solution was perfused via the aortic root **to induce cardiac arrest**.	A brain death determination was not performed (no apnea test). The heart was functioning.
Chen S et al. Chinese Journal of Cardiovascular Review. 2007 (07): 512-514]	Zhenjiang First People's Hospital	Heart transplant (n=4) (2005-2006)	供体均为男性，年龄 23-40 岁，均为**急性脑死亡患者**。**急性脑死亡后紧急插管**，吸尽呼吸道分泌物，纯氧通气。经胸骨正中切口，肝素化，切·心包，探查心脏，分离上、下腔静脉以及主动脉根部。	The 4 donors, aged 23-40 years, were all male **acute brain death patients**. **After acute brain death, intubation was performed immediately**, secretions in the respiratory were removed and mechanical ventilation was done with pure oxygen. A midline sternal incision was made, followed by heparinization and incision into the pericardium…	A brain death determination was not performed (no apnea test).

Publication	Hospital	Operation	Excerpt in Chinese	English translation	Comments
Chen T et al. Chinese Heart Journal 2011 (05): 699-700	Xijing Hospital of the Fourth Military Medical University	Combined heart-lung transplant (n=1) (2008)	供体来自一位男性脑死亡患者。首先吸净供体呼吸道分泌物·行气管插管通气，经外周静脉注射甲基强的松龙 500 mg 及2.5 mg /kg 肝素，无菌消毒铺单后行胸部正中切口，切除心包前壁… 阻断上下腔静脉，切断上腔静脉，数个心动 周期心脏排空后，阻闭升主动脉，灌注冷的心肌保护液 …	**The donor was male brain-dead patient.** Procurement procedure: First, secretions in the respiratory tract were removed. **Endotracheal intubation was performed for mechanical ventilation**, and 500 mg methylprednisolone and 2.5 mg/kg heparin were injected via a peripheral vein. A middle chest incision was made after skin disinfection… The superior and inferior vena cava were clamped, and the superior vena cava was cut. **The heart was emptied after several heartbeat cycles.** The ascending aorta was clamped …	Intubation and mechanical ventilation were directly followed by organ procurement. The heart was functioning.

In these cases, it was clear that a brain death determination was not performed because the donors were not on ventilator (thus no apnea test) before organ procurement. Moreover, in some cases, the organ procurement procedure indicates undoubtedly that the heart of the donor was functioning.

This means that the condition of these donors neither met the criteria of brain death nor that of cardiac death – the organs were harvest from living bodies.

Type	Incidence	Anesthesia
Organ harvesting from prisoners incompletely executed by shooting	unknown	no
Organ harvesting from prisoners after lethal injection	~ 100%	yes, but can be insufficient
Execution by organ explantation	unknown	very likely
Organ harvesting under the pretext of brain death	unknown	unclear

In conclusion, live organ harvesting has a history in China. The first type, organ harvesting from prisoners incompletely executed by shooting, is a brutal abuse with unknown incidence. The second type, organ harvesting from prisoners after lethal injection, is even legal in China because of the loopholes in the death determination criteria. The victims of the third type, death by organ removal, are very likely prisoners of conscience without death sentence. The identity of the fourth type, organ harvesting under the pretext of brain death, is unclear.

References
1. Paul NW, Caplan A, Shapiro ME, Els C, Allison KC, Li H. Human rights violations in organ procurement practice in China. *BMC Med Ethics* 2017; 18(1):11 [http://rdcu.be/o617].
2. Paul NW, Caplan A, Shapiro ME, Els C, Allison KC, Li H. Determination of Death in Execution by Lethal Injection in China. *Camb Q Healthc Ethics* 2018; 27(3):459-466 [https://www.ncbi.nlm.nih.gov/pubmed/29845916].
3. China Organ Harvest Research Centre (COHRC). "Abuse of Brain Death in China" (page 119) in COHRC 2018 Report. 2018 [Available from: https://www.chinaorganharvest.org/app/uploads/2018/06/COHRC-2018-Report.pdf.

Summary of oral testimony: 9th December 2018

[Expanding on warm ischaemia times] One can imagine that in the second type of live organ harvesting, organ harvesting from prisoners after lethal injection, anaesthesia is applied and the doctor performs the transplantation immediately. Here the short warm ischaemia time is understandable. In the third type, execution by organ explantation, the warm ischaemia time is of course short. This requires killing by organ removal and is unethical. Whereas, the second type of organ harvesting does not accord with international standards but is legal in China.

[Medical obligations] Perhaps it's beneficial to understand how my generation and the preceding generation were educated. I was born in the 1960s after the Cultural Revolution. We were taught to distinguish friends from enemies. The former should be treated warmly and enemies treated ruthlessly. In the Cultural Revolution, the people fought each other, many times with machine guns. In Qianxi alone 18,000 people were killed violently. Half of them were killed by the system, which means under certain conditions, killing became routine and was not punishable. Furthermore, there were documented instances of cannibalism.

In 2016, US Professor published a study about the Cultural Revolution and found that people ate their enemies. In particular, the most popular organs were hearts, livers and penises. There is a primitive understanding that these body parts, when consumed would enhance one's health and improve the function of their corresponding parts. In such a system, prisoners of conscience are no longer protected by the system. As you know that includes the Falun Gong. In summary, if there are enemies, kill them and take their organs.

[Whether other groups, like FG and Uyghur are treated as enemies of the state] This was only possible because of the hatred propaganda by the State. In 2004, an online survey amongst the young people posed the question of whether they would kill enemy women and children. 80% of respondents said they would.

[Drug use in a lethal injection] This is difficult as it's a secret. But there are hints that it's similar to the ones used in the US. These are drugs used to stop heart rate.

[Whether the population were divided into two groups as a result of the Cultural Revolution] Yes. If one considers the history of the Chinese Communist Party, landlords were eliminated for their lands; during the counter-revolution intellectuals were killed and so group after group were killed. Hence why the Falun Gong is being hunted because they are a peaceful albeit resistant group.

[State's intention towards the FG] The Chinese Communist Party always differentiates between the subgroups because they don't want to fight each group. The State has historically only cared about their power and will quash anyone, such as the Falun Gong that challenges that power.

Witness 38: Edward McMillan-Scott

Persecution of Falun Gong by the Beijing Regime
Evidence to the London Tribunal under Sir Geoffrey Nice QC, December 2018

My name is Edward McMillan-Scott, UK citizen. I enclose my CV as annex 1 to this statement.

It is nearly 20 years since the most systematic persecution of one group began in China in 1999.

As a European Parliament Vice-President 2004-2016 I campaigned since 2006 – my last visit to Beijing – to draw attention to the brutal and systematic persecution by the Chinese regime of practitioners of Falun Gong, a Buddha-school spiritual movement with 70 – 100 million adherents in 1999.

I welcome your inquiry into the systematic process of imprisonment without trial, torture and the murder of thousands of innocent people under torture, with the added horror that vital organs are removed from living Falun Gong prisoners for the organ transplant trade, conducted by the People's Liberation Army, usually resulting in death.

Falun Gong is a spiritual and meditation movement that echoes traditional Chinese beliefs that humans are connected to the universe through mind and body. The Chinese Communist Party describes it as a 'cult', whereas international jurisprudence suggests that a 'cult' should include financial commitment, alienation from family, disciplined organisation, brainwashing and anti-social behaviour, none of which apply to Falun Gong. Like all chi-gong (spiritual exercise) groups, Falun Gong has a 'master' whose book of exercises published in 1992 remains the only financial commitment for most of his followers.

On 25 April 1999, 10,000 Falun Gong practitioners spent a day in peaceful protest in Beijing after police brutality against fellow practitioners in Tianjin city. People who were there have told me that the police brutality was almost certainly organized by the security forces as a justification for the persecution which then began.

My campaign began in May 2006, when I visited China on a fact-finding mission in preparation for a report on human rights and democracy for the European

Parliament's Foreign Affairs Committee. In Beijing, at great personal risk to them, I interviewed two former prisoners, Falun Gong practitioners Cao Dong and Niu Jinping. Cao Dong was subsequently arrested and convicted of 'meeting a distinguished foreigner'. He was sent to Tianshui prison, being tortured to recant his religious convictions and to denounce his meeting with me. Niu Jinping appealed to me on behalf of his wife, Zhang Lianying, who had been in Beijing Forced Women's Labour Camp since June 2005, and so severely tortured that she suffered a coma in April 2007. The latter were subsequently re-imprisoned as part of Beijing's pre-Olympic round-up in early 2008.

Another of my contacts was Christian human rights attorney Gao Zhisheng, sometimes known as the 'conscience of China', who represented a number of Falun Gong practitioners after his investigation into their persecution in 2005. Manfred Nowak, then UN rapporteur for torture, met Gao at the US Embassy in Beijing in early 2006, after which a traffic accident involving Gao was staged by the regime. Well-known in China for publicly denouncing the regime, especially for corruption, Gao wrote an open letter to the European Parliament through me in September 2007 and another to the US Congress. He was then sentenced to prison on a charge of "subversion". After being temporarily released into house arrest, he was re-imprisoned and in 2008 so severely tortured that he twice tried to commit suicide. After his wife and children escaped through Thailand to the USA in January 2009, Gao was abducted by security forces. He has subsequently been released once again into the care of his brother.

According to The China Human Rights Lawyers Concern (CHRLCG), Gao is still in enforced disappearance (refer to its submission to the 31st Session of the UN UPR Working Group on China October/November 2018)[1]

During a series of parliamentary hearing, speaking tours and individual meetings with former torture victims from 2006 onwards, and in many countries, I can attest to the consistency of their testimony about the regime enforced on (usually anonymous) Falun Gong practitioners.

These are only a few examples drawn from my own experience, but they demonstrate the extent of the Communist regime's paranoia and brutality against any activity which could threaten or destabilise it.

I am in no doubt that the international publicity aroused by the denunciation of the CCP by "Annie" on the White House lawn, coupled with a growing political campaign in which I played a part, and the imminence of the 2008 Beijing Olympics led to the increased repression of FG, and of which practitioners were aware of. In most cases, individuals asked me to keep up the pressure for the sake of wider justice, even if they or those close to them suffered.

Falun Gong practitioners are usually imprisoned under 'administrative detention' with no trial: often they refuse to give their names to protect their families. As members of a banned 'evil cult' they suffer particularly harsh treatment, often at the hands of other prisoners and even Falun Gong who have recanted (to demonstrate their rejection of the practice). Ex-prisoners I have met outside China, having recanted, had suffered sleep deprivation for a period of weeks, then forced to stand motionless for several days, being prodded with sharp objects to keep them awake, followed by progressively brutal treatments involving electric prods – always including the genitals – excrement and general beatings. Zhang Lianying, who suffered a coma, wrote me a list of the 50 progressive tortures she suffered, which I submitted to the UN Rapporteurs on Torture and Religious Freedom, Dr Manfred Nowak and Mrs Asma Jahangir, both of whom I have met on a number of occasions.

Manfred Novak has stated following his 2006 visit to Beijing that some two-thirds of those undergoing 're-education through labour' in China's prison camps, are Falun Gong practitioners. In 2018, credible reports that some 1,000 new camps have been constructed to accommodate Uyghur dissidents amplify that crime, because Muslim Uyghurs, who renounce alcohol, are also organ-harvested.

In testimony to the US Congress in 2013, Mr Harry Wu, a former inmate and now director of New York's Laogai Research Center, estimated that there are some 900 such camps with between 3 – 6 million incarcerated. Falun Gong outside China maintain contact with prisoners and record their torture and torturers where either can be identified: records exist of more than 4,236 up to now are confirmed to have died in the persecution of Falun Gong since 1999.

Of particular concern is that only Falun Gong – who neither smoke nor drink – are routinely blood-tested and blood-pressure tested in prison: this is not for their well-being. They thus become the prime source for the live organ transplant trade: more than 40,000 additional unexplained transplants have been recorded recently in China since 2001 More recently, there is evidence that organ harvesting is being practised not only on Falun Gong and Uyghur prisoners, but also on Tibetans, following the 2013 uprising and repression there. (Kilgour/Matas reports).

Although using body parts from prisoners has been routine in China (in one province alone there are 16 specially converted evisceration buses) many believe, as I do, that live Falun Gong prisoners are quarried for their body parts. Indeed, Cao Dong told me that after his best friend disappeared from their prison cell one evening, the next day he saw his dead body in the morgue with holes where body parts had been removed.

The campaign of brutal repression of Falun Gong – once encouraged by Beijing for the wellbeing reportedly experienced by its adherents – shows no sign of easing.

There have been a number of initiatives to curb China's organ-harvesting trade, and I have taken part in numerous meetings, including with the Australian transplant profession, who attest to the low grade of surgical skills and poor outcomes in China.

Annex 1

I am a former Member of the European Parliament for Yorkshire & Humber UK (1984-2009 Conservative, then Independent: 2010-2014 Liberal Democrat) and 2004-2014 elected four times as European Parliament Vice-President, latterly holding the Democracy & Human Rights portfolio. In 1990 I founded the EU's Democracy and Human Rights Instrument, aimed at transforming E/Central Europe. Today it is the world's largest such programme with a budget of €165M and worldwide scope.

My EU involvement:

- Following my last visit to Beijing, in May 2006, all the dissidents and former prisoners-of-conscience with whom I had contact were arrested, imprisoned and in some cases tortured. These included the Christian human rights lawyer **Gao Zhisheng** and environmental activist **Hu Jia.**
- I successfully nominated **Hu Jia for the 2008 Sakharov Prize** for Freedom of Expression, awarded annually by the European Parliament.
- Further I was successful in nominating imprisoned Chinese dissident **Liu Xiaobo** for the 2010 Nobel Peace Prize. I represented the EU at the prize-giving ceremony, highlighting the empty chair the prize was awarded to due to Xiaobo's imprisonment.
- In November 2010 I met the dissident artist **Ai Weiwei**, co-designer of Beijing's 'Birds Nest' stadium, who made a highly critical series of comments about me on YouTube channel. Ai Weiwei later spent some

months under house arrest in Beijing. I authored a Parliamentary resolution on Ai WeWei's case in 2011.

- I have championed the **Falun Gong** Buddha-school spiritual movement, brutally persecuted after 1999 by the Beijing regime because of its popularity. I have met many former prisoners and published accounts of their torture. I have campaigned against the organ harvesting by the Chinese Peoples' Army, in which thousands of Falun Gong prisoners have been killed for body parts for the lucrative transplant business.

- On 29 January 2013, I organised a conference with the unrepresented Nations and People's Organization (UNPO) in the European Parliament, entitled 'Religious Persecution by China.[2] An international panel of experts shed light on live organ harvesting and re-education through labour camps, mainly targeting prisoners of conscience and religious groups. This included a personal testimony by a former surgeon in Xinjiang, China, who participated in live organ harvesting.

- I have written a key report for the European Parliament's foreign affairs select committee, of which, at the time, I was the longest-serving member, on a new EU–China strategy in 1997.

- I initiated a successful campaign aimed at an EU **political boycott of the August 2008 Beijing Olympic Games**. The Presidents of the European Parliament and European Commission boycotted the Games, as did the EU's external affairs Commissioner.

- I was the first politician to visit **Tibet** after a three-year blackout, in 1996. I have subsequently championed the cause of Tibetan independence, taking part in numerous activities to highlight oppression in Tibet. My staff and I have made many speeches and taken part in pro-democracy activities with Tibetan exiles. In March 2012, I organised a seminar entitled 'Tibet in Flames: the unfolding personal and collective tragedy of the Tibetan people" in the European Parliament examining the highlighting the spate of self-immolations in protest at China's cruel occupation. I also co-authored a Parliamentary resolution on the human rights situation in Tibet in June 2012.

- I was the first European politician to visit China for investigating the persecution of Falun Gong, including organ harvesting.

- Further I co-authored a 2006 EP resolution in EU-China relations, which put human rights at the centre for EU foreign policy with China.

- I co-authored 2013 European Parliament urgency resolution on organ harvesting in China.

- The EU holds a bi-annual Human Rights Dialogue with China, but the process is one which I have decried from the outset, because Beijing refuses to conform to the usual protocols, such as disallowing NGOs from attending as observers, exchanges of lists of alleged political prisoner etc., which usually accompany such EU HR Dialogues.

Summary of oral testimony: 9ᵗʰ December 2018

From 2006, I was Rapporteur for the European Parliament on new EU-China arrangement. I've maintained relations with the Falun Gong.

I will submit evidence of torture by torture victims. I've been in contact with about 200 – 300 Falun Gong Practitioners outside China who have been personal witnesses to organ harvesting. There's an exile route out of China for Falun Gong Practitioners.

There is a complete absence of fair judicial processes as far as Falun Gong Practitioners are concerned.

The origin of my allegation of genocide arose from an interview in Beijing with Cao Dong and Niu Jinping (two former prisoners). The video interview was available but was deleted. The only evidence of the interview is the written account I wrote.

Manfred Novak, a distinguished civil servant and lawyer mentioned Falun Gong Practitioners were victims of forced organ harvesting. I am not aware if his account has ever been challenged. The Minghui website also referenced FGPs that had died during persecution.

[In reference to evidence of Uyghurs and Tibetans being persecuted, what is the intention behind the state crack down] They were too popular, and the State wanted to crack down on them. In 2013, the State wanted to crack Tibetans following the uprising. I was struck by how Tibetans were a slave population; a subject people. Following, the 2013 uprising there was a repression. I believe Uyghurs are the most repressed groups in China. There is a BBC report of Uyghur-only camps, seen as a premium market for organs.

[Intent and purpose in relation to genocide] For Uyghurs, Tibetans and Falun Gong – their treatment is contrary to the provisions of Article 2 of the Genocide Convention, on the basis that other evidence is credible. There is no evidence that House Christians are persecuted as other groups. I believe that the intent against Falun Gong is criminal and the goal is death through evisceration.

References

1. https://www.chrlawyers.hk/sites/default/files/.%201.%20Revised_CHRLCG%20UPR%20full%20submission%202018.pdf
2. http://www.unpo.org/article/15404

Witness 39: Prof Wendy Rogers

Witness statement from Wendy Rogers[1]

I would like to offer two pieces of evidence to the Tribunal, followed by an opinion. The first piece of evidence concerns lack of compliance with international ethical standards in organ procurement in China and the second concerns attitudes and actions of some leading members of the international transplant community regarding evidence about procurement of organs from executed prisoners of conscience. The opinion proposes potential reasons for the second piece of evidence.

1. Lack of compliance with international ethical standards in organ procurement in China[2]

In my capacity as an expert in the ethics of organ donation, I led a team of researchers investigating whether publications reporting data from transplant recipients in China comply with international ethical standards.

The transplantation of organs procured from executed prisoners is widely condemned by the World Health Organisation, the World Medical Association, The Transplantation Society, Amnesty International and others. This condemnation extends to undertaking research and presenting results that involve the use of organs obtained from executed prisoners. In 2006, The Transplantation Society (TTS) explicitly stated that it would not accept conference papers based on research involving organs sourced from executed prisoners. The 2006 TTS policy statement led to calls for a boycott on publishing journal articles based on research involving organs from executed prisoners. Together, these statements by international bodies, professional societies, academics and journals constitute explicit ethical standards prohibiting the publication or presentation of research involving organs sourced from executed prisoners.

These ethical standards require peer-reviewers and journal editors to ask consistently whether the research:

1. involved any biological material sourced from executed prisoners;
2. received Institutional Review Board (IRB) (Research Ethics Committee) approval; and
3. required consent of donors.

To maintain these ethical standards, papers that do not comply should be rejected.

With a multi-disciplinary group of volunteer researchers, I performed a systematic analysis of articles reporting on lung, liver and heart transplants performed in mainland China, using scoping review methodology. We identified 445 relevant papers reporting on a total of over 85,000 transplants from 2000-2017.

Of these:

1. (7%) stated explicitly that no organs from executed prisoners were used in the research;
2. 33 324 (73%) reported research ethics approval
3. 6 (1%) reported that organ donors gave consent for donation

Overall, less than 1% of papers included all three pieces of evidence of ethical practice as mandated by international groups including TTS. However, the absence of this information had not been a barrier to publication, despite the failure to comply with ethical standards.

Furthermore, the claim in 33 papers that that no organs were procured from executed prisoners was demonstrably false in many cases. 19 of the 33 papers claiming that organs were not procured from executed prisoners reported on 2,688 transplants that took place prior to 2010, during which time there was a total of 120 volunteer donors across the whole of China, and all other organs were sourced, by Chinese admission, from executed prisoners.

This research shows that the majority of the published literature reporting research on transplants in China from 2000-April 2017 fails to comply with ethical standards regarding exclusion of research based on organs procured from prisoners and provision of consent by donors.

Of considerable concern, the research shows that the international transplant community (broadly construed), whose members reviewed the papers, and the journal editors who accepted papers for publication, failed to enforce their own professional ethical standards.

Another piece of research, performed with Prof Jacob Lavee and Prof Maria Fiatarone Singh, demonstrated that a paper published in the journal *Liver International* falsely claimed all of the transplanted organs were procured from volunteers. Our investigation, published in the form of two letters, led to a retraction of the paper by the journal.[3]

Overall, my conclusion from this research is that the international transplant community demonstrates little inclination to make even the most basic and cursory inquiries about the sources of organs reported in Chinese transplant research. This lack of concern is part of a broader failure to hold Chinese transplant researchers to widely agreed ethical standards. This is despite a proclaimed policy (of TTS) to refuse to engage with China or offer international acceptance as peers unless the Chinese transplant community complies with international ethical standards.

2. Attitudes and actions of members of the international transplant community regarding procurement of organs from executed prisoners of conscience

Over the three years in which I have been performing research on the topic of organ sourcing in China, I have noted that prominent members of the transplant community, two of whom reside in Sydney (Jeremy Chapman and Philip O'Connell) seem unwilling to make themselves familiar with evidence about forced organ harvesting from prisoners of conscience. Instead, their attitude is one of dismissal, repetition of official Chinese denials and claims that allegations of forced organ harvesting are a political strategy by what they describe as "the Falun Gong".

I offer the following evidence in support of my view.

When I first became aware of concerns about sourcing of organs from prisoners of conscience, I sent a message to Prof Jeremy Chapman (recent past president of TTS) through a mutual acquaintance. In the reply conveyed to me by my acquaintance, Prof Chapman indicated his view "Though some genuine humanitarians have an honest belief that the Chinese are persecuting innocent people by killing them for their organs, the stories are without substance. Those who travel to China and visit the wards of the transplant units looking for this activity have not found it." (personal communication, 27 Nov 2015, anonymised copy provided). However, the fact that visitors to China are not shown organ harvesting from prisoners of conscience is not proof that it does not occur.

In the time since then, Prof Chapman's rhetoric has become more dismissive of any reference to sourcing organs from prisoners of conscience. This is evident, in for example, his comments to the Joint Standing Committee on Foreign Affairs, Defence and Trade.[4] In that statement he says that the figure of 60,00-100,000 transplants per year (based on the research summarised in the *Update*) is a "concoction". On page 2 Prof Chapman provides details about the lengths of time that Chinese transplant patients spend in hospital, based upon which he concludes that if there were 60,000-100,000 transplants per year in China, there would need to be 30-40 times the amount of transplant infrastructure that there is in the US. His reasoning is hard to follow. I therefore sought clarification by email and was told that in China, patients stay in hospital for much longer than in the US or Australia – weeks compared to 4-6 days (Chapman, personal communication 6/6/2018, copy provided). This response indicates that Prof Chapman had failed to engage with the methodology in the *Update* and seemed unaware that in calculating the figure of 60,000-100,000 transplants per year, the authors allowed for a 4 week stay per person per transplant.

In that same transcript, Prof O'Connell (p 4) refers to the COTRS, the Chinese organ register, claiming that transplants recorded in this register are legitimate. However, this registry is not open to independent scrutiny therefore anything Prof O'Connell says about it is hearsay from Chinese sources. Like Prof Chapman, Prof O'Connell is "convinced there has been a profound change" but this conviction is based upon access to information and hospitals selected for visits by Chinese hosts, and in which information is provided via interpreters. These representatives of TTS have no independent way of knowing if the claims they make about sources of organs in China are true.

There is one further piece of evidence about reluctance to engage with credible research. In July 2016, shortly after the publication of the *Update*, one of the authors, Ethan Gutmann, visited Australia. I was keen to broker a meeting between Gutmann and members of the transplant community, so that they could become familiar with the evidence and methods used in the *Update*, and indicate any potential flaws or weaknesses. I contacted an acquaintance who is a transplant surgeon, to help arrange the meeting. Via this contact, Prof Chapman offered to organise it. I accepted his offer of help, but this was withdrawn on the grounds that he was concerned about who would be present at the meeting and that it might be "political". In a lengthy email chain, I sought to reassure him, and in the end organised the meeting myself. Despite his proclaimed interest, Prof Chapman did not attend the meeting and it is my view (although I do not have evidence of this) that he warned other transplant professionals not to attend it. In the end, only one surgeon attended, who was visibly shocked to find himself the only transplant person in the room, as several of his colleagues had previously indicated their intention to attend.

These and other experiences with members of the transplant community indicate to me that there is a significant determination by that community to deny all claims of organ harvesting. Denial is based upon largely upon unverifiable Chinese assurances combined with ignorance about detailed investigations and evidence amassed to date.

Opinion regarding attitudes amongst members of the transplant community
I have had little direct communication with members of the transplant community therefore can only speculate regarding the apparent general unwillingness to engage with evidence about forced organ harvesting from prisoners of conscience. There is one exception to this. In 2017 I had a lengthy conversation with one person associated with the international transplant community, who asked me to preserve their anonymity. This person expressed the strong view that if there were 60,000-100,000 transplants per year, then this volume would be obvious to external observers.

However, my informant was unable to explain how information about transplant volumes in China would become known in the absence of transparent organ tracing processes and admitted that the idea of forced organ harvesting was almost too terrible to contemplate.

Regarding apparent willful blindness about procurement of organs from executed prisoners of conscience, I offer the following potential explanations, but stress that I have no evidence regarding their accuracy or otherwise:

1. Huang Jiefu undertook several years of his transplant surgery training in Sydney, becoming colleagues with now senior clinicians including Jeremy Chapman. Given this strong professional and personal connection, it may be difficult for Australian transplant clinicians to believe that Huang Jiefu could preside over a system in which organ harvesting from prisoners of conscience (POC) takes place. Instead, it may have been easier for these clinicians to focus on the heroic narrative of assisting Huang to reform the unethical system of removing organs from prisoners who had received the death sentence. Huang vehemently denies any forced organ harvesting from POC, therefore any questioning of this by Australian clinicians would jeopardise their relationship and any potential good to be achieved by assisting with some degree of reform in China.

2. There are extensive research and other ties between Sydney hospitals and hospitals in China, some of which concern transplantation. For example, in 2011, a Memorandum of Understanding was established between the 2nd Xiangya Hospital of Central South University in Hunan Province and

Westmead Hospital in Sydney. I am not privy to the details of this MOU other than those details of the arrangements that have been published in the Chinese media, which indicate that exchanges included clinical and research activities involving transplantation. The Chinese research included xenotransplantation of animal tissue into humans, which at the time was not permitted in Australia. On a 2011 paper reporting on this research, one of the authors, Shounan Yi, reports his academic affiliation as Westmead.[5] 2016 Australian media articles[6] questioning the ethics of this research relationship led to forceful denials by Jeremy Chapman.[7]

3.   The final explanation I wish to canvas concerns ignorance about the freedom of Chinese transplant doctors to speak openly about their practices. The degree of surveillance and brutal repression in China is unfathomable by Western standards. At least some transplant clinicians have expressed the view that it would not be possible to conceal organ harvesting from POC because there would be whistleblowers. This view ignores the totalitarian system operating in China and the extent and gravity of the threat to anyone contemplating whistleblowing.

I am willing to provide more details on these matters should this be of assistance to the Tribunal.

Wendy Rogers
(Signature redacted)
17 Nov 2018

References
1. See Appendix 1 for my credentials.
2. This evidence is based upon Rogers WA, Robertson M, Ballantyne A, Blakely B, Catsanos R, Clay-Williams R & Fiatarone Singh M. Compliance with ethical standards in the reporting of donor sources and ethics review in peer-reviewed publications *involving organ* transplantation in China: A scoping review. *BMJ Open* (accepted 13 Nov 2018), and is provided to the Tribunal in confidence. Once the paper is published, it can be made available to the Tribunal members. Please do not cite or repeat any data from this statement without permission.
3. Rogers WA, Fiatarone Singh MA, Lavee J. Papers based on data concerning organs from executed prisoners should not be published. *Liver International* 2017; 37:769; and Rogers WA, Fiatarone Singh MA, Lavee J. Papers based on data concerning organs from executed prisoners should not be published:

Response to Zheng and Yan. *Liver International* 2017; 37: 771-772. Both letters are available from the Supplementary Reading list supplied to the Tribunal.

4. See Appendix 2 (with highlight on relevant sections)
5. Wang W1, Mo Z, Ye B, Hu P, Liu S, Yi S. A clinical trial of xenotransplantation of neonatal pig islets for diabetic patients. *J Cent South Unw (Med Scz)* 2011 Dec;36(12):1134-40. doi: 10.3969/j.issn.1672-7347.2011.12.002 (copy available on request).
6. See e.g. 'Chinese organ harvest furore', John Ross, *The Australian*, August 24, 2016.
7. 'Westmead Hospital rejects China link transplant 'benefits'' John Ross, *The Australian*, September 7, 2016.

CV: Prof Wendy Rogers
https://chinatribunal.com/wp-content/uploads/2019/04/ProfWendyRogers_
Appendix-to-witness-statement2.pdf

Summary of oral testimony: 10th December 2018

[Qualifications summarised] My evidence is based on my own research, paper based from Sydney, I have not travelled to China recently, and I have never travelled to China to speak to people about organ transplantation.

My evidence covers two points. First, I have found a lack of compliance with ethical standards in published research concerning recipients of transplanted organs in CCP. The second, of which I have personal experience, is a concerning lack of attentiveness or concern from the transplant community about allegations of FOH.

First, the lack of compliance is based on a project that I met with a group of other researchers. We looked at whether research in China conformed with the standards of TTS and WHO and world medical association. Those bodies have documents and statements that result in three widely accepted standards concerning data obtained from transplant recipients. First, research should not involve material sourced from executed prisoners, second research involving patients receiving transplants should be approved by a research ethics committee or review board, third research involving transplants should only proceed if there is consent from the donors. These standards became explicit in 2006 after CCP admitted that all donor organs were procured from executed prisoners. So I was testing to see whether these standards were maintained. In short, over a 12-month period with my volunteer researchers we used scoping methodology and found 445 relevant papers, reporting on research and the organs involved were livers, lungs and hearts. We couldn't do kidneys because it was not clear whether those donors were living. With these 445 papers, we then looked to see which stated exclusively that the organs were procured from executed prisoners were used in the research. We concluded that the majority of published literature, Jan – April 2017 fails to comply with ethical standards regarding exclusion of research based on data of organs procured from prisoners. Also, more concerning it shows that those involved in practice and research and editors seemed indifferent to compliance with ethical standards. So we really felt that the international community had little inclination to make the most basis scrutiny or enquiries into the source of organs in Chinese transplant research. That is a broad generalisation it could be that some journals were rejected but as a picture it seems that so much of the research failed to mention where the organs came from when it was publicly known that organs came from executed prisoners.

The second observation I want to make is that I found in personal experience that members of the transplant community do not seem to want to engage with research that has been done about FOH in China, and seem ignorant of that, whilst at the same time proclaiming that the system is ethical and it was only ever rumours about FOH and instead they have an attitude of dismissal and repetition of official denials that sound similar to denials made by Chinese official spokespersons. [Examples of such official statements given]. I found that response astonishing because there are 600 hospitals doing transplants, and just because you visit one hospital and haven't seen it, you wouldn't know whether it is going on. It seemed a dismissive reply. In fact, since then, November 2015, Professor Chatman's rhetoric has become more dismissive. Evidence in comments on public record to an enquiry made by the Joint standing committee on foreign affairs defence and trade, by the Australian Senate. In that statement he says that the figure which has been identified by the 2016 update (Gutmann, Matas Kilgour) that there are an estimate of 60-100,000 transplants a year, Professor Chapman calls those figures a "concoction". That seems disrespectful term to use. When you look the methodology in the update and that they ahem tried to triangulate make the data based on multiple sources with wide margin for errors but point to a much greater volume of transplant activity. (445 papers reviewed related to 85,000 transplants; can you transport these to items 1-3 of your report. For instance, how many relates to 6 papers referring to donors' consent?) Will provide the details later.

[Qualifications explained.] Appointed as a member of the Australian ethics committee and as a member of a working group who wrote the medical guidelines for transplants I became aware of this issue.

None of the authors of the papers we looked at were approached for further information, that was outside the scope of our research. But we hope that those papers have all been identified and believe we have identified those papers and that people will take it upon themselves to act on our findings. and the other two categories it is similar, open for them to choose to respond or investigators to approach them directly. I have had experience with one retraction, but it was a long process and took a lot of time and effort which is why we choose to approach this in a broad way and hope others would follow up the work as opposed to going one by one. The retraction did not identify the source of the organ, in the end the senior author claimed it was a junior person who had made a mistake of some sort. This was after two rounds of letters, the first response was very dismissive of our claims then it was reported that HJ had spoken to the author and told them it was a mistake although that is not what was said in writing, so that is what was said in the media.

In all of the papers there is almost no identification of where the organs come from.

I find it hard to explain. I don't have any evidence of insights people have given me; I have come to my own view. First, there is an Australian connection, HJ undertook some of his transplant surgery in Australia and is of the same cohort as Jeremy Chapman and they would have worked together so it is easy to take word from your friend as opposed to someone you consider to be hostile. It is a human tendency to believe the person you have worked closely with. In that situation you are more inclined to believe the person you know and then there must feel that there is an opportunity to transform China because it needs encouraging and help in turning around. Where I stand it seems they have been accepted with open arms, especially the two last transplant meetings but there has been no enforcement of ethical standard. Jeremy Chapman has said to me that he went through every paper at a Hong Kong seminar and I have no reason to disbelieve him but that is one in a sea of many. So each of the papers that were based on unethical practice are references around the world and the ripples start there.

Putting past behind rather than exploring it is part of what they do. I find that problematic because they have not acknowledged the depths of the badness and second why would you think the system can change overnight, it seems implausible.

The rest of the world varies a great deal. In Canada there is a significant cohort of transplant professionals who are concerned and will decline to take part in research agreements with Chinese universities that their own institutions are trying to push them to work with. In the UK the real bodies exhibition has had protests. Jacob Lavee was active in leading Israel to prevent insurance companies reimbursing those who travel for transplants. Sydney is an outlier. I was in Brisbane recently to give a lecture and there were so many people at the lecture that it was standing room only because the audience is interested. That makes it so much more tragic that it is O'Connell and Chapman who have each been TTS president have been leading the dismissals and reporting that these are misguided humanitarians who have been duped by a political movement trying to overthrow the CCP.

Whether it is possible that certain papers have been missed is hard to answer because we don't know what has been dismissed. There are some relatively significant journals there that had 20 papers in which a large proportion had not stated where the donors came from. So yes, it is possible that a lot of journal editors are on the board. I think there is a lot of room for improvement. My experience was that one editor who was horrified contacted the authors and went through with his intention to retract but we then had push back from the publishers and it took a lot of skilful negotiation with the editor to agree the retraction, and because they get a lot of income from China it takes a lot for them to retract and there is a lot of room for improvement and it would be helpful for the transplant community to agree standards to identify that there is a need to give details of the donor because if that was the standard it would be harder for the Chinese to put in a paper saying all donors were healthy young men between 20 and 40.

We don't have any consent forms and I haven't seen any I don't speak Mandarin so couldn't verify but have not seen any.

I don't know that it is a cover up, I think Chapman does believe that reform has taken place but what we know about unconscious and psychological tricks we play on ourselves is that we take the view that puts us in the far better light as opposed to being the person who has been fooled by the Chinese. I certainly don't believe he has firsthand knowledge of what is going on and is covering it up. I don't believe that for a minute.

I do not know of any whistle blowers in the research community, just the retraction I have mentioned which was apparently the mistake of a junior staff member. There is not a lot of publicly available information. I have had a lot of conversations with people in psychiatry who have tried to get retractions and it is very hard because processes are not easily identified and it is a hornet's nest to work through and it is rare for papers to be retracted.

In relation to motivation, so far as the wilful turning of the blind eye of professionals from multiple transplants may affect their ability to face up to what is obvious is possibility. I don't know whether the research is interesting, but they are at the leading edge of transplant techniques and that was part of the first response we got in relation to the retraction request, that they can retrieve more organs than anywhere else. In Australia it is hard to retrieve a liver from someone who has circulatory death because there is a period of low blood pressure so viability becomes difficult once they have died but they claim to retrieve 100% of livers which shows they are dying in a very different way in China than in Australia or America. Motivation can be to try and transform the system and if it doesn't work you are an enabler, so there are a number of reasons to influence what is going on and they may not all be overtly self-interested, I am not suggesting bribery but we fool ourselves that we are doing good and that can create tunnel vision.

Chapman's use of the word "concoction" was said at one point as claimed to be a political motivation, The FG with the intent of bringing down the Chinese government, and part of the attack is to promulgate FOH.

The team involved myself and six others. Academic and one medically qualified, several PhDs and a former journalist as well as bio ethics academic. I am not aware of others taking this work. It has been 18 months so far, and we formed at the end of 2016. The majority did not state where the organs came from but the only times there was reference was to state that the organs came from volunteers.

It is beyond my expertise to say whether the resistance to consider this is a result of Chinese proximity to Australia. We are very beholden to China in Australia and those who work with China have deep pockets with research collaboration so that does influence Australia and make it unusual compared to other English-speaking countries.

Witness 40: Yiyang Xia

Dear Members of the Independent Tribunal into Forced Organ Harvesting from Prisoners of Conscience in China,

I am the Director of China Policy at Human Rights Law Foundation ("HRLF"). I write first to commend the Tribunal on the Draft Findings and, second, to introduce myself to you should you decide to extend your mandate to include the overall persecutory acts carried out against Falun Gong believers and other dissident groups in China.

Human Rights Law Foundation was established in 2005 to hold human rights abusers accountable before courts of law; strengthen the legal framework through the key precedents we establish; and enable our clients to experience a sense of justice and find greater meaning connected to their struggles and courageous stances. For over a decade, HRLF has defended the Chinese religious and dissident communities through direct litigation in the United States and through global partnerships in Argentina, Australia, Belgium, France, Japan, Peru, Spain, the United Kingdom, as well as within China – to seek accountability for genocide, torture and other crimes against humanity. Our domestic and extraterritorial litigation continues to create a record of evidence, raise public awareness, and empower our clients. To date, many of these cases have been litigated successfully, including *Zhang et. al. v. China Anti-Cult World Alliance*, where Plaintiffs prevailed at the summary judgment phase in a case alleging religious- based attacks against Falun Gong practitioners by Chinese Communist Party-affiliated agents in the United States 311 F. Supp. 3d 514, 526 (E.D.N.Y. 2018);[1] *Doe v. Jiang Zemin and Chen Kuiyan*, where HRLF was instrumental in securing an indictment against former Chinese President Jiang Zemin and Party Chief of the Tibet Autonomous Region Chen Kuiyan for their role in the persecution of Tibetan Buddhists in China; and *Doe v. Liu Qi,* where the district court held the former Beijing City Mayor liable for torture and arbitrary arrest and detention of Falun Gong practitioners.[2] 349 F.Supp.2d 1258 (N.D. Cal. 2004).

As the Director of China Policy at HRLF, I have been responsible for research, investigation and reporting of the structure of the persecutory apparatus in China within the Chinese government and Chinese Communist Party systems. I have authored multiple reports on the role of ideological conversion through torture in extracting confessions from Falun Gong practitioners as part of a Chinese Communist

Party policy that has been carried out largely by Chinese security forces in China. I have studied the operation of the clandestine Office 610,[3] the use of propaganda and brainwashing in China, the role of the judicial branch of government in the persecution of Falun Gong, and others. These reports are available upon request.

I have also collected and analyzed evidence of torture as part of and in preparation for litigation filed against, for example, Li Lanqing, former Vice Premier and member of the Politburo Standing Committee, and Luo Gan, former member of the Politburo Standing Committee and Secretary of the Central Political and Legal Affairs Commission, both of whom Jiang appointed to run the Gestapo-like security apparatus, Office 610. I have also read hundreds of official secret documents that detail the well- orchestrated persecution of Falun Gong in China including the names of the major perpetrators, significant chains of command, and the impact specific perpetrators have had on victims who have filed suit against them. Some of these files have been sent from China by Falun Gong practitioners and other activists, at grave risk to their safety and liberty in China. Many are now serving lengthy prison terms as a result. These documents are an important basis of my expertise because the Chinese Communist Party conducts most of its business behind closed doors, in particular the persecution of Falun Gong, and is very careful not to leave a paper trail to avoid liability in China and abroad.

Based upon the cases we have filed and/or coordinated abroad, which have included interviews with Falun Gong believers, review of witness testimonials and evidence related to the role and conduct of many of the main perpetrators of the overall persecutory campaign, I offer the following statements in support of the Tribunal's Draft Findings:

1. Background Information
The Chinese Communist Party (the "Party") has a decades-long history of launching *"douzheng"* campaigns against particular groups, characterized by their systematic suppression and ostracism from society as well as subjection to various acts of Party-sponsored violence without due process of law. The word *douzheng* has taken on a specialized meaning in connection with the carrying out of such campaigns against an identified target.[4] While the word is also used in non-persecutory contexts, this semantic flexibility does not detract from its use for the purposes of political suppression campaigns. As a parallel, simply because the word "offensive" can be used to characterize either a hurtful comment or a violent military operation does not mean that it is unclear which is meant in any given context. Similarly, the term *douzheng* has acquired a specific meaning in the context of China's established

practice of crackdowns and political suppression campaigns against identified groups. That process is generally characterized by the following progression:

The decision to target any specific group as an enemy is always made by the highest levels of the Party. This practice extends from early suppression campaigns such as the Anti-Rightist campaign in 1957, which targeted at least 550,000 "rightists," through the Cultural Revolution of the 1960s and 1970s, the crackdown on "Spiritual Pollution" in the 1980s, the Tiananmen Square crackdown of 1989, and the targeting of Falun Gong and other religious groups from the 1990s through today, including the ongoing campaigns against Tibetan Buddhists and Uyghur Muslims.

Following such a decision, the group to be targeted is identified in official Party media and by Party affiliates with carefully crafted rhetorical language, branding the target as an enemy of both the Party and the "People," and as opposed to Party ideology as well as to social welfare in general. The initiation of the crackdown is signaled and implemented through society via the use of escalating hostile language by the Party, with the term "*douzheng*" being perhaps the most important such signal. Other persecutory terms like "*jiepi*" (to expose and criticize) and "*zhuanhua*" (to ideologically "transform") are also commonplace phrases used by the Party to single out groups and their members for exceptional aggression and abuse.

Flagship media in China, such as the People's Daily newspaper, the China Central Television evening news broadcast, and Party ideology journals, continually spread the word to inflame the masses and ensure that the designated group is broadly known to be a Party enemy.

Special and general security forces are mobilized to identify, round up, arbitrarily detain, and physically and mentally abuse individual members of the "group." The ideal aim is to force these so- called "enemies" to renounce their group identity and beliefs and "join forces" with the Party to attack other members of the targeted group, using the same methods.

The near-final step is what is referred to as "*zhuanhua*" or "forced conversion" (literally to ideologically "transform"). Individuals refusing to be converted are subjected to ever increasing violence and torture. At minimum, the term *zhuanhua* as used in the context of the Party's attempts to suppress Falun Gong signifies the call for members of the targeted group to be "re-educated" via coercion of various forms that extend from intense psychological pressure to physical abuse and torture. While the conditions for usage of the term are different overseas from those in China, widespread use of torture and arbitrary detention, and total lack of due process protections against or legal checks on the Party's use of such methods, is clearly understood to be a key feature of Party-initiated attempts to "*zhuanhua*" targeted groups or individuals.

2. The Prevalence of Torture

Notwithstanding international and Chinese legal prohibitions against torture, torture has been the Chinese Communist Party's "instrument" of choice in the persecutory campaigns it has waged against dissent. Since its inception it has implemented persecutory campaigns against members of groups that have appeared to undermine Party "rule." As noted, targets have ranged from entire social classes or professions (e.g. wealthy businesspeople, landlords) to individual Party members considered to have compromised their allegiance to the Party, and, as in the case of Falun Gong, Tibetan Buddhists, and Uyghur Muslims, to religious movements. Members of these and other disfavored groups have been and continue to be subjected to ideological conversion through torture and other forms of torture by Party agents. These agents operate with impunity, outside of and above the constraints of statutory law or precedent or government regulations largely due to the conspicuous absence of a rule of law in China and especially for politically sensitive cases such as Falun Gong.[5]

Torture is especially widespread and severe in politically sensitive, dissident cases due to the routine reliance on confession as evidence of "criminal conduct."[6] Coerced confessions are admissible at trial, and thus the application of torture at the pre-trial phase is especially widespread. A well-known housing activist, Ye Guozhu, who was sentenced to four-years in prison after he applied for permission to hold a demonstration against forced evictions in Beijing immediately prior to the Olympic Games, was suspended from the ceiling by the arms and beaten repeatedly by police in Dongcheng district detention center.[7] He was also repeatedly tortured in Qingyuan prison because he still refused to admit his "guilt."

Lawyers can do little to curtail incidents of torture. In fact, many lawyers who have filed complaints or attempted to protect their client's right to be free from torture under the Torture Convention that China has signed and ratified have themselves been subjected to persecution.[8] Notable examples include many once prominent members of the legal bar in China, such as Gao Zhisheng, Tang Jitian, Jiang Tianyong, Li Heping, and many others, who have been subjected to beatings, imprisonment, threats, disbarment, torture, and/or the shutting down of their law firms based on their (failed) attempts to advocate legally on behalf of dissidents in China.

3. Falun Gong

As a politically sensitive group targeted for persecution in China, Falun Gong believers are subjected to the same (and in many cases more intense) mistreatment meted out to Tibetan Buddhists and other politically sensitive groups. The authorities continue to use broad and vaguely defined provisions of Chinese law relating to social stability or state security as a political tool to silence dissent and restrict freedom of belief. Such basic due process rights as access to legal counsel, the right to a hearing, to freedom of appeal are similarly not available to Falun Gong believers in China.[9]

Lawyers representing Falun Gong practitioners are forced to discuss their cases with the relevant judicial departments and actively assist the persecutory authorities' use of the legal system to create the veneer of justice.[10] Indeed, lawyers in China have a duty to assist the authorities to promote solutions that are amenable to the Party. The courts in China are required to punish Falun Gong believers more severely than others. The courts are also required to dismiss all civil lawsuits filed on behalf of Falun Gong believers, curtailing their due process and other rights.[11]

The reports and testimonies of thousands of Falun Gong believers who have been persecuted in China illustrate how routine is the reliance on confession as evidence of "criminal conduct."

Chen Gang, an accomplished musician, was placed in a forced-labor camp for 18 months for practicing Falun Gong. While imprisoned, he was forcefully deprived of sleep by guards who punched or kicked him as soon as he closed his eyes. This sleep deprivation at one point extended for a duration of fifteen days. The police also shocked sensitive parts of his body (e.g., head, neck, and chest) using several high-voltage electric batons simultaneously. These electric shocks burned his skin black. The police even ordered more than ten other prisoners to beat Mr. Chen so savagely that his face became disfigured. Mr. Chen was also 'hog-tied' where his hands were tied behind his back and his neck to his legs behind him with tension. These and further atrocities were conducted by the police to force Mr. Chen to renounce his belief in Falun Gong until Mr. Chen could no longer bear the torture and gave in.[12]

The devastating effects of conversion through "brainwashing classes," which often also use torture is also well exemplified in James Ouyang's account – an electrical engineer who was forced by guards to stand facing a wall for nine days and then sent to a brainwashing camp.[13] He stated, "I am a broken man. I have rejected Falun

Gong. Now, whenever I see a policeman and those electric truncheons, I feel sick, ready to throw up."[14] Falun Gong practitioners are forced to remain in these classes until they renounce their beliefs in writing and then on videotape.

As Jennifer Zeng, an Australian Falun Gong believer featured in a recent documentary titled Free China noted, those who refuse to "confess" are subjected to further and more intense torture, those who have confessed are forced to share the names of other Falun Gong believers with the authorities and, in many instances, assist in their ideological conversion through torture.[15]

These findings are consistent with direct reporting from sources in China to the Minghui website,[16] that has named 1,680 Falun Gong adherents tortured during 2010, suggesting that a minimum of 7,000 to 8,000 Falun Gong practitioners were tortured between 2009 and 2013. Given the difficulty of reporting such incidents in China's censorship environment, the actual numbers are undoubtedly higher, reaching at least several million. These findings are also consistent with reports by other human rights observers and the U.N. Special Rapporteur for Torture.[17] In March of 2006, UN Special Rapporteur Dr. Manfred Novak reaffirmed findings that torture remained widespread.[18] UN Special Rapporteur, Sir Nigel Rodley, has reported that "[p]ractitioners are subjected to public humiliation for their membership in Falun Gong [m]any are said to have suffered torture or ill treatment."[19]

The United States Department of State has similarly described the widespread use of torture to coerce Falun Gong believers to renounce their religious beliefs. According to the US Department of State 2006 Human Rights Country Report,[20] "[t]he government continued its use of [torture] to force practitioners to renounce Falun Gong."

Several United States courts have indicated that torture is a widespread ongoing measure used against Falun Gong believers. For example, the Seventh Circuit Court of Appeals has made clear that membership in Falun Gong is a basis for fear of future persecution if deported to China. In particular, the Seventh Circuit found that "the [U.S.] government acknowledges that China persecutes adherents to Falun Gong. [and that] the Chinese government's determination to eradicate its root and branch is mysterious, but undeniable."[21]

U.S. courts have even found high-ranking Chinese officials liable for widespread persecutory campaigns that deprived Falun Gong practitioners of their right to be free from torture in China. In *Doe v. Liu Qi*, 349 F.Supp.2d 1258, 1334 (N.D. Cal.

2004), a case that HRLF led, the court concluded that "the People's Republic of China appears to have covertly authorized but publicly disclaimed the alleged human rights violations caused or permitted by Defendants Defendants Liu and Xia are responsible respectively for violations of the rights of [plaintiffs] to be free from torture cruel, inhuman, or degrading treatment [and] arbitrary detention." Similarly, in *Wei Ye et al. v. Jiang Zemin et al.*, 383 F.3d 620 (7th Cir. 2004), the Seventh Circuit Court of Appeals affirmed plaintiffs' widespread allegations of torture and ill treatment at the hands of Jiang Zemin. Although the court ultimately dismissed the case on head-of-state immunity grounds, it made several findings of fact supporting plaintiffs' allegations: "On June 10, 1999, President Jiang established, as part of the Party's apparatus, the Falun Gong Control Office. The office is known as 'Office 6/10' after the date of its creation. In July 1999, President Jiang issued an edict outlawing Falun Gong. This edict was followed by mass arrests torture, 're-education,' and the killing of members."[22]

On July 15, 2008, the Israeli Rabbinical Council likewise found that "on the basis of the accumulation of the various testimonies and indirect evidence there were unnumbered cases of killing of innocent Falun Gong practitioners through torture." Indictments issued by courts in Spain and Argentina have reached similar conclusions.[23]

Official third-party reports provide further support. In 2006, former U.N. Special Rapporteur on torture, Manfred Nowak, following a mission to China, reported that, of the cases of alleged torture he received in China, 66% involved the torture of Falun Gong practitioners.[24] Mr. Novak further noted that methods of torture were reported to include, among others: use of electric shock batons; cigarette burns, submersion in pits of water or sewage, suspension from overhead fixtures with handcuffs, "tiger bench" denial of medical treatment and medication.[25] Specific measures of torture widely used on Falun Gong practitioners have been summarized by a Minghui correspondent in Liaoning Province, China.[26] These findings were consistent with the statements of previous Special Rapporteurs that had addressed the issue. The previous Special Rapporteur on torture, Nigel Rodley, reported in 2001 that many Falun Gong practitioners "are said to have suffered torture or ill treatment."[27] The Special Rapporteur on violence against women likewise expressed concern about the use of violence against female Falun Gong practitioners.[28] The findings of international non-governmental organizations, such as Amnesty International, provide further evidence of the torture of the Falun Gong. For example, Amnesty International has reported that Falun Gong practitioners have been tortured in labor camps by fellow inmates, acting at the behest of camp guards, for attempting to practice their religion.[29]

These findings are also consistent with HRLF's review of Falun Gong believers' response to a questionnaire that specifically inquired as to their subjection to torture and interviews of Falun Gong believers in preparation of legal cases.[30]

HRLF lacks specific expertise in the area of organ harvesting per se. That said, in light of the goal of the widespread crackdown, to force targets to abandon their deeply held beliefs and align themselves instead with the Party's *douzheng* campaign, and the application of torture to virtually all detained Falun Gong believers, it would be an odd phenomena if those subjected to organ harvesting in various sorts of detention centers, were not also subjected to severe bouts of torture prior thereto. Or to put it differently, these operations appear to be the final stage of an ongoing systemic pattern of torture inflicted upon Falun Gong practitioners. As such, they would constitute the same international crimes, as is torture, including crimes against humanity.

In addition, insofar as the persecutory campaign has been described as inclusive of genocide by, among others, Professor Leisbeth Zegveld, a look at a translation of the body of the complaint she filed on behalf of Falun Gong believers, might be useful in sorting out the ways in which the practice of organ harvesting meets the definition of genocide in and of itself and as part of a larger genocide.[31]

Thank you for your attention and interest, and I look forward to providing whatever support I may. Please find enclosed a copy of the April 2018 Opinion of the Honorable Judge Weinstein, which Dr. Terri Marsh, the Executive Director of HRLF, asked that I include. It concludes, *inter alia,* that the beliefs and practice of Falun Gong meet the definition of a religion under the test of the Circuit Courts of Appeals in the United States.

/s/ Yiyang Xia
Sincerely,
Yiyang Xia

Human Rights Law Foundation Washington, D.C.

https://chinatribunal.com/wp-content/uploads/2019/05/HRLF_610_Office.pdf

https://chinatribunal.com/wp-content/uploads/2019/04/April_HRLF_02-Exhibit-B-Jiang-Zemin.pdf

https://chinatribunal.com/wp-content/uploads/2019/04/April_HRLF_03-Exhibit-C-EP-Hearing.pdf

https://chinatribunal.com/wp-content/uploads/2019/04/April_HRLF_04-Exhibit-D-Brainwashing.pdf

https://chinatribunal.com/wp-content/uploads/2019/04/April_HRLF_05-Exhibit-E-Zhang-Jingrong-v-Chinese-AntiCult-World-Alliance.pdf

https://chinatribunal.com/wp-content/uploads/2019/05/JiangZemin_DouzhengCampaignAgainst_FG_HRLC.pdf

https://chinatribunal.com/wp-content/uploads/2019/05/JiangZeminLiableForTortureOfFG_HRLF.pdf

https://chinatribunal.com/wp-content/uploads/2019/06/YiyangXia_How-does-610-work_en_YiyangXia.pdf

https://chinatribunal.com/wp-content/uploads/2019/06/YiyangXia_Reply-to-Questions_YiyangXia.pdf

https://chinatribunal.com/wp-content/uploads/2019/06/YiyangXia_Article-1_Liugezhuang_Shandong-Province_translated.pdf

https://chinatribunal.com/wp-content/uploads/2019/06/YiyangXia_Article-2_Door-knocking-harrassment_translated.pdf

https://chinatribunal.com/wp-content/uploads/2019/06/YiyangXia_Article-3_Xintai-City_Zhu-Xiulin_translated.pdf

References

1. 311 F. Supp. 3d 514, 526 (E.D.N.Y. 2018).
2. 349 F.Supp.2d 1258 (N.D. Cal. 2004).
3. For a discussion of Office 610, see Exhibit A. I have testified at the European Parliament Subcommittee on Human Rights, Congressional- Executive Commission on China ("CECC"), and the Ontario Superior Court of Justice as an expert on these issues.
4. While the word is also used in non-persecutory contexts, this semantic flexibility does not detract from its use for the purposes of political suppression

campaigns. As a parallel, simply because the word "offensive" can be used to characterize either a hurtful comment or a violent military operation does not mean that it is unclear which is meant in any given context. Similarly, the term *douzheng* has acquired a specific meaning in the context of China's established practice of crackdowns and political suppression campaigns against identified groups.

5. Indeed, after the establishment of the People's Republic of China and up through 1979, there was not even a criminal code, criminal procedure code, or comprehensive set of criminal laws and criminal procedure laws. Even now, twelve years after China's entry into the World Trade Organization in 2001, the Party used sham trials to appear as if to afford dissidents the due process rights they are routinely denied. Thus, as Amnesty International noted in its [4th periodic report Nov 2008], "the criminal justice system remains highly vulnerable to political interference. The police, procuratorate and courts are not independent and [deliberately kept] … under the supervision of the Chinese Communist Party." *See, e.g.*, Amnesty International, *Against The Law: Crackdown on China's Human Rights Lawyers Deepens*, June 2011, Index: ASA 17/018/2011. This lack of independence makes it impossible for torture victims and survivors to submit complaints with regard to allegations of torture without being subjected to persecutory retaliation that always includes torture.

6. Chinese Human Rights Defenders, *A Civil Report on China's Implementation of the United Nations Convention against Torture and Other Cruel, Inhuman or Degrading Treatment or Punishment, October 10, 2008*, page 5.

7. Amnesty International, *Briefing for the Committee against Torture in advance of their consideration of China's fourth periodic report*, at page 3.

8. *See, supra, Against The Law: Crackdown on China's Human Rights Lawyers Deepens.*

9. *See, e.g.*, Wang Bo's Defense: The Supreme Authority of the Constitution and Freedom of Belief, Li Heping, Li Xiongbing et al., The Epoch Times, March 27, 2007.

10. *See*, Statement of NYU Law Professor, Jerome Cohen, CECC Hearing: "Human Rights and Rule of Law in China," September 2006), available at: http://www.cecc.gov/pages/hearings/2006/20060920/cohen.php.

11. *See* Lu Botao's speech delivered at a meeting attended by heads of all Intermediate Courts in Guangdong Province on September 2, 1999 available at https://web.archive.org/web/20041214020535/http://www.gdcourts.gov.cn:80/fynj/1999/7/1/t20040816_5992.htm

12. Testimony available upon request.

13. John Pomfret, Torture is Breaking Falun Gong, Washington Post, Aug. 5, 2001 at A01.

14. Id.

15. The documentary, Free China, is available upon request.

16. Minghui is considered and treated as a reliable source for factual information relating to the persecution of Falun Gong by major human rights organizations and governmental research agencies; information available upon request.

17. Manfred Nowak, "Report of the Special Rapporteur on torture and other cruel, inhuman or degrading treatment or punishment, Mission to China," March 10, 2006, E/CN.4/2006/6/Add.6, pgs. 12-14

18. *See* March 10, 2006, "Mission to China" Report, available at http://ap.ohchr. org/documents/dpage_e.aspx?m=103. *See also* 2001 Report, United Nations Economic and Social Council, Commission on Human Rights Report, "Integration of the Human Rights of Women and the Gender Perspective: Violence Against Women," 57th Sess., E/CN.4/2001/73/Add.1 (13 February 2001) (reporting that Falun Gong practitioners are subjected to physical abuse, shocked with electric batons, including on the breasts and genitals of female practitioners, detained in solitary confinement and assigned intensive labor); 2001 Report of the Special Rapporteur of the UN, in issues of violence against women, Office of the High Commissioner on Human Rights, 57th Session, document number E/CN.4/2001/73/Add.1 at ¶¶ 15-16 (expressing grave concern at reported use of violence against women in China and in particular female Falun Gong practitioners (the vast majority of Falun Gong practitioners are women).

19. UN Special Rapporteur, Sir Nigel Rodley, E/CN.4/2001/66, January 2001, at ¶¶ 237, 238, ¶ 246.

20. Available at http://www.state.gov/g/drl/rls/hrrpt/2006/78771.htm.

21. See Iao v. Gonzales, C.A. 7, 2005 (No. 04-1700).

22. Id. at 622.

23. Available upon request.

24. See footnote 3, supra.

25. Id. ¶ 46.

26. Minghui.org, is a news platform run by Falun Gong believers who investigate on-the-ground conditions especially from China.

27. Commission on Human Rights, Report of the Special Rapporteur, Sir Nigel Rodley, U.N. ESCOR, 57th Sess., UN Doc. E/CN.4/2001/66 (2001).

28. Commission on Human Rights, Report of the Special Rapporteur on violence against women, Yakin Erturk, U.N. ESCOR, 61st Sess., UN Doc. E/CN.4/2005/72/Add.1 (2005).

29. Amnesty International, Annual Report 2010, available at URL: http://www. amnestyusa.org/research/reports/annual- report-china-2010.
30. Available upon request.
31. Available upon request

Summary of oral testimony: 6th April 2019

The Foundation has been collecting evidence of the persecution since 1999 and also collects the evidence of lawsuits brought against the Chinese authority officials by courts in different countries. The Foundation also helps other groups file lawsuits against Chinese officials.

The 610 Office is not under the control of the state authorities. It belongs to the Communist Party and it was established under the Commander Jiang Zemin. The Office is an extra judicial organ under the Party and can carry out persecution under the control of Jiang Zemin and the Communist Party.

The Office is able to employ a high number of staff and can obtain funding as the Party has the power to own organisations at every level. As everybody is aware, the Chinese Government structure is different to the structures of governments in the rest of the world; there is a parallel party system. The Party sits above the State and the 610 Office can obtain funding from the Government budget. The Office sits inside the Party and most of it is set within the Political and the Legal Affairs Committee which is a Party committee. This Committee was already established prior to the setting up of the 610 Office. Historically, the Party budget has never been disclosed to the public (not since the Communist Party took overpower in 1949). No one is able to ascertain or enquire about how they get their funding but it is clear that they have an endless source of funding. There is a specific budget called the "Maintain Stability Budget" and I believe the 610 budget forms part of this budget.

There were three offices under the Political and Legal Affairs Committee ("PLAC") which were similar to the 610 Office: one was the Office for Maintaining Political Stability and the other was the Comprehensive Social Order Management Office. The work of these two offices focused on the whole of Chinese society. The 610 Office however was the only office whose focus was specific to Falun Gong Practitioners. Once the 610 Office began to gain power, it expanded its focus to other religious groups. It did not, however, focus on other non-religious, dissident groups.

The Foundation has also assisted with lawsuits in Spain against high ranking Chinese officials. It assisted on a case brought by a pro-Tibetan rights group. It is helping on a case related to the Uyghur people now.

As regards "*Douzeng*", the campaign operates in such a manner that if anyone/ any group becomes the target of Douzeng, the public are made to feel that they should not help them. Groups that become subject to these campaigns are labelled as enemies of the state. The term "*Jiepi*" is also used and this is designed so that either members of the group itself or individuals outside the group will expose the activities of the group and criticize them. It is not that these groups will have committed any crimes; they are targeted simply because the government does not like them at the time.

"*Zhuanhua*" is used against religious beliefs. The Party believes that other beliefs cannot be tolerated so the belief has to be converted. This is used most widely against Falun Gong Practitioners and more recently the Uyghurs. There have been many reports of this.

There is evidence to show that even before the Communist Party came to power in the late 1940s, the Chinese State was already involved in using human bodies for unethical purposes. There were other cases in the 1970s of live organ harvesting. There was an author who investigated a particular incident that took place in 1978 and he located a witness (an armed police officer) who had been present during a live organ harvesting operation on a woman whose kidney was subsequently donated to the son of a high ranking official. This particular police officer testified. This was documented in a book. The Chinese Communist Party has never considered an "enemy of the state" as a human being.

Everything that is published is published by The Foundation and not by him personally. The communist party has never responded to him directly in respect of comments or allegations made nor does it ever respond to any allegation raised by the world against it.

The allegations surrounding organ harvesting was in fact first raised by the Party in 2005 during the time when the World Health Organisation held a meeting in Philippines. A Chinese official announced that most of the organs for transplantation were from executed prisoners. This statement seemed to have little impact on society. The following year however forced live organ harvesting was exposed. The reason the government itself first raised the issue of organ transplants in relation to executed prisoners was in an attempt to provide an explanation for the source of organs before the allegation came out that the source was from live organ harvesting. The Party has now established a so-called organ distribution system.

The establishing of the organ donation system seemed to happen overnight. The Chinese Government state that the organs are from volunteers. There has never been a voluntary organ donation culture in China. Such a culture would take years to develop and it therefore it does not follow that China should have been able to establish a voluntary system in such a short space of time.

The Chinese authorities have also discussed supplying organs to Taiwan. China therefore appears to have a significant supply of organs but no credible explanation as to their source. Therefore, organ harvesting is still continuing, and it appears to be increasing.

Recently the Chinese Government has announced the restructuring of the State and the three offices mentioned above. Two offices have been shut down, but the 610 Office has transferred to the PLAC. We do not know for certain whether the 610 Office still operates independently.

Two international human rights groups have internal documents sent to them by religious groups and the documents demonstrate that the persecution of Falun Gong remains ongoing. Falun Gong Practitioners are the Government's number one target. From 2013 – 2018, the number of Falun Gong prisoners increased rapidly. This was because the forced labour camps shut down in 2013.

The Foundation is aware that persecution of Falun Gong is still carried out by the by PLAC. The head of the leading group designated to deal with Falun Gong is the same individual responsible for the PLAC.

The difference between the Falun Gong minority and the Uyghurs and Tibetans is that the two latter groups are located in remote areas which mean they do not have as bigger an impact on the Han population as do Falun Gong; Falun Gong is widespread. Falun Gong are a threat for two main reasons: the first is that their ideas emanate from traditional Chinese culture. Christian and Catholics are also a threat to the Chinese Government, but it is easy for the Government to persuade the Chinese people against the beliefs of these minorities by using nationalism (their beliefs emanate from the West). There is also no aspect of Falun Gong which cooperates with the authorities. It is also very difficult for the Government to infiltrate Falun Gong. Previously, spies sent by the Government to investigate the Falun Gong converted to Falun Gong. Anything that the Government cannot control they will attempt to destroy.

Falun Gong is a political, religious and a social threat. At the beginning the State did not realise Falun Gong was a religion but as soon as they realised they began to arrest them. The Government is most threatened by the religious aspect of Falun Gong.

Tibetan Buddhists are handled by the Party Bureau Standing Committee Director. Several organisations are associated with this minority but none have a focus as specific as the 610 Office.

HRLF is neutral.

I am a Falun Gong Practitioner. Falun Gong already had many followers outside of China before the commencement of the persecutions. Lots of Falun Gong practitioners are able to send information out of the country regarding the persecution and there is a well-established database outside of China. The risk to the Uyghurs is high because it is easy to shut down the information systems available to the Uyghurs as they are located remotely. It is more difficult to do this in respect of Falun Gong.

There is evidence that blood samples are being collected directly from Falun Gong practitioners in their homes. There are many reports of this so this is another example that the practice is still ongoing and ongoing at high levels.

The reason that the levels of persecution appear to be decreasing is because the Government is spending more money on covering up the persecution.

Witness 41: Didi Kirsten Tatlow

Berlin, 23.02.2019

Dear Judges of the Independent Tribunal into Forced Organ Harvesting from Prisoners of Conscience in China.

Please note that some half a dozen stories I wrote about human organ transplant while working as a journalist in China (at the New York Times).

My research began without any preconceived idea about the situation. It was prompted by a report that Chinese airlines were not cooperating in getting organs to recipients in time. I followed where the reporting took me – the result was this series of articles.

I would like to submit the following observation, and four additional points:

Observation
While I personally believe there is an illegal organ trade, I remain unsure of its scale and the sources of organs. I think probably these are not "only" death row prisoners and prisoners of conscience but may also include e.g. missing persons, victims of murder gangs, mental health patients, otherwise healthy victims of accidents whose relatives are paid for the organs, soldiers who desert, and others. As for numbers: I don't know.

Additional Points
In early April 2016 1 attended a Red Cross Society of China event at "Beijing Hospital" (北京医院), where senior state health officials spoke about organ donation in China and commemorated organ donors. April 5th is Qing Ming, China's day of the dead. Following the morning event, I went to lunch with Dr. Chen Jingyu (陈静瑜) a lung transplant surgeon from the Wuxi People's Hospital, whom I had written about previously. Dr. Chen brought along a friend of his from Beijing Hospital, a lung surgeon called Dr. Tong (Dr. Tong said he had previously conducted lung transplants but was not doing so at that time as his hospital had stopped doing the procedure as it wasn't financially worth it.) Also present were a Chinese journalist from Global Times and a postgraduate student at Tsinghua University who said he was the head of a student organization there, researching medical issues. We were a party of 5. During the lunch Dr. Chen accused me of causing him a lot of

494

trouble with my reporting. Recently organizers at a major heart and lung transplant conference in Washington D.C. had rejected a poster of his after initially accepting it, on the grounds that the research was based on death row prisoners. Dr. Chen did not deny this but said it was my fault for having caused him "trouble" with my articles. I said, I had nothing to do with the poster, and if it was rejected due to involuntary donors such as death-row prisoners then that was his responsibility, not mine.

Dr. Chen then asked, "But what are we supposed to do?"

I replied, "Don't submit findings gathered from before you said you stopped using involuntary donors" (i.e. Dec. 2014.)

He looked at me as if to say, "that's impossible," but said nothing further to me on the topic.

During this conversation Dr. Tong was listening carefully. He turned to Dr. Chen and the following is a verbatim record of their brief conversation, from memory, which I wrote down immediately afterwards (the lunch was not a reporting event.)

Dr. Tong: "Prisoners can't be used?" (死囚不能用吗?)
Dr. Chen: "No (we) cannot use (them)." (不能用)
Dr. Tong: "What about prisoners of conscience?" (良心犯呢?)
Dr. Chen: "Can't use any of them." (都不能用)
Dr Tong looked down at the table and said nothing further. Dr. Chen also fell silent.

I drew three conclusions from this conversation:

- The use of prisoners of conscience for organ transplant has taken place (the state has itself admitted the use of death row prisoner organs.)
- It is common knowledge, at least among some medical specialists.
- The Dec. 2014 ban on using death row prisoner organs may not be effective or even real, since even a lung surgeon like Dr. Tong was apparently unaware of the ban. If it was a real ban it might be reasonable to assume he would know, since the state and party through their propaganda and information systems are able to transmit messages of importance very fast.

Point 2: Soon after the publication on Nov. 16, 2015, of a story in which I reported the use of death row prisoner organs was ongoing, a defamation campaign against me quickly began in state-run media. It went like this: the office of Dr. Huang Jiefu contacted me (they had not responded to previous requests for an interview,) and, surprisingly, agreed to allow me to interview Dr. Huang. When I arrived at the interview location there were already two journalists present from Chinese media (I was under the impression it would be just me and Dr. Huang, so this was an unexpected and unpleasant surprise, but I continued with the interview anyway.) During the 2-hour long interview these people barely spoke but observed the interview with Dr. Huang and took notes. The next day many identical reports began to appear in the Chinese media accusing me of erroneous reporting. This flood of reports continued for some time. I lost count how many there were.

Point 3: About a year later, I was required to go the Foreign Ministry for a warning, about an unrelated matter. While there I asked my interlocutor about the organs reporting, how the state viewed it. She replied, "You can do that reporting." I was a little taken aback and asked, "Don't you find it too sensitive?" She responded, "Just be sure you make clear that the leaders are going to deal with this" (within the context of our conversation I took this to mean Xi Jinping.) I asked her about the military hospital system and organ transplant practices there and she froze, saying only, "I know nothing about that."

Point 4: Finally, I'd like to say that it was my impression the New York Times, my employer at the time, was not pleased that I was pursuing these stories, and after initially tolerating my efforts made it impossible for me to continue. The newspaper made a hash of the edit of my story of Nov. 16th 2015, substantially changing its sense through an unfortunate cut at the end, and a senior colleague in Beijing blamed me for that (unfairly). The subsequent correction, which was not delayed due to needing to check anything (as it says), but simply due to inattention or overwork on the part of editors, shows that there were two editing errors only, not reporting errors (since I didn't actually make any reporting errors). So that was a kind of vindication. More broadly, I subsequently conducted several conversations in person or by email with senior editors but essentially my requests to continue this line of investigation – for which I'd need time – were ignored. Editors appeared to believe the organ donation issue in China had been solved by the state's admission that they had used prisoner organs, and its promise of Dec. 14 they no longer were doing so. I was told there was "nothing new" to the story. Another editor commented, when I tried to broaden the investigation from death row prisoners to prisoners of conscience (based on my conversation with Dr. Chen and Dr. Tong described above), that people who believed that prisoner of conscience organs were being used were on "the outer fringes of advocacy" – that is, not rational. The usual arguments were presented, for example that the Falun Gong are irrational and unreliable, and so on. It was clear to me the issue was unwelcome. I cannot be sure, but I suspect that this series of articles contributed to a decision by headquarters in February 2017 not to promote me, against the advice of regional editors. I left the paper in June 2017.

I hereby declare this all to be true and exactly as happened, according to the best of my memory and based on notes taken at the time.

Didi Kirsten Tatlow

https://chinatribunal.com/wp-content/uploads/2019/06/DidiKirstenTatlow_
Submission.pdf

https://chinatribunal.com/wp-content/uploads/2019/06/Debate-Flares-Over-
China%E2%80%99s-Inclusion-at-Vatican-Organ-Trafficking-Meeting-The-New-
York-Times.pdf

https://chinatribunal.com/wp-content/uploads/2019/06/DKT_Angry-Claims-and-
Furious-Denials-Over-Organ-Transplants-in-China-The-New-York-Times.pdf

https://chinatribunal.com/wp-content/uploads/2019/06/DKT_Choice-of-Hong-
Kong-for-Organ-Transplant-Meeting-Is-Defended-The-New-York-Times.pdf

https://chinatribunal.com/wp-content/uploads/2019/06/DKT_Debate-Flares-on-
China%E2%80%99s-Use-of-Prisoners%E2%80%99-Organs-as-Experts-Meet-in-
Hong-Kong-The-New-York-Times.pdf

Witness 42: Dr Zhiyuan Wang

Submission: https://chinatribunal.com/wp-content/uploads/2019/06/WOIPFG-Investigation-Report_NewEvidence_2018.pdf

Summary of oral testimony: 6ᵗʰ April 2019

As far as we know as a result of investigations of many Red Cross in China, I believe it [the Red Cross] is a pretence the CCP use and as far as I know in Beijing the Red Cross is not able to provide enough organs to sustain the number needed in China and it is not in operation at the moment. As far as we know there are 23 hospitals in Beijing involved in transplant. There is a large number of transplant surgeries but the CCP claimed that the source of organs is voluntary donation from general public. In fact, in Beijing there is no such organisation so I don't think it can sustain the need of the market.

The 17 phone call investigations are the most recent, which were published last year, we have more extensive reports in the form of phone investigation recordings which we published earlier. More than 290 phone investigations previously, 2015-18 we actually carried out 230 investigations in the form of telephone interview. Last year's report included 230 interview recordings.

This time we covered different interview recordings in different reports. Last year it covered 230 recordings, in this report, which is separate from last year, we focused on these 17 interviews because it is the latest part of our findings.

The investigation recently covered the major hospitals, 12 of them, in provinces and state-controlled municipalities including Beijing, and it span north to south across China. We also recorded the conversational interview with medical experts who are at the top level of these hospitals so I think my report can reflect the latest development in China.

The telephone interview carried out in a TV studio with commentators onside. I would like to play videos to show how these investigations were carried out.

CCP claimed that after 2015 they established the organ distribution system but according to our findings it is a hoax.

You have identified where donors were FG. Did you ever ask if they come from other Prisoners of Conscience or other prisoners?

Yes, definitely. For example, in Xiangxi there was a 6 year-old child whose eyes were taken out. And there was another case where a young person's organs were extracted. As far as I know there are only there 3 cases who are not Falun Gong who were the victim of live organ harvesting but we don't have that evidence because the issue and perception of FG has been made aware by a lot of people and it has to a certain extent had an impact on the whole of society.

[In response to the investigator asking leading questions]. As far as I know if the question was to be put in a more general way the medical professionals will become more vague and try to avoid the question. Normally they would just answer the question in a more unanimous way, such as saying it is a secret and they can't tell us. Or they would say that we can discuss this further after we come to them. Even a lot of hospitals won't disclose their telephone numbers to the public, but make patients visit them in person. I posed as a political official from the maintenance of the stability office in Sichuan Province, which is the equivalent to 610 office, so they are in charge of dealing with the cult of Falun Gong. The reason why I posed as political officers is because they took me as someone who knew the inside story so they would communicate with me in a more candid way. Also, I asked on behalf of my relatives who needs to do the transplant surgery and they were more willing to tell me the truth. Also, in another way, I provide financial source so they are more happy to talk to me about the details. I took advantage of how they think because I understand what they would worry about, for example disclosing information that puts them in trouble but if they think I was a political official they wouldn't worry about disclosing information because I already know.

Another reason was that I posed as someone from province, Sichuan Province, not the province they are based in so they don't feel pressure talking to me. I'd like to point out which is very important, most of the targets of the investigation, the extraction of organs was performed simultaneously so the source of the organ was in the operating room at that time. Also, the waiting time according to them is exceedingly short, one to two weeks or as fast as tomorrow so from this we can tell that these donors are very close to the hospital. Also the findings indicate that there is a live organ donor pool.

[In response to questions about why he chose to pose as a political officer]. Because my questions were prepared well, in this situation I think they were more likely to open up to me. So my questions were designed to make them expose information to me. Also, the officers based in 610 office are in charge of dealing with cult or Falun Gong persecution so the medical staff in the hospital would totally obey what we say. But I can say some of them who were investigated have certain reservations about my questions. Only 11 admitted openly that they use Falun Gong as organ donors, 6 evaded but did not deny that they use Falun Gong organs. They had to respond in a certain way because of my background.

So far I found during my investigation that by posing as the 610 officer is the most effective way to get the answer [not that it led them to the answers they gave]. Because of this the political power they have is enormous, and it is useful to pose as someone who has the power because they don't know how to get away and they have to answer my questions.

There were 17 phone calls in total, and I present them all.

The question I put to them was are you still using Falun Gong practitioners because if I ask where it is from, they will know I am not from 610 because if I am from there I will know where the organs are from and it is Falun Gong. Actually, I asked for something else rather than the source, so I first asked about the waiting time then the cost of the surgery.

[In relation to how he is certain that the answers would have been different if the questions had varied]. Because before me other investigators have conducted other investigations and posing as relatives or patients, they were not able to lure the answer out of them so we decided to put the question in another way. Based on my extensive experience we did it another way. Every year I make 1,000 phone calls, so these 17 are the recent investigation.

Witness 43: Yukiharu Takahashi

Transplant Tourism from Japan to China
By Yukiharu Takahashi

I am a freelance journalist in Japan. In 2007, I started to investigate the banning of restored kidney transplants[1] by the Japan Society for Transplantation without proper grounding. My research on transplant tourism from Japan to China started in 2010, and in 2015, I interviewed a staff member at a mediating organization arranging transplants for Japanese patients to China.

Three Japanese recipients from China

I interviewed three recipients face to face who had operations in China between April and June, 2018. They all stayed in Tianjin city, China, and had operations at the Oriental Organ Transplant Centre, at the First Central Hospital, between August and November, 2013. One had a liver and the other two had kidney transplants. When they arrived, five other patients had been waiting for their transplant operations at their hotel, and one of them passed away straight after their liver transplantation.

The costs of operations at the time in 2013 were \20 million (about US$200,000) for kidney and a range of \30 million (about US$300,000) for a liver.[2] In August 2018, a staff member at a mediating organization (who acts as a broker) I investigated stated "the trend in the cost of transplants is increasing every year by several million yen."

Three recipients I interviewed were told by a staff member of the mediating organization (the same one I investigated) that the waiting period would be about two weeks. However, they ended up waiting for three months. They don't know the exact reason for the delay, though they speculated that some political movements in China affected them. They went to China for transplants despite of the high fees, because it had been almost impossible to have transplants in Japan. The waiting time for a liver transplant is 15 years in Japan.

Once a patient decides to have a transplant in China, he/she pays a requested amount to their mediating organization. This is the starting point of everything. In a Japanese hospital designated by the mediating organization, the patient's blood sample is taken, and HLA and blood type are examined beforehand, and the information is sent to China. The two-week waiting time quoted by the mediating organization sounds reasonable, because the recipients' conditions and their necessary data for the transplants are sent to the Chinese hospital beforehand, providing enough time for them to select a matching donor in China.

The mediating organization used to be informed by their Chinese contact if the organ was from a death-row prisoner. Later, "organs from Beijing" became the commonly used euphemism, implying they were from death-row prisoners.

When the three recipients arrived in Tianjin, there were five other Japanese recipients waiting for their operations. The three recipients realized that operations using "organs from Beijing" tend to be carried out around midnight by observing the operation arrangements of the recipients waiting before them.

The liver operation for one of the three recipients started at around 8pm. He was in an acute condition, facing to death. He had an operation immediately after being informed an organ was available. From conversations with his interpreter and medical staff, this recipient had an impression that the donor was suddenly killed in a traffic accident. The kidney used for one of the recipients was donated from a 37 year-old man, so the hospital told him. He thought that the kidney must have come from a death-row prisoner based on the young age, but he did not dare to confirm it. Another recipient who had a kidney operation was told by a representative of the mediating organization that the donor was a death-row prisoner. He felt relieved when the mediating organization told him that a part of his payment would be paid to the prisoner's family.

Recipients from China Face Refusal of Aftercare from Hospitals in Japan
Japanese recipients coming back from China face the reality of "refusal by hospitals" for aftercare in Japan. When the recipients I interviewed left the Chinese hospital, they were prescribed with enough immunosuppressant medicine for three weeks. Two recipients who had kidney transplants visited F hospital in City A in Shizuoka for a check-up after the operation, treatment, and prescription of immunosuppressant medicine. They were told by the head of the hospital (at that time), Dr. T that "You are criminals. I will report you to the police." Dr. T is known as a former executive of the Japanese Society for Transplant. Cases like these have occurred in several hospitals. As a matter of fact, a kidney recipient from China filed an appeal against Hamamatsu Medical University Hospital (in Hamamatsu-city, Sizuoka, Japan) for their refusal of medical treatment.[3] Some doctors are treating recipients from China, believing that the recipients should be looked after on a humanitarian basis despite of having critical views against transplant tourism.

Lifting the Ban on Restored Kidney Transplant, and Statement at Meeting

On 13th September, 2018, a meeting to report the lifting of the ban on restored kidney transplantation by the "All Party Association of Restored Kidney Transplant", which consists of ruling and opposition MPs, was held at the Building for Members of Councillors (the Upper House) in Tokyo. Four MPs and members of the Japan Society for Transplantation, including Professor Hiroto Egawa, Chair of the Board of Trustees, the Japan Society for Transplantation, attended the meeting. Restored kidney transplantation is a technique developed by doctors led by Dr. Makoto Mannami of Uwajima Hospital (Tokushu Medical Association) in Japan. However, in 2007, five related medical associations led by the Japan Society for Transplantation declared the operation as "not medically appropriate", and banned the operation "on principle". However, the practice has been an accepted and established treatment in the US and Europe. In July 2018, the Japanese Ministry of Health and Labour recognised the practice as an advanced medical treatment so that it can be partially covered by medical insurance. Through banning the practice from 2007 till 2018, a numbers of kidney transplant opportunities had to be missed out in Japan.[4] The banning may have contributed Japanese patients to go abroad for kidney transplantations in places such as in China. At that meeting, Professor Egawa admitted the fact that doctors are saying to the transplant recipients from China that "we will see you if you don't mind us reporting you to the police". After the meeting, to find out his real motive behind the above statement about reporting patients to the police, I asked Professor Egawa directly. He replied "this is to stop patients going to China." He intends to prevent Japanese from going abroad for transplantation by spreading the information widely that there would be no hospitals in Japan who would look after the recipients from China. This is creating anxiety, fear, intimidation among patients who wish to go abroad for transplants. This is far from making appropriate efforts to improve the situation of organ transplantation in Japan.

Remuneration to Doctors

Several transplant mediating organizations are active on the internet, and arrange transplants in China for Japanese patients. Sometimes patients get information via word of mouth from other recipients who had transplants in China. Also, in some cases, doctors themselves, who learnt about a mediating organization, contact the mediator to confirm if they can arrange transplants in China. It appears that most of them are urologists or dialysis doctors. In October 2015, the mediating organization I interviewed told me that "When patients introduced by those doctors come back from China after having transplants there, most doctors contact us and ask for a kickback." This mediating organization has been paying "honorarium" to those doctors by handing out cash without any receipts, avoiding to leave evidences.

Doctors won't declare it to the tax office, regarding the cash as remuneration outside medical provisions.[5] The current Japanese situation of a severe shortage of organs for transplant operations is making transplantation into a business.

Summary

The Japan Society for Transplantation shows no indication of drastic reform plan. They banned restored kidney operations for 11 years, which made it inevitable that potential recipients would go to China. They intimidate recipients from China by saying "we will report you to the police" and create an environment where recipients from China suffer from being refused medical care after operations. Spreading this sort of information is their attempt at stopping transplant tourism from Japan. Meanwhile, there are doctors who introduce their patients to a mediating organization, and ask for a kickback when their patients come back from China. These doctors are urologists and dialysis doctors. The world of Japanese transplant medicine is extremely distorted. There is no sign of it being corrected.

References

1. "Restored kidney transplantation" refers to an operation where a patient suffering from chronic kidney failure receives a 'restored' kidney—meaning, a kidney that was removed from a living patient as a means of treatment of certain kinds of cancer. The cancerous portion of the explanted kidney is then removed on the operating bench, and transplanted to the new patient.
2. The liver recipient did not tell me the exact cost, but indicated a rough figure.
3. http://www.nishinippon.co.jp/nnp/medical/article/281777 "'Refusal of medical treatment is illegal': A man who had kidney transplant in China appealed" on Nishi- Nippon Newspaper dated 14th October, 2016. (Original text with English translation inserted.)
4. The number of usable kidneys being discarded due to the banning was estimated by Professor Hiroshi Tsutsumi in 2007, based on his analysis of the operations of removing cancerous cells from kidneys in Hiroshima Prefecture. His research was issued in "Microscopia" (Autumn Issue, 2007). Back number can be purchased: (The contents indicate the restored kidney transplant was featured in this issue): http://www.kokodo.co.jp/pub/shopping/naiyou.asp?ISBN=243
5. The organization was investigated for unreported tax on income from transplant abroad which amounts about \60 million (about US$600,000) in 2011. The organization revealed to me that in order to protect the names of the doctors, they paid penalties to the tax office. I was also told that this was not a large expense for them, considering potential income through doctors who introduce their patients.

Summary of oral testimony: 6th April 2019

I have discovered more and more that Japanese society is not doing enough so I felt compelled to testify.

There are many patients who are in need of transplants about 330,000 are going through dialysis currently but only a few are able to afford to travel to China for transplantation as of right now.

Usually money will be given to the families of those who are donating the organs.

I have only been able to interview three recipients of organs so far but I have no idea how many more have received organs.

Yes. I interviewed three recipients in August 2013. I have not had any subsequent interviews with the recipients since then. But in 2018 I interviewed people from the intermediary organisations not the recipients.

I have talked to the recipients face to face.

The recipients didn't know where the organs came from. Rather more than where the organs actually came from the fact that some of the fees that they paid for the transplantation went to the families of the donors made them feel good about it.

The recipients have heard from the mediating organisations that donating the organs to foreigners is acceptable in China.

Also, the recipients, whilst they were there, they witnessed many people from the Middle East even so they felt that receiving organs as foreigners was legal and that they were doing the right thing.

Restored kidney transplants are done in Japan where there is a shortage of healthy organs to be transplanted so they take kidneys for example that have less than 4cm of cancer cells and they treat the cancer and use the organs.

Donors had no idea what happened.

I personally would not participate in contacting the mediating organisations but if I had to I would go online and find a website for a mediating organisation that I could trust and go about contacting them in that way.

I do not have a list of the organisations but I have seen at least three or four organisations that are publicly advertising on the internet.

I spoke to those who had transplants directly.

The mediating organisations had information from the Chinese hospitals.

I interviewed just one mediating organisation in 2018.

Yes, there have been changes in Japan. Some hospitals do accept restored kidney transplants. This has not stopped people going to China for organ transplants at all.

Witness 44: Matthew Robertson
& Dr Raymond Hinde

Submission: https://osf.io/preprints/socarxiv/zxgec/
https://chinatribunal.com/wp-content/uploads/2020/02/Robertson_Hinde_Lavee_
AnalysisOfOfficialDeceased-OrganDonationDataCastsDoubtOnTheCredibilityOf
ChinasOrganTransplantReform.pdf

**Further the Tribunal received comments from Prof. Sir Spiegelhalter regarding
the above report:** https://chinatribunal.com/wp-content/uploads/2019/06/Comme-
ntary-on-Robertson-et-al-Spiegelhalter.pdf

Summary of oral testimony: 7th April 2019

Our paper is the first study of all of China's official voluntary deceased donor transport
data. We began the analysis by simply looking at China's COTRS data, the 'Computerised
Organ Transplant Response System', which is the official organ allocation system.
And then Dr Hinde discovered in the process of analysing that data that it conformed
extremely closely to something called a general quadratic equation. This was suspicious
because there was no reason that it should exhibit this behaviour and then we further
analysed other data to see whether there was anything odd or anomalous about it. That
included analysing the data produced by the Red Cross at the central level in China, the
Red Cross offices in every province or provincial unit in China, and also in a sampling
of provinces which were not random, but we chose because the data looks suspicious.
But in 5 provinces we looked at hospital data and compared it to Red Cross data. So, all
these different analyses were aimed at seeing whether the suspiciousness, so to speak,
of the data continued. When we looked at all those other data sets, we also found many
anomalies that are very difficult if not impossible to explain without concluding that the
data had been manipulated manually or, you know, was subject to human intervention in
an arbitrary way that resulted in nonsensical results. Our analysis found that according to
everything we'd looked at the data appeared to have been created from a mathematical
model so that it was centrally manufactured. And then data produced in each of the
provinces was then apportioned out, like assigned as quotas. That's the basic finding. It's
a long paper with many details associated with that.

Page 18 of your report these are the figures obtained from the COTRS quotas;
it shows the number of donors from 2010 – 2016 together with the number of
transplants that had been carried out from these donors. Is that right?

MR – Yes. That's right.

On opposite page you show this in a curve, which shows the donors in black colour and the kidneys and liver transplants that have been obtained from these donors. These figures produce a smooth curve which can be defined by a mathematical formula; therefore these cannot be random figures that would have been produced in a normal society with a normal body of donors and transplant activities. Is that a fair summary of your theory?

MR – Almost but it's a bit more subtle than that. Ray do you want to explain the intricacy of why we don't conclude directly from there that the data is falsified?

RH – What we are saying is not that it can't happen but that it would be unexpected to happen at such a smooth rate as that because we're talking about the infrastructure of a large sector that we would expect to grow more in fits and starts rather than conforming to such a smooth curve.

MR – The way I thought of it was that the finding of this super super smooth curve is kind of like our search warrant for then going and looking at the other data generated by this system. So, it doesn't prove that the data is falsified by itself. It's just highly suspicious and unexpected.

Page 21 of your report, the figures that are here are more or less the same as you had in the previous one except for the year 2017. These figures were provided by Dr Haibo Wang who is the director of COTRS in July 2018. Correct?

Yes. Correct.

The previous figures were produced by Dr Huang Jiefu. Correct?

MR – Yes and both subsequently appeared in official channels. So, they were both introduced by those officials, but they later appeared, you know, on public fora produced by the party state.

Would you or Dr Hinde be able to explain for people who do not understand quadratic formulas how these figures have been incorporated in your formula that is $y = ax^2 + bx + c$? But bear in mind that not everybody on the panel does understand mathematical formulas.

RH – Well the formula y = ax²+bx+c. The x with the 2 just means x times x. As in the data is going up with the square of the time plus there is the bx term and the cx term. It's simply a mathematical formula that defines a parabola which defines a well-known geometric shape and what you do is you have the parameters a, b and c are just numbers that you can pick however you like in order to get the best fit. So there are techniques for determining those values of a, b and c, which we give in other tables in the paper, there are techniques for finding what they call the 'optimal value'. The value that in some sense will draw a parabola that is collectively the closest to all the points.

MR – But also Ray, the significance of the simplification of the model from the 2016 to the 2017 data because that was important for our analysis, that the initial data set could be explained with a formula that had three parameters. But the 2017 data could almost totally be explained by a much simpler formula.

RH – The idea is that you can fit curves to any data you like but the simpler the curve is the more powerful it is as an explanation for the pattern in the data. And we've reproduced the 2 tables you referred to where the second one only has one extra row of numbers in it, which is the 2016 figures. The reason we separated them out was because we did the complete analysis when we only had the data up to 2015 and we put together…

MR – It's 16 and 17. 17 is the new one.

RH – Oh sorry. 17 is the new one. We had already done it up to 16 and found that it looked very very close to a parabola, a quadratic. We were then able to test the same thing with the new data point that came in and see if our previous conclusions were backed up by the new number that came in and it turns out that they were quite well backed up by it. So it became a predictive thing.

On this basis, you can predict what would be the result in 2018 and what would be the result in 2019 before even getting there. Is that correct?

RH – That's right. In principle you can. That's called an extrapolation. And extrapolations can be notoriously inaccurate. And so an extrapolation of one point did still conform quite well was reinforcing it. And then secondly, it also showed that we didn't even need the parameters B and C. We could throw that away and just use parameter A and have a much simpler formula so that it's an even more powerful statement that it closely fits it.

MR – However, its predictive power would not be unlimited because at a certain point because it's parabolic the numbers would just get far too big to be possible so at some point they have to deviate from this model. So we're not saying that… And especially now that it's published, we shouldn't expect that the behaviour that we identified continues now that they're aware that people are discussing that the data could have been falsified.

On page 23 of your report you use the factor of R-squared to adjust this. Can you explain this? And also there is some criticism of this.

RH – When a general quadratic was fitted to the addition of the new datapoint, the parameters B and C both became very small. This is another way of demonstrating that the parameters B and C are no longer needed. The graph here shows the difference in the sum of the squares of errors, which is simply the measure of how far away from the fitted line the points lie. So if the sum of the squares of the error are very small then it's a very close fit to the line. Now the graph shows the difference in the sum of squares of errors between fitting the general quadratic and fitting the quadratic without the B and C parameters, the simpler quadratic of $y = a.x^2$. The height of the curve is how much difference in goodness of fit there is between the general and the more specific one parameter. And as you can see it reaches a minimum actually of 5,160. That had been the value in 2017, that would have been the absolute best argument, the best possible number to support the statement that we can get rid of two parameters and just get $y = a.x^2$. And the actual value of 4, 146 is very close to that.

In other words, Dr Hinde, if the result of applying R-Squared is 1 then you have a 100% perfect fit?

RH – That's right.

The use of this method has been indirectly criticised by our expert Sir David Spiegelhalter in paragraph 5 of his report, which is at page 300 of our document. He says, "It should be noted that R^2 would not be the standard measure of agreement with a statistical model for such data". He agrees finally with you but he raises this issue with you that it's not the standard method.

RH – Yes. That's right. It's not the standard method because what we're doing here is not what you would normally do when you model data, you normally model data to try and get a handle on how the data behaves. And if you graph a person's height against their weight, it will tend to form a fairly straight line and so you can develop a relationship between two unknown variables, weight and height, and understand the behaviour that is happening. Now in this case we're not trying to do that, we're trying to say it unnaturally follows a parabola, the quadratic. The quadratic is a curve that there is no actual physical reason why this data should behave in that way and furthermore if it isn't real data then the random variations in it, the incidental inaccuracies, won't follow what you would expect them to do in real life, if it was real data. This is getting a bit technical. Data, which are counts of the number of donors successfully matched in a year, follows what they call a 'poisson distribution'. And the poisson distribution has well-known properties and so if you were going to fit a model, you would assume that the inaccuracies from the model would be poisson in nature.

MR – Ray, it means randomness in time over arrivals, right?

RH – No. Well in a sense. But it's randomness in the number of arrivals. If I can take a step back. The data that we're modelling changes from year to year and that change can logically be broken up into two parts. The first part is the change in infrastructure in the transplant sector. So that you would expect to get, as the infrastructure grows, you would expect to get a higher number of successful donor matches. The second part of the variability is what you call more random. Where it's the occurrence of a death that enables a possible match and that occurrence of a possible donor, a deceased donor, has just purely random fluctuations in it. And so the part of the variability that has those unpredictable randomness in it, they're the ones that are called 'poissant'. So if you were feeding the model normally you would assume poissant errors. But if you are looking at if from the point of the view that the data is not true data, then there is no reason to believe that they would behave like poissant variables. They would behave in some other way with an unknown origin.

I have provided you with a copy of the report of the of the Transplantation Society's China Relations Committee. They hired a statistician by the name of Jack Kalbfleisch. He also questions the use of R-Squared in Appendix 1 and is says it's "faulty in that in a country like China that has a growing transplant programme will always have a larger R-Squared than the other countries which are nearly in steady state"

RH – We make that point very clearly in the paper that we do expect China to have a higher R-Squared for a variety of reasons and in the paper we've attempted to allow for that as best way we can, it's difficult to do. But it should have higher values. But what we looked at was the pattern of, given the way that China is growing so quickly in size according to this data, we can get an estimate of how much better the R-Squared should be in the other countries. And we find that it looks like it is quite an outlier, it doesn't follow the progressive pattern. We expect it to be higher but not this high is the point.

There is a chart in page 26 of your report that shows certain abnormalities. These are the figures that Red Cross has provided. In this chart there are a number of abnormalities. Can you comment on them and why you consider them to be abnormalities?

MR – I also want to say, finishing off the previous point, the analysis of Dr Kalbfleisch's comments, they're on a particular part of the analysis. Our point is that the paper can't be viewed in separate parts because each part is important and contributes to the whole picture. So the Red Cross anomalies only take on more significance in light of the very close match to the formula. And similarly, if we only had one or the other we may not have had a paper. It's only when you put them all together that it starts to look like a Wizard of Oz kind of operation.

MR – To begin with, I think it's important to note that the only reason that we ended up with this data in the first place is because a researcher accessed the Red Cross website every couple of days and archived the data there. If not for that, there's no data series because the Red Cross website updates every few days or every few weeks or once a month, at random intervals, and all the previous figures are just wiped out. So they just put up a new number and they don't provide any historical series. So to begin with, there is a huge lack of transparency.

So all the figures on the Red Cross website are cumulative figures not showing the trend of the past. Is that what you're saying?

MR – Yes. And so the only reason we have a past trend is because we saved it.

Given that there may be very limited understanding of mathematics, statistics, and also people don't have the graphs before them. What is the underlying human assumption if these figures are said to be false? Is the underlying assumption that those producing false figures were making them according to a formula or is the underlying assumption that they were making them in some untrue way and the formulaic parabola that nearly matches the figures, in some other way shows that it's false?

The idea is that because the donor system was a new system that was established from 2010, in order for it to ramp up to a figure to a level that justifies the present day transplant numbers, then it had to go on a progressive curve to go to a level that is justifiable today. Is that correct Mr Robertson?

MR – Yes, essentially. I understand Sir Geoffrey to be asking basically, 'alright you guys are saying that the data conforms almost exactly to a mathematical model and basically they cooked the books and they made up this data.' Why on earth are you saying they used a formula? Why are you saying they used a formula in the first place? Is that your question Sir Geoffrey? In any case, I understand that to be the question. We thought about this and discussed it a great deal, because we're essentially trying to reverse engineer the process of creating the data, or what we think was their process for creating the data. I asked Dr Hinde, why might they use this rather than? Because you would think that it's quite non-intuitive. That's kind of the power of the finding. You would never expect that a high school equation would be used to create this data. Why wouldn't they just draw a nice curve just by hand that goes up and just randomly pick numbers, that you know, are growing fast, but they're not going to exhibit such a close relationship to any formula because they're just randomly picked, and you'd get kind of the same result. Ray do you want to respond. You mentioned that if you have a model then you can give the numbers out to the system.

RH – Specifically to answer the question. Yes. The implication is that they began with the model and then they continued to use that model to create the data but they added in some errors so it wouldn't be perfectly smooth and that's how it happened. If they're going to coordinate information coming out from different sources, then that would be an explanation of why they might use a formula. For example, the COTRS data which we figured $y = a.x^2$ to. The Red Cross data however which pretty much matches it is given at random points in time and so to know roughly where those points should be in order that the total for that year follows the $y = a.x^2$ pattern you would have to have some guidelines for all the bits of data that they might when they update their website every week or two weeks or how ever often. Because they've got the formula then you can actually derive the formula for the cumulative graph, and you've got a baseline for how the numbers should behave if they're going to match the COTRS annual totals.

MR – More generally, the Chinese authorities at this point have so many balls in the air, they have the actual number of transplants taking place which is a total state secret, they have the number of actual deceased voluntary legitimate transplants taking place, then they also have what we believe are the fake numbers. It's hard to keep track of everything I suppose and so they've probably got multiple data sets and they may not even have the actual real numbers. But at least having a model allows some internal consistency within the system. That's what we theorise. Of course, we don't know, we haven't seen the underlying data, we haven't had admissions from the people who we think created this.

Finally Mr Robertson, the anomalies in the chart that is at page 26 of your report it's called Figure 4, you were explaining these anomalies. At page 29 for instance, it shows for instance that in a period of 10 days, 30 donors passed away or became deceased and as a result of that they managed to get 640 organs from these donors which equates to 21 and one third per each donor. Is that a possible result, that each donor would give 21 organs?

MR – No that's not possible.

And the average in general remained constant at 2.75.

MR – Yes. So the point with these anomalies is that they it's… I mean an anomaly in the data just means something that doesn't make any sense. We observe that these 4 anomalies took place at a point when the cumulative data had deviated from a relationship of organs per donor of 2.75. And then an anomaly in the data appeared and that relationship was corrected or resumed. This is a highly suspicious pattern because the number of organs per donation fluctuates and the fact that an anomalous appearance in the data coincided with the correction of that ratio again suggests that there is some directive that this be maintained and that people manually manipulated the data to enforce a certain pre-determined outcome. That's what it's suggestive of, we argue.

And finally Mr Robertson, would you assist the Tribunal with your comments, which begin at page 33. This shows the registration of the donors, starting more or less from 0 and ramping up to quite a substantial number, but there are some anomalies here as well, can you explain what happens at the end of 2015 and the end of 2016?

MR – Yes. So first of all what this measures, the number of claim people who have said that if I become eligible to my donate organs I am willing to do so upon death. And so they are registered volunteers. This in the United States you put this on your driver's licence. That's the data that it is. Yes so in one day in 2015 it increased by exactly 25,000 and then subsequently it doubled in 2016, it doubled plus I believe exactly 7,800. So, in one day at the end of one year it increases by exactly 25,000 and then in the other year it doubles plus exactly 7,800. We didn't discover the latter until quite recently, Ray just saw that yesterday or recently. And so we don't have more data on this to be able check it against other things. For example, the way we checked the central Red Cross data was collecting the provincial Red Cross data across 31 or so provinces or municipalities and then we could cross check it and see if it held together and it didn't. But in this case we don't know what each province contributes to the total. So we can't say a lot more than it looks a bit suspicious. You could try to steelman the Chinese case and imagine that for example maybe they collect the data provincially and then at the end of the year they push it to the central data base however this still wouldn't really explain it because how likely is it that it would be exactly 25,000. And then the number grew throughout the year so… I'm sure there might be some scenario in which it could possibly be explained but in the context of all the other anomalies and the odd behaviour of the data, exactly 25,000, doubling plus 7,800, we would again suggest that it's indicative of human manipulation and that it's again another indication that it's not real data. But we can't prove that and we don't have as much evidence as for the other factors that we looked at.

And also you have comments about the rate of the donors that become deceased compared with the number of registered donors. Does it differ significantly from other countries in the world?

MR – Yes. China's is much, much higher.

By what ratio?

MR – I don't have those numbers with me. We didn't include that analysis because even though China's would be or is quite different from other countries. In other countries, when you consent to become a donor, that's binding. In China it's only the beginning of a negotiation between the hospital and the family. So even these registered donors… So Chinese officials had said that this is mostly for publicity purposes or to encourage the public to say "oh look how many people we've had come register". But even those registered donors, when the hospital wants to retrieve their organs, they have to engage in a prolonged negotiation with the family both direct and even extended families in some cases. So Chinese authorities could very easily say that this is not comparable to other countries and most of our donors are not registered volunteers in the first place and the family has to agree anyway and so on. So we didn't do along that but indeed if you just look at the number of donors in China versus the number of registered volunteers, it's much less as a ratio than other countries but I don't have those numbers with me but I've seen them.

Do you regard yourselves as being particularly close to/associated with Falun Gong as practitioners or otherwise? Mr Robertson?

MR – Well I have worked at a media that is commonly associated with Falun Gong, the Epoch Times, I worked there for 5 or 6 years until late 2016. Beyond that I decline to comment on my personal beliefs. I think it's quite interesting that for… I mean Falun Gong is a marginalised community and one of the issues that has come up is that evidence that is given by witnesses that are Falun Gong practitioners is sometimes dismissed because of their identity as Falun Gong practitioners. And so this is something that rarely occurs with other groups and so I think it is helpful to be ambiguous about my own beliefs.

Very well. That's fine. That's your answer. Doctor Hinde?

RH – I have no affiliation at all with Falun Gong.

Invert your numbers a bit just for the sake of lay people present and say what do you think the probability is that human manipulation of these data to generate the numbers you've described is? Is it, you know, 1/1000? 1000/1000? What would you put based on the numbers you've seen to the probability that these are kosher if you like?

RH – Well there's different parts of the data. I've been involved with the more government level data such as the COTRS data and so on. I've sort of thought long and hard on it. You can't make a conclusion one-way or the other. You actually can't. When I look at, say, the way the data follows a quadratic with one parameter, it's just worrying. It's difficult to really say "ah ok, well that's just happened, and you know, forget about it". That particular data, I would say, has it's power in the sense of being something that suggests something is going on that might then combine with other information. In fact it's only because of all the other information that it comes in, that something such as the adherence to a parabola really gets any traction anyway. Because it's all part of the big picture. So I see it is as sort of strong supportive evidence but not conclusive for the data at that level.

Could you expand on whether or not this matched the pattern of transplantation in other countries or in other centres of whether that quadratic equation could be seen in growth in other transplant communities? Because I think we need to understand fully by what extent China is an outlier in relation to other communities in the same era.

RH – It's an outlier in a few ways. It's presumably got a rapidly expanding infrastructure so that it will be increasing for that reason. I presume a lot of the physical infrastructure is already there and it's the more abstract infrastructure such as establishing the database of donors in the communicational levels to connect them and so on. So the way it's growing is quite different. It's growing super rapidly with part of the infrastructure already there. It's also starting from very small and going to very large. And so, for example, it's quite reasonable that it's going to increase with a general curve that is flat but then starts getting steeper at a faster rate for a while until it eventually levels off and it has to level off. So to really control for all of those. I guess another thing is they're coming in as a country with a large sector at a point where a lot of the technology, and I have no medical background, but presumably a lot of the technology has been developed and standard in certain situations and then they're tapping into that. And so that also makes it unique that there's not such a developmental stage involved, they just have to learn the techniques that are there. So it's actually quite a complex picture and there is no country that really matches all of those things. And if it is going to start off flat and then start increasing very quickly that will always be vaguely like a parabola. It will be vaguely like any increasing mathematical function. It just goes so closely to the quadratic and for example it doesn't fit an exponential growth as well. It's a much poorer fit.

Thank you that's very clear. I think the question for Mr Robertson is going back to the discussion about this curve, this growth in transplantation reaching a level associated with the existing, apparently large volume of transplantation going on in China, which could not be explained without donors coming from a different process than the one described here as voluntary organ donation system. Could you expand on that? In other words, does that match your calculations? Do they match some predicated volume that you observed in other data sets coming from other places. Was that clear? I didn't express it very well.

MR – Well, sort of. It's possible that someone said, "Look, we need 10,000 donors by a certain year" and then someone underneath came up with this model as a way of reaching there within the allotted time. So that's one possibility. Given that we're claiming that the number have been manufactured I don't think it bears any relation to the actual transplant volume that is happening. If I were, you know, to be speculating, it offers a useful explanation for the continued transplant activity that's happening but I don't see that there has to be any correspondence between the numbers. But I want to go back to your first question about essentially, "can we quantity the uncertainty of whether this data would have been fake?" and we couldn't because there is no natural model for the growth of a transplant system. If we have a coin that you flip you know the probability that it's a biased coin after a bunch of trials because you know that it should be 50/50. But you don't know the growth curve of what a transplant system should be so you can't say what is the probability that this was arrived at by chance. Because if it was $1/1,000,000,000$ (one in a billion) then you'd say that it was probably falsified. The way that I think of it is that the explanation that we have of, you know, a Wizard of Oz style data falsification arrangement appears to be the only explanation that accounts for the data being in the form that it is and that the official explanation doesn't account for that and there is no other plausible way of accounting for the data being as it is. What it would mean if the data was real would mean that they had opened organ procurement organisations, they had trained transplant coordinators, and that they had gained consent from donors, all at a rate that added up to exactly, or almost exactly, a quadratic equation. It's a very farfetched scenario. So we haven't even attempted to ascertain whether that's the case. Because it would mean that they needed 2 OPO's in the first year and then, you know, 5 in the second and then… According to what I've seen that's definitely not the case. Although we haven't tried to quantify that because it is so farfetched that all these factors could happen to match this very peculiar arbitrary mathematical model.

Just pressing you a little bit further on the COTRS 2017 data, I understand that it's very difficult to judge that you wouldn't end up at the final result in terms of where the parabolic curve gets to, it's the very smoothness of it is the bit I want to just kind of understand a bit more. Does that tell you anything other than the final destination?

RH – Well the model we've fitted doesn't tell us the final destination. I said before in principle you can extrapolate but the point is going to come when that just goes wildly different because you can't keep doing that. So we haven't made predictions of where it is going to go next. We've just observed it. So does that answer the question or not?

Yes.

Given the fact that the parabolic curve, sort of quadratic equation, would ultimately lead to a lot of difficulties as can be seen in page 19 of your report, because, you know, as time goes on you'll have to have far too many more donors being added. Why do you think then that it seems to have shifted to, as you point out, a simpler linear equation?

RH – It's not linear, it's single parameter. Well the only conclusion I could draw is that as we got an extra piece of data, we had more information on what the underlying curve is doing, but I can't give reasons why it would be parabolic.

MR – Well the issue is that it's probably what they used in the first place. They might have used not a general quadratic but a one parameter quadratic and then added random variation. And then in the first test it happened to most closely match a general quadratic with those parameters but when it got more data it appeared to more closely follow a simpler model. That's indicative that a simpler model was probably used in the first instance.

RH – Yes. We could go ahead and retrospectively fit a single parameter model to the earlier data. It just wasn't clear before.

Thank you both very much. We've taken your evidence comparatively swiftly, not least because we've got very detailed reports but also because we have pressures of time. Can I ask you if, in the event that members of the Tribunal have further questions, that they put to you in writing you'd be willing to respond? If they have such questions.

RH – Yes.

MR – Gladly.

In which case thank you very much for making yourself available today. Your evidence is now concluded.

Witness 45: Prof Maria Fiatarone Singh

Short Statement to the China Tribunal April 7, 2019
Prof Maria Fiatarone Singh, MD, FRACP

I am a physician, board certified in Internal Medicine and Geriatric Medicine in the USA and Australia, currently working full time as a Professor in the Faculty of Health Sciences and Sydney Medical School, University of Sydney. Brief CV is attached. My research, clinical, and teaching career has focused on the integration of exercise and nutrition into health care for the prevention and treatment of chronic disease and disability in older adults.

I became involved in the issue of organ harvesting after hearing data presented by Mr. David Matas at The Transplantation Society meeting in Sydney in 2008. My impetus was to bring awareness of this unethical medical practice to my colleagues in the Western medical community. Coincidentally, I discovered that the orchestrator of the entire transplant system in China and the then Assistant Minister for Health in China, Dr. Huang Jiefu, was actually trained at the University of Sydney and was still an honorary professor at our institution. Joining with colleagues in ethics, law and medicine internationally, we began efforts to investigate and to expose his personal involvement in the conduct, design and proliferation of unethical transplants, and to detail the extent of the organ harvesting of prisoners of conscience to the medical community, our academic institutions, editors of medical journals, as well as the broader public.

These efforts of myself and colleagues have led to, among other things:

- The University of Sydney not renewing the Honorary Professorship of Huang Jiefu in 2014 for a further 3-yr appointment
- a number of academic publications (shown below), including the most recent article in BMJ in which our research indicated that in 445 papers published in English-language transplant journals, in which 85,477 transplantation procedures were described between the years 2000 and 2017, and 84% of the papers did not provide evidence or a statement of ethical organ procurement. Only 33 papers explicitly stated that they did not use organs from executed prisoners, and in 19/33 cases, this was clearly a falsehood, as the transplants were performed prior to 2010, when *all* organs, by China's own admission, were sourced from executed prisoners.

- the establishment of an interest group among parliamentarians in Australia
- public forums and media coverage
- petitions to local government as well as to the UN, and
- the beginnings of legislative actions to hopefully ultimately bar transplant tourism to China and penalize any involvement in unethical procurement or receipt of organs harvested without consent or under coercion, with extraterritorial jurisdiction.

Academic publications on organ harvesting

1. Rogers, W., Robertson, M., Ballantyne, A. et al. 2019. Compliance with ethical standards in the reporting of donor sources and ethics review in peer-reviewed publications involving organ transplantation in China: A scoping review. *BMJ Open* 9.
2. Rogers, W., Fiatarone Singh, M.A. and Lavee, J. 2017. Papers based on data concerning organs from executed prisoners should not be published. *Liver International* 37 769-769.
3. Rogers, W., Fiatarone Singh, M.A. and Lavee, J. 2017. Papers based on data concerning organs from executed prisoners should not be published: Response to Zheng and Yan. *Liver International* 37 771-772.
4. Trey, T., Sharif, A., Schwarz, A. et al. 2016. Transplant Medicine in China: Need for Transparency and International Scrutiny Remains. *American Journal Of Transplantation* 1-6.
5. Sharif, A., Trey, T., Schwarz, A. et al. 2016. Truth and Transparency. *American Journal Of Transplantation* 2016 1-2.
6. Rogers, W., Trey, T., Fiatarone Singh, M.A. et al. 2016. Smoke and mirrors: unanswered questions and misleading statements obscure the truth about organ sources in China. *Journal of Medical Ethics* 42 552-553.
7. Trey, T., Sharif, A., Fiatarone Singh, M.A. et al. 2015. Organ transplantation in China: concerns remain. *The Lancet* 385 854-854.
8. Sharif, A., Fiatarone Singh, M.A., Trey, T. et al. 2014. Organ procurement from executed prisoners in China. *American Journal Of Transplantation* 14 2246-2252.
9. Lavee, J., Fiatarone Singh, M.A., Trey, T. et al. 2014. The uninvestigated factor behind the negative attitudes toward cadaveric organ donation in China. *Transplantation* 98 e78-e79.
10. Fiatarone Singh, M.A. 2012. *The Mission of Medicine*. Woodstock, Canada: Seraphim Editions.
11. Trey, T., Halpern, A. and Fiatarone Singh, M.A. 2011. Organ transplantation and regulation in China. *JAMA – Journal of the American Medical Association* 306 1863-1864.

CV of Prof Fiatarone Singh
https://chinatribunal.com/wp-content/uploads/2019/04/April_Prof-Maria-Fiatarone-Singh_CV-2018.pdf

Summary of oral testimony: 7th April 2019

[Background] Professor at University of Sydney, involved in 2008 after hearing David Matas speak. Had not known about this issue until then but felt more people needed to know. Huang Jiefu was not only trained at University of Sydney but was an Honorary Professor at the university which started a collaboration with lawyers and other ethicists to try and make the University of Sydney realise it is inappropriate given his background.

[Whether her work received resistance] Huge amount of resistance. Those with whom he had trained and current peers. He had been given the presidential medal of honour by TTS which is the highest honour they bestow and to this day they have never retracted it or taken away his membership although it is clear in their guidelines that no-one who has ever been involved in OH can be a member of the Transplantation Society. There has been a great reluctance on the part of transplant professionals to get to grips with what happens in China.

Their membership guidelines are clear, [they prohibit] both unethical transplant from prisoners but also other coercive means of transplantation like paying a family which is clearly going on in China with the Red Cross but none of that has been a reason to expel any of the members of China from TTS.

The Red Cross is a very different one from other parts of the world. They are, from what we know, which is even what TTS in China say, they are involved in things that are not ethical in other parts of the world. It means coercive payments to family members after somebody dies which basically means people who don't have a lot of money are unable to refuse so it is coercive which is against guidelines of UN, WHO TTS.

[Dialogue to challenge their behaviour] Not with me personally. There hasn't been any great move by anyone in the west to challenge what they are doing.

[Re BMJ paper about ethics in China] Those 33 papers stated that no organs were taken from executed prisoners yet in 19 of the 33 papers the dates of the transplant activity was prior to 2009 and we know that every pre 2009 was from executed prisoners.

The resistance to knowing about this, in 2008 HJ was reappointed twice until 2014. I think the reason he was not relieved of duties was an attempt to save face. I think that there was a tendency to believe him or believe he has changed in a way that would make it all ok, but by putting a bank robber in charge of the IMF is the same; he has lied to so many people for so long it is hard to believe he will stop lying, he denied use of executed prisoners, then admitted it and then no credible source of donors the numbers of which can't match the date and the blindness to it continues.

[Re call to retraction of papers] It has media attention. To my knowledge no journals have retracted, which would be the duty of the editor.

Yes [to liaising with WHO] and the UN. I have worked with DOFOH since 2008, we have a petition with 2million signatures but still reluctant to do anything but say that China is moving in the right direction. The UN requires transparency and that is not happening so to say it is within UN and WHO standards is completely false.

[Re knowledge of other doctors engaging in this practice and with TTS] I don't know how many. HJ has done 500 livers, including one day when he had spares delivered because they kept failing. He has said he doesn't object to the use of executed prisoners.

[Re why TTS are so unforthcoming] They have worked together for many years and belief that change is possible and through engagement as opposed to sanctions. But it doesn't make sense when you read the guidelines of what is ethical especially when you read their guidelines about what is ethical, they shouldn't have membership. Perhaps it is because they have worked so closely for so long and they don't want to admit that they didn't know their motives.

There has been a bill in New South Wales parliament to try to bring legislation to make it illegal to participate even extra territorially. But this is a federal not a state issue. There are close trade ties with China. So just as in other areas like publishing where there has been prohibition on books are critical of China that is unfortunate, but trade has superseded ethics.

Basically people have agreed that HJ set this system up and did it personally, but because he has been forced to change at least a little, he has been forced to change even though he has violated every medical ethic and should not be practicing medicine, or mentoring other medical and should have been stripped of this accreditation. The people who wrote about it 10 years ago are still leading the way.

I know that none in China involved in transplant have never been [expelled form TTS], but I don't know about others.

Witness 46: Dr Maya Mitalipova

Maya Mitalipova, PhD
Director of Human Stem Cell Laboratory, Whitehead Institute for Biomedical Research, MIT

We know now from credible sources that entire population of Uyghurs, Kazakhs and other Muslims in Xinjiang Autonomous Region Of China, had been forcefully health checked and the blood samples were withdrawn since 2016 to date. These procedures were not performed to Han Chinese population of Xinjiang, but only to Muslim population.

The entire Muslim's population blood was used for DNA sequencing.

DNA sequencing is a critical biological technique utilized in laboratories. By using this, we are capable of investigating various diseases and genetic illnesses. Additionally, many mutations are initiated by faulty genetic sequencing. Scientists can gain epidemiological data with multiple genomic candidates. Meaning, genomic sequencing (in clinical trials) can provide convenient information in treatment development. Below are specific advantages of DNA sequencing:

DNA sequencing has exhibited much importance in disease discovery, novel treatment, forensics, and human understanding. By using genetic sequencing, we are capable of exploring mysteries in many aspects of biology/life.

But the question remains unanswered: what for Chinese government is using million people's DNA sequenced data? It is very expensive procedure to perform DNA sequencing on such large scale. So, there has to be a very valid pay back outcome.

For successful organ transplantation doctors rely on several important criteria including three main blood tests, cell surface tests and limited DNA tests to determine if a patient and a potential donor are a match.

Now scientists have come up with a comprehensive DNA scoring system using many genes to predict long-term success of transplantation.

Current genetic tests detect differences in DNA sequences at just a few specific locations in the genomes of transplant recipients and their organ donor. The fewer differences, the better the chance of long-term acceptance of the new organ. But scientists reasoned that a much larger scale collection of DNA data for a large number of genes would give a better indication.

Group of researchers study it by taking large samples from 53 pairs of kidney donors and recipients, developed a computational method that assigned a DNA score to each pair based on mismatches in their DNA sequences. They followed the progress of the patients following transplantation surgery over several years and found that the score significantly predicted the success of the transplanted kidneys. These data showed that there is a need to more future studies to build on this new concept to confirm the initial observations which may lead to using this new concept of DNA sequencing in the clinic to optimise the matching of donor and recipients before transplantation.

The researchers say that any process that improves the success rate of transplants will also take pressure off the shortage of kidneys for transplantation. A major contributor to shortages are patients who have to go back on the waiting list after an organ has failed.

Over the last two decades, more than 300 000 solid organ transplantations have been performed in the United States alone. However, despite improvements in surgical techniques and the development of more effective immunosuppressant therapies, allograft rejection still affects 60% of transplanted individuals and remains one of the major risk factors of graft loss. Up to 40% of graft recipients experience some form of rejection within the first postoperative year, with lung and heart recipients showing the highest rates of rejection, with 55% and 25% of patients, respectively, and kidney and liver the lowest, with 10% and 17% of patients experiencing rejection, respectively. Rejection can occur where genetic disparities exist between donors and recipients, which may lead to presentation of polymorphic peptides that the recipient's immune system recognizes as non-self. Although key HLA loci have traditionally been considered to be the main contributor to the genetic variability of allograft rejection, some degree of rejection still occurs in HLA matched sibling transplantations, which may be the result of non- compatible loci beyond HLA between donor and recipient. Indeed, new findings indicate that non-HLA polymorphisms can impact upon transplantation outcomes since they have the potential of generating histo-incompatibilities influencing allograft rejection and impacting immunosuppressant responses. Approximately 3.5 million common and rare polymorphisms exist between two unrelated individuals of European ancestry and up to 10 million variants in individuals of African ancestry. However, investigations of non-HLA genetic determinants of clinical outcomes following organ transplantation have yet to be performed in any systematic fashion to date. Recent technological advances in genomics such as genome-wide association studies (GWAS) allow the characterization of hundreds of thousands to several million single nucleotide polymorphisms (SNPs) and copy number variants (CNVs) across the human genome rapidly and efficiently.

Furthermore, whole exome and whole genome sequencing, which interrogates the coding regions and the entire human genome, respectively, are quickly becoming commonly used tools within the clinical diagnostic arena. These second-generation sequencing technologies have the ability to extensively characterize genome-wide sources of histo-incompatibility between donors and recipients, potentially unraveling specific genetic risk factors influencing rejection and immunosuppressant responses or severe adverse effects.

In this article I tried to emphasize the current knowledge from existing genetics studies conducted for transplantation outcomes and therapeutic responses to immunosuppression therapies and bring to attention of the court the importance of using large cohort of DNA samples sequencing for the translational components from this genetic knowledge that may be rapidly implemented in organ transplantation field.

There is a huge direct link between DNA sequencing and organ transplantation outcome! We know that Chinese government favors forced organ harvesting from prisoners of conscience and this has been practised for a substantial period of time involving a very large number of victims. It is beyond doubt on the evidence presently received that forced harvesting of organs has happened on a large scale by state-supported or approved organisations and individuals. And State approved DNA sequencing of entire Muslim population of Xinjiang without informed consent is another proof of evidence that the knowledge obtain from genomic data analysis will be used to determine if a patient and a potential donor are a better match for a long-term success of transplantation.

Uyghurs detained in secretive "political re-education" camps in China's northwestern Xinjiang region may have their organs harvested for profit by the Chinese Communist Party (CCP), a former medical surgeon who was forced to carry out the procedure in 1995 told The Epoch Times.

Not surprisingly, China has the second-highest transplant rate in the world, with amazingly short transplant wait times of just two-to-three weeks.

Summary of oral testimony: 7ᵗʰ April 2019

I am a stem cell scientist. My point was that DNA sequencing by itself is playing a major role in many diseases, but also in organ transplantation. So given the fact that the entire population of Xinjiang area Muslims, Uyghurs, Kazakhs, and other ethnic minorities, Muslim minorities, where withdrawn the blood and where DNA sequencing was performed and this is the major reason why DNA sequencing occurred. Because DNA sequencing itself is not a very cheap procedure per se.

The conclusion is that blood and DNA sequencing was performed on this entire population in order to have a better outcome of organ transplant. This is my conclusion between the link of DNA sequencing and organ transplant in the population of Xinjiang.

Organ transplant is performed in every developed country. One of the reasons why it was a very limited number of people. We need a huge population of donors in order to really sequence. You need 100,000's of sequences.

This has been difficult with the low number of donors in US. China has a good chance of matching donors with recipients. This is why they have done it with 10 million Muslims. It is a very expensive procedure.

As a scientist we usually use DNA sequencing in order to know if there are any inherited mutations for disease study. For example, if the person has diseases so we would actually do a DNA sequencing to see if this person has any mutation. And another thing will be used in forensic; for example, to see in a crime scene if a person committed the crime is actually matching his DNA too. And the third option would be an ancestry, for example if you want to know your ancestors or if you want to know whether the relationship between your relatives and so on, so you would to a DNA sequencing.

So I would say in this case, when they did it on such a large scale … I believe that if the Chinese government put such a large population, up to 3 million into a concentration camp and then actually does a DNA sequencing of an entire population, then it is very unlikely that the Chinese government would be actually worried about diseases and this population or the curing of these diseases. Because it's really an expensive procedure to do so.

Unlikely [to be used to define ethnic purity or relations]. It's too extensive a procedure to do so. Organ transplant procedure would benefit it. For best matching of donors and sequencing. This is my expert opinion. I don't have access to direct evidence. It's still very expensive. I am 99% sure it's being used to match the best organs to the recipients.

There are many reasons why they can use the DNA sequencing [database]. This region has become a police state. It's hard to believe that these people can do any terrorist attack under such surveillance. They have dragonflies, phones being checked etc. It's very hard to imagine they could do this. In order to own a kitchen knife, they have to register in 5 different government places. Chef knives are chained so they can't use it for anything. I hardly believe they would go to such expense unless they wanted to suspect them as terrorists.

[The cost] In the Royal Institute, it cost 5000 USD to test my mother. Not the whole genome, just the sequencing. You can imagine what the cost would be. One US company refused to keep selling to region.

Witness 47: Dr Torsten Trey

Submission: https://chinatribunal.com/wp-content/uploads/2019/04/April_2019-DAFOH-Report-on-Forced-Organ-Harvesting-in-China.pdf

Summary of oral testimony: 7th April 2019

In order to understand the table [page 21 of report], we need to compare the group of registered donors and the group out of this pool that passes away every year. You find in the second line the number of actual eligible donors. Now there is a discrepancy between those who pass away and become eligible organ donors and those who eventually become eligible organ donors. For example, in the UK, only one percent of the people who pass away in the UK become organ donors. We have compared that figure to the entire pool of registered donors. In the last line you see that it is typical that 0.01% of the registered organ donors become eligible organ donors. But in China this ratio is 140 times as large as in many other countries. We consider this an inconsistent ratio.

Our conclusion is that the explanation of the organ source does not follow the official explanation. It is complex because, before 2015, the explanation for the organ source was that they were from the executed prisoners. But we found that before 2015, executed prisoners could not explain the exponential increase of transplantations in China. After 2015, the pattern has changed because executed prisoners were no longer officially the source. After 2015, the public organ donation programme was used as an explanation for the organ source. We found inconsistencies in this programme also. In both scenarios, the explanation of the organ source is not sufficient. We postulate that there is an undisclosed organ donor pool.

[Re how one can draw conclusions without direct evidence] It is very rare that any type of crime or murder takes place with a camera in the room with witnesses around, so in most cases the hard evidence is not present. In this case we are even talking about a political system with all the facilities to conceal the crime. If hard evidence is the only acceptable criteria to accept force organ harvesting as a reality, it will be very difficult. However, the amount and complexity of circumstantial evidence and indirect evidence is tremendous and it is sufficient to trigger independent international investigations.

This table [report page 6, transplant tourism figures] is part of a publication which was published in 2016. It is a review of 86 medical papers which were published over

15 years- 2000-2015. It is a summary of transplant tourism which was documented in paper. Question: So these are cumulative figures not annual figures? Answer: Yes. Question: So it cannot help us with transplant tourism for each year? Answer: no. But if we would look at the 86 medical papers we could find out to which years these individuals publications refer to.

[Infrastructure and transplant industry] There are individual cases where transplant centres were followed. In the report there is an example of the Tianjin 9 hospital. There are other centres that were followed over the course of the years and their expansion was followed at different times. I cannot give an answer right now to the number of beds, or comparisons with the UK or USA.

[Report page 14 covers the observation that the allegations of FOH of the FG population was initially not put forward by the FG community itself.

[Re 60% of all organ donors being registered in only 7 days]. See figure 9 – by the end of 2016, numbers were around 200,000. Yet in the last week on 31 December 2015, 25,000 of those numbers were added and in the last week of December 2016, 88,000 were added. So take these numbers, it is higher than 150,000. That's how you get to the statement.

[Whether the figures are false] If you take the number in 2015, in one day 25,000 donors were added. This is unusual that so much in one day and more unusual that number ends on three zeros. We are not talking about numbers that you can round up or round down. It is incomprehensible to have exactly 25,000 with a real name, real individuals being added on one day.

[Reference to page 30 and the chart showing Falun Gong, Christians, Uyghurs and Tibetans, and whether there evidence that FOH is happening to the Christian community] We have too little data on this. We rely on data reported to us and we get almost no reports from Christians being targeted for organ harvesting. But it is too vague to come to a conclusion on this. But we see a high risk in this group. Data comes from medical papers, sometimes newspapers, media.

Similar [for Uyghurs and Tibetans] but there is more information but to provide this information it requires a network to convey the information, and there is less information being reported (in respect of the Christians). Less for Christians than the Uyghurs and the Tibetans but not enough being reported for all groups.

Within these three groups, we believe the risk for the Uyghurs is increasing. There is more systematic categorising that allows for the screening and there are signs in airports which allows for fast track of organ harvesting.

Between 2012 and 2018 we have organised global petitions to the UN where we have highlighted this issue and asked for international investigations. So far we have not had any action on this. We have had parliamentary hearings and publications where we asked for investigations. The resonance to look into forced organ harvesting that is focussed on China is extremely difficult. There is a layer that does not want to look into this. If this had happened in a different country, something would have happened much earlier.

The medical profession is known for its medical oath to not do harm. If every doctor remembered this there would be the drive to find out what is happening. A gold standard for transplant medicine is transparency. In the United States each hospital publishes its transplant figures. In China this does not occur; you get a national transplant number. You cannot find out which hospital contributed and by how much to the transplant figures. If the medical community would make it a standard that each country has to report transplant numbers by individual transplant hospitals, then this would create transparency and would allow for scrutiny. Transparency does not do any harm; it only helps to reveal where harm is being done. Another approach would be, and something that has been missed for a long time, that is there is hard evidence in the transplant patients that travel to China. When they leave the country, they have the hard evidence in their bodies. If globally, the individuals travelling to China agreed to have a biopsy and then we could build up a DNA database of these organs, then we could collect the DNA of persecuted prisoners of conscience in China for example of Falun Gong practitioners, then we could compare the results the DNA from the transplanted organs and those who went missing who were tortured to death. Then you could medically establish the organs that were taken from Falun Gong practitioners. But because of the cover up in China, this would be difficult to get this information but by doing this method we could prove it outside China.

Before 2000, transplant medicine was not well established, but knowledge and infrastructure has increased and this is being built on the blood and the bodies of prisoners of conscience, mainly Falun Gong practitioners. If you look at this picture, the inviting of transplant surgeons to the west is equal to educating them on how to commit crimes against humanity better, so until there is 100% guarantees that forced organ harvesting is not taking place in China, it is unethical in training and helping transplant surgeons from China.

[Whether they investigate in other countries] The mission of our association is forced organ harvesting; taking organs without consent. This is different to commercial trafficking. We don't find this in other countries. What we have seen in 2016 is that ISIS is meeting this criterion otherwise we do not find this because it is including the killing of the organ source and this is not seen in other countries.

[Whether official rebuttals are genuine ignorance or willful] That is difficult as you ask me about the intent but in my opinion, it is wilful. When we provide data, information, reports for years and in communications with the TTS, I often hear that they have not even read the reports. And when there are visits to hospitals, this is only to preselected hospitals which is meaningless and if we ask them to look into detention camps, they say things such as that they are not in position to investigate, that they are professional organisations, and that they do not have the means to investigate the camps. My problem here is that whilst I understand they are not in the position to investigate detention camps however at the same time there is also the expertise that China has developed and follows ethical standards in transplant medicine and I find this is a discrepancy; on one side to establish that they follow ethical rules and then on the other side decline to conduct investigations in detention camps to look into hospitals that were not preselected. There is a bias. That is why I think it is wilful.

Our members are from all over the world and have all sorts of belief systems and there are members who practice Falun Gong.

Witness 48: Dr David Matas

Submission: https://chinatribunal.com/wp-content/uploads/2019/04/April_Matas_
Kilgour_Gutmann_ResponseMarkField.pdf

Summary of oral testimony: 7th April 2019

Your statement makes reference to a debate that took place at Westminster, in the Houses of Parliament, in London on 26th March. In that debate Mark Field MP [and Foreign and Commonwealth Minister for Asia] spoke about your initial report and the 2016 update.

He said his officials had studied the update. Did they approach you before or after [the debate] to identify what that study was?

No he did not.

He stated that as authors you acknowledge the following about your report and we will take each in turn shortly:
As authors you acknowledge that there is a lack of incontrovertible evidence of wrongdoing;
The authors made clear that they had no smoking gun;
That there is a less than rigorous research technique applied;
That you still make assumptions;
that you have to infer the scale of organ transplant systems from hospital promotional material.
Do you acknowledge that there is a lack of incontrovertible evidence of wrong doing?

We made no such acknowledgement. I word searched the report, there is nothing similar to that. In fact we had over 2,400 footnotes, 2,200 coming from official Chinese sources. I would say it is the revers of incontrovertible evidence and it certainly hasn't been controverted.

No smoking gun?

The point we were making was smoking gun or smoking scalpel, but the point was we drew conclusions from a number of pieces of evidence, rather than from one, we certainly didn't say there is nothing to prove what happened conclusively but rather that we accumulated different pieces of evidence rather than one single piece, it is a distortion of what we said, when we say it came from not one but many sources.

Less than rigorous research techniques?

Human Rights Watch did a similar research report. They were also prepared to rely on secondary evidence. we were not.

Assumptions?

I appreciate it is a long statement [our report of 7th April].
We made assumptions that people were meeting requirements, but that sort of assumption does not mean that our report made assumptions.

Relying on hospital data, you say you did not rely on that alone?

It is a question of whether all evidence justified the conclusion not just whether one piece of it does, so they [the FCO] had misrepresented it. I don't refute any of it. I would say I have no reservations. In a legal context I have no doubt.

With what strength do you hold your view on the first report and the update?

I don't refute any of it.

How strong is your conclusion?

As strong as ... I had no reservations and no hesitations. In a legal context I have no doubt.

You and Ethan Gutmann and Kilgour feature prominently. What was the first trigger for your interest?

It was a simple request to investigate and I was asked to do it to determine whether it a true or not. I had been involved in a lot of human rights work [reference to Annie] and knew it involved a large amount of evidentiary work to determine whether it was true or not.

How soon did you start working with Mr Gutmann and Mr Kilgour?

Do you personally have any proximity to FG as a belief system?

No, I am not a practitioner and I never have been. I have no proximity to FG, no associations with that or China, for me this is strictly a professional interest.

What do you think the motive for the UK government putting up a smoke screen is?

I attribute it to the fact that it is diplomatically awkward for governments.

Witness 49: Ethan Gutmann

Submission: https://chinatribunal.com/wp-content/uploads/2019/04/April_Matas_Kilgour_Gutmann_ResponseMarkField.pdf

Summary of oral testimony: 7th April 2019

Questions as put to Mr Matas, namely

Your statement makes reference to a debate that took place at Westminster, in the Houses of Parliament, in London on 26th march. In that debate Mark Field MP [and Foreign and Commonwealth Minister for Asia] spoke about your initial report and the 2016 update.

He said his officials had studied the update. Did they approach you before or after [the debate] to identify what that study was?
No he did not.

He stated that as authors you acknowledge the following about your report and we will take each in turn shortly:
As authors you acknowledge that there is a lack of incontrovertible evidence of wrongdoing;
The authors made clear that they had no smoking gun;
That there is a less than rigorous research technique applied;
That you still make assumptions;
that you have to infer the scale of organ transplant systems from hospital promotional material.

No I was not contacted before or after the debate on 26th March. However, I did speak to the main fellow at the FCO who would be responsible, a staffer not the MP. We had heated words because I had bought up the idea, by asking him publicly how good his Chinese was. You see 2,400 footnotes and notes in the update and the fact is unless you have very, very good Chinese ability it is awfully difficult to go through these. And so I mentioned that there were three Chinese who work at the Congressional executive commission on China who spent 5 weeks going through our end notes and there is a friendly relationship with the US and UK and nothing preventing him from picking up the phone and talking to them about their assessment to discuss the end notes. That is the only contact on this, extrapolating from what he said, I don't think he was even claiming that he had gone through the evidence.

Have you heard allegations about your work in those terms before?

Not the "promotional material". The smoking gun is taken out of context if you read what we actually said, we threw in that phrase. It seems to me that he is quoting from a movie "Hard to Believe" where they say there is no smoking gun or scalpel. I had nothing to do with that movie, although I'm in it a lot, but it seems to me that is what he is quoting from, not from our report. It is clear to me that what we are saying is that we have a series of smoking guns and there is so many points of evidence and put together there is the killing ton of evidence, so that was surprising that it was mentioned quite that way.

I think the assumptions is the fairest point. We have to make assumptions, we are not in a war with China, we're not overrunning their positions, we can't examine the hospitals on the ground. We can look at what the Ministry of Health puts out as a minimal requirement for every hospital permitted to do transplants. Those minimum requirements are 40 beds and dedicated transplant teams and beds. If you put that together, and think that we're not there with a clip board, people cut corners in China so you have to make some assumptions but they are reasonable on data.

You say some of the assumptions of the use of facilities is an underestimate?

There are two ways it is an underestimate. One is that if we actually ran the numbers, I'm the main one responsible for the numbers, I actually lowered them from what I was coming with which is 125,000, that's the highest range. I went on what I know people in China do, which is exaggerate output by 20%, like they exaggerate resumes, exaggerate the time they spent at company by about 20%. So the assumptions were made to lower them because there is a tendency to claim over production on a local level. On a national level they're trying to keep numbers down, nationally they're trying to keep them up.

Comparisons with other countries responses?

In terms of comparisons with other countries, refer to our response of 7th April, as drafted by Matas.

Do you consider it a misrepresentation?

We welcome critique. the problem, for instance the Congressional committee came back with questions after they'd read the report. And I think that is legitimate. The problem here is that is it being used as a recipe for inaction. I understand this is a country with a Brexit concern, and there are many economic uncertainties I live here, and I know people don't want to add to that but it is also true that this has been going on for 12 years, or significantly more in fact, so something to say transplant volumes is a real problem in china would have been a more legitimate response because there are so many evidence trails leading to that same conclusion. We only have one piece of evidence against it which is China, which are the official data China comes up with.

In that debate, there was reference to few UK travelling to China for transplants. Do you have any data or know where he would have got that from?

All we know is we did FOIA requests, a fellow I know did them, to over 50 hospitals in this country, asking if they had transplant patients who'd gone to China, all of them replied to say medical confidentiality, 5 said the equivalent of medical confidentiality but "we tried to tell them not to go". How many didn't put that statement in we don't know. I spoke to one man in Birmingham who received a kidney in China.

With what strength do you hold your opinions?

My opinions have grown stronger and stronger because of the Uyghur situation. It is a speedier version of the Falun Gong situation, it is just happening faster.

The first trigger to investigate?

I was in China when the persecution took place. I remember the day vividly because sound trucks appeared on the streets. I was working at Beijing TV and several people started weeping it was like watching a big family erupt at a dinner table. The first trigger came when I was interviewing a witness who said she had had received an exam for corneas but not eyesight. She didn't know about the organ harvesting issue, but that meant I knew she couldn't be talking about it because she didn't know.

In 2006 I met David Kilgour in New York. A few years later they asked me to write Bloody Harvest with them, I said no I wanted to do my own study then after my own book came out, we worked together more closely.

I am agnostic, my wife is a militant atheist.

(Panel quote from The Slaughter). In my book, The Slaughter, I do mention a smoking gun, specifically which is the interview I did with the Mayor of Taiwan, now mayor, who gave a very explicit interview because he was looking into the prices of organs for his clinic.

Targeting of other groups?

Don't agree that there is lack of evidence that House Christians have been targeted for this. Christian Solidarity Worldwide are not getting a lot of reports of this, but I get other stories. In terms of Tibetans, the community is not cooperative because the Dali Lama is concerned it will lead to an end of discussion with Beijing. We do know that the hospital facilities are far greater than they were in 2010. In terms of Uyghurs, they are 1.5m people who have been blood tested, in detention and their families have lost them. We have other evidence, such as crematoriums and the dedicated transplant lane at airports so it is impossible, you can made estimates a few years after it has happened, like looking at a star, with the Uyghur situation this is the catastrophe I'd like to see governments act upon which is why this Minister's response is so disappointing.

Blood testing at home. What does that indicate?

The minister said (in response to blood testing, transplant lanes etc) that it is not that there is no evidence, but that they don't believe it is state sponsored. It is impossible to test 15m people without it being state sponsored, it is not a private initiative. There is just no way this is a private initiative; it has to be state sponsored. It was done in record time, in malls, public places, at home as they did to FG the three years before to practitioners who had been in detention but were no longer. So, there is a precedent for it.

Witness 50: Dr James Shapiro

January 10, 2019

Sir Geoffrey Nice
Chair, China Tribunal
Independent Tribunal into Forced Organ Harvesting from Prisoners of Conscience
in China

Via email as PDF to Susie Hughes (email redacted)

Dear Sir Geoffrey:

Re: China Tribunal Statement of Contribution

Thank you for providing this opportunity to provide representation of our position at the University of Alberta in Edmonton, Canada with respect to collaborations in islet cell transplantation in China.

By way of background, I serve as the Director of the Clinical Islet Transplant Program at the University of Alberta, and hold a Tier 1 Canada Research Chair in Transplantation Surgery and Regenerative Medicine. I was the lead investigator that developed the Edmonton Protocol for transplantation of human islets into the livers of patients with unstable forms of type 1 diabetes, and published our findings in the first seven treated patients in the New England Journal of Medicine in the year 2000. Since then we have treated almost 300 patients in Edmonton, and up to 2,000 patients have received similar treatments internationally with variants of the Edmonton Protocol since 2000. The islets we transplant are derived from human organ donors across Canada that have previously expressed their wish before their unexpected death to become organ donors. They further informed their family members, and family members of the deceased provided written approval to proceed with organ donation under the accepted ethical standards set out by all of the Provinces in Canada and validated by Health Canada and Canadian Blood and Transplant Services. Donors include brain dead organ donors (neurological determination of death (NDD) as well as deceased cardiac death donors (DCD)).

I was approached in 2017 to help train scientists and clinicians from Zhejiang University Fourth Affiliated Hospital set up a clinical islet transplant program to

541

treat patients with diabetes with cells that make insulin, taken from organ donors. This process was not initiated by me, but came through the Dean of Medicine and Chair of Surgery at the University of Alberta. A delegation went to visit the President and team at Zhejiang University First Affiliated Hospital. I was not party to that visit. I was then asked to train scientists and physicians in the process of islet extraction and clinical care of transplant recipients. The President of Zhejiang University First Affiliated Hospital came to Edmonton in 2017.

I subsequently discovered that Zhejiang University First Affiliated Hospital clearly was, and likely still is, actively engaged in 'forced organ harvest.' (as reported in the Guardian newspaper, BMI report, and retractions in the journal Liver International as of 2017). I was concerned based on the data available that Zhejiang University Fourth Affiliated Hospital continued to access donated organs that far exceeded expected rates for this region, and source their organs from an organ donor pool that overlaps with the First Affiliated Hospital. It is therefore remained highly likely in my mind that at least a majority of donated pancreas organs continued to be derived from forced organ harvest. While I understand that organ donation practice in China had supposedly changed (computerized registry system and new prohibitive laws), it is clear from extensive US congressional hearings held in June 2016 that this practice was continuing unchecked in China

(https://www.youtube.com/watch?v=fXXihdjo_jo).

Further, I was in communication with the past president of the International Transplantation Society (Professor Frank Delmonico), an expert and WHO representative involved in assessment of Chinese organ donation practice, and with David Matas who wrote the Kilgour-Matas report on organ harvest from Falun Gong practitioners in China, both of whom underline ongoing concerns in this region. It was abundantly clear that we in Alberta are incapable of monitoring organ donation practice at the Fourth Affiliated Hospital with sufficient resolution to be absolutely certain that not even a single organ used for islet isolation could have been derived from any unethical source. I felt that if there was any possibility whatsoever that Albertan transplant professionals could end up collaborating, training and aiding transplant practice in a country where unethical forced organ harvest is actively practiced, that this would be unethical and would have serious potential knock on impact to our own ethical transplant programs in Canada. I therefore made the choice that the Clinical Islet Transplant Program would not comply with the Dean and Chair's request, and to refuse to collaborate with the Fourth Affiliated Hospital of Zhejiang University in any areas that involved transplantation science of clinical practice. The University of Alberta has continued collaborations in the area of teaching and education in General Surgery, but not in any areas that involve transplantation surgery or research to the best of my knowledge.

Clearly my decision was based on hearsay evidence, and I do not pretend to have direct knowledge of current practice of transplantation in China. I just felt that the weight of evidence was so concerning that I could not personally justify knowingly or unknowingly crossing this ethical line.

I trust this letter and testament is helpful to your committee, and I applaud the contributions that your team are making internationally to this issue. I further hope that with the pressure of public awareness that Chinese officials will change their practice and ensure that transplantation surgery in China meets internationally recognized ethical standards.

Yours sincerely

A.M. James Shapiro
(signed on PDF copy)

Professor of Surgery, Medicine and Surgical Oncology, University of Alberta

https://chinatribunal.com/wp-content/uploads/2019/04/April_DrJamesShapiro.pdf

Summary of oral testimony: 7th April 2019

In 2017 there was some interest to set up an islet cell transplant programme at this new university. As I mentioned I was not involved. And then there was an invitation sent to me to go visit Zhejiang University, I think in around November 2017, I can't be sure of the exact date. I couldn't go, I am a busy liver transplant and hepatobiliary surgeon here and I didn't want to take the time off to go there at the time. And colleagues of mine went, not on my behalf, but were also invited. Dr Ray Rajotte, who has since retired from the university, accompanied the Chair of Surgery and others. And during that visit they discussed the design and implementation of an islet cell transplant laboratory and discussed the possibility that they might come to Edmonton for training. And only after that visit did I hear about what had gone on.

The next thing I knew I was invited to a meeting in the Dean's Office where the President of the Fourth Affiliated Hospital attended with a delegation of around 10 to 12 of his colleagues, that was Professor Chen. So I was invited to that meeting.

It was a very friendly meeting, very nice people, very enthusiastic about what we'd achieved with the islet cell transplant Edmonton Protocol and I enjoyed the discussion with them didn't really commit to anything but there was a memorandum of understanding that was supposed to be written between the University of Alberta and the Fourth Affiliated Hospital.

And I didn't sign that and I was reviewing the documents for that and across my email appeared some details about forced organ harvest and I didn't know much about that. I mean I'd seen the FG demonstrations that occur weekly outside of our local farmer's market downtown but other than that I hadn't really been aware of that issue so that caught my eye. And I contacted the organiser of that this is still going on in China and she sent me the retracted papers from the liver transplant journals from 2017, an editorial by Professor Wendy Rogers, the piece that was written about this in the Guardian, and the piece that was written in the British Medical Journal. I read these, I realised that Zhejiang University was linked to this area where there had been retractions of these papers and for me that was a red flag.

And so I sent those four documents to the Dean and to the Chairman of Surgery and said I have concerns about this based on what I have just learned and I don't feel that I can be involved in any way nor my programme with the cooperation with this particular university until we can be absolutely sure that there is no possibility of any unethical practice with forced organ harvest.

So that led to some further discussion with the university and then they really came back to me and said would there be any way that I could find to work with this university and I said I would need to know with absolute certainty that there was no line that was being crossed in terms of unethical organ harvest and how could I be sure of that?

So I contacted Professor Frank Delmonico from the Transplantation Society who I knew from my work in liver transplantation surgery and I'd lectured at Harvard previously so I knew him. And I talked to him about this and the answers that I got back were really not to my satisfaction. The bottom of line of it all was that there was no way that I would be able to police the organ harvesting details in any way that would allow me to know with absolute certainty that there was no line being crossed and no unethical organ harvest. So I said no. I cannot work with this university until that occurs.

I tried to see if we could set up with the Vatican the links there to see if we could have some third party that could act as an intermediary, again to police it for me. And I didn't feel that would be adequate. There were no clear answers for me.

So I have never cooperated with this university in terms of training for islet cell transplantation and I won't do so, and my team won't do so, until we can be certain that there is no possibility of unethical harvesting of organs.

I'd have to dig that up [the date he spoke to Francis Delmonico]. I've got emails back and forth from him. It would have been in… If the process began in 2017 it would have probably been within the six months following that. So into early 2018 I suppose.

And then I also saw the paper that was released in preliminary from Matthew Robertson and Jacob Lavee showing where the data essentially had, to my eye, been massaged, in terms of the numbers of organ donors following mathematical curves and formulae. And I felt that again that there was sufficient concern in my mind that his was a real and ongoing activity that I could not ethically collaborate with.

[Whether his university is under commercial pressure to take Chinese students or engage with the Chinese medical community] So I can't comment on that directly because I don't have direct knowledge of that. I can tell you that our faculty of medicine is short of money. I am sure one component of their desire to collaborate with the Chinese is financial, but I don't know that for sure. But I think it's exceedingly likely based on our position. I think some of it is altruistic on the university's behalf from my Chairman of Surgery and from the Dean's Office. But there is clearly some financial component. And there would have been some further financial benefit I presume coming to the university if we'd agreed to train this team in islet cell transplantation.

[What the medical community engaged in transplant should do in response to events that you perceive in China] First and foremost, at least in western society, my concern is around the free will and altruistic activity of organ donation. And I think if any of our leading centres, any centre in the western world, is seen to collaborate with centres where forced organ harvesting is going on, I think from the general public's perspective it would really jeopardise the ability to continue to derive altruistic organ donation. And we rely heavily on that. And even with that. Today our relationship for altruistic donation is tenuous. We have many patients that die on our waiting list waiting for transplant. And we desperately need more organs to go around. That's why I do a fair number of living donor liver transplants in Edmonton. But I think if we cross that line, and if others cross that line, it will jeopardise our relationship with the general public. That I think is number one for me.

In terms of science, I think where there is unethical practice that science should not be presented in the public domain, that's my own personal feeling. And I know over previous years, I have been to meetings where there have been retraction of papers from China, where it's believed that there has been unethical practice, and I think that should continue to occur until we can be certain that their practice is aligned with the rest of the world.

Yes I am [a member of TTS].

[Why TTS have been reticent to comment to us on these allegations] I can't answer that. I'm not in the higher echelons of the Transplantation Society. However, I must say that I was very surprised by the response that I got back from Frank Delmonico and from others that I knew or had been affiliated with the Transplantation Society. They seem to reassure me that there had been a seismic shift in the practice in China and they were relying heavily upon assurances that I really couldn't see data for and I don't know why that is. I know Frank Delmonico has spent a lot of time in China and has travelled there, as I am sure his delegates and team have. I was expecting, and in fact relying upon the Transplantation Society, as our representative international society to take a higher moral high ground than perhaps even I would myself. So I feel a little bit left out on a wing on that one.

[Turning a blind eye to the practices alleged would be turning a blind eye to murder. How can medics do that?] I don't know. They must somehow be able to disconnect their day-to-day practice of surgery and transplantation from their own ethics. And I don't quite know how that happens. I think we have to be very careful as professionals and as physicians not to cross that line. And when others do so, I think it may be through ignorance, through a belief that such a practice couldn't be possibly occurring in China. I think it's probably it more. The belief that mass murder wouldn't be occurring and that this is somehow being trumped up by groups that are being franchised somehow. That's all that I can take from that. It's difficult to understand, clearly. But I think it must be based on a disbelief that this is occurring.

Witness 51: Dr Charles Lee

Academic Papers and Publications Inside China Confirm That a Huge Living Donor Pool Exists

March 7th, 2019

Charles Lee, M.D., Director of Public Awareness,
World Organization to Investigate the Persecution of Falun Gong (WOIPFG)

My testimony would involve information in five aspects. Since Dr. Wang from WOIPFG has testified in front of the tribunal regarding much of the content, I would just elaborate on the second part, the liver emergency transplants.

1)   Very short waiting times.

2)   Large portion of liver emergence transplant operations. The China Liver Transplant Registration (CLTR) project was started in February, 2005. 9,610 cases have been collected as of May, 2007. Among 4,331 cases with available data for timing manner, 1,150 cases were emergency operations, which was as high as 26.6%. The very same database provides that 97.7% of the liver donors were cadavers, living (relatives) donors accounted for only 2%. By contrast, out of 919 liver transplants performed at Multi-Organ Transplant Programme, London Health Sciences Centre in Canada from 1994 to 2008, 60 were performed on patients for acute liver failure (ALF), which was only 6.5%. Emergency liver transplant is needed for those who have ALF and transplantation should be performed in 48-72 hours. Canada has a waiting list/donor registration system; those with ALF are assigned with the highest priorities, the system is supposed to be much more efficient than the one in China, where there's no waiting list system or donation system available for matching up. A more plausible explanation is that it is the donors waiting for the recipients in China, which is an evidence supporting that a large living donor pool exists in China.

3)   Abundance of donors provides multiple standby donors

4)   An abundance of donors results in hospitals promoting the organs in the market and offering "free" transplant operations.

5)   The abundance of donors has even made Chinese medicine hospitals, forensic hospitals, psychiatric hospitals to conduct organ transplant operations.

Thank you.

https://chinatribunal.com/wp-content/uploads/2019/06/CharlesLee_Supple-mataryMaterial.pdf

https://chinatribunal.com/wp-content/uploads/2019/06/Charles-Lee_English_PLA_HHRG-114-FA16-20160623-SD002.pdf

https://chinatribunal.com/wp-content/uploads/2019/06/Charles-Lee_liver.annual.2006.report.pdf

https://chinatribunal.com/wp-content/uploads/2019/06/Charles-Lee_PLA.2%E7%82%AE%E5%8C%BB%E9%99%A2.01.pdf

Summary of oral testimony: 7ᵗʰ April 2019

[Comments on the report of Dr Wang]. We have studied thousands of academic papers by doctors in China regarding organ transplant procedures and we find that more than 300 papers talk about donor situations, health, procuring organs. We found a lot of procedures and the papers approved that they have conducted a mass murder and these donors and these donors were killed. Some of the academic papers say that they would inject Heparin two hours before the organ was obtained. They say these were "cadavers" which are like conflicted by itself.

More specifically they have some data from the Ministry of Public Health from China. They studied a collection of liver transplant procedures from 26 hospitals and another 11 hospitals. The 26 hospitals are all the prominent hospitals in China. They are very good at doing these organ transplants procedures. They have collected 8,645 cases from February 2005 – December 2006 and they had two reports published and one of the reports published in December 2006 they say they have data on 4,341 cases regarding the timing manner. Among them 1150 of them were emergency cases which was as high as 26.6%. So more than a quarter of these were conducted as emergency liver transplants. This means there is a large donor pool readily available. For regular societies for example, Canada, we had data showing that for the year 1994 – 2008 there were only 60 transplants for acute liver failure which was only 6.5%. So for the large portion of these emergency donor liver transplants in China it means they have the donors waiting for the recipients. They have a system which means they can procure the donors in a very fast way. So this is some of the evidence showing that the living donor pool does exist in China. For acute liver failure, patients only have 72 hours before they need the transplant, so the liver has to be readily available. China has such a high rate of emergency liver transplant and this is not usual and not seen in other countries.

We have some other academic papers. They have very young healthy donors. In China there is no legal procedure to determine what brain death is. In most of the academic papers they claim that the patients are brain dead. They say there is a very short warm ischemia time. Many of them claim that there are zero-minute warm ischemia time. So they can literally take the organ from the donor which still has circulation, a heartbeat and that kind of thing. We have a table published in the China transplant journal in 2011. It shows that they had 298 cardiac transplants. Among these only 60 of them had the heartbeat stopped or in a kind of vibration state. For all the others, the heart was taken whilst it was still beating. So clearly this is a mass murder conducted by the doctors.

The tissue typing and blood type would have been done beforehand so that is why they can do this, the transplant quickly and if you call the doctors beforehand, they can always promise you the organs can be available in 2 weeks or 1 month. The database is available. These academic papers published by a hospital in Shanghai have done emergency liver transplant and the shortest waiting time was 4 hours after the patient was admitted. In normal societies it is not that fast so the tissue type and blood type is already done and that is why it can be done that fast.

[Whether there has been a relaxation of tissue matching regulations, and that they were not taking imperfectly matched organs] We do not have data on this in the papers. And I don't think we have access to this kind of data regarding the tissue matching.

Warm ischemia is the time when you have organs with the blood supply stopped or reduced. When you take organs out and immediately transfer them into the recipient's body or into an ice box to preserve the organ. When you have this zero-time warm ischemia it means you take the organ when it still has full blood supply meaning the circulation and heartbeat is still going. That is how they practice. At the moment they have something called brain death centre in central hospitals and they can conduct procurement of the organs with zero warm ischemia time, so we believe that the donors were killed and killed right away.

[Re significance if warm ischemic times] There is a paper from 2006 in [Guangshee] province which talks about two multi organ donor transplants (June 2003 and June 2005). In these two cases Heparin was injected intramuscular into the bodies 2 hours before which means the donors were still alive as there needs to be heartbeat and circulation in order for the Heparin to be circulated and to be effective. Therefore, the people were still alive. This is from the academic papers themselves; they explain how they procure the organs themselves. There have been phone interviews from investigators and the doctors admit that the transplants can be done right away and from very close by. It is still going on. Question: So just to be clear, this is a different practice – a different mode – for multi organ retrieval than is practised elsewhere. Answer: Yes of course – you mean the donors were still alive when the organs were taken.

[In a cardiac retrieval procedure, in a patient who is known to be brain dead it would be normal for the heart to still be beating until cardioplegia is given at the very last moment to retrieve the heart.] Yes, it is normal in other places that the heart still is beating but in China there is no legal definition of brain death and the doctors do not know the definition of brain death and they do not care if the person is dead. There was an academic paper published in 2011 and still there was nothing at that time about how the doctors monitor the patients as to whether they are brain dead. These donors are all very young – 18 – 45 and they have no history of disease and this is why we believe that the patient is not dead. The brain death concept in China does not exist at that time.

No [other statistics from around the world]. We have obtained these figures from the London Science Health Centre in Canada. But for normal society, even if they have a very mature donation system, you can only get this percentage (6.5%) because of donor.

No [rates from other countries].

[Whether there can be an explanation from the conclusion that there is a donor pool in China] There is no other explanation: you have a very warm ischemic time, you have a high percentage of emergency organ transplants, and all the people going for the transplants you can get an organ in two weeks or less than a month. These organs are readily available – you can just come to schedule the operation instead of waiting for someone to be terminally ill or an accident to happen somewhere which is what happens in other parts of the world. There is only one possibility: you have a pool of donors.

[The figures come from 2007, are there more recent figures] We do not because the Government of China is always trying to cover this up. They have done a lot of things to mislead people. It is difficult to obtain figures such as percentages of emergency liver transplants from China itself. This data was from 10 years ago.

[Direct question: A zero-time warm ischemia transplant essentially involves the murder of somebody adjacent to the recipient, the murder conducted by the extraction of their organs. Is it as simple as that?] There are two possibilities: one is that the recipient is nearby in the next room or something like that or the organ is placed into the ice solution in order to preserve the organ. But when you have zero-time warm ischemia it means the organ is obtained when the blood circulation is normal. The point is they can get these organs with zero warm ischemia time. organ extraction is the cause of death.

[Direct question: I really want to go through this again. In my experience, you are always aiming for the shortest possible warm ischemic time. It is not an indication that I have murdered the donor just because I have a short ischemic time; that is the aim. I want the organs cold and, in a bag, as quickly as possible. I do not see the relationship between the zero warm ischemic time and the certainty that the donor has been killed specifically for those organs] I believe there is a lot of legal criteria in other countries to determine brain death. So they would always want to wait for at least five minutes to confirm that the patient is brain dead. This is a legal procedure. You have to wait for at least five minutes before you can procure the organs. You cannot get organs with zero warm ischemic time legally. It is not possible for normal medical hospitals. If you get an organ from a car accident, then it is an even longer time. It isn't possible literally zero time.

[The issue being brain death not ischemic time] Yes. You have to wait for five minutes, everything is clear, the patient is dead. Occasionally it is possible to have a short warm ischemic time. In these procedures discussed in the papers, there is no legal procedure to ensure the patient is dead.

[Direct question: We have to understand that the warm ischemia definition that you are implying takes place in Chinese practice is different in some way to the warm ischemic terminology that we would use in other centres wherever they may be. What you have been describing seems more to be about how you define the time of death/or the type of death i.e. brain death rather than warm ischemic time] Yes. The key point here is about the brain death; the definition and how you practice the brain death. There is an expert doctor in China on this brain death issue. He conducted the first ever heart transplant in the country using a brain-dead donor on 1 July 2006. All the academic papers that we collected between the years 2000 – 2006 said that said there had been transplants conducted using brain dead donors can therefore not be correct because [the doctor] announced that the first ever transplant using a brain-dead donor occurred in July 2006.

[Absent a definition of brain death, it is cardia death] It could be. When they claim that the death was brain death this is not possible because is China there is no such practice. We still see this happening; they claim brain death, but we do not see any evidence.

I am not practising at the moment. I am a businessman. But I have been involved in WOIPFG for many years. I am a Falun Gong Practitioner. I was also imprisoned between 2003 and 2006. Because I went to China to review the truth of persecution of people in China.

[In relation to anaesthesia] I have a paper relating to heart and lung extraction. It says the donors were put under anaesthesia and after a few hours after the anaesthesia took effect they opened the chest and they took the heart and lung together. The donors were breathing well when they entered the room and the fact that they needed anaesthesia shows that they had good brain function. The point is that the two donors were alive and well when they entered the room.

[In other evidence that we had before patients were breathing normally and intubated endrotracheally and then operated on for a donor operation and therefore they were not and could not have been in any way said to be brain dead by any conventional definition] That's right.

[Recent data] Is not readily available.

Answer: No other [information evidential material available that would confirm my conclusions].

We do not have anything in the last couple of years because they are always trying to cover it up.

Witness 52: Dolkun Isa

http://www.uyghurcongress.org/en/?p=33706

Speech to Roundtable Meeting at the UK Parliament – submitted to China Tribunal

Thank you all for inviting me to speak at this roundtable on the very important topic of organ harvesting. It has been great to hear from all of the speakers here today; their words have been equally shocking and informative.

My statement today will focus on putting the practice of organ harvesting in the context of the Chinese government's repressive policies towards Uyghurs. Organ harvesting must be viewed in the context of a widespread campaign of repression and control against the Uyghur people, resulting in the wrongful mass incarceration and enforced disappearances of many Uyghurs.

Organ harvesting is a particularly egregious crime. It violates the victims and causes further pain and distress to their families. It strips the humanity of the victims, who are treated as a collection of parts to bought and sold for profit. Even after death, it disrespects the victims and deprives them of the right to decide what is done with their remains. At its core, organ harvesting is dehumanizing and brutal crime.

As was mentioned by previous speakers, prisoners are the most at risk for organ harvesting in China. This is dangerous for the Uyghur people, who are experiencing an unprecedented crackdown on their right to peacefully practice their own religion, use the Uyghur language in schools and freely express themselves. Mass arrests of Uyghurs, on unfounded or unspecified charges, have put thousands in prisons and re-education centres. Invasive and overbearing new security measures such as 'predictive policing', constant surveillance online and through security cameras and countless roadblocks and checkpoints in cities in East Turkestan, ethnically profile Uyghurs and further exacerbate the problem.

Relatives of those arrested are often not informed of what their loved one is charged with, what prison they are being held in, or when they are set to be released.

In this uncertainty and vacuum of information, with no meaningful accountability or notice about the prisoner's well-being, that organ harvesting is carried out with impunity.

We are also deeply disturbed by reports of the Chinese authorities collecting blood samples from the Uyghur population in East Turkestan. There is a dual purpose to this. On the one hand, collecting blood samples allows the Chinese government to establish a genetic database of the Uyghur people to further monitor, control and repress them. This genetic information also facilitates organ harvesting, making it easier to compare blood types and compatibility of potential Uyghur victims.

Even more concerning are the hundreds of Uyghurs who have disappeared at the hands of the Chinese police. After unrest in Urumqi in 2009, hundreds of Uyghurs disappeared in Chinese custody. Despite efforts by their families and the international community to find out what happened to the disappeared, the Chinese government has not released any information or acknowledged their disappearances. Recently, the Chinese government has been pressuring other governments to return Uyghur refugees and asylum seekers. When they are forcibly returned to China, many of them disappear. Most recently, this was the case with 23 Uyghur students, who were returned to China from Egypt and have since disappeared. We have strong reason to believe that many of those who have disappeared have died in Chinese custody and have had their organs harvested and sold.

These people are subjected to a final indignity of having their organs harvested without their consent, like stripping a car for its parts. Not only were they subjected to one of these most serious human rights violations, deprived of their freedom and had their lives taken from them, even after death they are not permitted to rest in peace. Their bodies and physical integrity are desecrated for profit.

Therefore, organ harvesting remains a major issue for the World Uyghur Congress. As long as the Chinese government, police and security forces are able to act with impunity and detain thousands of Uyghurs without procedure or accountability, the practice of organ harvesting of Uyghur people will continue. It is the hope of those who engage in this barbaric practice that the Uyghurs who disappear or who die in prison are forgotten. In response, we must continue to raise their cases and to demand justice and accountability.

To do this, we need the help of national governments and the international community. We therefore call of the government of the United Kingdom and the international community to continue to publicly raise the cases of those who have disappeared, to denounce the repression of the Uyghur people and to demand answers from the Chinese government.

China is sensitive to criticism and the words and acknowledgement of other states has an impact. When the international community remains silent, organ harvesting flourishes and the cycle of violence, dehumanisation and impunity continues. The Uyghur people look to you, the international community, to speak up on their behalf and help to end the horrific crime of organ harvesting.

Summary of oral testimony: 6th April 2019

My name is Dolkun Isa. I am the current President of the World Uyghur Congress based in Munich, Germany. World Uyghur Congress is an umbrella organisation and the united voice of the Uyghurs in exile.

Today the situation of the UG has really deteriorated, particularly since 5 years we have witnessed the Chinese Government's strategy to eliminate all Uyghur identity really clearly. Since Xi Jing Ping took power 5 years ago he really implemented and eradicated Uyghur identity. And in August 2016, Chen Quanguo, former Chinese Communist Party Secretary in Tibet, was appointed Party Secretary in Xinjiang Uyghur Autonomous Region. When he was the Party Secretary in Tibet, Chen Quanguo, did a brutal crackdown on the Tibetan and after he was appointed Party Secretary in Xinjiang Uyghur Autonomous Region he used a brutal way and his experience in Tibet really implemented a new restriction rule and started in October 2016 he had all the communication between transportation particularly direct flight from Ürümqi to Istanbul, Dubai, some other country. Because before this, each week, five days, there was a direct flight from Ürümqi to Istanbul. After Chen Quanguo came to Ürümqi he stopped all transportation and in October he started to collect all passports of all the Uyghurs.

And slowly slowly, in 2017, at the beginning of March or April, he implemented a so-called eradication camp. Today some resources say more than two million people are suffering in the camp, some say possibility is three million, but it is really difficult to comprehend how many, but it is definitely more than one million people in the camp. And Radio Free Asia, Uyghur Service, confirm until now 40 deaths, one of them was my mum.

On 12th June 2018 I got the heart-breaking news that my mum Ia Memet, she was 78 years old, she was a retired woman, she passed away, died in the camp. I didn't know in what conditions she passed away. Actually, my mother passed away on 17th May 2018 but I got this news nearly three weeks later. Then a lot of media called me and asked me what the situation was, in what conditions did my mother died, but I had no idea. I had tried to communicate with my family members, my friends,

I tried to call all telephone numbers, which I had, but no I couldn't access. Then some international media, randomly went to the police office and local government and later, maybe it was a few weeks later, I learnt my mother was put in the camp nearly one year before, it was around maybe June, May 2017. And one year later she died in the camp. This I learnt from the media. This is just an example. It is exact evidence of what is going on in the camp and another big thing was Mohammed Sali who was an 80-year-old Islamic Scholar, he translated the Quran from the Arabic language into the Uyghur language.

[Whether there is any information about Uyghurs being DNA tested and news about the FOH of that population] Around 2017 and 2018 they were already taking the blood of 11 million people. Of course, it is impossible to provide evidence of exactly why the Chinese Government took the blood samples and DNA tests. But so many Uyghurs since 2016 escaped from my country to Europe and the US, they are saying, and some of them have given reports that the Chinese government took blood samples and conducted DNA tests as well. It is also the Chinese government and some family members also reported this, so today we don't know the exact number.

Since October 2018 the Chinese government stopped all the transportation from Beijing and from other provinces to Ürümqi. Then they transport detainers to inland China, we don't know the exact number, but some reports say 200,000 to 300, 000, some reports say 400,000, 500,000 Uyghurs detainers being transported to inland China. This is all we can work on. Maybe the Chinese government is using these people for organ harvesting.

Because in 2009, a peaceful uprising was cracked down, that time also a few thousand Uyghurs disappeared. World Uyghur Congress, we documented 43 cases, but still already 10 years have passed, and these people have disappeared. So it's possible these people were used for organ harvesting, maybe.

And in 1997 in Ghulja one uprising occurred, and that time Amnesty International and other international organisations reported that around 300 people died this time and there were so many death sentences were happening. There were also so many disappearances. No news. So many people were arrested but most of them disappeared. Possibly these people were used for organ harvesting.

Yes [FG have always been peaceful].

Yes, some groups [in Northwest China] have such [separatist] ambitions. Some people really want to separate from China. Some organisations, some people, do this in a peaceful way. I believe self-determination is not a crime.

Well yes. Some violence has happened. It is true. But I don't say it is linked with terrorism. Because no one is safe. Uyghurs have no right to express...

Well there are Uyghurs in the camps who are subject to political indoctrination and mental torture and physical torture. So, there is evidence suicide is happening. It is impossible to get information from the camps.

We have interviews with several witnesses [to get the information about brain washing]. It is reported around 2000 Kazakh and Uyghurs but is a Kazakh citizen. They were in the camps and the Chinese government because of the Kazakhs they are released and came to Kazhstan. Most of the evidence is based on those people who have spent time in the camps and what they have witnessed, and we also received some anonymous letters about what is happening there. Most of these anonymous letters came from Turkey, Kazhstan, Kyrgystan. We had about two letters actually come from people inside China, and they said they are inside mainland China.

[Whether information has been received about medical testing] We have received consistent information. Some said that medical examination is widespread. Some said that there was death in the camp. And there were people taken away from the cell and never returned to the cells. Even unknown medication injections.

It is very difficult to estimate the numbers [taken away from the camp for an unknown reason] because we know there are many many camps in the country at the moment. As far as I know the people who told us about the disappearance of cell mates are those who spent time inside. So it is very difficult for me to give you any estimation.

[Whether there are reports detailing the numbers who disappear or the use of medical tests] I can't really explain it to you because of the difficulties in obtaining information within the region. It created huge difficulties to produce a detailed report with evidence. But we have general information regarding what is happening there. Also the estimation by some experts that we know, at least over one million or up to two million people are held in the camp at the moment but we don't know how many people are alive how many have died already how many people have been transferred to prisons in mainland China.

Yes, there are many different ethnic groups in East Turkistan, my country; there are Uzbek people, Kazakh people, Katar, Kyrgyz. They are all Muslims. Also, another very large Muslim group, they are Hui and although they are not persecuted to the exact same level lately they are also being targeted.

[Whether all groups are treated the same] It is not treated exactly the same, the Hui Muslims are relatively free to practise their religion but they are also in the last two years being targeted, although not putting them into camps, the situation as severe in East Turkistan, and in my country, the victimised race are the Uyghur Muslims and the Kazakhs.

[How samples were taken and where blood testing occured, by whom and whether forced] In 2016 the Chinese government actually made an announcement for the people to go to their local clinics, the hospitals, all in East Turkistan, from the town, village, city, level and at that time they made the announcement that they were giving this free health check and also in order to prevent some contagious disease.

If someone refused to go to their local clinic would that result in a sanction?
[Consequences if someone refused to go to their clinic for testing] I don't have any information regarding that.

Witness 53: David Kilgour

Organ Pillaging in China
Submission by Hon. David Kilgour, J.D.,

To China Tribunal headed by Sir Geoffrey Nice,
London, United Kingdom
9 Jan 2019

Honourable members of the China Tribunal,

Organ pillaging/trafficking/tourism has targeted and victimized innocent people for almost twenty years across China.

In mid-2006, the Coalition to Investigate the Persecution of Falun Gong in China (CIPFG) asked David Matas and me as volunteers to investigate claims of organ trafficking from Falun Gong practitioners. We released two reports and a book, *Bloody Harvest*, and have continued to investigate (Our revised report is available in 18 languages from www.david-kilgour.com). We concluded that for 41,500 transplants done in the years 2000-2005 in China, the sourcing beyond any doubt was Falun Gong prisoners of conscience.

Evidence
Here are two of the 18 kinds of evidence that led to our finding:

Investigators made many calls to hospitals, detention centres and other facilities across China claiming to be relatives of patients needing transplants and asking if they had organs of Falun Gong for sale. We obtained on tape and then transcribed and translated admissions that approximately 15 such facilities across the country were then trafficking in Falun Gong organs.

Falun Gong prisoners, who later got out of China, indicated that they were systematically blood-tested and organ-examined while in forced-labour camps across the country. Since they were tortured, this could not have been for their health, but was necessary for successful organ transplants and for building a bank of live "donors".

The Slaughter
Ethan Gutmann

Nobel Peace Prize nominee and co-founder of the International Coalition to end Organ Abuse in China Ethan Gutmann's 2014 book, *The Slaughter,* places the persecution of the Falun Gong, Tibetan, Uyghur, and Eastern Lightening Christian communities in context. He explains how he arrived at his "best estimate" that organs of 65,000 Falun Gong and "two to four thousand" Uyghurs, Tibetans and Christians were "harvested" in the 2000-2008 period

The closing words of *Slaughter* are addressed to responsible governments, organizations and persons: "No Western entity possesses the moral authority to allow the (P)arty to impede the excavation of a crime against humanity in exchange for promises of medical reform. As a survival mechanism of our species, we must contextualize, evaluate, and ultimately learn from every human descent into mass murder … The critical thing is that there is a history. And only the victims' families can absolve the (P)arty from its weight."

Mid-2016 Update
Matas, Gutmann and I released an *Update* on our two books in June 2016 in Washington, Ottawa and Brussels (accessible from the International Coalition to End Transplant Abuse in China www.endtransplantabuse.org).

- It provides a thorough examination of the transplant programs of hundreds of hospitals across China, drawing on medical journals, hospital websites, and deleted websites found in archives. It analyzes hospital revenues, bed counts and utilization rates, surgical personnel, state funding and other factors.
- We conclude cautiously that a minimum of 60,000 transplants per year are being done across China as of mid-2016, not the approximately 10,000 the government claims. There is a very small pool of 'volunteer donors' plus a few thousand convicted prisoners. This means that about 150 persons daily are killed for their organs.
- We provide much evidence of a state-directed organ transplantation network, controlled through national policies and funding, and implicating both the military and civilian healthcare systems.

The party-state's current narrative asserts that all transplantation organs since Jan 2015 are voluntarily provided through the semantical trick of reclassifying prisoner organs as "voluntary donations".

Professionals who should know better, including the World Health Organization, the Transplantation Society (TTS) and the Pontifical Academy of Sciences, have accepted the party line, skipping over, as Louisa Greve of the International Coalition to End Transplant Abuse in China puts it (www.endtransplantabuse.org), "the admission that China's billion-dollar transplant industry was built on prisoners' organs".

Last fall, after a screening of the Peabody award-winning film *Human Harvest* at a theatre in Boston's Harvard Square, I stressed points made earlier by my colleague David Matas (http://endtransplantabuse.org/party-profession-organ-transplant-abuse-china/):

- Mental health professionals globally faced the abuse of psychiatry in the Soviet Union and acted strongly against it. Today, international transplant professionals face the abuse of transplant surgery in China, but their response differs.
- The global transplantation profession today can be broken into three groups.
  - The aware who have read the research and realize that what is going on in China with transplantations is mass killing of innocents and cover up. They react accordingly, distancing themselves from the Chinese transplant profession and encouraging others to do likewise.
  - The naive do not consider the research and argue that doing so falls outside their area of responsibility. They hear research conclusions on the one hand and party-state propaganda on the other and draw no conclusions.
  - The foolish buy Chinese party-state propaganda. They parrot its line that the research demonstrating mass killing of innocents is based on rumour. They echo the Party line that the research is unverifiable, though it is both verifiable and verified. They repeat its claim that abuses are in the past, when they are not.
- The global transplant leadership does not have the time to read research into transplant abuse in China, or the grace to invite researchers to the events they help organize, but they might at least listen to what they themselves are saying.
- People in China, especially state officials, who deviate from the Party line get arrested. That is pervasive across all areas of policy, and not just something which happens in the transplantation field. They are released only if they undertake, after release, to conform to the Party line. There is no other basis for release, except for extreme illness. For foreign transplant leaders

to take at face value what a released official says, without investigation or verification, means that they too are adopting the Party line.

- Outside China, organ sources are either dead (at least brain dead) before the sourcing or alive both before and afterwards. China is the only country where sources are killed by organ extraction, and where sources are alive before and dead afterwards.

There is an equation here of Chinese law and policy with practice, showing a lack of awareness that the law in China cannot be enforced against the Party, since it controls all aspects of the enforcement of the legal system... The four organizations (World Health Organization (WHO), the Vatican's Pontifical Academy of Sciences (PAS), The Transplantation Society (TTS) and the Declaration of Istanbul Custodian Group (DICG)) are pleased that the Party says what they want to hear.

Beijing has no credible answers to the work of independent researchers who have demonstrated the mass killings of innocents. Given the scale of the transplantation industry in China, it is impossible to deny this research in any credible manner. Party propaganda, denying official data, pretending what is there is not there, can persuade only the gullible or the willfully blind. One can only hope that a willingness to confront the truth about China will prevail generally in the transplantation profession before many more innocents are killed for their organs.

Forced Labour Camps

David Matas and I visited a dozen countries to interview Falun Gong practitioners who had managed to leave both the camps and China. These prisoners of conscience have been the major source of organs since 2001 across China. They told us of working in appalling conditions for up to sixteen hours daily in these camps with no pay and little food, crowded sleeping conditions and torture. Inmates make a range of export consumer products as subcontractors to multinational companies. This constitutes gross corporate irresponsibility and a violation of WTO rules, calling for an effective response by all trading partners of China.

The Honourable David Kilgour, J.D.

(www.david-kilgour.com)

David Kilgour is the former Secretary of State for Latin America and Africa (1997-2002) and Asia-Pacific (2002-2003) in the cabinet of Prime Minister Jean Chretien. He represented south-east Edmonton in the House of Commons from 1979 to 2006 during eight Parliaments. He was born in 1941 in Winnipeg. Graduating from high school with the Governor General's medal, he studied economics at the University of Manitoba and graduated from the University of Toronto Faculty of Law. He later did doctoral studies in constitutional law at the Faculty of Law at the Sorbonne in Paris.

Mr. Kilgour's passion for multi-party democracy, human rights and justice for all began in community service. He stepped down as a Member of Parliament in 2006 to become an advocate for human dignity and good governance internationally. He and David Matas were nominated in 2010 for the Nobel Peace Prize for their book, *Bloody Harvest*, and campaign to end party-state-run organ abuse across China.

He is a volunteer at the Ottawa Mission for homeless men and a member of its Foundation. He is co-chair of the NGO Canadian Friends of a Democratic Iran, a Senior Fellow of both the Raoul Wallenberg Centre for Human Rights and the Macdonald Laurier Institute. He also sits on the boards of the Helsinki-based First Step Forum, Ethiopiaid Canada, the Educational Foundation of the Canadian Association of Former Parliamentarians, and the session of Westminster Church. He is married to Laura Scott Kilgour. They have three daughters and a son and live in Ottawa.

https://chinatribunal.com/wp-content/uploads/2019/04/April_Matas_Kilgour_Gutmann_ResponseMarkField.pdf

Summary of oral testimony: 6th April 2019
I was asked by a group in Washington if I would take an independent look at FG in China. Matas and I did a report in 2006 and concluded to our horror that 41,000 FG had been killed between 2001 and 06 for their organs. We then wrote Bloody Harvest

I was a prosecutor for 10 years so I should know something about the evidence and in my view a jury in Britain or any place hearing the evidence we have amassed with Ethan Gutmann as well is overwhelming and it is increasing across China. So it is dismaying when people ignore [it] and your Prime Minister is not the only one to say they don't have enough evidence.

[How the report identifies that 150 people are killed each day in China] We believe on a cautious minimum that 60,000 human beings are being killed a year. We think it is very much higher than that. And that is happening to prisoners of conscience in

China today. We know it from day one that we have to be extremely cautious and have to have proof of absolutely everything. We have looked at Tianjin hospital and estimate that it is a minimum of 5,000 transplant operations a year. We have said, based on the update, that it is a minimum of 60,000 a year.

[How the report authors know that this is the only country where it is happening] We explain clearly that there is back alley transplant, but in all 196 countries that exist there is only one that is run by the government, and that is China. The doctors get a lot of money, so there is a fee system and we explain clearly that the fee system is run by China.

Your joint statement of 7th April 2019 (with Matas and Gutmann).

I have seen the text of the debate. There is reference to his officials studying the report carefully. No I don't think any of us were [approached for comment]. It was not just Britain where this happens where they say there is not enough evidence. We ask if they have read the update and they say they have not. As soon as they say it is happening, they have to do something so they have to say there isn't enough evidence. If you look at the update you would have no doubt that it is happening so it hurts when people of good will say there is not enough evidence because there is an abundance of evidence. The only thing that the Embassy of China in Ottawa could rebut was a city in the wrong province so they can't rebut the rest of the evidence so they say that because there is a city in the wrong place and that is all they can say.

[Direct question: Mr Field, in the debate on 26th March, stated that as authors you acknowledge the following about your report and we will take each in turn shortly: As authors you acknowledge that there is a lack of incontrovertible evidence of wrongdoing;
The authors made clear that they had no smoking gun;
That there is a less than rigorous research technique applied;
That you still make assumptions;
that you have to infer the scale of organ transplant systems from hospital promotional material.]

Yes, people make these statements when we're not around. What they want is a smoking scalpel. The "donor" is dead, and their body is incinerated, and the doctor has committed murder, the scalpel has been cleaned. This is not television we are talking about.

[to Characterise the comments made] I try to be polite about it. I was a minister for 7 years and I know how departments have to work. Saying it is incontrovertible they can say they don't have enough evidence. Anyone who has read the book and the update has no doubt. There are still people in some ministries who have to say they haven't seen enough evidence and if you ask them they will say that they haven't read the report, they are intellectually lazy or don't want to see it.

You were not just a minister, but a Secretary of State which matches the same level of seniority in this country?

Correct.

Mark Field, who made the observations in parliament, a junior ranking minster made comments about your work. As a western democrat, before a minister makes a statement criticising conclusions of this gravity, would you expect a detailed analysis of the evidence?

Yes, the very least.

If as is the case here we have written to him asking him to provide the written analysis, would you count it as his duty?

Yes but I am sure 6 months will go by and it won't be done. I don't believe study of the evidence has been done since 2006.

And further, given a minister of that rank says these things in a public setting, would you expect him to be available to give evidence to a tribunal of this admittedly formal character?

The last thing on earth he is going to do is appear in this tribunal because you will make him look lazy, foolish irresponsible whatever, but trust me in my 7 years in the ministry, he is doing what someone on the China desk is telling him to do, Minister, say it is inconclusive. We are doing our best to ask him to study it and telling him he has a duty to Britain and his constituents to study it.

You would accept that bad behaviour by a government in what it says about OH is no evidence in itself contrary to China?

Yes, indeed, of course it is just, I wish I could tell you some of the things we have heard. You have to be honest; I am ashamed that a Minister from Britain would make a statement like that.

But it doesn't add to evidence of malpractice in China?

No, it doesn't.

Your evidence, the first book and the update. You have explained how you got involved but tell us what is the strength of your conclusions that you have drawn in the update.

Your tribunal will know this. The Government of China put out the narrative that it stopped in 1st January 2015. Our update was September 2016. If you go through it, it shows escalating industry, number of hospitals increasing so it is preposterous to say it stopped in January 2015. The momentum has kept growing, the traffic is increasing. I presume that you will be looking at the Uyghur community. I believe Ethan Gutmann has identified the number who have been tested and I shudder to think what is happening to that community.

When you finished the update what was the strength of your opinion?

Overwhelming evidence that it is increasing.

Any doubt?

None whatsoever. I believe most juries would be out for 10 minutes looking at this.

Have you stayed in close contact with these materials?

I was in Greece recently, we travel talking about this, write articles, give speeches always seeking to obtain new witnesses. As I said I am terrified about what is happening to the Uyghur community. Enver Tohti in 1995 was asked to take the heart out of a prisoner and I can't prove it but I am very worried about that community now.

Since your conclusions in 2016, in the update, have you been aware of material that could justify a diminution in your opinion?

Noting other than that this vastly human organ industry is growing in China.

Since you started working on this have China engaged you on the issue?

Yes, once someone came to the university, read out from a piece of paper something he had from the local Consulate. But no serious attempt to refute what we have said; they have nothing to say. They accuse us of being anti-China, but we are trying to get this thing to stop. That is how feeble their intellectual argument is.

From April 3rd China news headlines, for example "China sees more body donors", is that a response to this issue or a trend in China?

This is propaganda; we all know that very few people in China will donate organs. In 2010 it was about a few hundred that were donated and given the volumes of transplants that barely makes a dent in the need for organs in China.

The allegation is of mass murder on a significant scale, you describe it as an inconvenient truth. Is the failure by the UK government, amongst others, a deliberate attempt not to engage on this, in other words, is it wilful ignorance?

Yes. It is a sad thing to say but I am absolutely convinced that it is a wilful ignorance. It is choosing not to say anything. I think when our update came up we are accused of being stooges of the FG community. Well, none of us is FG, we are independent people who did this as volunteers. We have applied the skills we have to the evidence and have come to this conclusion. In a democratic world, governments are supposed to look at evidence and have the courage and intellectual vigour to read it. But instead they say they aren't satisfied that there is enough evidence. We could give them Mount Everest and they would say it would not be enough. At some stage it becomes good faith and it is a shame that your government has not shown the sort of good faith that one expects from one of the great democracies of the world.

Which governments are doing the best?

I get asked that a lot. I give full credit to European Parliament; their motion was unanimous. The House of Representatives in USA. Canadian Senate bill if before election will make organ tourism illegal, the Czech Senate has just passed a measure dealing with this. The leader is Taiwan, and a lot of people from Taiwan were traveling there. Israel did it first, to their credit, Norway has done something, Spain are quite good. Britain and Canada are two of the major democracies doing the least. And that makes me very sad.

We have heard from people who pose as someone looking for a transplant or as an official from the 610 Office to get information. What credibility do you attach this?

We were concerned so we engaged an independent interpreter to go over the tapes. We didn't use them all of course but we have enough that anyone who has time to look at them will see a clear pattern to get FG who are healthy and considered the best so-called donors. That is one of the major 30 types of evidence we have. Annie, who sort of blew the whistle on this, whose husband had removed corneas, then if you don't like that evidence look at the phone calls and if you don't like the phone calls look at the Update and at some stage you will see the evidence is overwhelming.

Witness 54: Kim Hyunchul

On October 20th 2017, I met an ethnic Korean Chinese nurse at the lobby located on the first floor of Tianjin First Central Hospital. She brought us to the tenth floor for VIPs, opened a door manipulating by security cards given to specially authorized people, and introduced a kidney transplant surgeon to us in the room located at the end of the 10th floor's hall. She showed the documents that we prepared from Korea on behalf of a patient to check the possibility of transplant in their hospital. We asked the doctor the possibility, the waiting length of time, the method shortening waiting time. The nurse answered that the transplant is possible, the average of waiting time, and informed us that we can shorten the waiting time to a maximum of three months and minimum of two weeks by donating money to the hospital.

She also said that a Korean patient took a liver transplant and was admitted in the hospital for recovery and a Korean patient is waiting for kidney plus pancreas transplants at the same time as many foreigners came and took transplants. In addition, she showed us a hotel through a window which was prepared across the street from the hospital for patients and their families during the period for the pre & post-transplant care. She let us enter a room where a Middle East Asian patient and family members stayed to wait for transplants and said that currently many patients came from Middle East.

On October 21st 2017, we could meet a Korean patient and his wife waiting for transplant at a room in the hotel building showed to us by the nurse.

The nurse introduced them to us. They said that they came from Korea since the husband needed a kidney and pancreas transplant at the same time.

On October 23rd 2017, we met a patient who took a liver transplant and was recovering with her son. She said that she could take the transplant two months later after she arrived in the hospital.

Our documentary team was possibly able to pass all these procedures and produced the documentary because we were provided a patient's real documents who is in the waiting list for transplants in Korea who was asking about the possibility for the patient to take a transplant in the Tianjin hospital as we showed in medical reports on blood exams, CT, and a Doctor's note.

https://chinatribunal.com/wp-content/uploads/2019/04/April_Submission_-Kim-Hyun-Chul.pdf

https://vimeo.com/280284321

https://chinatribunal.com/wp-content/uploads/2019/06/KoreanWebpages
WhereTheDocumentaryTeamHadClues.pdf

https://chinatribunal.com/wp-content/uploads/2019/06/The-letter-from-the-online-club-to-Shen-Zhongyang.pdf

https://chinatribunal.com/wp-content/uploads/2019/06/The-reply-from-Shen-Zhongyang-to-the-online-club.pdf

Summary of oral testimony: 7th April 2019

On 21 October 2017, I started to investigate the First Central Hospital in [Shenzhen/Tgianjin] because I found a particularly large number of Korean patients going to this particular hospital for organ transplants. The numbers of people going there had started to increase and this is why I started to investigate. I met three Korean patients in there. One was recovering from a kidney transplant and another was waiting for surgery and was in need of a pancreas and kidney. I heard of another patient who also came to receive surgery, but I never met him.

[Conditions of patients and how they got transplants] One elderly lady I met was in recovery and seemed well. Her family were introduced to the hospital by unknown personnel and that is how she became connected to the hospital.

The patients were unaware of origins [of the organs] and I and my team were unaware. None of us actually asked.

[Waiting time for] I consulted a Chinese nurse and she said any time between two weeks and longest would be three months. I asked the patients and they said it would not take more than 3 months.

[Information required by the patient before transplant, blood type etc] My team acquired a medical chart from a patient who had his name on a waiting list in Korea and they used it and when asking the hospital for information. In general, I know that Korean patients would go over there first and then have a physical examination then they check if the organs are available.

Yes [they have to wait two weeks to three months from when they arrive in China].

[How is it paid for] The expenses are paid for by the patients. Before they go, they have a rough idea of cost of the organs and then get consulted in China. Before receiving surgery, they have to pay. When I was investigating, I heard that there were lots of people coming from the Middle East. Their own embassies pay for the patients' transplants.

[Cost to a Korean family of a transplant] US$170,000 for a liver transplant and there are living costs to pay for whilst they wait for the surgery and afterwards.

[Waiting time for a liver transplant in Korea] Minimum five years.

I am not certain that it is widely known in South Korea [that organs are available] but the Korean patients who are waiting for surgery are aware and are going over to China.

It seems like doctors make recommendations and the recipients then spread the word after their surgeries [that is how they become aware of organ availability in China]. The patients that have come back to Korea have made their own group and they have regular meetings and a website.

I cannot estimate [the scale of people going to China] but in October 2017 when I visited the hospital there were 3 patients so if someone can do the maths, this will give an indication of the scale.

I am not sure if [the website that patients were on] still exists especially after my own investigation and documentary came out. It is more like a social network. I still think they have regular offline meetings to this day.

I think that the patients would not have bothered to ask [about the origin of the organ] but when I asked the medical staff they did not tell me the source.

During my trip to the hospital and while we were investigating, I saw Middle Eastern people and whilst I saw them being shown to their rooms the nurse mentioned that there were lots of people coming from the Middle East and, unlike Korea, their own embassies were paying. She also mentioned that the way they handled business was very neat.

[How he knew that Korean patients were going to the First Central Hospital inShenzhen/Tianjin] The information came from the AEIOT which is a group in Korea. The President of the AEIOT informed me about the [Shenzhen/Tianjin] hospital and said that a lot of Korean patients were going there. I then went there and confirmed this.

I did ask the medical staff [at Shenzhen/Tianjin where the organs came from] but they did not give me a clear answer. At the beginning they didn't want to answer the question and later they said it was by donation.

I did meet two Korean doctors who were sending their patients to China. They said they were unaware of the origin of the source of the organs. They then said they are not doing that anymore. The doctors said they were unwilling to answer that question [why they were not doing that any more] and stated they did not want to participate in the interview anymore. It is too difficult to say whether I did or not [feel that the doctors were suspicious about the sources].

[My documentary came out] After October 2017. There was no direct [public] feedback, so this is difficult to answer [the question of how the public responded]. [The indirect feedback] The public was surprised at the number of Korean patients travelling to receive surgery and they were wondering about the source of the organs.

I regret that I cannot express my personal conclusion, and this is because I am still representing the media organisation.

[What research revealed before visiting China] I understand that this counsel is very interested in the source of the organs and we too were interested in that, but we were also interested in a machine called the "brain killer/brain striker": we wanted to know if this still existed. We were able to meet in person the partner of a company who co-developed this machine. We also found out from this interview that the machine still exists in China, but the partner said he did not have the authority to show us. They said they did human experiments whilst they were developing the machine, but they were not able to confirm any facts about the source of the organs.

The people who participated in the interviews all cut all ties with me and the team other than a lady who appears at the end of the program. She was a Falun Gong practitioner's daughter and now she has also cut ties. There are a few people still in touch who helped with the research.

I am unsure [whether availability of organs in China has changed] but I think that the group who received the organs in China and the Head of the Organ Transplant Centre are still in touch.

It is difficult to conclude that it [the machine causing brain death] is still being used but it still exists.

Appendix 2B. Expert Witnesses: Documents Submitted

W. No.	Name	Document	Date	Link
29	Dr David Matas	Bloody Harvest	2009	http://endtransplantabuse.org/2006-report/
		An Update – 2016	2016 March	www.endtransplantabuse.org/an-update
		Magnitsky Act Submission	2018	https://chinatribunal.com/wp-content/ uploads/2019/06/MagnitskySubmission_ OfficialsSurgeons_Final.pdf
		Crossborder Transplant Abuse	2018	https://chinatribunal.com/wp-content/ uploads/2019/06/MatasPPT.pdf
				https://chinatribunal.com/wp-content/ uploads/2019/03/A10_Submission_ DrDavidMatas_PD.pdf
30	Dr Zhiyuan Wang	Submission to the Tribunal	Dec 2018	https://chinatribunal.com/wp-content/ uploads/2019/04/WOIPFG_DrWang.zip
31	Dr Jacob Lavee	The Impact of Use of Organs	Nov 2018	https://chinatribunal.com/wp-content/ uploads/2019/03/A02_B_State-Organs-Prof-Jacob-Lavee-.pdf
				https://chinatribunal.com/wp-content/ uploads/2019/03/A02_A_Submission_ ProfJacobLavee_PD.pdf
32	Clive Ansley	China Legal System	Dec 2018	https://chinatribunal.com/wp-content/ uploads/2019/04/Clive-Ansley_Submission_ Report.pdf
		Response to the Tribunal's questions	April 2019	https://chinatribunal.com/wp-content/ uploads/2019/05/CliveAnsley_response_ May_.pdf

W. No.	Name	Document	Date	Link
33	Sarah Cook	Freedom House Report	Feb 2017	https://freedomhouse.org/report/china-religious-freedom https://chinatribunal.com/wp-content/uploads/2019/04/Cook-Freedom-House-Organ-Transplant-Abuse-letter-11.20.2018.pdf
34	Matthew Robertson	Profiles of Chinese Transplant Surgeons	Oct 2018	https://chinatribunal.com/wp-content/uploads/2019/06/12_SurgeonProfileOne_ZhengShusen.pdf https://chinatribunal.com/wp-content/uploads/2019/03/A04_Submission_MatthewRobertson_PD.pdf
35	Ethan Gutmann	The Slaughter An Update – 2016	2014 2016	https://endtransplantabuse.org/2014-report/ www.endtransplantabuse.org/an-update https://chinatribunal.com/wp-content/uploads/2019/04/EthanGutmann.pdf
36	David Li Dr Huige Li (COHRC)	Medical Genocide	28 Nov 2018	https://chinatribunal.com/wp-content/uploads/2019/04/COHRC_SubmissionCover-Letter_COHRC-DavidLi.pdf https://chinatribunal.com/wp-content/uploads/2019/04/COHRC_Independent-Tribunal-_Statement-of-Facts-Application-to-Law_20181128_Submited.pdf
37	Dr Huige Li	Live Organ Harvesting	Dec 2018	https://chinatribunal.com/wp-content/uploads/2019/03/A11_Submission_DrHuigeLi_PD.pdf

W. No.	Name	Document	Date	Link
38	Edward McMillan-Scott	Interview with a victim	9 Dec 2013	https://chinatribunal.com/wp-content/ uploads/2019/06/Edward-McMillan-Scott-supplementary-material-submitted-to-the-Tribunal.pdf
		Original interview – torture survivor	13 Sep 2007	https://chinatribunal.com/wp-content/ uploads/2019/06/Edward-McMillan-Scott-supplementary-material-submitted-to-the-Tribunal.pdf
		Gao Zhisheng Interview	12 Dec 2007	https://chinatribunal.com/wp-content/ uploads/2019/06/Edward-McMillan-Scott-supplementary-material-submitted-to-the-Tribunal.pdf
		EMS slamming Chinese envoy	31 Oct 2010	https://chinatribunal.com/wp-content/ uploads/2019/06/Edward-McMillan-Scott-supplementary-material-submitted-to-the-Tribunal.pdf
		EMS / EU Parliament	20 Jun 2013	https://chinatribunal.com/wp-content/ uploads/2019/06/Edward-McMillan-Scott-supplementary-material-submitted-to-the-Tribunal.pdf
		Gao Zhisheng's daughter appeals to EU	5 Dec 2013	https://chinatribunal.com/wp-content/ uploads/2019/06/Edward-McMillan-Scott-supplementary-material-submitted-to-the-Tribunal.pdf
				https://chinatribunal.com/wp-content/ uploads/2019/06/Edward-McMillan-Scott-supplementary-material-submitted-to-the-Tribunal.pdf
				https://chinatribunal.com/wp-content/ uploads/2019/04/McMillan-Scott_ PERSECUTION_OF_FALUN_GONG_BY_ THE_BEIJING_REGIME_FINAL.pdf
39	Prof Wendy Rogers	Additional information on the number of transplants	2 Jan 2019	https://chinatribunal.com/wp-content/ uploads/2019/04/ProfWendyRogers_Witness-statement3.pdf
				https://chinatribunal.com/wp-content/ uploads/2019/04/ProfWendyRogers_ Appendix-to-witness-statement2.pdf
			5 Feb 20190	https://chinatribunal.com/wp-content/ uploads/2019/06/Additional-information-supplied-to-the-China-Tribunal-by-Wendy-Rogers.pdf
		BMJ Open, Scoping Review Compliance of Chinese Transplant Articles with Ethical Standards		https://chinatribunal.com/wp-content/ uploads/2019/06/BMJ_Open_ ComplianceEthicalStandardsIn ReportingDonorSourcesPeerReviewed PublicationsInvolvingOrganTransplantation InChina.pdf

W. No.	Name	Document	Date	Link
40	Yiyang Xia	Treatment of FG Appendices	April 2019	https://chinatribunal.com/wp-content/uploads/2019/04/April_HRLF_01-Letter-to-Independent-Tribunal.pdf
		A.610 office		https://chinatribunal.com/wp-content/uploads/2019/05/HRLF_610_Office.pdf
		B. Role of Jiang Zemin		https://chinatribunal.com/wp-content/uploads/2019/04/April_HRLF_02-Exhibit-B-Jiang-Zemin.pdf
		C. Illegality of crackdown		https://chinatribunal.com/wp-content/uploads/2019/04/April_HRLF_03-Exhibit-C-EP-Hearing.pdf
		D. Brainwashing		https://chinatribunal.com/wp-content/uploads/2019/04/April_HRLF_04-Exhibit-D-Brainwashing.pdf
		E. Anti-cult alliance		https://chinatribunal.com/wp-content/uploads/2019/04/April_HRLF_05-Exhibit-E-Zhang-Jingrong-v-Chinese-AntiCult-World-Alliance.pdf
		F. Campaign against FG		https://chinatribunal.com/wp-content/uploads/2019/05/JiangZemin_DouzhengCampaignAgainst_FG_HRLC.pdf
		G. JZ liable for torture		https://chinatribunal.com/wp-content/uploads/2019/05/JiangZeminLiableForTortureOfFG_HRLF.pdf
		H. How 610 Office works		https://chinatribunal.com/wp-content/uploads/2019/06/YiyangXia_How-does-610-work_en_YiyangXia.pdf
		Reply to Tribunal questions		https://chinatribunal.com/wp-content/uploads/2019/06/YiyangXia_Reply-to-Questions_YiyangXia.pdf
		Blood testing in police station		https://chinatribunal.com/wp-content/uploads/2019/06/YiyangXia_Article-1_Liugezhuang_Shandong-Province_translated.pdf
		Door knocking harassment		https://chinatribunal.com/wp-content/uploads/2019/06/YiyangXia_Article-2_Door-knocking-harrassment_translated.pdf
		Forced blood samples in homes		https://chinatribunal.com/wp-content/uploads/2019/06/YiyangXia_Article-3_Xintai-City_Zhu-Xiulin_translated.pdf

W. No.	Name	Document	Date	Link
41	Didi Kirsten Tatlow	Submission	Feb 2019	https://chinatribunal.com/wp-content/uploads/2019/06/DidiKirstenTatlow_Submission.pdf https://chinatribunal.com/wp-content/uploads/2019/06/Debate-Flares-Over-China%E2%80%99s-Inclusion-at-Vatican-Organ-Trafficking-Meeting-The-New-York-Times.pdf https://chinatribunal.com/wp-content/uploads/2019/06/DKT_Angry-Claims-and-Furious-Denials-Over-Organ-Transplants-in-China-The-New-York-Times.pdf https://chinatribunal.com/wp-content/uploads/2019/06/DKT_Choice-of-Hong-Kong-for-Organ-Transplant-Meeting-Is-Defended-The-New-York-Times.pdf https://chinatribunal.com/wp-content/uploads/2019/06/DKT_Debate-Flares-on-China%E2%80%99s-Use-of-Prisoners%E2%80%99-Organs-as-Experts-Meet-in-Hong-Kong-The-New-York-Times.pdf
42	Dr Zhiyuan Wang	New Evidence of Live Organ Transplant	April 2019	https://chinatribunal.com/wp-content/uploads/2019/06/WOIPFG-Investigation-Report_NewEvidence_2018.pdf
		Instructions to check the phone calls (ETAC)	May 2019	https://chinatribunal.com/wp-content/uploads/2020/02/Phone-call-content-verification-report.pdf
		Phone call verification report – independent academics (ETAC)	May 2019	https://chinatribunal.com/wp-content/uploads/2020/02/PhoneCallsVerification_AcademicCommentators_15May.pdf
43	Yukiharu Takahashi	Japanese Organ Tourism to China	April 2019	https://chinatribunal.com/wp-content/uploads/2019/04/April_Yukiharu-Takahashi-Submission_-Japan.pdf https://chinatribunal.com/wp-content/uploads/2019/06/Yukiharu_Takshashi_Correction-on-my-testimony.pdf

W. No.	Name	Document	Date	Link
44	Matthew Robertson & Dr Raymond Hinde	Analysis of China Organ Donation	Jan 2019	https://chinatribunal.com/wp-content/uploads/2020/02/Robertson_Hinde_Lavee_AnalysisOfOfficialDeceased-OrganDonationDataCastsDoubtOnTheCredibilityOfChinasOrganTransplantReform.pdf
		Comments by Prof. Spiegelhalter	June 2019	https://chinatribunal.com/wp-content/uploads/2019/06/Commentary-on-Robertson-et-al-Spiegelhalter.pdf
	Matthew Robertson	VOC report on WOIPFG Phone Calls	May 2019	https://chinatribunal.com/wp-content/uploads/2020/02/Authentication-and-Analysis-of-Purported-Undercover-Telephone-Calls-Made-to-Hospitals-in-China-on-the-Topic-of-Organ-Trafficking_MatthewRobertson_VOCWorkingPaper.pdf
45	Prof Maria Fiatarone Singh	Organ Transplantation	April 2019	https://chinatribunal.com/wp-content/uploads/2019/04/April_Prof-Maria-Fiatarone-Singh-MD-FRACP.pdf
		CV		https://chinatribunal.com/wp-content/uploads/2019/04/April_Prof-Maria-Fiatarone-Singh_CV-2018.pdf
46	Dr Maya Mitalipova	DNA Sequencing of Uyghurs	April 2019	https://chinatribunal.com/wp-content/uploads/2019/06/April_Submission_Maya-Mitalipova.pdf
47	Dr Torsten Trey	Forced Organ Harvesting	Jan 2019	https://chinatribunal.com/wp-content/uploads/2019/04/April_2019-DAFOH-Report-on-Forced-Organ-Harvesting-in-China.pdf
48	Dr David Matas	Response to Mark Field MP	April 2019	https://chinatribunal.com/wp-content/uploads/2019/04/April_Matas_Kilgour_Gutmann_ResponseMarkField.pdf
		Response to Australian Parliament Inquiry	2017	https://chinatribunal.com/wp-content/uploads/2019/06/Response_-CompassionNotCommerce_AustGovtReport_Rogers_Matas_Hughes.pdf
49	Ethan Gutmann	Response re Mark Field MP	April 2019	https://chinatribunal.com/wp-content/uploads/2019/04/April_Matas_Kilgour_Gutmann_ResponseMarkField.pdf
50	Dr James Shapiro	Alberta University & Zhejiang University Fourth Affiliated Hospital	Jan 2019	https://chinatribunal.com/wp-content/uploads/2019/04/April_DrJamesShapiro.pdf

W. No.	Name	Document	Date	Link
51	Dr Charles Lee	Source of Organ Donation in China China Liver Transplant Registry 2006 Report PLA Article – English/Chinese	March 2019	https://chinatribunal.com/wp-content/uploads/2019/04/April_CharlesLee_Testimony.London.Tribunal.pdf https://chinatribunal.com/wp-content/uploads/2019/06/CharlesLee_SupplemataryMaterial.pdf https://chinatribunal.com/wp-content/uploads/2019/06/Charles-Lee_English_PLA_HHRG-114-FA16-20160623-SD002.pdf https://chinatribunal.com/wp-content/uploads/2019/06/Charles-Lee_liver.annual.2006.report.pdf https://chinatribunal.com/wp-content/uploads/2019/06/Charles-Lee_PLA.2%E7%82%AE%E5%8C%BB%E9%99%A2.01.pdf
52	Dolkun Isa	FOH of Uyghurs	Dec 2017	https://chinatribunal.com/submissions/world-uyghur-congress-_-wuc-president-speaks-on-organ-harvesting-at-roundtable-in-the-uk-parliament/
53	David Kilgour	Bloody Harvest Response re Mark Field MP An Update 2016	April 2019	https://chinatribunal.com/wp-content/uploads/2019/04/April_Tribunal_Submission_DavidKilgour_-jan-2019.pdf PDF Download – http://endtransplantabuse.org/2006-report/ https://chinatribunal.com/wp-content/uploads/2019/04/April_Matas_Kilgour_Gutmann_ResponseMarkField.pdf www.endtransplantabuse.org/an-update
54	Kim Hyunchul	Documentary – The dark side of transplant tourism in China: Killing to live Korean Webpages and letters Letter from the online club to Shen Zhongyang Reply from Shen Zhongyang	April 2019	https://chinatribunal.com/wp-content/uploads/2019/04/April_Submission_-Kim-Hyun-Chul.pdf https://vimeo.com/280284321 https://chinatribunal.com/wp-content/uploads/2019/06/KoreanWebpagesWhereTheDocumentaryTeamHadClues.pdf https://chinatribunal.com/wp-content/uploads/2019/06/The-letter-from-the-online-club-to-Shen-Zhongyang.pdf https://chinatribunal.com/wp-content/uploads/2019/06/The-reply-from-Shen-Zhongyang-to-the-online-club.pdf

Appendix 3. Prereading Material Submitted by ETAC

Category	Title	Description/Pages to View	Date	Author	Link
Pre-reading materials submitted by ETAC to the China Tribunal					
Category 1: Introductory Material					
1. Overview/ Introduction	Organ Procurement and Extrajudicial Execution: A Summary of the Evidence	Overview Document: The introduction of this paper was provided to the Tribunal as a draft before publication	2018	Matthew Robertson	https://victimsof communism.org/ publication/china-organ-procurement-report-2020/
2. Introduction Video	Hard to Believe Documentary	Hard to Believe is a multi-award winning documentary that examines the issue of forced live organ harvesting from Chinese prisoners of conscience, and the response-or lack of it-around the world. Includes interviews with numerous experts and investigators including Dr Enver Tohti and Prof Jacob Lavee. NOTE – this film was released before the 'Update' report in 2016.	2015	Two-time Emmy Award winning director/ producer, Ken Stone and Irene Silber	www. hardtobelievemovie. com
3. Introduction Video	Medical Genocide – 10 min version (20 min version also available)	A short documentary providing information on the 'Update' report released in 2016	2017	China Organ Harvest Research Centre	https://www. youtube.com/ watch?v=-I5QDPQbEjo &feature =youtu.be
4. Investigation	The Slaughter: Mass Killings, Organ Harvesting, and China's Secret Solution to Its Dissident Problem	8-year investigation – includes extensive witness testimony and provides a comprehensive overview	2014	Ethan Gutmann	hard copy provided https:// endtransplantabuse. org/2014-report/

		Pre-reading materials submitted by ETAC to the China Tribunal				
Category	**Title**	**Description/Pages to View**	**Date**	**Author**	**Link**
5. Investigation Video	Harvested Alive: 10 Year Investigation	Harvested Alive includes audios of a number of important telephone investigations. Indicated are timecodes for viewing the phone call investigation excerpts. Excerpts – 15 mins – Timecodes to watch are: 7:00 to 8:55; 9:53 to 10:39; 11:19 to 12:03; 37:26 to 47:00; 56:43 to 58:42	2017	Deer Park Productions	http://harvestedalive.com/?page_id=351&lang=en (scroll down on this page)
6. Investigation	A Hospital Built for Murder	Investigative report into transplant volumes at Tianjin First Central Hospital, the self-proclaimed largest transplant center in Asia, located in Tianjin city, about 100 miles southeast of Beijing	2016	Matthew Robertson	https://www.theepochtimes.com/china-hospital-built-for-murder_1958171.html
7. Investigation	An Update to Bloody Harvest and The Slaughter	**We have chosen 65 pages of essential reading (the remainder of the 680 p report can be used as a reference document)** **Volume Indicators section includes explanation of:** Media reports, hospital reports on volume, multiple transplant for the same patient, multiple transplants conducted simultaneously, short waiting times for organs, all types of transplants, experience of transplant patients, donors seeking recipients, high bed utilization waiting for beds, capacity expansion, overworked doctors and nurses, continued growth since 2006. **State Crime** section includes a few examples of phone call evidence. audios also available. Additional phone call examples are in Bloody Harvest, WOIPFG report and the documentary Harvested Alive: 10 Year Investigation. TO ACCESS THE FULL REPORT VISIT LINK ON RIGHT – scroll through the full report online to see the number of transplant facilities in China. Excerpts (72 pages) – Indicators – p 279 – 318; Wang Lijun's Human Body Experiments p 387 – 391; A State Crime p.400 – 423; Closing Recommendations/Conclusions p. 428 – 434 *(For examples of two hospitals see People's Liberation Army No '309' Hospital p.24 – 26; Shanghai Changzheng Hospital Affiliated with the Second Military Medical University p. 34-35)*	2016	David Kilgour, David Matas and Ethan Gutmann	https://endtransplantabuse.org/wp-content/uploads/2017/05/Bloody_Harvest-The_Slaughter-2016-Update-V3-and-Addendum-20170430.pdf

		Pre-reading materials submitted by ETAC to the China Tribunal			
Category	**Title**	**Description/Pages to View**	**Date**	**Author**	**Link**
8. Documentary Investigation Video	South Korean Documentary: The Dark Side of Transplant Tourism in China: Killing to Live	The "Investigative Report 7" team travelled to an unnamed hospital in Tianjin, China with the medical documents of a Korean man in need of a kidney to inquire about obtaining an organ for him. With hidden cameras they interviewed the head nurse and an elderly Korean patient who was recovering from a recent transplant operation. This documentary shows that organs are still readily available in China for transplant tourists. It also shows the brain stem killing machine continues to be developed. Excerpts – 14 mins – Interview with Korean transplant patient 1:44 to 2:30; Nurse explains availability of organs for Koreans 9:50 to 18:15	2017	TV Chosun	https://vimeo.com/280284321
9. Journal Article	Cold Genocide: Falun Gong in China	This article argues that the eradication campaign against Falun Gong is a cold genocide as it is: (1) multi-dimensional – the destruction of Falun Gong Practitioners is not only physical but psychological, social and spiritual; (2) subtle in terms of visibility; and it is (3) normalized in the society in which it takes place. INCLUDES: information on the 610 Office: *"The 610 Office is the primary entity responsible for organizing the eradication campaign against Falun Gong. The 610 Office operates extra-judicially; it is not an organ of the Chinese State, but rather of the Chinese Communist Party. The 610 Office directs all levels of State institutions including the judiciary, the civil service, business and education. It has overarching power and authority over all other Party entities and all State bodies. All State agencies and all other Party agencies have to comply with the 610 Office's directives and orders."*	2018	Cheung, Maria; Trey, Torsten; Matas, David; and An, Richard	http://scholarcommons.usf.edu/cgi/viewcontent.cgi?article=1513&context=gsp
10. Investigation	Bloody Harvest: The Killing of Falun Gong for their Organs –	The first investigation that took place in 2006	2006; book 2009	Dr David Matas, David Kilgour	PDF Download – http://endtransplantabuse.org/2006-report/

Pre-reading materials submitted by ETAC to the China Tribunal					
Category	Title	Description/Pages to View	Date	Author	Link
11. Journal Article Excerpt	State Organised Forced Organ Harvesting	Journal article (p.1 – 10) An overview of organ harvesting in China. Provides information on the Ethical Guidelines in Transplant Medicine, an overview of organ trafficking, an explanation on the difference between 'black market' and 'state organised' organ trafficking in China Excerpt: pages 1 – 10	2017	Dr David Matas and Dr Torsten Trey	https://www.uitgeverijparis.nl/scripts/read_article_pdf.php?id=1001349943
12. Report	Profiles on Chinese surgeons/ official: Zheng Shusen, Huang Jiefu	Backgrounders on Chinese surgeons/ officials implicated in forced organ harvesting	2018	Various	https://chinatribunal.com/wp-content/uploads/2019/10/12_SurgeonProfileOne_ZhengShusen.pdf https://chinatribunal.com/wp-content/uploads/2019/10/12_SurgeonProfileTwo_HuangJiefu.pdf
Category 2: Published Reports					
13. Report – NGO	Transplant Abuse Continues in China Despite Claims of Reform	See Foreword, Introduction, and Chapter IX (the final chapter, from p. 164) for comment on recent developments; the report condenses much of the evidence in the 2016 Update See the Overview (pp. 11-22) for a brief summary	2018	Grace Yin et al. (China Organ Harvest Research Center)	https://www.chinaorganharvest.org/app/uploads/2018/06/COHRC-2018-Report.pdf
14. Report – US Government	U.S. Commission on International Religious Freedom (USCIRF) Report	This 2018 report by the US Commission on International Religious Freedom (USCIRF) documents ongoing persecution of Falun Gong practitioners, and discusses the Vatican summit including statements made by Huang Jiefu (page 34)	2018	USCIRF	www.uscirf.gov/sites/default/files/2018 USCIRFAR.pdf
15. Report – NGO	Religious Revival, Repression, and Resistance under Xi Jinping: The Battle for China's Spirit.	Page 21: General reference to organ harvesting from prisoners of conscience; Section V (pp. 109-135,) describes the status of the persecution of the practice and its scale and significance with estimates of 20+ million Falun Gong in China, also contains some corroborative points on organ harvesting and a piece of new evidence	2017	Sarah Cook (Freedom House)	https://freedomhouse.org/report/china-religious-freedom

Category	Title	Description/Pages to View	Date	Author	Link
16. Report – UK Political Organisation	Forced Organ Harvesting in China	A general summary of the evidence and third party reporting on the issue	2016	UK Conservative Party Human Rights Commission	http://conservative humanrights.com/ reports/CPHRC_ ORGAN_ HARVESTING_ REPORT.pdf
17. Report – UK Political Organisation	The Darkest Moment: The Crackdown on Human Rights in China 2013-16	A compilation of human rights abuses in China with a section on organ harvesting	2016	UK Conservative Party Human Rights Commission	www.conservative humanrights.com/ reports/submissions/ CPHRC_China_ Human_Rights_ Report_Final.pdf
18. Report – US Government	Organ Harvesting: An Examination of a Brutal Practice	Lengthy testimony to US Congress by researchers and Dr. Francis Delmonico (for a guide to this episode, see "At Congressional Hearing, China's Organ Harvesting Seen Through Rose-Colored Glasses", Matthew Robertson, The Epoch Times: https://www.theepochtimes.com/ at-congressional-hearing-chinas-organ-harvesting-seen-through-rose-colored-glasses_2103475.html also listed below)	2016	US Committee on Foreign Affairs Joint Hearing	http://docs.house.gov/ meetings/FA/FA16/ 20160623/105116/ HHRG-114-FA16-20160623-SD006.pdf
19. Report – NGO	China: The Crackdown on Falun Gong and Other So-called "Heretical Organizations"	General background/reference material comprising one of the earliest pieces of human rights reporting on the anti-Falun Gong campaign	2000	Amnesty International	http://www.refworld. org/docid/3b83b6e00. html
20. Report – UN	Concluding Observations of the Committee Against Torture	UNCAT report presented to the Special Rapporteur on Torture regarding the persecution of Falun Gong practitioners and its coincidence with increases in China's transplant rates, with calls for investigation of claims regarding the torture and organ procurement from some Falun Gong practitioners and for measures to ensure that those responsible for such abuses are prosecuted and punished	2008	United Nations Committee Against Torture	https://drive.google. com/file//0Byxw XcZlX2dXdmtaS DNYVTlyR3c/ view?usp=sharing
21. Report – UN	Report of the Special Rapporteur on Torture and Other Cruel, Inhuman or Degrading Treatment or Punishment, Manfred Nowak	Excerpts from Manfred Nowak's key report on the anti-Falun Gong campaign and the extent of torture and other abuses. Includes references to organ harvesting	2006	Manfred Nowak (United Nations)	https:// endtransplantabuse. org/wp-content/ uploads/2017/07/ Torture-UN-07.pdf

	Pre-reading materials submitted by ETAC to the China Tribunal					
Category	Title	Description/Pages to View	Date	Author	Link	
22. Report – UN	Report of the Special Rapporteur on Extrajudicial, Summary or Arbitrary Executions	pp. 63-68 have some deaths of Falun Gong in custody	2008	Philip Alston, (United Nations)	https://chinatribunal. com/wp-content/ uploads/2019/01/ UNCAT-2008-comment-on-organ-harvesting.pdf	
23. Report – US Government	US Congressional – Executive Commission on China Annual Report	General background/ reference material	2016	US Congress	https://www.cecc. gov/publications/ annual-reports/2016-annual-report	
23. Report – NGO	The Origins and Long-Term Consequences of the Communist Party's Campaign against Falun Gong	General background/ reference material	2012	Sarah Cook (Freedom House)	https://freedomhouse. org/article/China-communist-party-campaign-against-falun-gong	
25. Report – NGO	Amnesty International Human Rights Report 2016/2017	General summary of human rights issues around the world	2017	Amnesty International	https://www.amnesty. org/en/documents/ pol10/4800/2017/en/	
26. Report – UK Political Organisation	Human Rights Report on Persecution of Falun Gong in China 2013-2016	Summary of statistics in the anti-Falun Gong campaign gathered on Minghui	2016	UK Conservative Party Human Rights Commission	http://conservative humanrights.com/ reports/submissions/ Falun_Gong_ Submission_Human_ Rights.pdf	
27. Report – NGO	Human Rights in China: Part 3; Part 4	General background/reference material	2016	Gao Zhisheng	http://www.csw. org.uk/2017/10/16/ report/3754/article. htm	

Category	Title	Description/Pages to View	Date	Author	Link

Pre-reading materials submitted by ETAC to the China Tribunal

Category 3: Published Research and Expert Statements

Category	Title	Description/Pages to View	Date	Author	Link
28. Additional reporting/ research	Analysis of Official Data Casts Doubts on Credibility of China's Organ Transplant Reform	Forensic statistical methods were used to examine key deceased organ donation datasets from 2010 to 2018. Two central-level datasets — published by the China Organ Transplant Response System (COTRS) and the Red Cross Society of China — are tested for evidence of manipulation, including conformance to simple mathematical formulae, arbitrary internal ratios, the presence of anomalous data artefacts, and cross-consistency. Provincial-level data in five regions are tested for coherence, consistency, and plausibility, and individual hospital data in those provinces are examined for consistency with provincial-level data.	2018	Matthew P. Robertson, Raymond L. Hinde, Jacob Lavee (BMC Medical Ethics)	https://chinatribunal.com/wp-content/uploads/2020/02/Robertson_Hinde_Lavee_Analysis OfOfficialDeceased-OrganDonationData CastsDoubtOnThe CredibilityOfChinas OrganTransplant Reform.pdf
29. Additional reporting/ NGO submission	Canadian Magnitsky Act Submission	Profiles of a number of key individuals involved in the anti-Falun Gong campaign and organ transplantation in China, prepared by the Falun Dafa Association of Canada in their submission on the Canadian Magnitsky Act	2018	Falun Dafa Association of Canada and David Matas (with one profile prepared by Matthew Robertson included)	https://chinatribunal.com/wp-content/uploads/2019/06/Magnitsky Submission_Officials Surgeons_Final.pdf
30. Additional reporting/ research (docu-mentary)	Who To Believe? Discovery: China's Organ Transplants Episode 1 of 2	Part 1 of a recent BBC radio documentary on the topic containing relevant witness testimony	2018	Matthew Hill, (Discovery, BBC)	https://www.bbc.co.uk/programmes/w3csxyl3
31. Additional reporting/ research (docu-mentary)	Tourism and Transparency Discovery: China's Organ Transplants Episode 2 of 2	Part 2 of a recent BBC radio documentary on the topic containing relevant witness testimony. Interviews with Huang Jiefu and Prof Jeremy Chapman. Prof Wendy Rogers explains the Liver International retraction	2018	Matthew Hill, (Discovery, BBC)	https://www.bbc.co.uk/programmes/w3csxyl4
32. Additional reporting/ published research	State Organs: Transplant Abuse in China	An important compilation of essays on the topic	2012	David Matas & Torsten Trey	ISBN: 9781927079119 Seraphim Editions (2012)

Pre-reading materials submitted by ETAC to the China Tribunal

Category	Title	Description/Pages to View	Date	Author	Link
33. Additional reporting/ research – peer reviewed	Transplant Medicine in China: Need for Transparency and International Scrutiny Remains	A critical analysis of the debate on China's claims of reform within the mainstream transplant profession, published in the leading international transplantation journal	2016	T.Tray, A.Sharif, A.Schwarz, M. Fiatarone Singh, J Lavee. (American Journal of Trans-plantation)	http://onlinelibrary. wiley.com/ doi/10.1111/ ajt.14014/full
34. Additional reporting / research – peer reviewed	Engaging with China on Organ Trans-plantation	Peer-reviewed editorial reporting on Huang Jiefu's call for two spare livers	2017	W Rogers, M Robertson, J Lavee (BMJ)	https://www.bmj. com/content/356/bmj. j665
35. Additional reporting/ research – peer reviewed	Cold Genocide: Falun Gong in China	Paper arguing that the eradication campaign against Falun Gong is a cold genocide as it is: (1) multi-dimensional; (2) subtle in terms of visibility; and (3) normalized in the society in which it takes place	2018	M Cheung, T Trey, D Matas, R An. (Genocide Studies and Prevention: An International Journal)	https:// scholarcommons. usf.edu/cgi/view content.cgi?article =1513&context=gsp
36. Additional reporting/ research – peer reviewed	Smoke and Mirrors: Unanswered Questions and Misleading Statements Obscure the Truth About Organ Sources in China	General commentary on Chinese official lack of transparency on the issue	2016	W. Rogers, T. Trey, M. Fiatarone Singh, M. Bridgett, K. Bramstedt, J. Lavee. (Journal of Medical Ethics)	https://jme.bmj.com/ content/42/8/552
37. Additional reporting/ research – peer reviewed	Engaging With China on Organ Trans-plantation	Argument about the need for more robust engagement with Chinese officials on organ sourcing practices	2017	Wendy Rogers, Matthew Robertson, Jacob Lavee (The BMJ)	https://www.bmj. com/content/356/bmj. j665
38. Additional reporting/ research – peer reviewed	Papers Based on Data Concerning Organs from Executed Prisoners Should Not Be Published	Letter calling for retraction of research by Zheng Shusen	2016	Rogers, Fiatarone Singh and Lavee. Liver International	https://onlinelibrary. wiley.com/ doi/10.1111/liv.13348

		Pre-reading materials submitted by ETAC to the China Tribunal				
Category	Title	Description/Pages to View	Date	Author	Link
39. Additional reporting/ research – peer reviewed	Papers Based on Data Concerning Organs from Executed Prisoners Should Not Be Published: Response to Zheng and Yan	Follow-up letter arguing that Zheng and his colleague's response raised more questions than it answered and failed to demonstrate the ethical origin of the organs in his publication (which was eventually retracted)	2016	Wendy Rogers, Jacob Lavee *research by Matthew Robertson* Liver International	https://onlinelibrary. wiley.com/doi/ abs/10.1111/liv.13366
40. Additional reporting/ research/ academic dissertation	Genocide in the People's Republic of China: Violations of International Criminal Law in the Suppression of Falun Gong	Argument and analysis using a framework of international law that the CCP campaign against Falun Gong constitutes a genocide	2017	Caylan Ford	https://chinatribunal. com/wp-content/ uploads/2019/01/ Caylan-Ford-Oxford-IHRL-Dissertation-Falun-Gong-genocide.pdf
41. Additional reporting/ expert statement	The Party and the Profession: Organ Transplant Abuse in China	Summary of the history of interactions between Western transplant professionals and Chinese officials on the transplant question	2017	David Matas	https:// endtransplantabuse. org/party-profession-organ-transplant-abuse-china/
41a. Additional reporting/ expert statement	Organ Sourcing in China: The Official Version	An analysis of the debate on China's claims of reform within the mainstream transplant profession	2015	David Matas	http:// endtransplantabuse. org/organ-sourcing-in-china-the-official-version/
42. Additional reporting/ expert statement	Learning about the Communist Party of China	General background/reference material	2017	David Matas	https:// endtransplantabuse. org/learning-about-the-communist-party-of-china/
43. Additional reporting/ expert statement	World Uyghur Congress president speaks on organ harvesting at roundtable in the UK Parliament	General background/reference material. Relevant for considering the potential exploitation of Uyghurs as an organ source	2017	Dolkun Isa	http://www. uyghurcongress.org/ en/?p=33706

	Pre-reading materials submitted by ETAC to the China Tribunal					
Category	**Title**	**Description/Pages to View**	**Date**	**Author**	**Link**	
44. Additional reporting/ statement to US Government committee	Statement of the Hon. Frank R. Wolf, a Rep in Congress from the State of Virginia. Testimony before the Subcommittee on Trade of the House Committee on Ways and Means Hearing on Renewal of Normal Trade Relations with China	Contains testimony by Wang Guoqi, former doctor at a Chinese PLA hospital recounting his involvement in removing skin from the bodies of executed prisoners. see pp. 13-15	2001	Frank Wolf	https://www.gpo.gov/ fdsys/pkg/CHRG-107hhrg75054/ pdf/CHRG-107hhrg75054.pdf	
45. Additional reporting/ expert statement	Human Rights in China: Part 3; Part 4	General background/reference material	2016	Gao Zhisheng	http://www.csw. org.uk/2017/10/16/ report/3754/article. htm	
46. Additional reporting/ research (docu-mentary)	Human Harvest	A documentary on the topic that won the Peabody Award. (Note: the sequence of the guard has been edited slightly out of sequence)	2015	Leon Lee (Flying Cloud Productions Inc)	https://vimeo. com/ondemand/ humanharvestdoc	
47. Additional reporting/ expert statement	Independent Tribunal into Forced Organ Harvesting of Prisoners of Conscience in China: Why the Focus on Prisoners of conscience	Remarks by David Matas on the need for a focus on prisoners of conscience as organ sources	2018	David Matas	https://chinatribunal. com/wp-content/ uploads/2019/01/ POC_TribunalFocus-FinalDraft.pdf	
Category 4: Statements and Policy of Transplant Community						
48. Statements and/or policy of international transplant community	TTS Ethics Committee Policy Statement: Chinese Tran-splantation Program	First official statement by TTS in relation to organ harvesting from prisoners in China	2006	The Tran-splantation Society Ethics Committee	https://www.tts.org/ images/stories/pdfs/ StatementMembs-ChineseTXProg.pdf	

		Pre-reading materials submitted by ETAC to the China Tribunal				
Category	**Title**	**Description/Pages to View**	**Date**	**Author**	**Link**	
49. Statements and/or policy of international transplant community	TTS Interactions with China – July 31, 2016	The official position of The Transplantation Society (TTS) (updated) on organ transplantation in China question	2016	Dr Phillip J. O'Connell	https://www.tts. org/newstts-world/ member-news/2174-tts-interactions-with-china-july-31-2016	
50. Statements and/or policy of international transplant community members	Congressional testimony by F. Delmonico	Offers a clear summary of the official TTS stance and relations with China, delivered to Congress by Dr Frances Delmonico in 2016	2016	Dr Francis Delmonico	https://chinatribunal. com/wp-content/ uploads/2019/01/ Organ-harvesting-in-China-an-examination-of-a-brutal-practice-Congressional-hearing-June-2016-Delmonico-testimony. pdf	
50a. Statements and/or policy of international transplant community members	Dr Frances Delmonico's response to questions by Congress, plus his testimony	Short extract of supplementary comments by Dr Frances Delmonico (in response to Congressional questions, in 2016)	2016	Dr Francis Delmonico	https://chinatribunal. com/wp-content/ uploads/2019/10/ Additional-comments-by-Dr.-Delmonico.pdf	
Category 5: Media and Blogs						
51. Media and blogs	China's Organ Transplant Problem	A general summary of the argument of extrajudicial organ sourcing in China	2017	Dr Jacob Lavee & Matthew Robertson (The Diplomat)	https://thediplomat. com/2017/03/chinas-organ-transplant-problem/	
52. Media and blogs	China's Semantic Trick with Prisoner Organs	Analysis of China's claims of transplant reform	2015	Kirk C Allison, Norbert W Paul, Michael E Shapiro, Charl Els, and Huige Li (BMJ)	http://blogs.bmj.com/ bmj/2015/10/08/ chinas-semantic-trick-with-prisoner-organs/	
53. Media and blogs	Debate Flares Over China's Inclusion at Vatican Organ Trafficking Meeting	Reporting of concerns about Chinese involvement in the Vatican's 2017 organ trafficking meeting	2017	Didi Kirsten Tatlow (New York Times)	https://www.nytimes. com/2017/02/07/ world/asia/china-vatican-organ-transplants.html	

	Pre-reading materials submitted by ETAC to the China Tribunal				
Category	Title	Description/Pages to View	Date	Author	Link
54. Media and blogs	At Congressional Hearing, China's Organ Harvesting Seen Through Rose-Colored Glasses	Summary of the key points and ideas in the 2016 congressional session following release of The Update, by Kilgour, Matas and Gutmann	2016	Matthew Robertson, (The Epoch Times)	https://www.theepochtimes.com/at-congressional-hearing-chinas-organ-harvesting-seen-through-rose-colored-glasses_2103475.html
55. Media and blogs	Acrimony Mars Transplant Conference in Hong Kong	The 2016 TTS conference in Hong Kong was a controversial event; the first TTS conference after China's claim of reform in 2015, where hundreds of Chinese surgeons were present	2016	Matthew Robertson (The Epoch Times)	https://www.theepochtimes.com/acrimony-mars-transplant-conference-in-hong-kong_2142209.html
56. Media and blogs	A Transplant Conference Plays Host to China, and its Surgeons Accused of Killing	Article presenting evidence about complicity and ignorance on the part of TTS about transplant abuse in China	2016	Matthew Robertson (The Epoch Times)	https://www.theepochtimes.com/a-transplant-conference-plays-host-to-china-and-its-surgeons-accused-of-killing_2130297.html
57. Media and blogs	Call for Correction to Washington Post article	Response to the Simon Denyer/ Washington Post article in which Denyer claimed the evidence of high transplant volumes in China is based on flawed assumptions; this assumption is rebutted in this article	2017	Multiple	https://endtransplantabuse.org/call-correction-washington-post/
58. Media and blogs	A Darkly Sinister Accusation. Response to Washington Post article by Ethan Gutmann	Gutmann's rebuttal of Denyer's Washington Post article, together with a detailed history of interaction between the international transplant professionals and China's organ transplant officials	2017	Ethan Gutmann	https://endtransplantabuse.org/darkly-sinister-accusation-response-washington-post-article-ethan-gutmann/
59. Media and blogs/ Official China media source	Various	A compilation of relevant comments made by Chinese officials, and some TTS and WHO officials	2015-2018	Various, Chinese state media	https://chinatribunal.com/wp-content/uploads/2019/01/Compilation-of-Chinese-media-reports-and-comments-on-organ-transplant-reform-Tribunal.pdf

	Pre-reading materials submitted by ETAC to the China Tribunal				
Category	Title	Description/Pages to View	Date	Author	Link
Category 6: Persecution of Uyghurs					
60. Persecution of Uyghurs	Eradicating Ideological Viruses. China's Campaign of Repression Against Xinjiang's Muslims	Summary of a report that presents new evidence of the Chinese government's mass arbitrary detention, torture, and mistreatment of Turkic Muslims in Xinjiang	2018	Human Rights Watch	https://www.hrw.org/report/2018/09/09/eradicating-ideological-viruses/chinas-campaign-repression-against-xinjiangs
61. Persecution of Uyghurs	China: Police DNA Database Threatens Privacy	General background/reference material	2017	Human Rights Watch	https://www.hrw.org/news/2017/05/15/china-police-dna-database-threatens-privacy
62. Persecution of Uyghurs	Uyghurs Forced to Undergo Medical Exams, DNA Sampling	General background/reference material, relevant for considering the potential exploitation of Uyghurs as an organ source	2017	Eset Sulayman, Gulchehra Hoja, and Jilil Kashgary (Radio Free Asia)	http://www.rfa.org/english/news/uyghur/dna-05192017144424.html
63. Persecution of Uyghurs	China: Minority Region Collects DNA From Millions	General background/reference material, relevant for considering the potential exploitation of Uyghurs as an organ source	2017	Human Rights Watch	https://www.hrw.org/news/2017/12/13/china-minority-region-collects-dna-millions
64. Persecution of Uyghurs	Xinjiang Authorities Secretly Transferring Uyghur Detainees to Jails Throughout China	Recent media report of mass movements of Uyghur detainees around prisons in China	2018	Radio Free Asia	https://www.rfa.org/english/news/uyghur/transfer-10022018171100.html
Category 7: Official Statements					
65. Official statements / Government	European Parliament Resolution of 12 December 2013 on organ harvesting in China	Self-explanatory	2013	European Parliament	http://www.europarl.europa.eu/sides/getDoc.do?pubRef=-//EP//TEXT+TA+P7-TA-2013-0603+0+DOC+XML+V0//EN

Pre-reading materials submitted by ETAC to the China Tribunal					
Category	Title	Description/Pages to View	Date	Author	Link
66. Official statements / Government	Written declaration on stopping organ harvesting from prisoners of conscience in China	An EP declaration against organ harvesting in China	2016	European Parliament	www.europarl. europa.eu/sides/ getDoc.do?pubRef=- %2f%2fEP%2f%2f NONSGML%2bW DECL%2bP8-DCL- 2016-0048%2b0%2b DOC%2bPDF%2bV 0%2f%2fEN
67. Official statements / Government	H. Res. 343 – 114th Congress (2015-2016)	A Congressional resolution against organ harvesting in China	2016	Representative Ileana Ros-Lehtinen	https://www. congress.gov/ bill/114th-congress/ house-resolution/343/ text

Appendix 4. Additional Material Submitted

Ref	Title	Author	Date	Link
1	Parliamentary questions	Professor the Lord Alton of Liverpool	December 2018 to February 2019	https://chinatribunal.com/wp-content/uploads/2019/06/Lord-Alton_China-Tribunal-Submission.pdf
2	The extent to which Falun Gong constitutes a "religious group" under the Genocide Convention 1948, and customary international law	Professor Peter Edge, Professor of Law & Dr M. John-Hopkins, Senior Lecturer in Law Oxford Brooks University Submitted at the invitation of Counsel to the Tribunal	15th January 2019	https://chinatribunal.com/wp-content/uploads/2019/06/Edge-and-John-Hopkins-letter.pdf
3	An open invitation by Gao Zhisheng to the Canadian international independent investigation team	Sent to the Tribunal by: Dr David Matas and David Kilgour	30th June 2007	https://chinatribunal.com/wp-content/uploads/2019/06/Response-regarding-Gao-Zhisheng_MatasKilgour.pdf
4	Opinion for the Independent Tribunal into Forced Organ Harvesting from Prisoners of Conscience in China on the religious groups protected against genocide Professional profile of Professor Szpak	Professor Agnieszka Szpak Nicolaus Copernicus University in Torin, Poland Submitted at the invitation of ETAC	23rd March 2019	https://chinatribunal.com/wp-content/uploads/2019/06/ProfAgnieszkaSzpak_SubmissionForChinaTribunal.pdf https://chinatribunal.com/wp-content/uploads/2019/06/ProfAgnieszkaSzpak_CV.pdf
5	Panel discussion: Organ Transplantation Medical, Technological and Ethical Challenges	Harvard T.H. Chan, School of Public Health Video featuring: David Freeman, Dr Francis Delmonico & Dr Daniel Wikler ETAC submission	20th May 2016	https://chinatribunal.com/wp-content/uploads/2019/06/VideoComment-of-Dr-Francis-Delmonico-_Harvard-forum_20-May2016.pdf

Ref	Title	Author	Date	Link
6	610 Office point system English translation and original Chinese text	ETAC submission	5th December 2002	https://chinatribunal.com/wp-content/uploads/2019/06/610-Point-System-English1.pdf https://chinatribunal.com/wp-content/uploads/2019/06/610-Points-system-page-1_originalChinese.jpg.pdf https://chinatribunal.com/wp-content/uploads/2019/06/610-Points-system-page-2_original_Chinese.jpg.pdf
7	Sydney General Consulate: Work List of Anti-Falun Gong Foreign-related Struggle Special Group. English translation and original Chinese text	ETAC submission	Various dates in February 2001	https://chinatribunal.com/wp-content/uploads/2019/06/Work-List-of-Anti-Falun-Gong-Foreign-related-Struggle-Special-Group.pdf https://chinatribunal.com/wp-content/uploads/2019/06/Work-List_page1-_original_-2007-8-1-baoguang-01.jpg.pdf https://chinatribunal.com/wp-content/uploads/2019/06/Work-List_page2-_original_2007-8-5-baoguang-02a.jpg.pdf https://chinatribunal.com/wp-content/uploads/2019/06/Work-List_page3-_original_2007-8-5-baoguang-02b.jpg.pdf https://chinatribunal.com/wp-content/uploads/2019/06/Work-List_page4-_original_2007-8-5-baoguang-02c.jpg.pdf
8	Organ Transplants Video presentation made available on youtube by Casina Pio IV	Professor Francis L. Delmonico, MD Chair, Organ Donation and Transplantation Task Force World Health Organisation Pontifical Academy of Sciences ETAC submission	26th November 2018	https://chinatribunal.com/wp-content/uploads/2019/09/Video_DrDelmonico2018_Pontifical_AcademyForum_FalunGongOnPowerpoint.pdf

Ref	Title	Author	Date	Link
9	Excerpts from China's Responses to the Committee Against Torture's List of Issues	Provided to the Tribunal by Counsel	October 2015	https://www.hrichina.org/en/excerpts-chinas-responses-committee-against-tortures-list-issues
10	Dr. Haibo Wang's public response to the 2016 update report by Kilgour, Gutmann and Matas (see appendix 2B)	ETAC submission	13th February 2017	https://www.youtube.com/watch?v=flhSY0evT0o
11	Witness statements provided by Falun Gong practitioners who were not asked to provide evidence at either hearing	Provided to the Tribunal by Counsel	Various. Provided to the Panel in advance of the April hearings.	https://chinatribunal.com/submissions/submissions_notcalled_falungongfactwitnesses/
12	The Transplant Society China Relations Committee meeting considering the report of Lavee, Robertson, Hinde (Appendix 2 item Q)	Provided to the Tribunal by Counsel, who received it in error from by DICG	25th February 2019	https://chinatribunal.com/submissions/tts_chinarelationscommitteenotes_feb25_2019/
13	Compilation of information about 610 Office, various open sources	Requested by the Tribunal and provided by ETAC	Various dates.	https://chinatribunal.com/submissions/610_office_information/
14	Legal Opinion\n\nSupplementary Legal Opinion\n\nVideo recording of Tribunal's questions to Edward Fitzgerald QC regarding first legal opinion	Edward Fitzgerald QC, Doughty Street Chambers\n\nProvided to the Tribunal by Counsel	22nd January 2019\n\n3rd June 2019	https://chinatribunal.com/wp-content/uploads/2019/06/LegalAdvice_EdwardFitzgeraldQC_January2019.pdf\n\nhttps://chinatribunal.com/wp-content/uploads/2019/06/LegalAdvice_2-of-2_EdwardFitzgeraldQC_2019.pdf\n\nhttps://chinatribunal.com/submissions/china-tribunal-video-of-questioning-edward-fitzgerald-qc-regarding-written-legal-advice-1/
15	ETAC's position on Uyghurs as prisoners of conscience in China	ETAC's China Tribunal Steering Committee\n\nETAC Submission	8th May 2019	https://chinatribunal.com/wp-content/uploads/2019/06/ETAC_PoC_Uyghurs-Statement.pdf
16	ETAC statement – call for submissions process	ETAC Submission	May 2019	https://chinatribunal.com/wp-content/uploads/2019/09/ETAC_Statement_CallForSubmissionsProcess.pdf
17	Chart containing a compilation of links to various Chinese commentaries on Falun Gong	Compiled and submitted by ETAC at the request of the Tribunal	Various dates 1993 – 2006	https://chinatribunal.com/wp-content/uploads/2019/06/OfficialChineseDocumentsAndCommentsOnFalunGong_Final.pdf

Ref	Title	Author	Date	Link
18	Correspondence	Louisa Greve, Director of External Affairs Uyghurs Human Rights Project Link to CNN article by Matt Rivers and Lily Lee	30th May 2019 10th May 2019	https://chinatribunal.com/wp-content/uploads/2019/06/Correspondence-from-Louisa-Greve-Director-of-External-Affairs-Uyghur-Human-Rights-Project-UHRP.pdf
19	Memo to County Economic Commission and Party Committee from Tianjin Re-education-through-labour Management Committee Decision on Re-education-through-labour for Hong Chen	Tianjin Re-education-through-labour Management Committee Submitted to the Tribunal by Hong Chen	28th April 2000	https://chinatribunal.com/wp-content/uploads/2019/06/HongChen_Decision-on-Re-education-through-Labour-English.pdf https://chinatribunal.com/wp-content/uploads/2019/06/HongChen_Decision-on-Re-education-through-Labour-Chinese.jpg.pdf https://chinatribunal.com/submissions/hongchen_decision-on-re-education-through-labour-chinese-jpg-2/ https://chinatribunal.com/submissions/hongchen_instructionsonremovingchenhongspartymembershipenglish-jpg-2/ https://chinatribunal.com/submissions/hongchen_list-of-withheld-articles-english-jpg-2/ https://chinatribunal.com/submissions/hongchen_list-of-withheldarticleschinese-jpg-2/
20	CCP decision on handling Hong Chen mistakes Chinese and English translations	Submitted to the Tribunal by Hong Chen	May 2019 Various dates	https://chinatribunal.com/wp-content/uploads/2019/06/HongChen_Instructions-on-the-Handling-of-CHEN-Hong%E2%80%99s-Mistakes-English.jpg.pdf https://chinatribunal.com/wp-content/uploads/2019/06/HongChen_Instructions-on-the-Handling-of-CHEN-Hong%E2%80%99s-Mistakes-Chinese.jpg.pdf

Ref	Title	Author	Date	Link
21	Legal Opinion	Datuk N. Sivananthan Of Lincoln's Inn Provided to the Panel by Counsel to the Tribunal	23rd May 2019	https://chinatribunal.com/submissions/china-tribunal-opinion-sgd/
22	Various screenshots and links from/to Korean webpages identifying organ availability for transplant purposes	Witness submission to Tribunal	2005 onwards	https://chinatribunal.com/submissions/koreanwebpages wherethedocumentar yteamhadclues/
23	Correspondence concerning Korean patients visiting transplant centres in China	Letter to Dr Shim, Chong Yang from Mr Choi, Soo Jin, Leader of Liver Transplantation Gathering In Korea Reply from Shen Zhongyang Tainjin First Central Hospital, Orient Organ Transplant Center Witness submission to Tribunal	27th April 2007	https://chinatribunal.com/submissions/the-letter-from-the-online-club-to-shen-zhongyang/ https://chinatribunal.com/submissions/the-reply-from-shen-zhongyang-to-the-online-club/
24	Dr David Matas; in response to Chinese doctor Lu Guoping's denial of legitimacy of the phone call investigation of May 2006	ETAC Submission	Phone call 2006 Response 2015	https://chinatribunal.com/submissions/phonecalle videncecomments_matas/
25	Senate Committee Proceedings from the Australian Parliament – Foreign Affairs Defence and Trade	Senators Rice and Abetz questioning Mr. Fletcher on Organ Harvesting in China and the 2016 *Update* report ETAC Submission	20th October 2016	https://chinatribunal.com/wp-content/uploads/2019/06/AustralianDFAT_Senate EstimatesQuestionsOnForced OrganHarvesting.pdf

Ref		Title	Author	Date	Link
26	1.	Selected information on 610 Office and articles in Chinese and English translation	Yiyang Xia Human Rights Law Foundation	28th April 2019	1. https://chinatribunal.com/wp-content/uploads/2019/06/YiyangXia_How-does-610-work_en_YiyangXia.pdf
	2.	Response to questions from the Tribunal			2. https://chinatribunal.com/wp-content/uploads/2019/06/YiyangXia_Reply-to-Questions_YiyangXia.pdf
	3.	Details of allegations that at the police station of Liugezhuang Town, Haiyang City, Yantai City, Shandong Province, Falun Gong practitioners were forced to have blood tests			3 – translated https://chinatribunal.com/wp-content/uploads/2019/06/YiyangXia_Articcle-1_Liugezhuang_Shandong-Province_translated.pdf 3 – original Chinese https://chinatribunal.com/submissions/yiyangxia_article-1_original/
	4.	Account of door knocking operation in Xinbin Country and the harassment of 162 Falun Gong practitioners			4 – translated https://chinatribunal.com/wp-content/uploads/2019/06/YiyangXia_Article-2_Door-knocking-harrassment_translated.pdf 4 – original Chinese https://chinatribunal.com/wp-content/uploads/2020/02/YiyangXia_Article-2_original.pdf
	5.	Blood samples at home by State Security Police who broke into his home			5 – translated https://chinatribunal.com/wp-content/uploads/2019/06/YiyangXia_Article-3_Xintai-City_Zhu-Xiulin_translated.pdf 5 – original Chinese https://chinatribunal.com/wp-content/uploads/2020/02/YiyangXia_Article-3_original.pdf

Ref	Title	Author	Date	Link
27	Supplementary documents about liver transplant	Various authors, submitted to the Tribunal by Dr Charles Lee	Various dates	https://chinatribunal.com/wp-content/uploads/2019/06/CharlesLee_SuplemataryMaterial.pdf https://chinatribunal.com/wp-content/uploads/2019/06/Charles-Lee_English_PLA_HHRG-114-FA16-20160623-SD002.pdf https://chinatribunal.com/wp-content/uploads/2019/06/Charles-Lee_liver.annual.2006.report.pdf https://chinatribunal.com/wp-content/uploads/2020/02/Charles-Lee_PLA.pdf
28	Response prepared by ETAC to comments contained within Compassion, Not Commerce: An Inquiry into Human Organ Trafficking and Organ Transplant Tourism by the Human Rights Sub-Committee of the House of Representatives Joint Standing Committee on Foreign Affairs, Defence and Trade Compassion Not Commerce Full Report	ETAC Submission	Drafted and submitted May 2019	https://chinatribunal.com/submissions/response_-compassionnotcommerce_austgovtreport_rogers_matas_hughes/ https://chinatribunal.com/wp-content/uploads/2020/02/CompassionNotCommerce_AnInquiryintoHuman OrganTraffickingOrgan TransplantTourism_HumanRightsSub-Committee_Australian GovttReport.pdf
29	Video: Harvard professor praises China's organ transplant efforts	CGTN (China Global Television Network) ETAC Submission	9th May 2019	https://news.cgtn.com/news/3d59444d35637a4d/share_p.html
30	Invitations to participate, sent to authorities and physicians/correspondence	Sent by Counsel, on behalf of the Tribunal	Various	https://chinatribunal.com/wp-content/uploads/2020/03/InvitationsCorrespondence_withIndex_2020.pdf
31	Opinion provided by expert statistician on the Robertson, Hinde, Lavee report	Professor Sir David Spiegelhalter FRS OBE Submitted at the invitation of Counsel to the Tribunal	19th March, 2019	https://chinatribunal.com/wp-content/uploads/2019/06/Commentary-on-Robertson-et-al-Spiegelhalter.pdf

Ref	Title	Author	Date	Link
32	Phone call verification report by independent academics	Submitted by ETAC at the request of the Tribunal	2019	https://chinatribunal.com/wp-content/uploads/2020/02/PhoneCallsVerification_AcademicCommentators_15May.pdf https://chinatribunal.com/wp-content/uploads/2020/02/Phone-call-content-verification-report.pdf
33	Does Chinese terminology indicate religion or cult	Clive Ansley (China Law expert/ Mandarin speaker) & Dr David Matas Submitted by ETAC	2019	https://chinatribunal.com/wp-content/uploads/2019/06/ETAC_Question_ChineseTerminology_ReligionORCult.pdf
34	WOIPFG 2016 phone call report – Final Harvest Translation check of 5 calls in Chapter 6 (2020)	WOIPFG at request of the Tribunal	2016 2020	https://chinatribunal.com/submissions/woipfg_finalharvest_april22_2016/ https://chinatribunal.com/wp-content/uploads/2020/02/TranslationCheck_5-calls-from-WOIPFG-Final-Harvest_-translator-comment.pdf
35	WOIPFG research notes from Chongqing Southwest Hospital, Third Military Medical University —Liver Transplantation Center	WOIPFG at request of the Tribunal		https://chinatribunal.com/submissions/woipfg_files_southwest_googletranslation/ https://chinatribunal.com/wp-content/uploads/2020/02/WOIPFG-files-Southwest-original.pdf
36	Audio recording of a witness regarding 'halal' organs	Submitted by ETAC	February, 2020	https://chinatribunal.com/wp-content/uploads/2020/02/Statement_HalalOrgans.pdf
37	Statement regarding Chinese Communist Party harvesting Uyghur organs	Professor Erkin Sidick Submitted by ETAC	February, 2020	https://chinatribunal.com/wp-content/uploads/2020/02/Statement_ProfessorSidick_UyghursFOH.pdf

Ref	Title	Author	Date	Link
38	Organ Procurement and Judicial Execution in China – investigation	Human Rights Watch Submitted by ETAC	1994	https://www.hrw.org/reports/1994/china1/china_948.htm#N_104_
39	Report on Forensic Examination of WOIPFG Recording	Professor Peter French Professor of Forensic Speech Science Submitted at the invitation of Counsel to the Tribunal	February, 2020	https://chinatribunal.com/wp-content/uploads/2020/02/Report-on-Forensic-Examinations-of-Recordings_Prof-French_A.pdf

China Tribunal Video Footage

Video footage of the December 2018 Public Hearings – chinatribunal.com/the-hearings/
Video footage of the April 2019 Public Hearings – chinatribunal.com/the-hearings-april-2019/
China Tribunal Judgment Documentary – chinatribunal.com/final-judgement-film/
China Tribunal Final Judgment – chinatribunal.com/final-judgement-video/

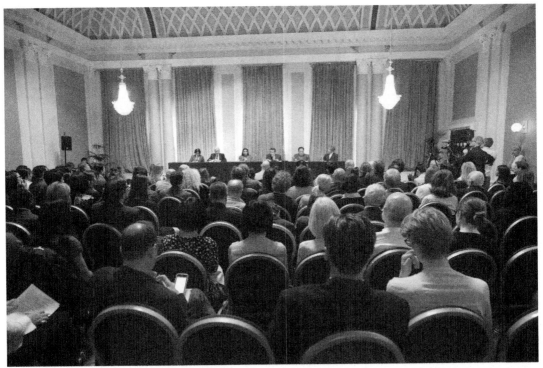

Final Judgment, London, 17 June, 2019

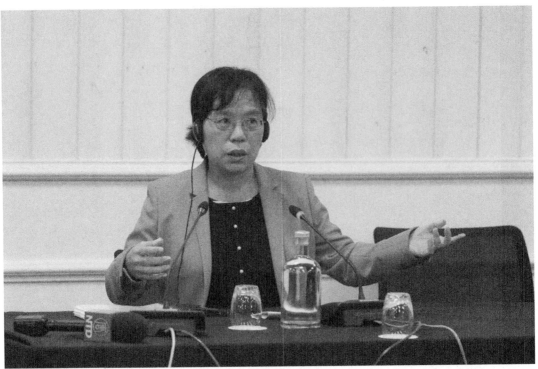

Dai Ying, Falun Gong Practitioner, Witness, Public Hearings, London, December 2018.

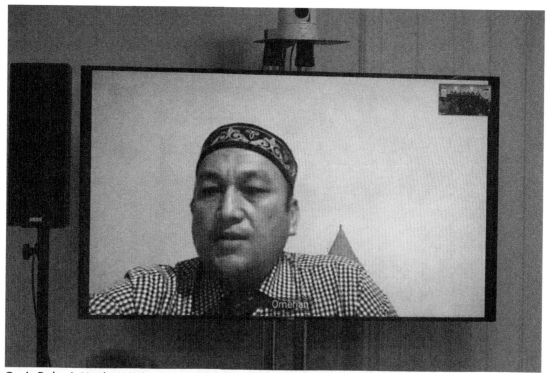

Omir Bekari, Uyghur, Witness, Public Hearings, London, December 2018.

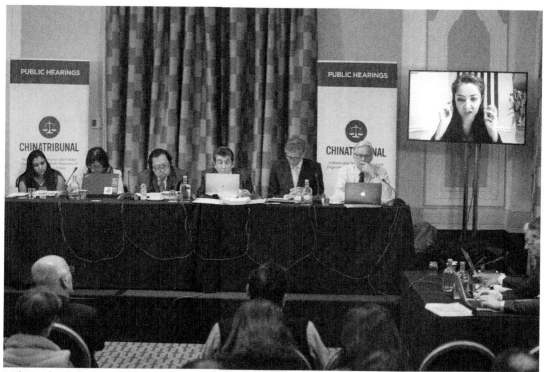

Mihrigul Tursun, Uyghur, Witness, Public Hearings, London, April 2019.

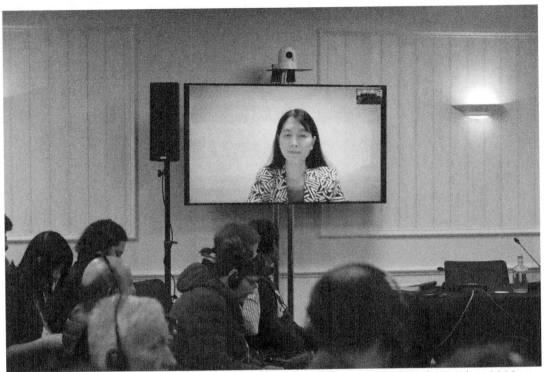

Liu Huiqiong, **Falun Gong Practitioner, Witness, Public Hearings, London, December 2018.**

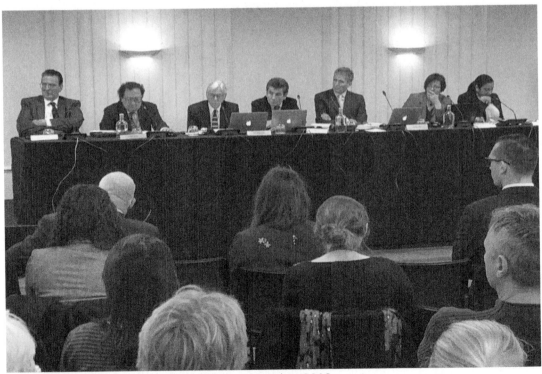

China Tribunal, Public Hearings, London, December 2018.

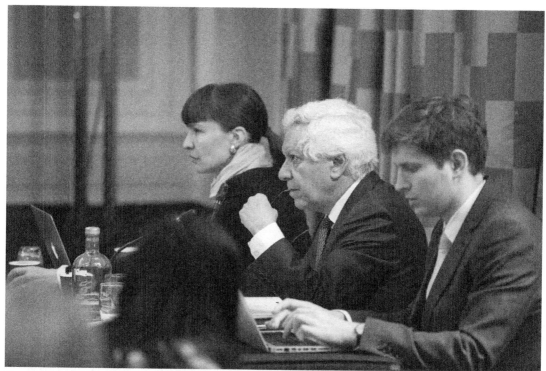

Counsel to the Tribunal – Hamid Sabi and Tabitha Nice. Junior Counsel - Markus Findlay.

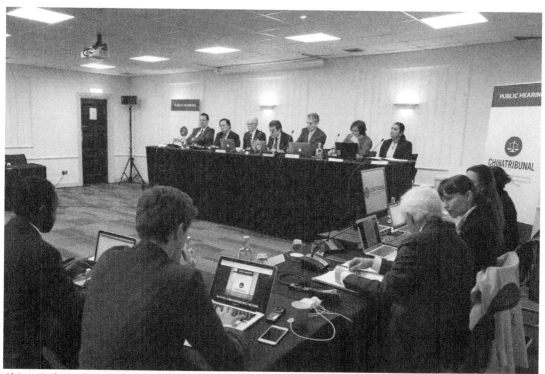

China Tribunal, Public Hearings, London, December 2018.

China Tribunal Members

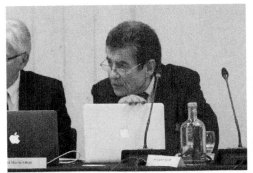

Sir Geoffrey Nice QC (Chair)

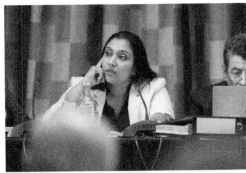

Regina Paulose

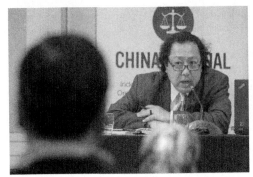

Andrew Khoo

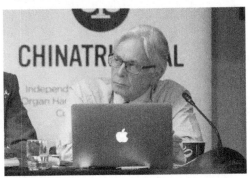

Prof Martin Elliott

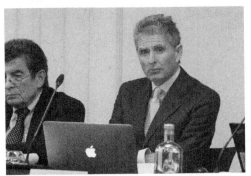

Nicholas Vetch

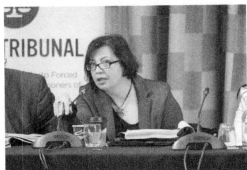

Shadi Sadr

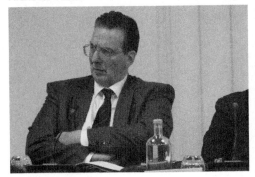

Prof Arthur Waldron

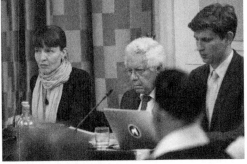

Counsel: Tabitha Nice, Hamid Sabi, Markus Finlay

Printed in Great Britain
by Amazon

77989869R00359